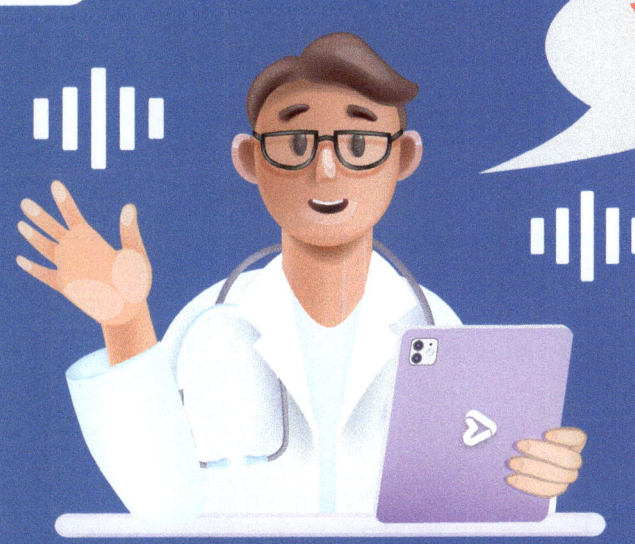

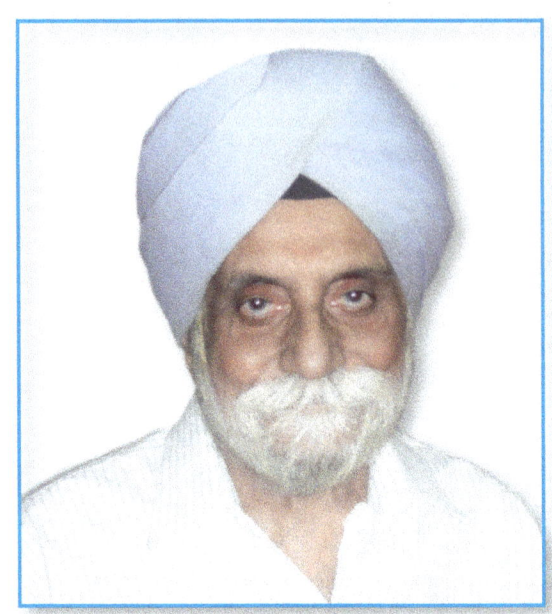

Late Professor Inderbir Singh
(1930–2014)

Tribute to a Legend

Professor Inderbir Singh, a legendary anatomist, is renowned for being a pillar in the education of generations of medical graduates across the globe. He was one of the greatest teachers of his time. He was a passionate writer who poured his soul into his work. His eagle's eye for details and meticulous way of writing made his books immensely popular amongst students. He managed his lifetime to become enmeshed in millions of hearts. He was conferred the title of Professor Emeritus by Maharshi Dayanand University, Rohtak.

On 12th May, 2014, he was awarded posthumously with Emeritus Teacher Award by National Board of Examination for making invaluable contribution in teaching of Anatomy. This award is given to honour legends who have made tremendous contribution in the field of medical education. He was a visionary for his time, and the legacies he left behind are his various textbooks on *Gross Anatomy*, *Histology*, *Neuroanatomy* and *Embryology*. Although his mortal frame is not present amongst us, his genius will live on forever.

Inderbir Singh's
HUMAN EMBRYOLOGY

A Clinically Integrated Approach with Case Scenarios and Clinical Applications

As per the Competency-based Medical Education Curriculum (NMC)

FOURTEENTH EDITION

Edited by

Raveendranath Veeramani MBBS MD (Anatomy)
Additional Professor
Department of Anatomy
Jawaharlal Institute of Postgraduate Medical Education and Research (JIPMER)
Puducherry, India

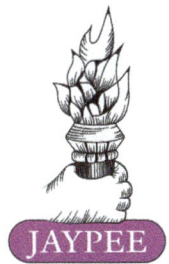

JAYPEE BROTHERS MEDICAL PUBLISHERS
The Health Sciences Publisher
New Delhi | London

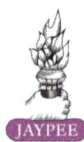
Jaypee Brothers Medical Publishers (P) Ltd

Headquarters

Jaypee Brothers Medical Publishers (P) Ltd
EMCA House, 23/23-B
Ansari Road, Daryaganj
New Delhi 110 002, India
Landline: +91-11-23272143, +91-11-23272703
+91-11-23282021, +91-11-23245672
Email: jaypee@jaypeebrothers.com

Overseas Office

J.P. Medical Ltd
83 Victoria Street, London
SW1H 0HW (UK)
Phone: +44 20 3170 8910
Email: info@jpmedpub.com

Corporate Office

Jaypee Brothers Medical Publishers (P) Ltd
4838/24, Ansari Road, Daryaganj
New Delhi 110 002, India
Phone: +91-11-43574357
Phone: +91-11-43574357
Fax: +91-11-43574314
Email: jaypee@jaypeebrothers.com

EU GPSR Authorised Representative

Logos Europe, 9 rue Nicolas Poussin
17000, La Rochelle, France
Phone: +33 (0) 6 67 93 73 78
E-mail: Contact@logoseurope.eu

Website: www.jaypeebrothers.com
Website: www.jaypeedigital.com

© 2025, Jaypee Brothers Medical Publishers

The views and opinions expressed in this book are solely those of the original contributor(s)/author(s) and do not necessarily represent those of editor(s) and publisher of the book.

All rights reserved. No part of this publication may be reproduced, stored or transmitted in any form or by any means, electronic, mechanical, photocopying, recording or otherwise, without the prior permission in writing of the publishers.

All brand names and product names used in this book are trade names, service marks, trademarks or registered trademarks of their respective owners. The publisher is not associated with any product or vendor mentioned in this book.

Medical knowledge and practice change constantly. This book is designed to provide accurate, authoritative information about the subject matter in question. However, readers are advised to check the most current information available on procedures included and check information from the manufacturer of each product to be administered, to verify the recommended dose, formula, method and duration of administration, adverse effects and contraindications. It is the responsibility of the practitioner to take all appropriate safety precautions. Neither the publisher nor the author(s)/editor(s) assume any liability for any injury and/or damage to persons or property arising from or related to use of material in this book.

This book is sold on the understanding that the publisher is not engaged in providing professional medical services. If such advice or services are required, the services of a competent medical professional should be sought.

Every effort has been made where necessary to contact holders of copyright to obtain permission to reproduce copyright material. If any have been inadvertently overlooked, the publisher will be pleased to make the necessary arrangements at the first opportunity.

Inquiries for bulk sales may be solicited at: jaypee@jaypeebrothers.com

Inderbir Singh's Human Embryology

First to Ninth Editions published by Macmillan Publishers India Ltd (1976-2013)
Tenth Edition published by Jaypee Brothers Medical Publishers (P) Ltd (2014)
Eleventh Edition: 2018
Reprint: 2019
Twelfth Edition: 2021
Thirteenth Edition: 2023, Revised Reprint: 2023
Fourteenth Edition: 2025
ISBN: 978-93-5696-748-9

Dedicated to

'My Beloved Students'

Preface to the Fourteenth Edition

Embryology, the study of the fascinating journey of life, has long captivated scientists and scholars, all striving to unravel the mysteries of human development, growth, and organ formation.

In this 14th edition, I embark on a comprehensive exploration of embryology, delving into the latest advancements in molecular regulation and discoveries in the field while maintaining the legacy and simplicity of Prof. Inderbir Singh. This book is designed to serve as a thorough resource for students, researchers, and healthcare professionals, providing an in-depth understanding of the principles and mechanisms that govern embryonic development.

Each chapter is enriched with cutting-edge information, beginning with competencies and flowing seamlessly into core content, supported by engaging illustrations and flowcharts. I have integrated molecular regulation and clinical correlations throughout the chapters to maintain readers interest and foster a deeper understanding. At the end of each chapter, summaries and self-assessment questions are provided to aid students in their examination preparation.

The following pedagogical features and updates in this 14th edition are designed to facilitate student learning:
1. NMC competencies
2. Organized updated contents
3. Student-friendly images to follow the content step-by-step
4. Clinical correlations
5. Molecular regulation insights
6. Timelines of developmental events
7. Summary and flowcharts for rapid revision
8. Chapter highlights
9. Reasoning and review questions
10. Self-assessment multiple choice questions (MCQs)

May this book inspire you to embrace your own journey of discovery, to ask questions, seek answers, and to never stop learning.

Raveendranath Veeramani

Preface to the First Edition

This book on human embryology has been written keeping in mind the requirements of undergraduate medical students. The subject of embryology has traditionally been studied from imported textbooks of anatomy or of embryology. Experience has shown that the treatment of the subject in most of these books is way above the head of the average medical students in India. The difficulty has increased from year to year as there has been, and continues to be, progressive deterioration in the standards of the teaching of English in our schools and colleges. The combination of unfamiliar sophistications of language and of an involved technical subject, has very often left the student bewildered.

In this book, care has been taken to ensure that the text provides all the information necessary for an intelligent understanding of the essential features of the development of various organs and tissues of the human body. At the same time, several innovations have been used to make the subject easy to understand.

Firstly, the language has been kept simple. Care has been taken not to compress too many facts into an involved sentence. New words are clearly explained.

Secondly, simultaneous references to the development of more than one structure have been avoided as far as possible. While this has necessitated some repetition, it is hoped that this has removed one of the greatest factors leading to confusion in the study of this subject.

Thirdly, almost every step in development has been shown in a simple, easy to understand, illustration. To avoid confusion, only structures relevant to the discussion are shown. As far as possible, the drawings have been oriented as in adult anatomy to facilitate comprehension.

Fourthly, the chapters have been arranged so that all structures referred to at a particular stage have already been adequately introduced.

In an effort of this kind it is inevitable that some errors of omission, and of commission, are liable to creep in. To obviate as many of these as possible a number of eminent anatomists were requested to read through the text. Their suggestions have greatly added to the accuracy and usefulness of this book. Nevertheless, scope for further improvement remains, and the author would welcome suggestions to this end both from teachers and from students.

Rohtak
January 1976

Inderbir Singh

Acknowledgments

First and foremost, I would like to express my profound gratitude to the Almighty for granting me the opportunity and strength to complete this work.

I extend my deepest thanks to all the faculties of the Department of Anatomy at JIPMER for their unwavering support and encouragement throughout this project. Your guidance and expertise have been invaluable.

I am particularly grateful to **Dr Gomathi**, Senior Resident, for her assistance during critical moments. Your help has been instrumental in the successful completion of this book.

My heartfelt gratitude goes to my fellow seniors and anatomy faculties for their constructive feedback and insights. Your contributions have significantly enhanced the quality of this edition.

I am profoundly grateful to **Dr Piyush Gupta**, Professor, Department of Pediatrics, UCMS, New Delhi, India, and **Dr Hiralal Konar**, Professor and Senior Consultant, Department of Obstetrics and Gynecology, Ramakrishna Sarada Mission Matri Bhavan, Kolkata, West Bengal, India, for their contributions to clinical images to this book. Their generosity in granting permission to use these invaluable visual aids has greatly enriched the content. This contribution will undoubtedly enhance the learning experience for medical students, providing them with clearer, more engaging visual representations of complex concepts. Thank you for your invaluable support and dedication to medical education.

Special acknowledgment to **Dr Aditya Tayal** (Editorial Manager–Content Strategy) of M/s Jaypee Brothers Medical Publishers Ltd, New Delhi, India, for his exceptional contribution towards the editing of this book, showcasing his profound content knowledge and unparalleled skills in content editing and reviewing. His meticulous attention to detail has greatly enhanced the quality of this work.

I would also like to thank **Shri Jitendar P Vij** (Group Chairman), **Mr Ankit Vij** (Managing Director), **Mr MS Mani** (Group President), **Dr Madhu Choudhary** (Director–Educational Publishing), **Ms Pooja Bhandari** [Director–Production (Books and Journals)], **Mr Ajay Kumar Sharma** [Deputy General Manager (Books and Journals)] and **Dr Aditya Thakur** (Development Editor) of M/s Jaypee Brothers Medical Publishers Ltd, New Delhi, India, for their unwavering support and commitment to this project. Your leadership and dedication to advancing medical education are truly appreciated.

Last but not the least, **Mr Rajesh Sharma** (Production Coordinator), **Ms Seema Dogra** (Cover Visualizer), **Ms Neha Verma** (Graphic Designer–Cover), **Ms Geeta Barik** and **Mr Anil Singh** (Proofreaders), **Mr Kulwant Singh** and **Mr Kapil Dev Sharma** (Typesetters) & **Mr Manoj Pahuja** (Graphics Designer) of M/s Jaypee Brothers Medical Publishers (P) Ltd, New Delhi, India, for their help in the formatting and their experienced technical assistance in developing this project.

Thank you all for your continuous support and encouragement.

National Advisory Board

ANDHRA PRADESH

Hema
Professor
Department of Anatomy
Narayana Medical College
Nellore, Andhra Pradesh, India

Narayan Rao
Professor and Head
Department of Anatomy
KIMS Medical College
Amalapuram, Andhra Pradesh, India

Parimala M
Professor and Head
Department of Anatomy
NRI Medical College
Mangalagiri, Andhra Pradesh, India

Sucharita
Professor
Department of Anatomy
NRI Medical College
Mangalagiri, Andhra Pradesh, India

Swathi Poornima
Professor and Head
Department of Anatomy
PSIMS
Vijayawada, Andhra Pradesh, India

Uma Maheshwara Rao S
Professor and Head
Department of Anatomy
Government Medical College
Ananthapuram, Andhra Pradesh, India

Vasantha Lakshmi
Assistant Professor
Department of Anatomy
NRI Medical College
Mangalagiri, Andhra Pradesh, India

ASSAM

Himamoni Deka
Associate Professor
Department of Anatomy
Guwahati Medical College
Guwahati, Assam, India

Jyotirekha Gogoi
Assistant Professor
Department of Anatomy
Jorhat Medical College & Hospital
Jorhat, Assam, India

Malamoni Dutta
Head
Department of Anatomy
Kokrajhar Medical College
Kokrajha, Assam, India

Mousumee Saikia
Assistant Professor
Department of Anatomy
Jorhat Medical College and Hospital
Jorhat, Assam, India

Shobhana Medhi
Assistant Professor
Department of Anatomy
Tezpur Medical College
Tezpur, Assam, India

Vinay G
Associate Professor
Department of Anatomy
All India Institute of Medical Sciences
Guwahati, Assam, India

BIHAR

Md Jawed Akhtar
Additional Professor
Department of Anatomy
Indira Gandhi Institute of Medical Sciences
Patna, Bihar, India

Padamjeet Panchal
Additional Professor
Department of Anatomy
All India Institute of Medical Sciences
Patna, Bihar, India

Rakesh Ranjan
Assistant Professor and Head
Department of Anatomy
Government Medical College and Hospital
Purnea, Bihar, India

Ranjit Guha
Principal
Department of Anatomy
Indira Gandhi Institute of Medical Sciences
Patna, Bihar, India

Rashmi Prasad
Head
Department of Anatomy
Nalanda Medical College and Hospital
Patna, Bihar, India

CHHATTISGARH

Bithika Nel Kumar
Associate Professor and Head
Department of Anatomy
Government Medical College
Jagdalpur, Chhattisgarh, India

Manik Chatterjee
Professor
Department of Anatomy
Shri Balaji Institute of Medical Science
Raipur, Chhattisgarh, India

Mrinal Biswas
Assistant Professor
Department of Anatomy
Late Smt Indra Gandhi Memorial Government Medical College
Kanker, Chhattisgarh, India

Praveen Kurrey
Associate Professor
Department of Anatomy
Pt. Jawaharlal Nehru Medical College
Raipur, Chhattisgarh, India

Sumedha Anjankar
Professor and Head
Department of Anatomy
Shri Balaji Institute of Medical Science
Raipur, Chhattisgarh, India

Surajit Kandu
Associate Professor
Department of Anatomy
Late Shri Lakhiram Agrawal Memorial Government Medical College
Raigarh, Chhattisgarh, India

GUJARAT

Bharat Patel
Dean
Department of Anatomy
Bhagyoday Medical College
Kadi, Mehsana, Gujarat, India

Dilip V Gohil
Professor
Department of Anatomy
MP Shah Government Medical College
Jamnagar, Gujarat, India

Hina B Rajput
Associate Professor
Department of Anatomy
Baroda Medical College
Vadodara, Gujarat, India

Kanan Shah
Associate Professor
Department of Anatomy
NHL Medical College
Ahmedabad, Gujarat, India

Mayank Kumar Javia
Professor and Head
Department of Anatomy
GMERS Medical College
Porbandar, Gujarat, India

Padma Hirpara
Head
Department of Anatomy
GMERS Medical College
Sola, Gujarat, India

Sarzoo Girish Bhai Desai
Associate Professor
Department of Anatomy
Narendra Modi Medical College
Ahmedabad, Gujarat, India

Shalom Elay Phillip
Assistant Professor
Department of Anatomy
Dr MK Shah Medical College
Ahmedabad, Gujarat, India

Sonal H Govindwar
Associate Professor
Department of Anatomy
Kiran Medical College
Surat, Gujarat, India

HARYANA

AP Batra
Head
Department of Anatomy
Bhagat Phool Singh Government Medical College
Khanpur Kalan, Haryana, India

Ashima Das
Professor
Department of Anatomy
Government Medical College
Mewat, Haryana, India

Jaswinder Kaur
Professor and Head
Department of Anatomy
MM Institute of Medical Sciences & Research
Sadopur, Haryana, India

Kirandeep Kaur Aulakh
Professor and Head
Department of Anatomy
Maharishi Markandeshwar Medical College
Ambala, Haryana, India

Meetu Agarwal
Associate Professor
Department of Anatomy
Amrita Medical College
Faridabad, Haryana, India

Monika Jain
Professor
Department of Anatomy
Maharaja Agrasen Medical College
Agroha, Haryana, India

Nibedita Pandey
Head
Department of Anatomy
NC Medical College
Panipat, Haryana, India

Prachi Aneja
Head
Department of Anatomy
SGT University
Gurugram, Haryana, India

Shavi Garg
Assistant Professor and In-charge Head
Department of Anatomy
Shri Atal Bihari Vajpayee Government Medical College
Faridabad, Haryana, India

Shveta Swami
Head
Department of Anatomy
Kalpana Chawla Medical College
Karnal, Haryana, India

Virender Budhiraja
Professor
Department of Anatomy
Kalpana Chawla Medical College
Karnal, Haryana, India

HIMACHAL PRADESH

Anju Partap
Professor and Head
Department of Anatomy
Indira Gandhi Medical College and Hospital
Shimla, Himachal Pradesh, India

Bhagya Shree
Assistant Professor
Department of Anatomy
All India Institutes of Medical Sciences
Bilaspur, Himachal Pradesh, India

Nidhi Puri
Professor
Department of Anatomy
All India Institutes of Medical Sciences
Bilaspur, Himachal Pradesh, India

Prabhjot Kaur
Associate Professor
Department of Anatomy
Shri Lal Bahadur Shastri Government Medical College & Hospital
Mandi, Himachal Pradesh, India

JAMMU & KASHMIR

Arsh Nazir Shora
Assistant Professor and Head
Department of Anatomy
Government Medical College
Handwara, Jammu & Kashmir, India

Berjina Farooq Naqshi
Assistant Professor and IC Head
Department of Anatomy
Government Medical College
Baramulla, Jammu & Kashmir, India

Nusrat Jabeen
Professor
Department of Anatomy
Government Medical College
Jammu, Jammu & Kashmir, India

National Advisory Board   **XV**

Reeha Mahajan
Associate Professor
Department of Anatomy
All India Institutes of Medical Sciences
Jammu, Jammu & Kashmir, India

Sajad Hamid Khan
Professor
Department of Anatomy
SKIMS Medical College
Srinagar, Jammu & Kashmir, India

Sangeeta Gupta
Professor and Head
Department of Anatomy
Government Medical College
Jammu, Jammu & Kashmir, India

JHARKHAND

Ruchi Ratnesh
Assistant Professor
Department of Anatomy
All India Institute of Medical Sciences
Deoghar, Jharkhand, India

KARNATAKA

Ajay Udyavar
Professor and Head
Department of Anatomy
AJ Institute of Medical Sciences
Mangaluru, Karnataka, India

Anitha MR
Professor and Head
Department of Anatomy
Chikkaballapura Institute of Medical Sciences
Chikkaballapura, Karnataka, India

Asha KR
Professor and Head
Department of Anatomy
Siddaganga Medical College and Research Institute
Tumakuru, Karnataka, India

Ashwini C Appaji
Professor and Head
Department of Anatomy
MS Ramaiah Medical College
Bengaluru, Karnataka, India

Bindurani MK
Professor
Department of Anatomy
Sri Siddhartha Medical College
Tumakuru, Karnataka, India

Deepa Bhat
Associate Professor
Department of Anatomy
JSS Medical College
Mysuru, Karnataka, India

Dinanath Pujari
Professor and Head
Department of Anatomy
ESIC Medical College
Kalaburgi, Karnataka, India

Divya C
Professor
Department of Anatomy
Yenepoya Medical College
Mangaluru, Karnataka, India

GC Poornima
Professor and Head
Department of Anatomy
Mysore Medical College and Research Institute
Mysuru, Karnataka, India

Gangadhara
Professor and Head
Department of Anatomy
Chikkamagaluru Institute of Medical Sciences
Chikkamagaluru, Karnataka, India

Geethanjali BS
Professor
Department of Anatomy
Chandramma Dayananda Sagar Institute of Medical Education and Research
Bengaluru, Karnataka, India

Geethanjali HT
Associate Professor
Department of Anatomy
Mandya Institute of Medical Sciences
Mandya, Karnataka, India

Girish V Patil
Professor and Head
Department of Anatomy
Chamarajanagar Institute of Medical Sciences
Chamarajnagar, Karnataka, India

Harsha Mishrikoti
Assistant Professor
Department of Anatomy
Belagavi Institute of Medical Sciences
Belagavi, Karnataka, India

Kavyashree
Professor and Head
Department of Anatomy
Sri Siddhartha Medical College
Tumakuru, Karnataka, India

Komala B
Professor and Head
Department of Anatomy
BGS Global Institute of Medical Sciences
Bengaluru, Karnataka, India

Lakshmiprabha Subhash
Professor and Head
Department of Anatomy
Sri Siddhartha Institute of Medical Sciences and Research Centre
Bengaluru, Karnataka, India

Lohit Shaha
Associate Professor
Department of Anatomy
SR Patil Medical College
Badagandi, Karnataka, India

Mallikarjun Morigero
Professor
Department of Anatomy
Vijaynagar Institute of Medical Sciences
Bellary, Karnataka, India

Manisha Sachin Chougule
Professor and Head
Department of Anatomy
Jagadguru Gangadhara Mahaswamigalu Moorusaviramath Medical (JGMM) College
Hubballi, Karnataka, India

Manjunath
Associate Professor
Department of Anatomy
Koppal Institute of Medical Sciences
Koppal, Karnataka, India

Martin Lucas
Professor and Head
Department of Anatomy
Chandramma Dayananda Sagar Institute of Medical Education and Research
Mangaluru, Karnataka, India

Mavis Clarrybel
Assistant Professor
Department of Anatomy
Karwar Institute of Medical Sciences
Karwar, Karnataka, India

National Advisory Board

Meenakshi
Professor and Head
Department of Anatomy
Shri Atal Bihari Vajpayee Medical College and Research Institute
Bengaluru, Karnataka, India

Meera Jacoob
Professor and Head
Department of Anatomy
Yenepoya Medical College
Mangaluru, Karnataka, India

Mohandas Rao KG
Professor
Department of Anatomy
Manipal Academy of Higher Education
Manipal, Karnataka, India

Mohankrisna N
Tutor
Department of Anatomy
KVG Medical College
Sullia, Karnataka, India

NM Suresh
Professor and Head
Department of Anatomy
Sri Chamundeshwari Medical College & Research Institute
Channapatna, Karnataka, India

Nagashree MV
Professor and Head
Department of Anatomy
BGS Medical Sciences & Hospital
Bengaluru, Karnataka, India

Naveen NS
Professor and Head
Department of Anatomy
Raichur Institute of Medical Sciences
Raichur, Karnataka, India

Nirmala D
Professor and Head
Department of Anatomy
JJM Medical College
Davangere, Karnataka, India

Patil Shrish
Professor and Head
Department of Anatomy
Basaveshwara Medical College and Hospital
Chitradurga, Karnataka, India

Prakash BS
Professor and Head
Department of Anatomy
Hassan Institute of Medical Sciences
Hassan, Karnataka, India

Praveen Shenoy
Associate Professor
Department of Anatomy
Kasturba Medical College
Mangaluru, Karnataka, India

Premakumari CR
Assistant Professor
Department of Anatomy
Karwar Institute of Medical Sciences
Karwar, Karnataka, India

Pretty Rathnakar
Professor and Head
Department of Anatomy
KS Hegde Medical Academy
Mangaluru, Karnataka, India

Priya Ranganath
Professor
Department of Anatomy
Bengaluru Medical College
Bengaluru, Karnataka, India

Pushpalatha K
Professor
Department of Anatomy
JSS Medical College
Mysuru, Karnataka, India

Pushpalatha M
Professor and Head
Department of Anatomy
Bengaluru Medical College
Bengaluru, Karnataka, India

Qudusia Sultana
Professor
Department of Anatomy
Yenepoya Medical College
Mangaluru, Karnataka, India

Raghavendra
Professor
Department of Anatomy
JJM Medical College
Davangere, Karnataka, India

Rajanigandha
Professor and Head
Department of Anatomy
Kasturba Medical College
Mangaluru, Karnataka, India

Rajapur Parashuram
Professor
Department of Anatomy
Mysore Medical College and Research Institute
Mysuru, Karnataka, India

Rajkumar
Professor and Head
Department of Anatomy
Gulbarga Institute of Medical Sciences
Kalaburgi, Karnataka, India

Rashmi Bhat
Professor and Head
Department of Anatomy
Srinivas Institute of Medical Sciences & Research
Mangaluru, Karnataka, India

Ravikumar
Professor and Head
Department of Anatomy
Subbaiah Institute of Medical Sciences
Shivamogga, Karnataka, India

Ravindra Patil
Professor and Head
Department of Anatomy
Vijaynagar Institute of Medical Sciences
Bellary, Karnataka, India

Rekha Hiremath
Associate Professor
Department of Anatomy
S Nijalingappa Medical College
Bagalkot, Karnataka, India

Rohini
Associate Professor
Department of Anatomy
BGS Global Institute of Medical Sciences
Bengaluru, Karnataka, India

Roopasree Ramakrishna
Professor and Head
Department of Anatomy
East Point Medical College
Bengaluru, Karnataka, India

Roshan S
Professor and Head
Department of Anatomy
Kanachur Institute of Medical Sciences and Research
Mangaluru, Karnataka, India

National Advisory Board **xvii**

Roshni Bajpe
Professor and Head
Department of Anatomy
Kempegowda Institute of Medical Sciences
Bengaluru, Karnataka, India

Sangeeta M
Professor and Head
Department of Anatomy
MVJ Medical College
Bengaluru, Karnataka, India

Seema
Professor and Head
Department of Anatomy
ESIC Medical College
Bengaluru, Karnataka, India

Shailaja C Math
Professor and Head
Department of Anatomy
SS Institute of Medical Sciences
Davangere, Karnataka, India

Shashi Rekha M
Professor and Head
Department of Anatomy
Vydehi Institute of Medical Sciences
Bengaluru, Karnataka, India

Sheetal Pattanshetti
Professor and Head
Department of Anatomy
Jawaharlal Nehru Medical College
Belagavi, Karnataka, India

Shilpa Madhukar
Assistant Professor
Department of Anatomy
Karwar Institute of Medical Sciences
Karwar, Karnataka, India

Shivarama Bhat
Professor
Department of Anatomy
Yenepoya Medical College
Mangaluru, Karnataka, India

Shruthi BN
Professor and Head
Department of Anatomy
Rajarajeshwari Medical College and Hospital
Bengaluru, Karnataka, India

Somesh MS
Professor and Head
Department of Anatomy
Father Muller Medical College
Mangaluru, Karnataka, India

Sridevi NS
Professor and Head
Department of Anatomy
PES University Institute of Medical Sciences & Research
Bengaluru, Karnataka, India

Sucharitha
Professor and Head
Department of Anatomy
Sapthagiri Institute of Medical Sciences
Bengaluru, Karnataka, India

Suma MP
Professor and Head
Department of Anatomy
The Oxford Medical College and Hospital
Bengaluru, Karnataka, India

Sunil O
Assistant Professor
Department of Anatomy
BR Ambedkar Medical College
Bengaluru, Karnataka, India

Tanveer Ahamed Khan
Associate Professor
Department of Anatomy
Shivamogga Institute of Medical Sciences
Shivamogga, Karnataka, India

Tejaswi HI
Professor and Head
Department of Anatomy
Adichunchanagiri Institute of Medical Sciences
BG Nagara, Karnataka, India

Trinesh Gowda
Professor and Head
Department of Anatomy
Mandya Institute of Medical Sciences
Mandya, Karnataka, India

Vanadan Blossom
Tutor
Department of Anatomy
Kasturba Medical College
Mangaluru, Karnataka, India

Varalakshmi
Professor
Department of Anatomy
KS Hegde Medical Academy
Mangaluru, Karnataka, India

Varsha Shenoy
Professor
Department of Anatomy
Father Muller Medical College
Mangaluru, Karnataka, India

Vasuda Kulkarni
Professor and Head
Department of Anatomy
Akash Institute of Medical Sciences
Bengaluru, Karnataka, India

Veerabhadra Nandyal
Professor and Head
Department of Anatomy
Mahadeva Rampure Medical College
Kalaburgi, Karnataka, India

Venkatesh
Professor and Head
Department of Anatomy
Sri Devaraj Urs Medical College
Kolar, Karnataka, India

Vidhya R
Assistant Professor and Deputy Registrar (Examination)
Department of Anatomy
International Medical School
MS Ramaiah Group of Institutions
Bengaluru, Karnataka, India

Vidya CS
Professor and Head
Department of Anatomy
JSS Medical College
Mysuru, Karnataka, India

Vishal Kumar
Professor and Head
Department of Anatomy
Kodagu Institute of Medical Sciences
Madikeri, Karnataka, India

Vishal M Salve
Professor and Head
Department of Anatomy
Navodaya Medical College
Raichur, Karnataka, India

National Advisory Board

Yogesh D
Associate Professor
Department of Anatomy
Shridevi Institute of Medical Sciences
Tumakuru, Karnataka, India

Yogitha R
Professor and Head
Department of Anatomy
St John's Medical College
Bengaluru, Karnataka, India

KERALA

Abdul Waheed Ansari
Professor
Department of Anatomy
MES Medical College
Perinthalmanna, Kerala, India

Ashalatha
Head
Department of Anatomy
Malabar Medical College
Calicut, Kerala, India

Beena
Head
Department of Anatomy
Government Medical College
Kannur, Kerala, India

Benjamin W
Professor
Department of Anatomy
PK Das Institute of Medical Science
Palakkad, Kerala, India

Harilal T
Assistant Professor
Department of Anatomy
Sri Sankara Dental College
Thiruvananthapuram, Kerala, India

Indira CK
Head
Department of Anatomy
Government Medical College
Ernakulam, Kerala, India

Jikend
Assistant Professor
Department of Anatomy
Azeezia Medical College
Kollam, Kerala, India

Lola Das
Head
Department of Anatomy
Amala Institute of Medical Science
Thrissur, Kerala, India

Minnie Pillay
Head
Department of Anatomy
Amrita Institute of Medical Science
Ernakulam, Kerala, India

Nandagopalan
Head
Department of Anatomy
Jubilee Mission Medical College
Thrissur, Kerala, India

PK Ramakrishnan
Head
Department of Anatomy
PK Das Institute of Medical Science
Palakkad, Kerala, India

Ranjith S
Professor
Department of Anatomy
Jubilee Mission Medical College
Thrissur, Kerala, India

Sandhya Kurup
Head
Department of Anatomy
Sree Narayana Institute of Medical Science
Ernakulam, Kerala, India

Sathidevi
Head
Department of Anatomy
Government Medical College
Thrissur, Kerala, India

Sheela Sivan
Head
Department of Anatomy
MES Medical College
Perinthalmanna, Kerala, India

Suma Thomas
Professor and Head
Department of Anatomy
Believers Church Medical College
Thiruvalla, Kerala, India

Susan Varghese
Professor and Head
Department of Anatomy
Government Medical College
Kollam, Kerala, India

TK Kumari
Professor and Head
Department of Anatomy
Azeezia Medical College
Kollam, Kerala, India

Usha Devi KB
Professor and Head
Department of Anatomy
Government Medical College
Thiruvananthapuram, Kerala, India

Vandana LR
Assistant Professor
Department of Anatomy
Government Medical College
Thiruvananthapuram, Kerala, India

Vijayamma KN
Professor
Department of Anatomy
Believers Church Medical College
Thiruvalla, Kerala, India

MADHYA PRADESH

Ashutosh Mangalgiri
Professor
Department of Anatomy
Chirayu Medical College
Bhopal, Madhya Pradesh, India

AS Parmar
Professor
Department of Anatomy
Shyam Shah Medical College
Rewa, Madhya Pradesh, India

Israr Ahemad
Assistant Professor
Department of Anatomy
Government Medical College
Shahdol, Madhya Pradesh, India

Manjunath V Motagi
Professor and Head
Department of Anatomy
SAMC & PGI
Indore, Madhya Pradesh, India

Naresh Thaduri
Associate Professor
Department of Anatomy
LN Medical College
Bhopal, Madhya Pradesh, India

Natwar Agrawal
Professor and Head
Department of Anatomy
Netaji Subhash Chandra Bose Medical College
Jabalpur, Madhya Pradesh, India

National Advisory Board   **xix**

Neha Rai
Professor
Department of Anatomy
LN Medical College & JK Hospital
Bhopal, Madhya Pradesh, India

Shema Nair
Professor
Department of Anatomy
LN Medical College & JK Hospital
Bhopal, Madhya Pradesh, India

MAHARASHTRA

Aditya Tarnekar
Professor and Head
Department of Anatomy
All India Institute of Medical Sciences
Nagpur, Maharashtra, India

Ajit Holkunde
Professor and Head
Department of Anatomy
Ashwini Rural Medical College
Solapur, Maharashtra, India

Amol Ashok Shinde
Professor
Department of Anatomy
DY Patil Medical College
Pune, Maharashtra, India

Anita Rahul Gune
Professor
Department of Anatomy
DY Patil Medical College
Kolhapur, Maharashtra, India

Anjali Patil
Professor and Head
Department of Anatomy
Government Medical College
Baramati, Maharashtra, India

Anupama Sawal
Professor
Department of Anatomy
Jawaharlal Nehru Medical College
Wardha, Maharashtra, India

Archana D Kannamwar
Associate Professor and Head
Department of Anatomy
Shri Vasantrao Naik Government Medical College
Yavatmal, Maharashtra, India

Archana Kalyankar
Professor and Head
Department of Anatomy
Government Medical College and Hospital
Chhatrapati Sambhajinagar, Maharashtra, India

Archana Shekokar
Professor and Head
Department of Anatomy
Smt Kashibhai Navale Medical College
Pune, Maharashtra, India

Arun S Karmalkar
Professor
Department of Anatomy
DY Patil Medical College
Kolhapur, Maharashtra, India

Ashalata Deepak Patil
Professor
Department of Anatomy
DY Patil Medical College
Kolhapur, Maharashtra, India

Ashwini Jadhav
Professor
Department of Anatomy
Grant Government Medical College
Mumbai, Maharashtra, India

Brijesh Singh
Professor and Head
Department of Anatomy
Datta Meghe Medical College
Nagpur, Maharashtra, India

Col Debashish Bandyopadhyay
Head and Professor
Department of Anatomy
Armed Force Medical College
Pune, Maharashtra, India

Deepali Gaurav Vidhale
Professor and Head
Department of Anatomy
Panjabrao Deshmukh Memorial Medical College
Amravati, Maharashtra, India

Deepali Omkar
Professor and Head
Department of Anatomy
NKP Salve Institute of Medical Sciences
Nagpur, Maharashtra, India

Dhapate SS
Dean
Department of Anatomy
Swami Ramanand Teerth Rural Government Medical College
Ambajogai, Maharashtra, India

Eva Marker
Assistant Professor
Department of Anatomy
Mimer Medical College
Talgeon, Maharashtra, India

Gautam Shroff
Professor and Head
Department of Anatomy
MGM Medical College
Chhatrapati Sambhajinagar, Maharashtra, India

Jaideo Manohar Ughade
Professor and Head
Department of Anatomy
Parbhani Medical College
Parbhani, Maharashtra, India

Jwalant Waghmare
Professor and Head
Department of Anatomy
Mahatma Gandhi Institute of Medical Sciences
Wardha, Maharashtra, India

K Shyamkishore
Professor and Head
Department of Anatomy
TN Medical College
Mumbai, Maharashtra, India

Kanchan Pandurang Wankhede
Professor
Department of Anatomy
Government Medical College
Nagpur, Maharashtra, India

Kirti Solanke
Assistant Professor
Department of Anatomy
Smt Kashibhai Navale Medical College
Pune, Maharashtra, India

Mahesh Taru
Associate Professor
Department of Anatomy
BJ Medical College
Pune, Maharashtra, India

National Advisory Board

Maitreyee Muthalic
Professor and Head
Department of Anatomy
SSPM Medical College
Kasal, Maharashtra, India

Mandar Ambike
Professor and Head
Department of Anatomy
Symbiosis Medical College for Women
Pune, Maharashtra, India

Mangesh Selukar
Professor and Head
Department of Anatomy
Dr Vaishampayan Memorial
Government Medical College
Solapur, Maharashtra, India

Manoj Ambali
Professor and Head
Department of Anatomy
Krishna Vishwa Vidyapeeth
Karad, Maharashtra, India

Meenakshi Borkar
Additional Professor
Department of Anatomy
HBT Medical College
Mumbai, Maharashtra, India

Nambrata Marate
Assistant Professor
Department of Anatomy
Vikhe Patil Medical College
Ahmednagar, Maharashtra, India

Neelesh Kanskar
Professor
Department of Anatomy
DY Patil Medical College
Pune, Maharashtra, India

Nitin R Mudiraj
Head and Professor
Department of Anatomy
Bharati Vidyapeeth (Deemed to Be University) Medical College and Hospital
Sangli, Maharashtra, India

Pallavi Bajpaye
Professor
Department of Anatomy
DY Patil Medical College
Pune, Maharashtra, India

Pathan FT
Professor and Head
Department of Anatomy
MIMSR Medical College
Latur, Maharashtra, India

Pradeep Bokariya
Assistant Professor
Department of Anatomy
Mahatma Gandhi Institute of Medical Sciences
Wardha, Maharashtra, India

Praful Nikam
Professor
Department of Anatomy
Jawaharlal Nehru Medical College
Swangi Wardha, Maharashtra, India

Prafulla Sahebrao Dakhane
Professor and Head
Department of Anatomy
Vasantrao Pawar Medical College
Nashik, Maharashtra, India

Pratima Kulkarni
Professor and Head
Department of Anatomy
Government Medical College
Latur, Maharashtra, India

Preeti Sonja
Professor and Head
Department of Anatomy
DY Patil Medical College
Pune, Maharashtra, India

Priya P Roy
Professor
Department of Anatomy
Krishna Vishwa Vidyapeeth
Karad, Maharashtra, India

Pushpa Burute
Professor and Head
Department of Anatomy
BKL Walawalkar Rural Medical College
Chiplun, Maharashtra, India

Rajani Joshi
Professor and Head
Department of Anatomy
Government Medical College
Miraj, Maharashtra, India

Rajesh Dehankar
Professor
Department of Anatomy
NKP Salve Institute of Medical Sciences
Nagpur, Maharashtra, India

Rashmi Patil
Professor Additional
Department of Anatomy
GS Medical College
Mumbai, Maharashtra, India

Ritika Gaddewar
Associate Professor
Department of Anatomy
Indira Gandhi Government Medical College & Hospital
Nagpur, Maharashtra, India

Rupali Atul Gajare
Associate Professor
Department of Anatomy
Rajiv Gandhi Medical College
Thane, Maharashtra, India

Rupali Kavitake
Assistant Professor
Department of Anatomy
Government Medical College
Alibaug, Maharashtra, India

Ruta Bapat
Professor
Department of Anatomy
DY Patil Medical College
Navi Mumbai, Maharashtra, India

Sadiq Sayed
Associate Professor
Department of Anatomy
Government Medical College
Miraj, Maharashtra, India

Sandeep Pakhale
Professor and Head
Department of Anatomy
Rural Medical College
Loni, Maharashtra, India

Santosh Dope
Associate Professor and Medical Superintendent
Department of Anatomy
Government Medical College
Latur, Maharashtra, India

National Advisory Board

Shailendra Jadhav
Professor and Head
Department of Anatomy
RCSM Government Medical College
Kolhapur, Maharashtra, India

Sharadkumar P Sawant
Professor and Head
Department of Anatomy
KJ Somaiya Medical College
Mumbai, Maharashtra, India

Shashank Vedpathak
Professor and Head
Department of Anatomy
Maharashtra Institute of Medical
Education and Research
Pune, Maharashtra, India

Shilpa Gosawi
Professor and Head
Department of Anatomy
Bharati Vidyapeeth Medical College
Pune, Maharashtra, India

Sonali Khake
Professor
Department of Anatomy
SSPM Medical College
Kasal, Maharashtra, India

Srividya Sreenivasan
Professor and Head
Department of Anatomy
DY Patil Medical College
Navi Mumbai, Maharashtra, India

Sudhir Pawar
Professor and Head
Department of Anatomy
Vikhe Patil Medical College
Ahmednagar, Maharashtra, India

Sumedh Ganpat Sonavane
Additional Professor
Department of Anatomy
TN Medical College
Mumbai, Maharashtra, India

Sunita Bharti
Professor
Department of Anatomy
MGM Medical College
Navi Mumbai, Maharashtra, India

Sunita Sawant
Professor and Head
Department of Anatomy
Bharatratna Atal Bihari Vajpayee
Medical College
Pune, Maharashtra, India

Surekha Jadhav
Professor
Department of Anatomy
Vikhe Patil Medical College
Ahmednagar, Maharashtra, India

Suruchi Singhal
Assistant Professor
Department of Anatomy
KJ Somaiya Medical College
Mumbai, Maharashtra, India

Suvarna Gulanikar
Associate Professor
Department of Anatomy
Shri Ramchandra Institute of Medical
Sciences
Chhatrapati Sambhajinagar,
Maharashtra, India

Swapna A Ambekar
Associate Professor
Department of Anatomy
Government Medical College
Chhatrapati Sambhajinagar,
Maharashtra, India

Swati Patil
Professor
Department of Anatomy
Prakash Institute of Medical Science
Islampur, Maharashtra, India

TD Golghate
Professor and Head
Department of Anatomy
Government Medical College
Chandrapur, Maharashtra, India

Ujwala Gajbe
Professor and Dean
Department of Anatomy
Datta Meghe Medical College
Nagpur, Maharashtra, India

Vaishali B Bhagwat
Associate Professor
Department of Anatomy
Vilasrao Deshmukh Government
Medical College
Latur, Maharashtra, India

Vaishali Inamdar
Professor and Head
Department of Anatomy
Government Medical College
Nanded, Maharashtra, India

Vaishali Sushil Anturlikar
Professor
Department of Anatomy
ACPM Medical College
Dhule, Maharashtra, India

Varsha Dahiphale
Associate Professor
Department of Anatomy
SRTR Government Medical College
Ambajogai, Maharashtra, India

Vatsalaswami
Director Academy
Department of Anatomy
DY Patil Medical College
Pune, Maharashtra, India

Vasudha Nikam
Professor and Head
Department of Anatomy
DY Patil Medical College
Kolhapur, Maharashtra, India

Vidya Kharat
Associate Professor
Department of Anatomy
Bharati Vidyapeeth Medical College
Pune, Maharashtra, India

Vijaya Sagar T
Dean
Department of Anatomy
Symbiosis Medical College for Woman
Pune, Maharashtra, India

Vilas Chimurkar
Professor and Head
Department of Anatomy
Jawaharlal Nehru Medical College
Wardha, Maharashtra, India

Yashwant Kulkarni
Professor and Head
Department of Anatomy
Government Medical College
Satara, Maharashtra, India

Yuvaraj Jayprakash Bhosale
Additional Professor
Department of Anatomy
T N Medical College
Mumbai, Maharashtra, India

NAGALAND

Arun Sharma
Assistant Professor
Department of Anatomy
Nagaland Institute of Medical Sciences
and Research (NIMSR)
Kohima, Nagaland, India

NEW DELHI

Anjoo Yadav
Professor and Head
Department of Anatomy
Lady Harding Medical College
New Delhi, India

Gourav Dadarao Thakre
Associate Professor
Department of Anatomy
BSA Medical College and Hospital
Rohini, New Delhi, India

Hitendra Loh
Professor
Department of Anatomy
Vardhman Mahavir Medical College and
Safdarjung Hospital
New Delhi, India

Kusum Singla
Associate Professor
Department of Anatomy
Army College of Medical Science
New Delhi, India

Minakshi Malhotra
Professor
Department of Anatomy
Lady Harding Medical College
New Delhi, India

Preeti Shrivastava
Professor
Department of Anatomy
North DMC medical College and Hindu
Rao Hospital
New Delhi, India

Shaifaly Madan Rustagi
Professor and Head
Department of Anatomy
Army College of Medical Sciences
New Delhi, India

Sarika Rachel Tigga
Assistant Professor
Department of Anatomy
University College of Medical Sciences
New Delhi, India

Saba Yaseen
Assistant Professor
Department of Anatomy
Hamdard Institute of Medical Sciences
New Delhi, India

ODISHA

Geetanjali Arora
Head
Department of Anatomy
Hitech Medical College
Bhubaneswar, Odisha, India

Gyanaranjan Nayak
Professor
Department of Anatomy
IMS and SUM Hospital Siksha 'O'
Anusandhan (Deemed to be University)
Bhubaneswar, Odisha, India

Prajna Parimita Samanta
Professor
Department of Anatomy
Kalinga Institute of Medical Sciences
Bhubaneswar, Odisha, India

Rajashree Bisoi
Professor and Head
Department of Anatomy
SCB Medical College
Cuttack, Odisha, India

Ramakrishna Sahu
Professor and Head
Department of Anatomy
Pandit Raghunath Murmu Medical
College
Baripada, Odisha, India

Santosh Kumar Sahu
Professor and Head
Department of Anatomy
Bhima Bhoi Medical College
Bolangir, Odisha, India

Saurjya Ranjan Das
Professor
Department of Anatomy
IMS and SUM Hospital SOA University
Bhubaneswar, Odisha, India

Smruti Rekha Mohanty
Head
Department of Anatomy
Kalinga Institute of Medical Sciences
Bhubaneswar, Odisha, India

PUDUCHERRY

Arul Moli
Professor and Head
Department of Anatomy
Mahatma Gandhi Medical College and
Research Institute
Puducherry, India

Aruna S
Professor and Head
Department of Anatomy
Indira Gandhi Medical College and
Research Institute
Puducherry, India

Ilankathir
Professor and Head
Department of Anatomy
Aarupadai Veedu Medical College
Puducherry, India

Malar
Professor and Head
Department of Anatomy
Sri Venkateswaraa Medical College
Hospital and Research Centre
Puducherry, India

Prabavathy
Professor
Department of Anatomy
Mahatma Gandhi Medical College and
Research Institute
Puducherry, India

Ratnasamy
Director and Professor
Department of Anatomy
Sri Venkateshwaraa Medical College
Hospital and Research Centre
Puducherry, India

Rema Devi
Professor and Head
Department of Anatomy
Pondicherry Institute of Medical
Sciences and Research
Puducherry, India

National Advisory Board   **xxiii**

Suba Ananthi
Professor
Department of Anatomy
Indira Gandhi Medical College and Research Institute
Puducherry, India

Suriyakumari KVP
Professor and Head
Department of Anatomy
Sri Manakula Vinayagar Medical College and Hospital
Puducherry, India

Vijisha
Professor and Head
Department of Anatomy
Sri Laskhmi Narayana Institute of Medical Sciences
Puducherry, India

PUNJAB

Ajay Kumar
Professor
Department of Anatomy
Dayanand Medical College and Hospital
Ludhiana, Punjab, India

Anjali Jain
Professor
Department of Anatomy
Christian Medical College
Ludhiana, Punjab, India

Anterpreet Kaur
Head
Department of Anatomy
Shri Guru Ram Dass Medical College
Amritsar, Punjab, India

Anu Sharma
Professor
Department of Anatomy
Dayanand Medical College & Hospital
Ludhiana, Punjab, India

Gursharan Singh Dhindsa
Associate Professor
Department of Anatomy
Guru Gobind Singh Medical College
Faridkot, Punjab, India

Harpreet Singh Gulati
Associate Professor
Department of Anatomy
Punjab Institute of Medical Sciences
Jalandhar, Punjab, India

Harsimarjit Kaur
Associate Professor
Department of Anatomy
Government Medical College
Patiala, Punjab, India

Jyoti Rohila
Assistant Professor
Department of Anatomy
BR Ambedkar Medical College
Mohali, Punjab, India

Jyotsna Singh
Associate Professor
Department of Anatomy
Government Medical College and Hospital
Chandigarh, Punjab, India

Kanchan Kapoor
Professor
Department of Anatomy
Government Medical College
Chandigarh, Punjab, India

Kulbir Kaur
Assistant Professor
Department of Anatomy
Government Medical College
Amritsar, Punjab, India

Kuntal Vashishtha
Head
Department of Anatomy
National Dental College
Dera Bassi, Punjab, India

Manisha
Professor and Head
Department of Anatomy
BR Ambedkar State Institute of Medical Sciences
Mohali, Punjab, India

Monika Gupta
Professor and Head
Department of Anatomy
Adesh Institute of Medical Sciences and Research
Bathinda, Punjab, India

Navjot Kaur
Associate Professor
Department of Anatomy
Adesh Institute of Medical Sciences and Research Center
Bathinda, Punjab, India

Priti Chaudhary
Professor and Head
Department of Anatomy (Additional)
All India Institute of Medical Sciences
Bathinda, Punjab, India

Seema
Professor
Department of Anatomy
Shri Guru Ram Das Medical College
Amritsar, Punjab, India

Vandana Sidhu
Assistant Professor
Department of Anatomy
Government Medical College
Amritsar, Punjab, India

RAJASTHAN

Aarushi Jain
Professor and Head
Department of Anatomy
Government Medical College
Kota, Rajasthan, India

Abha Bharadwaja
Senior Professor and Head
Department of Anatomy
Jawaharlal Nehru Medical College
Ajmer, Rajasthan, India

Abhijeet Joshi
Associate Professor and Head
Department of Anatomy
Government Medical College
Barmer, Rajasthan, India

Ajay R Nene
Professor and Head
Department of Anatomy
ESIC Medical College
Alwar, Rajasthan, India

Anjali Jain
Associate Professor
Department of Anatomy
American International Institute of Medical Sciences
Udaipur, Rajasthan, India

Anita
Professor and Head
Department of Anatomy
SJP Medical College
Bharatpur, Rajasthan, India

National Advisory Board

Anoop Singh Gurjar
Professor and Head
Department of Anatomy
Government Medical College
Pali, Rajasthan, India

Aprajita Raizada
Professor and Head
Department of Anatomy
American International Institute of Medical Sciences
Udaipur, Rajasthan, India

Ashish Sharma
Professor and Head
Department of Anatomy
Government Medical College
Chittorgarh, Rajasthan, India

Charu Sharma
Professor
Department of Anatomy
Geetanjali Medical College and Hospital
Udaipur, Rajasthan, India

Dharmendra Choudhary
Assistant Professor
Department of Anatomy
National Institute of Ayurveda
Jaipur, Rajasthan, India

GN Trivedi
Professor and Head
Department of Anatomy
S S Tantia Medical College and University
Sri Ganganagar, Rajasthan, India

Heena Sharma
Professor
Department of Anatomy
Pacific Medical College and Hospital
Udaipur, Rajasthan, India

Isha Shrivastava
Associate Professor
Department of Anatomy
Pacific Medical College and Hospital
Udaipur, Rajasthan, India

Kalpana Sharma
Assistant Professor
Department of Anatomy
Pacific Institute of Medical Sciences
Udaipur, Rajasthan, India

Kavita Pahuja
Professor
Department of Anatomy
SP Medical College
Bikaner, Rajasthan, India

Monali Sonawane
Professor
Department of Anatomy
Geetanjali Medical College and Hospital
Udaipur, Rajasthan, India

Neha Vijay
Associate Professor
Department of Anatomy
Government Medical College
Alwar, Rajasthan, India

Nikha Bhardwaj
Associate Professor
Department of Anatomy
All India Institute of Medical Sciences
Jodhpur, Rajasthan, India

Parvéen Kumar Sharma
Director Academic and Research
Department of Anatomy
Tantia university
Sri Ganganagar, Rajasthan, India

Pooja Gangrade
Professor and Head
Department of Anatomy
Government Medical College
Bhilwara, Rajasthan, India

Prakash KG
Professor and Head
Department of Anatomy
Geetanjali Medical College and Hospital
Udaipur, Rajasthan, India

Pratima Jaiswal
Professor
Department of Anatomy
Government Medical College
Kota, Rajasthan, India

Praveen Ojha
Professor and Head
Department of Anatomy
RNT Medical College
Udaipur, Rajasthan, India

Rasalika Miglani
Assistant Professor
Department of Anatomy
SS Tantia Medical College Hospital and Research Centre
Sri Ganganagar, Rajasthan, India

Rekha Gahlot
Associate Professor
Department of Anatomy
Sardar Patel Medical College
Bikaner, Rajasthan, India

Ritu Agarwal
Professor
Department of Anatomy
Government Medical College
Pali, Rajasthan, India

Sachendra Mittal
Assistant Professor
Department of Anatomy
NIMS
Jaipur, Rajasthan, India

Saryu Sain
Associate Professor and Head
Department of Anatomy
Shri Kalyan Government Medical College
Sikar, Rajasthan, India

Sajan Sakaria
Associate Professor
Department of Anatomy
American International Institute of Medical Sciences
Udaipur, Rajasthan, India

Sami Ahmed
Assistant Professor
Department of Anatomy
JNU Jaipur Institute for Medical Sciences and Research Centre
Jaipur, Rajasthan, India

Sanjay Sharma
Professor and Head
Department of Anatomy
Government Medical College
Sri Ganganagar, Rajasthan, India

Seema Prakash
Senior Professor
Department of Anatomy
RNT Medical College
Udaipur, Rajasthan, India

Shweta Asthana
Associate Professor
Department of Anatomy
RNT Medical College
Udaipur, Rajasthan, India

Stuti Srivastava
Professor and Head
Department of Anatomy
Ananta Institute of Medical Sciences
and Research Centre
Udaipur, Rajasthan, India

Sumeet Gupta
Professor
Department of Anatomy
Government Medical College
Kota, Rajasthan, India

Sushma Kushal Kataria
Senior Professor and Head
Department of Anatomy
Sampurnanand Medical College
Jodhpur, Rajasthan, India

TAMIL NADU

Amudha G
Professor and Head
Department of Anatomy
PSG Institute of Medical Science
Coimbatore, Tamil Nadu, India

Anandthi
Professor and Head
Department of Anatomy
KAP Viswanthan Government Medical
College
Trichy, Tamil Nadu, India

Anitha
Professor and Head
Department of Anatomy
Government Villupuram Medical
College
Villupuram, Tamil Nadu, India

Anjana TSR
Associate Professor
Department of Anatomy
Government Medical College
Omandurar
Chennai, Tamil Nadu, India

Anupama
Professor and Head
Department of Anatomy
St Peter Medical College
Hosur, Tamil Nadu, India

Archana
Associate Professor
Department of Anatomy
Government Chengalpattu Medical
College
Chengalpattu, Tamil Nadu, India

Arul Santhini
Professor and Head
Department of Anatomy
Vinayaka Missions Medical College
Karaikal, Tamil Nadu, India

Bharathi Rani
Associate Professor
Department of Anatomy
Government Sivagangai Medical
College
Sivaganga, Tamil Nadu, India

Chithra
Professor and Head
Department of Anatomy
Dhanalakshmi Srinivasan Medical
College
Siruvachur, Tamil Nadu, India

Dhanalakshmi V
Professor
Department of Anatomy
Thoothukudi Medical College
Thoothukudi, Tamil Nadu, India

Dharani
Professor and Head
Department of Anatomy
Government Medical College
Nagapattinam, Tamil Nadu, India

Dhivya
Associate Professor
Department of Anatomy
Government Medical College
Namakkal, Tamil Nadu, India

Duraipandian
Professor and Head
Department of Anatomy
Karpaga Vinayaka Institute of Medical
Sciences and Research Center
Kanchipuram, Tamil Nadu, India

Durga Devi
Professor and Head
Department of Anatomy
Sree Balaji Medical College and Hospital
Chennai, Tamil Nadu, India

Ezhilarasn
Professor and Head
Department of Anatomy
Government Medical College
Theni, Tamil Nadu, India

Gayathri
Professor and Head
Department of Anatomy
Government Medical College
Ariyalur, Tamil Nadu, India

Gnanavel A
Professor
Department of Anatomy
Meenakshi Medical College and
Research Institute
Kanchipuram, Tamil Nadu, India

Gnanavelraja C
Professor and Head
Department of Anatomy
SRM Medical College and Hospital and
Research Centre
Tiruchirappalli, Tamil Nadu, India

Guna Priya
Professor and Head
Department of Anatomy
Annai Medical College and Hospital
Sri Perumbadur, Tamil Nadu, India

Janaki
Professor
Department of Anatomy
Bhaarat Medical College and Hospital
Chennai, Tamil Nadu, India

Jeyanthi
Professor and Head
Department of Anatomy
Tirunelveli Medical College
Tirunelveli, Tamil Nadu, India

Jose Hemalatha
Professor and Head
Department of Anatomy
Government Medical College
Virudhunagar, Tamil Nadu, India

Jothi Ganesh
Assistant Professor
Department of Anatomy
Government Medical College
Dindigul, Tamil Nadu, India

KC Shanthi
Professor and Head
Department of Anatomy
Vinayaka Missions Kirupananda Variyar
Medical College
Salem, Tamil Nadu, India

National Advisory Board

Kafeel Hussain
Professor and Head
Department of Anatomy
Bhaarat Medical College and Hospital
Chennai, Tamil Nadu, India

Kalai Anbusudar
Associate Professor
Department of Anatomy
Government Mohan Kumaramangalam Medical College
Salem, Tamil Nadu, India

Kalaivani
Associate Professor
Department of Anatomy
VELS Medical College and Hospital
Thiruvallur, Tamil Nadu, India

Kalaiyarasi S
Professor and Head
Department of Anatomy
Government Medical College
Pudukkottai, Tamil Nadu, India

Kalpana
Senior Assistant Professor
Department of Anatomy
Government Medical College and Hospital
Krishnagiri, Tamil Nadu, India

Kalpana
Professor and Head
Department of Anatomy
Sri Ramachandra Institute of Higher Education and Research
Chennai, Tamil Nadu, India

Kanagavali
Professor and Head
Department of Anatomy
Government Medical College
Tiruvallur, Tamil Nadu, India

Kavipriya
Assistant Professor
Department of Anatomy
Government Medical College
Pudukkottai, Tamil Nadu, India

Lokanayaki
Professor and Head
Department of Anatomy
Kilpauk Medical College
Chennai, Tamil Nadu, India

Mahajan
Professor and Head
Department of Anatomy
Indira Medical College and Hospital
Tiruvallur, Tamil Nadu, India

Mahima Sophia
Professor and Head
Department of Anatomy
Panimalar Medical College Hospital and Research Institute
Chennai, Tamil Nadu, India

Margaret
Professor and Head
Department of Anatomy
Thiruvarur Government Medical College
Thiruvarur, Tamil Nadu, India

Muthu Kumar
Professor
Department of Anatomy
Sri Lalithambigai Medical College and Hospital
Chennai, Tamil Nadu, India

Muthuprasad P
Associate Professor
Department of Anatomy
Government Medical College
Karur, Tamil Nadu, India

Nedunchezhiyan
Associate Professor
Department of Anatomy
Government Medical College
Ariyalur, Tamil Nadu, India

Nirmala Devi
Professor and Head
Department of Anatomy
Karpagam Faculty of Medical Sciences and Research
Coimbatore, Tamil Nadu, India

Nisha Manual
Professor and Head
Department of Anatomy
Government Tiruvannamalai Medical College
Tiruvannamalai, Tamil Nadu, India

Padmasrini S
Professor
Department of Anatomy
Madha Medical College and Hospital
Chennai, Tamil Nadu, India

Parthiban
Professor
Department of Anatomy
Madurai Medical College
Madurai, Tamil Nadu, India

Perumal
Associate Professor
Department of Anatomy
Srinivasa Medical College
Trichy, Tamil Nadu, India

Prabavathi
Professor and Head
Department of Anatomy
Government Dharmapuri Medical College
Dharmapuri, Tamil Nadu, India

Pratheepa
Professor
Department of Anatomy
SRM Medical College Hospital and Research Centre
Chengalpattu, Tamil Nadu, India

Prefulla
Associate Professor
Department of Anatomy
Government Medical College
Nagapattinam, Tamil Nadu, India

Radha
Professor
Department of Anatomy
Dhanalakshmi Srinivasan Institute of Medical Sciences
Perambalur, Tamil Nadu, India

Rajapriya
Professor and Head
Department of Anatomy
Government Medical College
Chennai, Tamil Nadu, India

Rajesh
Professor
Department of Anatomy
Dhanalakshmi Srinivasan Institute of Medical Sciences
Perambalur, Tamil Nadu, India

Rajeswari
Professor and Head
Department of Anatomy
Government Medical College
Tiruppur, Tamil Nadu, India

National Advisory Board | **xxvii**

Rajila
Assistant Professor
Department of Anatomy
Chettinad Hospital and Research Centre
Kanchipuram, Tamil Nadu, India

Ramesh
Associate Professor
Department of Anatomy
Dhanalakshmi Srinivasan Institute of Medical Sciences
Perambalur, Tamil Nadu, India

Ramesh P
Associate Professor
Department of Anatomy
St Peter Medical College
Hosur, Tamil Nadu, India

Rohini Devi
Professor and Head
Department of Anatomy
Coimbatore Medical College
Coimbatore, Tamil Nadu, India

Samuel Frank
Senior Assistant Professor
Department of Anatomy
Government Medical College
Nilgiris, Tamil Nadu, India

S Sumathi
Associate Professor
Department of Anatomy
Thanjavur Medical College
Thanjavur, Tamil Nadu, India

Sarah
Professor and Head
Department of Anatomy
All India Institute of Medical Sciences
Madurai, Tamil Nadu, India

Sasikala
Professor and Head
Department of Anatomy
Swamy Vivekanandha Medical College Hospital and Research Institute
Namakkal, Tamil Nadu, India

Sasirekha M
Professor and Head
Department of Anatomy
ACS Medical College and Hospital
Chennai, Tamil Nadu, India

Sathish Kumar
Professor and Head
Department of Anatomy
Government Medical College
Kalakuruchi, Tamil Nadu, India

Sivakami
Professor and Head
Department of Anatomy
Thanjavur Medical College
Thanjavur, Tamil Nadu, India

Sowjanya
Professor and Head
Department of Anatomy
Shri Sathya Sai Medical College
Thiruporur, Tamil Nadu, India

Sreevidhya
Professor and Head
Department of Anatomy
Chengalpattu Government Medical College
Chengalpattu, Tamil Nadu, India

Subadha
Associate Professor
Department of Anatomy
Government Dharmapuri Medical College
Dharmapuri, Tamil Nadu, India

Subbulakshmi G
Professor and Head
Department of Anatomy
Government Erode Medical College
Erode, Tamil Nadu, India

Sudha R
Professor and Head
Department of Anatomy
Annapoorna Medical College and Hospital
Salem, Tamil Nadu, India

Suganthy Rabi
Senior Professor
Department of Anatomy
Chirstian Medical College
Vellore, Tamil Nadu, India

Sujatha
Professor and Head
Department of Anatomy
Government Stanley Medical College
Chennai, Tamil Nadu, India

Sumana
Professor and Head
Department of Anatomy
Velammal Medical College Hospital and Research Institute
Madurai, Tamil Nadu, India

Sundarapandian
Professor and Head
Department of Anatomy
SRM Medical College Hospital & Research Centre
Chengalpattu, Tamil Nadu, India

Suresh
Professor and Head
Department of Anatomy
Government Vellore Medical College and Hospital
Vellore, Tamil Nadu, India

Thilagavathy
Professor
Department of Anatomy
Madras Medical College
Chennai, Tamil Nadu, India

Udhaya K
Professor and Head
Department of Anatomy
Swamy Vivekanandha Medical College, Hospital and Research Institute
Namakkal, Tamil Nadu, India

Vidulatha
Professor
Department of Anatomy
Government Medical College
Ramanathapuram, Tamil Nadu, India

Vijaianand M
Professor and Head
Department of Anatomy
KMCH Institute of Health Science and Research
Coimbatore, Tamil Nadu, India

Vijaya
Associate Professor
Department of Anatomy
All India Institute of Medical Sciences
Madurai, Tamil Nadu, India

Vijaya Kumar
Professor and Head
Department of Anatomy
Sri Ramachandra Institute of Higher Education and Research
Chennai, Tamil Nadu, India

Vijayalakshmi
Professor and Head
Department of Anatomy
Melmaruvathur Adhiparasakthi Institute
of Medical Sciences
Melmaruvathur, Tamil Nadu, India

Vinnarasie
Associate Professor
Department of Anatomy
Government Chengalpattu Medical
College
Chengalpattu, Tamil Nadu, India

Vinoth S
Professor and Head
Department of Anatomy
Madha Medical College and Hospital
Chennai, Tamil Nadu, India

Vishali N
Professor
Department of Anatomy
VELS Medical College and Hospital
Thiruvallur, Tamil Nadu, India

TELANGANA

C Kishan Reddy
Professor and Head
Department of Anatomy
Prathima Medical College
Karimnagar, Telangana, India

Chandi Priya
In-Charge and Head
Department of Anatomy
Government Medical College
Khammam, Telangana, India

Chandrasekhar
Professor
Department of Anatomy
Government Medical College
Sangareddy, Telangana, India

Gouri
Professor
Department of Anatomy
PMRIMS College
Chevella, Telangana, India

Naveen Kumar S
Professor and Head
Department of Anatomy
Mallareddy Institute of Medical
Sciences
Hyderabad, Telangana, India

Sumalatha T
Professor and Head
Department of Anatomy
Osmania Medical College
Hyderabad, Telangana, India

Zafar Sultana
Professor
Department of Anatomy
Deccan Medical College
Hyderabad, Telangana, India

UTTARAKHAND

AK Singh
Head
Department of Anatomy
Soban Singh Jeena Medical College
Srinagar, Uttarakhand, India

Brijendra Singh
Head
Department of Anatomy
All India Institute of Medical Sciences
Rishikesh, Uttarakhand, India

Deepa Deopa
Head
Department of Anatomy
Government Medical College
Haldwani, Uttarakhand, India

Jolly Aggarwal
Assistant Professor
Department of Anatomy
Government Doon Medical College
Dehradun, Uttarakhand, India

Kishore Chand
Head
Department of Anatomy
Graphic Era Medical College
Dehradun, Uttarakhand, India

Pant MK
Head
Department of Anatomy
Doon Medical College
Dehradun, Uttarakhand, India

Richa Niranjan
Head
Department of Anatomy
VCSG Government Medical College
Srinagar, Uttarakhand, India

Sadakat Ali
Head
Department of Anatomy
Shri Guru Ram Rai Medical College
Dehradun, Uttarakhand, India

Shashi Munjal
Head
Department of Anatomy
Gautam Budha Chikitsa
Mahavidhyalaya
Dehradun, Uttarakhand, India

Suchit Kumar
Head
Department of Anatomy
Gautam Budha Medical College
Dehradun, Uttarakhand, India

Vandana Sharma
Assistant Professor
Department of Anatomy
Government Medical College
Haldwani, Uttarakhand, India

UTTAR PRADESH

Abhinav Kumar Mishra
Assistant Professor
Department of Anatomy
KMC Medical College and Hospital
Maharajganj, Uttar Pradesh, India

Aditya Pratap Singh
Professor
Department of Anatomy
United Institute of Medical Sciences
Prayagraj, Uttar Pradesh, India

Alok Kumar Singh
Head
Department of Anatomy
Rajkiya Medical College
Jalaun, Uttar Pradesh, India

Alok Tripathi
Associate Professor and Head
Department of Anatomy
Mahatma Vidur Autonomous State
Medical College
Bijnor, Uttar Pradesh, India

Amit Saxena
Professor and Head
Department of Anatomy
Government Medical College
Shahjahanpur, Uttar Pradesh, India

National Advisory Board

Anand Kumar Mishra
Assistant Professor
Department of Anatomy
Maharshi Vashishtha Autonomous Medical College
Basti, Uttar Pradesh, India

Archana Singh
Professor and Head
Department of Anatomy
Government Medical College
Pilihibit, Uttar Pradesh, India

Anshu Gupta
Head
Department of Anatomy
SN Medical College
Agra, Uttar Pradesh, India

Avinash Thakur
Professor
Department of Anatomy
ESIC Medical College and Hospital
Faridabad, Uttar Pradesh, India

Farah Ghaus
Professor and Head
Department of Anatomy
KD Medical College
Mathura, Uttar Pradesh, India

Fateh Mohammad
Professor and Head
Department of Anatomy
Kalyan Singh Government Medical College
Bulandshahr, Uttar Pradesh, India

Hari Narayan Yadav
Associate Professor
Department of Anatomy
KM Medical College and Hospital
Mathura, Uttar Pradesh, India

Hasmatullah
Associate Professor
Department of Anatomy
Madhav Prasad Tripathi Medical College
Siddarthnagar, Uttar Pradesh, India

Hina Kaushar
Professor and Head
Department of Anatomy
Rajshree Medical College and Research Centre
Bareilly, Uttar Pradesh, India

Kamal Bhardwaj
Professor
Department of Anatomy
SN Medical College
Agra, Uttar Pradesh, India

Krishna Gopal
Professor and Head
Department of Anatomy
Shri Ram Murti Smarak Institute of Medical Sciences
Bareilly, Uttar Pradesh, India

Muktyaz Hussain
Associate Professor
Department of Anatomy
Government Medical College
Budaun, Uttar Pradesh, India

Munish Khanna
Professor
Department of Anatomy
Autonomous State Medical College
Firozabad, Uttar Pradesh, India

Nirupma Gupta
Dean and Professor
Department of Anatomy
School of Medical Sciences & Research
Sharda University
Greater Noida, Uttar Pradesh, India

Nisha Kaul
Professor and Head
Department of Anatomy
Rama Medical College
Hapur, Uttar Pradesh, India

Nidhi Sharma
Associate Professor
Department of Anatomy
Kalyan Singh Government Medical College
Bulandshahr, Uttar Pradesh, India

Pratishtha Potdar
Professor and Head
Department of Anatomy
Noida International Institute of Medical Science
Noida, Uttar Pradesh, India

Punita Manik
Head
Department of Anatomy
King George's Medical University
Lucknow, Uttar Pradesh, India

Rajni Patel
Professor and Head
Department of Anatomy,
Veerangana Avanti Bai Lodhi Autonomous State Medical College
Etah, Uttar Pradesh, India

Rakesh Gupta
Professor and Head
Department of Anatomy
Rohillkhand Medical College
Bareilly, Uttar Pradesh, India

Rakesh Kumar Verma
Additional Professor
Department of Anatomy
King George's Medical University
Lucknow, Uttar Pradesh, India

Ram Prakash Gupta
Professor and Head
Department of Anatomy
School of Medical Sciences & Research
Sharda University
Greater Noida, Uttar Pradesh, India

Ramkumar Singhal
Professor
Department of Anatomy
SJP Medical College
Bharatpur, Uttar Pradesh, India

Ratesh Kumar Munjal
Professor and Head
Department of Anatomy
ESIC Medical College and Hospital
Faridabad, Uttar Pradesh, India

Raveena Singh
Assistant Professor
Department of Anatomy
ASJSATDS Medical College
Fatehpur, Uttar Pradesh, India

Shikha Sharma
Professor and Head
Department of Anatomy
FH Medical College
Tundla, Uttar Pradesh, India

Shikky Garg
Professor and Head
Department of Anatomy
Autonomous State Medical College
Firozabad, Uttar Pradesh, India

Shivani Dhingra
Assistant Professor
Department of Anatomy
Bhimrao Ramji Ambedkar Medical College
Kannauj, Uttar Pradesh, India

Shubha Srivastava
Head
Department of Anatomy
NCR Institute of Medical Sciences
Hapur, Uttar Pradesh, India

Soniya Gupta
Assistant Professor
Department of Anatomy
Rama Medical College
Hapur, Uttar Pradesh, India

Sumita Shukla
Assistant Professor
Department of Anatomy
Rajarshi Dashrath Autonomous Medical College
Ayodhya, Uttar Pradesh, India

Swati Yadav
Assistant Professor
Department of Anatomy
Santosh Medical College
Ghaziabad, Uttar Pradesh, India

Srishti Pal
Head
Department of Anatomy
Madhav Prasad Tripathi Medical College
Siddharth Nagar, Uttar Pradesh, India

Vanita Gupta
Head
Department of Anatomy
GS Medical College
Hapur, Uttar Pradesh, India

Vipin Kumar
Assistant Professor
Department of Anatomy
Sone Lal Patel Autonomous State Medical College
Pratapgarh, Uttar Pradesh, India

Vivek Parashar
Associate Professor
Department of Anatomy
Veerangna Awantibai Lodhi Autonomous State Medical College
Etah, Uttar Pradesh, India

Yogesh Yadav
Professor and Head
Department of Anatomy
Saraswati Medical College
Hapur, Uttar Pradesh, India

WEST BENGAL

Anirban Sadhu
Professor
Department of Anatomy
North Bengal Medical College
Darjeeling, West Bengal, India

Hiranmoy Roy
Professor
Department of Anatomy
IPGME & R and SSKM Hospital
Kolkata, West Bengal, India

Kalyan Bhattacharya
Head
Department of Anatomy
Medical College and Hospital
Kolkata, West Bengal, India

Satyajit Saha
Associate Professor
Department of Anatomy
Murshidabad Medical College
Murshidabad, West Bengal, India

Sukanya Palit
Professor
Department of Anatomy
Jhargram Government Medical College
Jhargram, West Bengal, India

Contents

Chapter 1: Some Preliminary Considerations 1
- What is Embryology? 1
- Reproduction 1
- Development and Stages of Human Life 2
- Pregnancy/Gestation, Trimesters, Viability 2
- Basic Processes in Embryology 4

Chapter 2: Molecular Aspect of Embryology 7
- Chromosomes 7
- Karyotyping 10
- Lyon Hypothesis and Sex Chromatin 11

Cell Cycle and Cell Division 12
- Cell Cycle 12
- Cell Division 12
- Mitosis 12
- Meiosis 14
- Molecular Control of Development of Embryo 15

Chapter 3: Gametogenesis, Ovarian and Menstrual Cycle 19
- Structure of a Mature Spermatozoon 19
- Spermatogenesis 20
- Oogenesis 22
- Ovarian Cycle 23
- Menstrual Cycle 26
- Hormonal Control of Ovarian and Uterine Cycles 29

Chapter 4: First Week of Development 35
- Overview of First Week of Development 35
- Fertilization 35
- Test Tube Babies/In Vitro Fertilization 39
- Sex Determination 39
- Cleavage 39
- Implantation 41
- Changes in the Endometrium of the Uterus 44

Chapter 5: Second Week of Development 48
- Events of Second Week of Development 48
- Changes in the Embryoblast 48
- Changes in the Trophoblast 50

Chapter 6: Third Week of Development 58
- Overview of Third Week of Development 58
- Changes in the Germ Disc or Embryonic Area 58
- Formation of Primitive Streak 59
- Gastrulation 60
- Formation of Notochord 60
- Formation of the Neural Tube 62
- Formation of Intraembryonic Mesoderm (Third Germ Layer) 63
- Changes in the Trophoblast 66

Chapter 7: Embryonic Period (Fourth to Eighth Week) of Development 68
- Growth of the Embryo and its Age Determination 68

Embryonic Period 69
- Folding of Embryo 69
- Derivatives of Germ Layers 73

Chapter 8: Fetal Period of Development, Prenatal Diagnosis and Teratology 77
- Fetal Period 77
- Determining the Age of a Living Fetus 78
- Teratology and Birth Defects 79
- Prenatal Diagnosis of Fetus 80
- Fetal Therapy 81

Chapter 9: Fetal Membranes, Placenta and Twinning 85
- Fetal/Extraembryonic Membranes 85
- Placenta 88
- Mutual Relationship of Amniotic Cavity, Extraembryonic Coelom and Uterine Cavity 93
- Multiple Births and Twinning 94

Chapter 10: Basic Tissues of the Body 101
- Epithelia 101
- Connective Tissue 102
- Muscular Tissue 111
- Nervous Tissue 113

Chapter 11: Integumentary System (Skin and its Appendages, Mammary Gland) 118
- Skin 118
- Appendages of Skin 120
- Mammary Glands 122

Chapter 12: Branchial Apparatus (Pharyngeal Arches, Endodermal Pouches and Ectodermal Clefts) 126
- Pharyngeal or Brachial Arches 126

- Derivatives of the Skeletal Elements   128
- Nerves and Muscles of the Arches   128
- Fate of Ectodermal Clefts   130
- Fate of Endodermal Pouches   131
- Pharyngeal Membranes   132
- Development of Palatine Tonsils   132
- Development of the Thymus   132
- Development of Parathyroid Glands   132
- Development of the Thyroid Gland   133

Chapter 13: Skeletal and Muscular System   138

Skeletal System   138
- Axial Skeleton   138
- Appendicular Skeleton   143

Muscular System   145
- Skeletal Muscle   145
- Development of Muscular System   146

Chapter 14: Face, Nose and Palate   150
- Development of Face   150
- Development of Nose   155
- Development of the Palate   156

Chapter 15: Alimentary System—I: Oral Cavity, Salivary Glands and Pharynx   161
- Development of Mouth   161
- Development of Teeth   162
- Development of Tongue   165
- Development of Salivary Glands   167
- Development of Tonsils   168
- Development of Pharynx   168

Chapter 16: Alimentary System—II: Gastrointestinal Tract   171
- Derivatives of All Three Segments of the Primitive Gut   173
- Development of Individual Parts of Gut   173
- Rotation of the Gut   183
- Fixation of the Gut   184

Chapter 17: Liver and Biliary Apparatus; Pancreas and Spleen   189

Liver and Biliary Apparatus   189
- The Liver   189
- Gallbladder and Biliary Passages   191

Pancreas and Spleen   192
- Pancreas   192
- Spleen   195

Chapter 18: Body Cavities and Diaphragm   200
- Body Cavities   200
- Diaphragm   206

Chapter 19: Respiratory System   211
- Overview of Respiratory System Development   211
- Development of Larynx   212
- Development of Trachea   213
- Development of Lungs   214

Chapter 20: Cardiovascular System   219

Heart   219
- Development of Heart Tube   219
- Development of Various Chambers of Heart   220
- Exterior Shape of Heart   228
- Layers of Cardiac Wall   229
- Valves of the Heart   230
- Conducting System of Heart   231
- Pericardial Cavity   231

Development of Blood Vessels   233
- Development of Arteries   233
- Development of Veins   240

Fetal Circulation   248
- Changes in the Circulation at Birth   250

Lymphatic System   251

Chapter 21: Urogenital System   258
- Intermediate Mesoderm   258
- Cloaca   259

Urinary System   259
- Development of Kidneys   259
- Absorption of Lower Parts of Mesonephric Ducts into Cloaca   262
- Development of the Ureter   262
- Development of the Urinary Bladder   262
- Development of Urethra   264
- Development of the Prostate   266

Genital System   266
- Female Genital System   266
- Development of External Genitalia   269
- Development of Gametes Producing Organs   272
- Fate of Mesonephric Duct   277

Chapter 22: Nervous System   283
- Neural Tube and its Subdivisions   283
- Development of Brain   283

- ❖ Neural Crest Cells 285
- ❖ Spinal Cord 288
- ❖ Medulla Oblongata 290
- ❖ Pons 291
- ❖ Midbrain 292
- ❖ Cerebellum 293
- ❖ Cerebral Hemisphere 293
- ❖ Autonomic Nervous System 301

Chapter 23: Pituitary, Pineal and Adrenal Glands 306
- ❖ Hypophysis Cerebri/Pituitary Gland 306
- ❖ Pineal Gland/Epiphysis Cerebri 307
- ❖ Adrenal Gland/Suprarenal Gland 307

Chapter 24: The Eye and Ear 310
- ❖ Development of the Eye 310
- ❖ Development of the Ear 317

Chapter 25: Chromosomal and Genetic Abnormalities 325
- ❖ Chromosomal Abnormalities 325
- ❖ Allele 328
- ❖ Gene Polymorphism and Mutation 328
- ❖ Punnett Square 329
- ❖ Inheritance of Genetic Disorders 329
- ❖ Genetic Counseling 333

Index 335

Competency Table

Number	Competency: The student should be able to	Core (Y/N)	Chapter number	Page number
AN9.3	Describe development of breast.	N	11	118
AN13.8	Describe development of upper limb.	N	13	138
AN20.10	Describe basic concept of development of lower limb.	N	13	138
AN25.2	Describe development of pleura, lung and heart.	Y	19, 20	211, 219
AN25.3	Describe fetal circulation and changes occurring at birth.	Y	20	219
AN25.4	Describe embryological basis of: (1) atrial septal defect, (2) ventricular septal defect, (3) Fallot's tetralogy and (4) tracheo-esophageal fistula.	Y	19, 20	211, 219
AN25.5	Describe developmental basis of congenital anomalies, transposition of great vessels, dextrocardia, patent ductus arteriosus and coarctation of aorta.	Y	20	219
AN25.6	Mention development of aortic arch arteries, SVC, IVC and coronary sinus.	N	20	219
AN26.6	Explain the concept of bones that ossify in membrane.	N	10	101
AN39.1	Describe and demonstrate the morphology, nerve supply, embryological basis of nerve supply, blood supply, lymphatic drainage and actions of extrinsic and intrinsic muscles of tongue.	Y	15	161
AN43.4	Describe the development and developmental basis of congenital anomalies of face, palate, tongue, branchial apparatus, pituitary gland, thyroid gland and eye.	Y	12, 14, 15, 23, 24	126, 150, 161, 306, 310
AN52.1	Microanatomical structure of suprarenal gland.	Y	23	306
AN52.4	Describe the development of anterior abdominal wall.	Y	18	200
AN52.5	Describe the development and congenital anomalies of diaphragm.	Y	18	200
AN52.6	Describe the development and congenital anomalies of—foregut, midgut and hindgut.	Y	15, 16, 17	161, 171, 189
AN52.7	Describe the development of urinary system.	Y	21	258
AN52.8	Describe the development of male and female reproductive system.	Y	21	258
AN64.2	Describe the development of neural tube, spinal cord, medulla oblongata, pons, midbrain, cerebral hemisphere and cerebellum.	Y	22	283
AN64.3	Describe various types of open neural tube defects with its embryological basis.	N	22	283
AN65.1	Identify epithelium under the microscope and describe the various types that correlate to its function.	Y	10	101
AN65.2	Describe the ultrastructure of epithelium.	N	10	101
AN66.1	Describe and identify various types of connective tissue with functional correlation.	Y	10	101
AN66.2	Describe the ultrastructure of connective tissue.	N	10	101
AN67.1	Describe and identify various types of muscle under the microscope.	Y	10	101
AN67.2	Classify muscle and describe the structure-function correlation of the same.	Y	10	101
AN67.3	Describe the ultrastructure of muscular tissue.	N	10	101
AN68.1	Describe and Identify multipolar and unipolar neuron, ganglia, peripheral nerve.	Y	10	101

Number	Competency: The student should be able to	Core (Y/N)	Chapter number	Page number
AN68.2	Describe the structure-function correlation of neuron.	Y	10	101
AN68.3	Describe the ultrastructure of nervous tissue.	N	10	101
AN70.1	Identify exocrine gland under the microscope and distinguish between serous, mucous and mixed acini.	Y	10	101
AN71.1	Identify bone under the microscope; classify various types and describe the structure-function correlation of the same.	Y	10	101
AN71.2	Identify cartilage under the microscope and describe various types and structure-function correlation of the same.	Y	10	101
AN72.1	Identify the skin and its appendages under the microscope and correlate the structure with function.	Y	11	118
AN73.1	Describe the structure of chromosomes with classification.	Y	2	07
AN73.2	Describe technique of karyotyping with its applications.	Y	2	07
AN73.3	Describe the Lyon's hypothesis.	Y	2	07
AN74.1	Describe the various modes of inheritance with examples.	Y	25	325
AN74.2	Draw pedigree charts for the various types of inheritance and give examples of diseases of each mode of inheritance.	Y	25	325
AN74.3	Describe multifactorial inheritance with examples.	Y	25	325
AN74.4	Describe the genetic basis and clinical features of achondroplasia, cystic fibrosis, vitamin D resistant rickets, hemophilia, Duchene's muscular dystrophy and sickle cell anemia.	N	25	325
AN75.1	Describe the structural and numerical chromosomal aberrations.	Y	25	325
AN75.2	Explain the terms mosaics and chimeras with example.	N	25	325
AN75.3	Describe the genetic basis and clinical features of Prader Willi syndrome, Edward syndrome and Patau syndrome.	N	25	325
AN75.4	Describe genetic basis of variation—polymorphism and mutation.	Y	25	325
AN75.5	Describe the principles of genetic counseling.	Y	25	325
AN76.1	Describe the stages of human life.	Y	1	01
AN76.2	Explain the terms—phylogeny, ontogeny, trimester, viability.	Y	1	01
AN77.1	Describe the uterine changes occurring during the menstrual cycle.	Y	3	19
AN77.2	Describe the synchrony between the ovarian and menstrual cycles.	Y	3	19
AN77.3	Describe spermatogenesis and oogenesis along with diagrams.	Y	3	19
AN77.4	Describe the stages and consequences of fertilization.	Y	4	35
AN77.5	Enumerate and describe the anatomical principles underlying contraception.	Y	4	35
AN77.6	Describe teratogenic influences; fertility and sterility, surrogate motherhood, social significance of "sex-ratio".	N	4	35
AN78.1	Describe cleavage and formation of blastocyst	Y	4	35
AN78.2	Describe the development of trophoblast.	Y	4, 5	35, 48
AN78.3	Describe the process of implantation and common abnormal sites of implantation.	Y	4	35
AN78.4	Describe the formation of extraembryonic mesoderm and coelom, bilaminar disc and prochordal plate.	Y	5, 6	48, 58
AN78.5	Describe in brief abortion; decidual reaction, pregnancy test.	Y	4	35
AN79.1	Describe the formation and fate of the primitive streak.	Y	6	58
AN79.2	Describe formation and fate of notochord.	Y	6	58
AN79.3	Describe the process of neurulation.	Y	6, 22	58, 283
AN79.4	Describe the development of somites and intraembryonic coelom.	Y	6, 7, 18	58, 68, 200

Number	Competency: The student should be able to	Core (Y/N)	Chapter number	Page number
AN79.5	Explain embryological basis of congenital malformations, nucleus pulposus, sacrococcygeal teratomas, neural tube defects.	N	6, 13, 22	58, 138, 283
AN79.6	Describe the diagnosis of pregnancy in first trimester and role of teratogens, alpha-fetoprotein.	N	7, 8	68, 77
AN80.1	Describe formation, functions and fate of chorion: amnion; yolk sac; allantois and decidua.	Y	7, 9	68, 85
AN80.2	Describe formation and structure of umbilical cord.	Y	7, 9	68, 85
AN80.3	Describe formation of placenta, its physiological functions, fetomaternal circulation and placental barrier.	Y	9	85
AN80.4	Describe embryological basis of twinning in monozygotic and dizygotic twins.	Y	9	85
AN80.5	Describe role of placental hormones in uterine growth and parturition.	Y	9	85
AN80.6	Explain embryological basis of estimation of fetal age.	N	8	77
AN80.7	Describe various types of umbilical cord attachments.	N	9	85
AN81.1	Describe various methods of prenatal diagnosis.	Y	8	77
AN81.2	Describe indications, process and disadvantages of amniocentesis.	Y	8	77
AN81.3	Describe indications, process and disadvantages of chorion villus biopsy.	Y	8	77

CHAPTER 1

Some Preliminary Considerations

COMPETENCIES COVERED/LEARNING OUTCOMES

The student should be able to:

AN76.1	Describe the stages of human life.
AN76.2	Explain the terms—phylogeny, ontogeny, trimester, viability.

WHAT IS EMBRYOLOGY?

Human development is a continuous process which starts from fertilization of gametes, ovum and sperm. This includes the initial stages of cell division, the formation of the blastocyst, implantation in the uterine wall, and the subsequent differentiation of cells into various tissues and organs.

Early stage of human development from fertilization to the end of the eighth week, during which major organs and structures begin to form is called as *embryo* and from the ninth week to birth, embryo undergoes significant growth and maturation of the structures and is referred to as *fetus*.

Embryology is the study of the development of an embryo from the fertilization of the ovum to the fetus stage or up to the time it is born as an infant. It also involves the study of the genetic, molecular, and environmental factors that influence normal development, as well as the mechanisms underlying developmental disorders and congenital anomalies.

Embryology is also referred to as *developmental anatomy*.

Subdivisions of Embryology

- **General embryology:** It is the study of development during pre-embryonic and embryonic periods (first 8 weeks after fertilization). During this period, the single celled zygote is converted by cell multiplication, migration and reorganization into a miniature form of an individual with various organs and organ systems of the body.
- **Systemic embryology:** It is detailed study of formation of primordia and their structural and early functional organization into various organs and systems of the body. It is further subdivided into development of cardiovascular system, digestive system, urinary system, genital system, etc.
- **Comparative embryology:** It is the study of embryos in different species of animals.
- **Experimental embryology:** It is for understanding the effects of certain drugs, environmental changes that are induced (exposure to radiation, stress) on the growth and development of embryos and fetuses of lower animals. The knowledge gained from these experiments can be used for avoiding the harmful effects of these factors in the human development. It is a vigorous and promising branch of embryology.
- **Biochemical and molecular aspects in embryology:** Chromosomes, gene sequencing and regulation play an important role in the development of embryo.
- **Teratology:** This is a branch of embryology that deals with abnormal embryonic and fetal development, i.e., congenital abnormalities or birth defects.

Role of Embryology in Medicine

- This subject tells us how a single cell (the fertilized ovum) develops into a newborn, containing numerous tissues and organs.
- This knowledge helps us to understand many complicated facts of adult anatomy.
- Embryology helps us understand why some children are born with organs that are abnormal. Appreciation of the factors responsible for maldevelopment assists us in preventing, or treating, such abnormalities.
- Cells forming tissues in the embryo are called *stem cells*. These cells are capable of treating certain diseases in postnatal life.

REPRODUCTION

Reproduction is the biological process by which new individuals of a species are produced, ensuring the continuation of genetic material from one generation to the next. In vertebrates, this involves the combination of male and female gametes, which are produced by the gonads and are essential for sexual reproduction.

Gonads and Gametes

* The cells that carry out the special function of reproduction are called *gametes*. The development of a new individual begins at the movement when one male *gamete* (*sperm* or *spermatozoon*) meets and fuses with one female gamete (*ovum* or *oocyte*).
* The process of fusion of male and female gametes is called *fertilization*. The fused ovum and spermatozoon form the *zygote*. The zygote later develops into an embryo and then into a fetus.
* The male sex cells (spermatozoa) are produced in the *male gonads* (testes) while the female sex cells (ova) are produced in *female gonads* (ovaries). The formation of spermatozoa in testis is called *spermatogenesis*, while the formation of ova in the ovary is called *oogenesis*. The two are collectively referred to as *gametogenesis*.

DEVELOPMENT AND STAGES OF HUMAN LIFE

Definition: Development is a process where someone or something grows or changes and becomes more advanced.

Period: Human development is a continuous process that does not stop at birth. It continues after birth for increase in the size of the body, eruption of teeth, etc.

Phases

* Development before birth is called *prenatal development*.
* Development after birth is called *postnatal development.*

Each period is further subdivided into several stages **(Flowchart 1.1)**. We are going to study the prenatal development in detail in this book.

Ontogeny and Phylogeny

* **Ontogeny** refers to the complete life cycle of an organism involving both prenatal and postnatal period of development. It involves processes such as cell division, differentiation, morphogenesis, and organogenesis.
* **Phylogeny** refers to the evolutionary history and the relationships among different species or groups of organisms. It traces the lineage and the diversification of species over time, often represented in a phylogenetic tree. Phylogeny helps in understanding how different species are related and how they have evolved from common ancestors.

PREGNANCY/GESTATION, TRIMESTERS, VIABILITY

Pregnancy/Gestation

Definition: The process or period of development during which one or more offspring develop inside the uterus (womb). This is the time between conception and birth.

FLOWCHART 1.1: Different stages of development of human being.

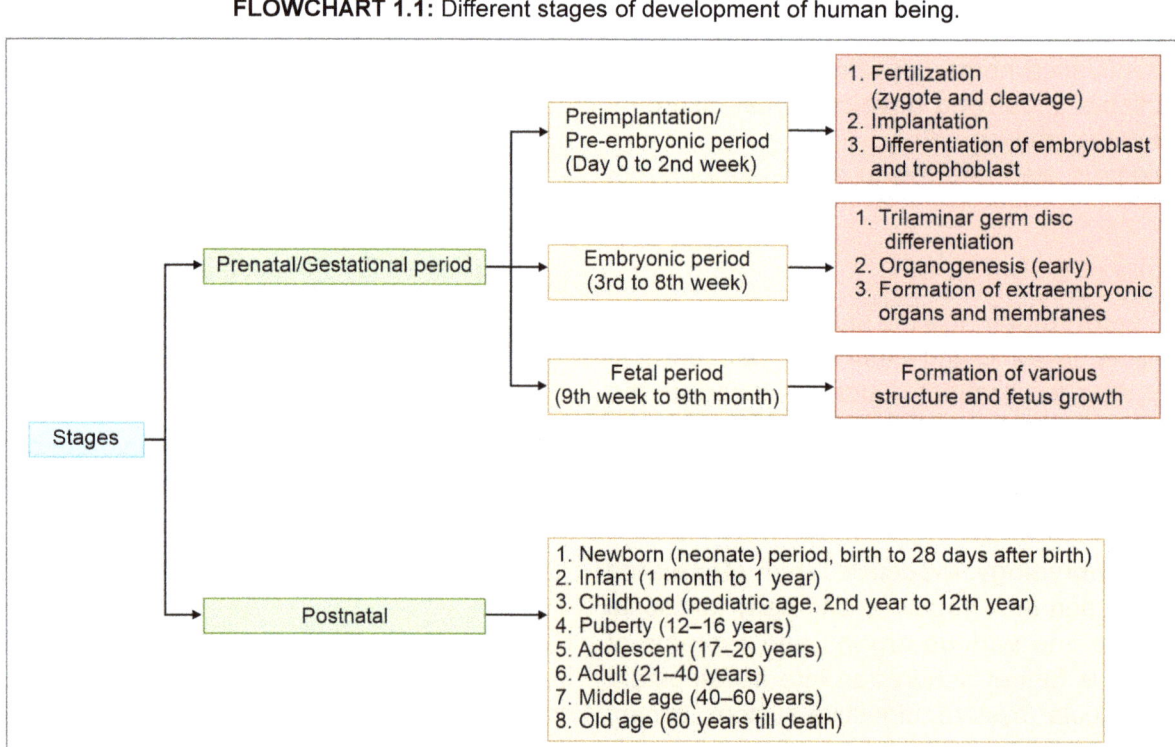

Duration: The length of gestation is 280 days/40 weeks/9 months +/–7 days.

Division of period of gestation: It is divided into three trimesters.

- **First trimester** is from *week 1 to the end of 12th week*. It is the most critical period in the development. This is the period of crucial events, such as implantation, differentiation of germ layers, early organogenesis and functioning of certain organs, such as heart.
- **Second trimester** is from *13th week to 26th week*. It is the *golden period or honey moon period* as most of unpleasant effects of pregnancy disappear and the pregnant woman starts enjoying the fetal movements.
- **Third trimester** is from *27th week to the end of pregnancy*, i.e., delivery of the fetus (newborn). The final stage in the overall growth of the fetus and its preparation for delivery.

This is a *physically and emotionally challenging period* (frequency in movements of the baby and urination, swollen ankles, sleeping difficulties, anxiety about the delivery, etc.)

Premature delivery: If the baby is delivered before 37 weeks of pregnancy, it is called preterm or premature delivery. The chances for breathing problem are more in preterm babies. The causes for preterm birth are many. Some of the causes are diabetes and high blood pressure in the mother; overweight or underweight of the fetus; smoking, alcohol and use of certain medications by the mother.

Viability of Fetus

Fetal viability is the ability of the fetus to survive outside the uterus. The chances of viability of fetus increases if it is born after 28 weeks of gestation (>95%) than if it is between 24 and 28 weeks (4–90%) and between 21 and 24 weeks (0–40%).

Table 1.1 summarizes the events and processes of human prenatal development that we are going to study in this book on human embryology.

TABLE 1.1: Key events in prenatal development period.

Day/week of development	Key events and organ development
Day 0	**Fertilization:** Fusion of sperm and egg to form a zygote
Week 1	• **Cleavage:** Rapid cell division of the zygote leading to formation of a morula • **Blastocyst formation:** Differentiation into trophoblast and inner cell mass • **Implantation:** Attachment of blastocyst to uterine wall • Formation of the amniotic cavity and yolk sac
Week 2	• **Bilaminar germ disc:** Formation of epiblast and hypoblast layers • Formation of extraembryonic mesoderm and initiation of chorionic villi • Development of the amniotic cavity and yolk sac
Week 3	• **Gastrulation:** Formation of trilaminar germ disc (ectoderm, mesoderm, endoderm) • **Neurulation:** Formation of neural tube and neural crest cells • **Beginning of organogenesis:** Primordial heart tube starts to beat • Formation of notochord and early limb buds • Establishment of primitive streak and intraembryonic coelom
Week 4	• Completion of neurulation and closure of neural tube • Formation of somites and differentiation into sclerotome, myotome, and dermatome • Development of pharyngeal arches and early brain structures • Formation of heart chambers and initiation of vascular development • Formation of the foregut, the midgut and the hindgut • Upper limbs appear as paddle-shaped buds • Otic pits and the lens placodes become visible
Weeks 5–8	• **Continued organogenesis:** Development and differentiation of major organs and systems including brain, heart, lungs, gastrointestinal tract, and kidneys • Limb development progresses with formation of digits • External genitalia differentiation begins • Formation of facial features and sensory organs (eyes, ears) • Placenta fully forms and takes over hormone production
Weeks 9–12	• Transition from embryonic to fetal period • Rapid growth and maturation of body structures • Intestinal loops that had herniated out of the abdominal cavity now return into it • Formation of external genitalia becomes distinguishable • Skeleton ossification begins

Day/week of development	Key events and organ development
	• Fetal movement starts • Urine formation begins
Weeks 13–16	• Proportion of the size of the head relative to the rest of the body is less as compared to that in the third fetal month • Fetal movement more pronounced and felt by the mother • Development of lanugo (fine hair) and vernix caseosa (protective covering) • Development of facial muscles and fine movements
Weeks 17–20	• Length of fetus increases. Increase in weight is however slow • Fetal heartbeat audible via stethoscope • Formation of meconium in intestines • Skin covered with vernix caseosa for protection • Rapid eye movement begins
Weeks 21–24	• Substantial weight gain and maturation • Continued development of lungs with surfactant production showing sign of the maturity of the respiratory system • Fetus develops sleep-wake cycles • Eyelids begin to open • Brain continues to develop rapidly • Fetus now starts gaining body weight rapidly
Weeks 25–29	• Significant brain development and continued growth • Lungs continue maturation with increased surfactant production • Fetus more active with stronger movements felt by the mother • Continued development of sensory organs (taste buds, hearing) • Increased subcutaneous fat deposition for temperature regulation • Fetus has reached age of viability • Blood formation now begins to shift from spleen to bone marrow
Weeks 30–34	• Rapid weight gain and final maturation of organ systems • Increased brain activity and development of reflexes • Skin is smooth due to deposition of subcutaneous fat. It is pink due to increase in blood supply • Continued growth of nails and hair
Weeks 35–38	• At the end of the fetal period, the skull has the largest circumference of all parts of body • The testes usually lie in the scrotum • Immune system maturation with development of antibodies • Continued lung maturation and surfactant production • Fetus moves into head-down position for birth • Fetus considered full-term by week 37
Weeks 39–40	• Final maturation and preparation for delivery • Continued weight gain and fat deposition • Formation of vernix caseosa thickens • Placenta aging begins as it prepares for delivery • Full development of fetal organs and systems for independent survival outside the womb

BASIC PROCESSES IN EMBRYOLOGY

Growth and *differentiation* are the two basic processes involved in the conversion of a single cell zygote into a multicellular human newborn.

Growth

It is a quantitative change, i.e., increase in the bulk. Growth of cells is either by synthesizing new protoplasm in the interphase (G1, S, and G2) of cell cycle or reproduction of individual cells of body by mitotic cell divisions. There are four types of growth.

1. **Multiplicative:** This is predominantly seen during prenatal period. There is increase in cell number through mitotic divisions without cell size increase. *Examples:* Blastomeres, cells in epidermis, intestinal epithelium, and blood cells.
2. **Auxetic:** Increase in cell size due to increase in cytoplasmic content, altering nuclear-cytoplasmic ratio without gene changes. *Examples:* Satellite cells around neurons, follicular cells around oocytes.
3. **Accretionary:** Accumulation of intercellular substance leading to overall structure growth. *Examples:* Bone and cartilage lengthening.
4. **Appositional:** Addition of new layers to existing structures, seen in rigid structures like bones for width increase.

Differentiation

It is a qualitative change in structure with an assigned function. Different types of differentiation are:
* **Chemo-differentiation:** It is an invisible differentiation that takes place at molecular level. The substances producing this type of differentiation are called *organizers.*
* **Histo-differentiation:** It takes place at tissue level.
* **Organo-differentiation/organogenesis:** This is at organ level and is the basis for organ remodeling.
* **Functional differentiation:** Hemodynamic changes in blood vessels.

Organizer

An organizer refers to a specialized group of cells of embryo which exerts a morphogenetic stimulus on an adjacent part or parts. They secrete signaling molecules or growth factors that induce nearby cells to differentiate into specific cell types or to undergo particular developmental pathways. There are 3 types of organizers: *primary, secondary and tertiary.*

Primitive streak —Primary→ Notochord —Secondary→
Neural tube —Tertiary→ Paraxial mesoderm to somites

Stem Cells

These are undifferentiated (raw material) cells that are capable of giving rise to more number of cells of same type (new stem cells) by replication from which some other kinds of specialized cells with more specific function (neurons, cardiac muscle cells, bone cells, blood cells) arise by differentiation.

There are three sources from which stem cells are derived:
1. Embryonic
2. Fetal/neonatal
3. Adult/somatic

Embryonic stem cells are tabulated in **Table 1.2**.

TABLE 1.2: Embryonic stem cells.

Type of stem cell	Features	Examples
Pluripotent stem cells	• Derived from the inner cell mass of blastocysts • Capable of differentiating into cells of all three germ layers (ectoderm, mesoderm, endoderm)	Embryonic stem cells (ESCs)
Multipotent stem cells	• Derived from specific tissues or organs • Can differentiate into a limited range of cell types related to their tissue of origin	Hematopoietic stem cells (found in bone marrow)
Totipotent stem cells	• Found in early embryos at the zygote stage • Can differentiate into all cell types, including both embryonic and extra-embryonic tissues	Zygote (fertilized egg)

Clinical Importance

Stem Cell Therapy
* **Regeneration of tissues and organs:** Use of stem cells underneath the skin for skin grafting in burns cases.
* **Treatment of diseases:** Regeneration of blood vessels; use of embryonic stem cells in treating Alzheimer's and Parkinson's diseases, healing of damaged tissue and replace damaged tissue in rheumatoid arthritis and osteoarthritis, insulin producing cells in type I diabetes, cardiac muscles and treatment of leukemia, sickle cell anemia.
* **Drug trials:** To test the safety and quality of newer drugs.

HIGHLIGHTS

* **Embryology** is the study of the development of an individual before birth.
* During the first two months, we call the developing individual an *embryo*. After that, we call it a *fetus*.
* The *testis* is the male sex organ or male gonad. The *ovary* is the female sex organ or gonad. They produce *gametes*.
* **Gametogenesis:** This is the process of production of gametes in gonads or sex organs. In males it is known as *spermatogenesis* and in females as *oogenesis*.
* **Prenatal development** is development before birth.
* **Postnatal development** is development after birth.
* **Ontogeny** refers to complete life cycle of an organism.
* **Phylogeny** is evolutionary history of a group of organisms.
* **Pregnancy/gestation:** Time during which one or more offspring develop in the uterus.
* **Viability of fetus** is an ability of the fetus to survive outside the uterus.
* **Zygote** is single cell that results from fertilization.
* **Organizer:** Any part of the embryo which exerts stimulus on an adjacent part.
* **Stem cells** are undifferentiated cells which capable of renewing and giving rise to new cell types.

Chapter 1: Some Preliminary Considerations

TEST YOUR UNDERSTANDING

REVIEW QUESTIONS

1. Define embryology and discuss its subdivisions.
2. Explain the terms ontogeny and phylogeny.
3. Describe various stages of human life.
4. Explain the term gestation and viability.
5. Explain the types of growth and differentiation.
6. What are stem cells? Discuss embryonic stem cells.

MULTIPLE CHOICE QUESTIONS

1. Which period of pregnancy is termed as "golden period"?
   A. 1–5 weeks
   B. 13–26 weeks
   C. 6–8 weeks
   D. 20–24 weeks
2. The process of production of gametes in male gonads is called:
   A. Spermiogenesis
   B. Oogenesis
   C. Spermatogenesis
   D. Gametogenesis
3. Which of the following represents the correct sequence of stages in human development, from earliest to latest?
   A. Embryo, fetus, zygote, neonate
   B. Zygote, embryo, fetus, neonate
   C. Neonate, embryo, zygote, fetus
   D. Fetus, embryo, zygote, neonate
4. Which of the following statements about embryonic viability is correct?
   A. Viability is achieved immediately after fertilization
   B. Viability is primarily determined by the number of cells in the embryo
   C. Viability refers to the ability of the embryo to survive outside the uterus
   D. Viability is determined by the presence of specific genes
5. Ontogeny refers to:
   A. Evolutionary history
   B. Ancestral history
   C. Complete life cycle of an organism
   D. Prenatal development
6. During which trimester of pregnancy does the majority of fetal organogenesis occur?
   A. First trimester
   B. Second trimester
   C. Third trimester
   D. Organogenesis is evenly distributed across all trimesters
7. Which type of stem cell is typically used in regenerative medicine due to its ability to differentiate into a limited range of cell types?
   A. Totipotent stem cells
   B. Pluripotent stem cells
   C. Multipotent stem cells
   D. Unipotent stem cells

Answers: 1. B   2. C   3. B   4. C   5. C
         6. A   7. C

Molecular Aspect of Embryology

CHAPTER 2

COMPETENCIES COVERED/LEARNING OUTCOMES

The student should be able to:

AN73.1	Describe the structure of chromosomes with classification.
AN73.2	Describe technique of karyotyping with its applications.
AN73.3	Describe the Lyon's hypothesis.

Before we move on the details of embryonic development, we must study about the cell division and chromosomes. These concepts are fundamental to the complexities of prenatal development, providing insights into genetic inheritance, developmental disorders, and their clinical implications.

CHROMOSOMES

A chromosome is a thread-like structure composed of DNA and proteins found in the nucleus of cells. It carries genetic information in the form of genes, which determine hereditary traits and direct cellular functions.

- **Genetic information:** Chromosomes contain DNA, which stores the genetic instructions necessary for growth, development, and functioning of organisms.
- **Structure:** Each chromosome consists of a single DNA molecule tightly coiled around histone proteins, forming a compacted structure that is visible under a microscope during cell division.

Haploid and Diploid Chromosomes

- The number of chromosomes in each cell is fixed for a given species and in human beings, it is 46. This is referred to as the *diploid* (or double) number.
- However, in spermatozoa and ova, the number of chromosomes is only half the diploid number, i.e., 23. This is called the *haploid* (or half) number.
- After fertilization, the resulting zygote has 23 chromosomes from the sperm (or father), and 23 from the ovum (or mother). The diploid number is thus restored.

Autosomes and Sex Chromosomes

- The 46 chromosomes in each cell can be divided into 44 *autosomes* and two *sex chromosomes*. The sex chromosomes may be of two kinds, X or Y. In a man, there are 44 autosomes, one X-chromosome and one Y-chromosome; while in a woman, there are 44 autosomes and 2 X-chromosomes in each cell **(Fig. 2.1)**.
- When we study the 44 autosomes, we find that they really consist of 22 pairs, the two chromosomes forming a pair being exactly alike *(homologous chromosomes)*.
- In a woman, the two X-chromosomes form another such pair; in a man this pair is represented by one X-and one Y-chromosome.
- One chromosome of each pair is derived from the mother and the other from the father.

Significance of Chromosomes

The entire human body develops from the fertilized ovum. It is, therefore, obvious that the fertilized ovum contains all the information necessary for formation of the numerous tissues and organs of the body, and for their orderly assembly and function. Each cell of the body inherits from the fertilized ovum, all the directions that are necessary for it to carry out its functions throughout life. This tremendous volume of information is stored within the chromosomes of each cell.

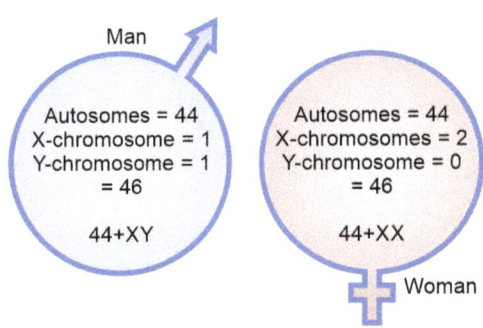

FIG. 2.1: Number of chromosomes in the somatic cells of a man and of a woman.

- Each chromosome bears on itself a very large number of structures called *genes*.
- Genes are made up of a nucleic acid called *deoxyribonucleic acid* (or *DNA*) and all information is stored in the molecules of this substance. Genes are involved in synthesis of proteins.
- Thus genes play an important role in the development of tissues and organs of an individual.
- **Traits (characters)** of an individual are determined by genes carried on his (or her) chromosomes. As we have seen half of these are inherited from the father and half from mother.

To summarize, chromosomes are made up predominantly of a nucleic acid, DNA, and all information is stored in molecules of this substance. When the need arises, this information is used to direct the activities of the cell by synthesizing appropriate proteins. To understand how this becomes possible, we must consider the structure of DNA in some detail.

Basic Structure of DNA

DNA in a chromosome is in the form of very fine fibers. Each fiber consists of two strands that are twisted spirally to form what is called a *double helix*. The two strands are linked to each other at regular intervals.

Each strand of the DNA fiber consists of a chain of *nucleotides*. Each nucleotide consists of a sugar, deoxyribose, a molecule of phosphate and a base (Fig. 2.2). The phosphate of one nucleotide is linked to the sugar of the next nucleotide. The base that is attached to the sugar molecule may be *adenine, guanine, cytosine* or *thymine*. The two strands of a DNA fiber are joined together by the linkage of a base on one strand with a base on the opposite strand.

This linkage is peculiar in that adenine on one strand is always linked to thymine on the other strand, while cytosine is always linked to guanine. The reason why adenine on one strand is always linked to thymine on the other strand is that the structure of these two molecules is complementary and hydrogen bonds are easily formed between them. The same is true for cytosine and guanine.

Ribonucleic Acid (RNA)

In addition to DNA, cells contain another important nucleic acid called *ribonucleic acid* or *RNA*. The structure of a molecule of RNA corresponds fairly closely to that of one strand of a DNA molecule, with the following important differences.
- RNA contains the sugar ribose instead of deoxyribose.
- Instead of the base thymine, it contains uracil.

RNA is present both in the nucleus and in the cytoplasm of a cell. It is present in three main forms, namely *messenger RNA (mRNA)*, *transfer RNA (tRNA)* and *ribosomal RNA*. Messenger RNA acts as an intermediary between the DNA of the chromosome and the amino acids present in the cytoplasm and plays a vital role in the synthesis of proteins from amino acids.

Synthesis of Protein

Every protein is made up of a series of amino acids; the nature of the protein depending upon the amino acids present, and the sequence in which they are arranged which is determined by the order of bases in DNA.
- **Triplet code:** DNA has four bases: adenine (A), cytosine (C), thymine (T), and guanine (G), which form triplet codes to encode amino acids. Each amino acid is represented by multiple triplet codes, allowing for variation in DNA sequences.
- A *structural gene (cistron)* on a chromosome carries the code for a complete polypeptide chain.

The main steps in the synthesis of a protein are as follows:
- The two strands of a DNA fiber separate from each other (over the area bearing a particular cistron) so that the ends of the bases that were linked to the opposite strand are now free.
- A molecule of messenger RNA is synthesized using one DNA strand as a guide (or *template*), in such a way that one guanine base is formed opposite each cytosine base of the DNA strand, cytosine is formed opposite guanine, adenine is formed opposite thymine, and uracil is formed opposite adenine. In this way, the code for the sequence in which amino acids are to be linked is passed on from DNA of

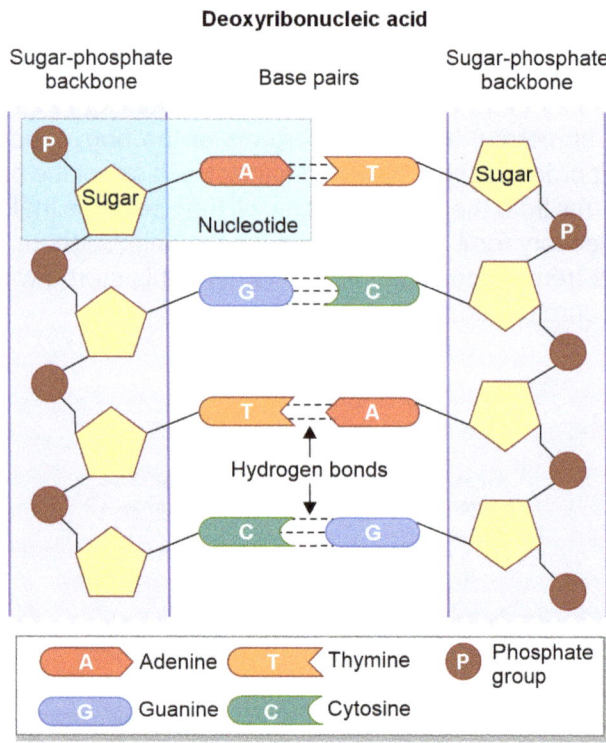

FIG. 2.2: Structure of DNA.

the chromosome to mRNA. This process is called *transcription*. That part of the mRNA strand that bears the code for one amino acid is called a *codon*.
- mRNA carries the code from DNA to ribosomes in the cytoplasm via nuclear pores. mRNA attaches to ribosomes in the cytoplasm.
- On one side, tRNA becomes attached to an amino acid. On the other side, it bears a code of three bases *(anticodon)* that are complementary to the bases coding for its amino acid on mRNA. Under the influence of the ribosome several units of tRNA, along with their amino acids, become arranged alongside the strand of mRNA in the sequence determined by the code on mRNA. This process is called *translation*.
- The amino acids now become linked to each other to form a polypeptide chain. Proteins are formed by union of polypeptide chains.

The flow of information from DNA to RNA and finally to protein has been described as the "central dogma of molecular biology".

Duplication of Chromosomes

One of the most remarkable properties of chromosomes is that they are able to duplicate themselves. From the foregoing discussion on the structure of chromosomes it is clear that duplication of chromosomes, involves the duplication (or replication) of DNA. This takes place as follows **(Fig. 2.3)**:
- The two strands of the DNA molecule to be duplicated unwind and separate from each other so that their bases are 'free'.
- A new strand is now synthesized opposite each original strand of DNA in such a way that adenine is formed opposite thymine, guanine is formed opposite cytosine, and vice versa.
- This new strand becomes linked to the original strand of DNA to form a new molecule.
- As the same process has taken place in relation to each of the two original strands, we now have two complete molecules of DNA.
- It will be noted that each molecule has one strand that belonged to the original molecule and one strand that is new. It will also be noted that the two molecules formed are identical to the original molecule.

Structure of Fully Formed Chromosomes

Each chromosome consists of two parallel rod-like elements that are called *chromatids* **(Fig. 2.4)**. The two chromatids are joined to each other at a narrow area that is light staining and is called the *centromere* (or *kinetochore*). In this region, the chromatin of each chromatid is most highly coiled and, therefore, appears

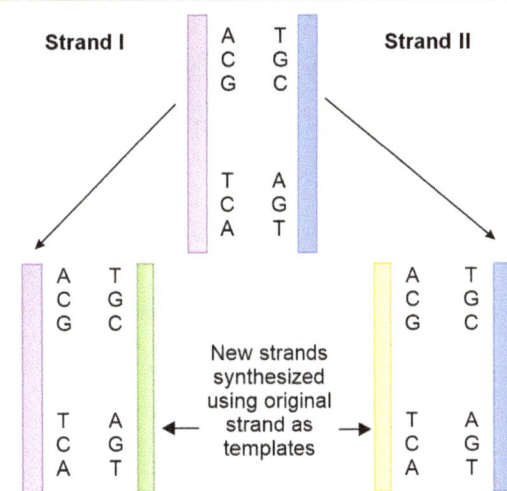

FIG. 2.3: Scheme to show how a DNA molecule is duplicated.

to be thinnest. The chromatids appear to the 'constricted' here and this region is called the *primary constriction*.
- Typically, the centromere is not midway between the two ends of the chromatids, but somewhat towards one end.
- As a result, each chromatid can be said to have a *long arm* and a *short arm*. Such chromosomes are described as being *submetacentric* (when the two arms are only slightly different in length); or as *acrocentric* (when the difference is marked) **(Fig. 2.5)**.
- In some chromosomes, the two arms are of equal length: such chromosomes are described as *metacentric*.
- Finally, in some chromosomes the centromere may lie at one end: such a chromosome is described as *telocentric*.

Differences in the total length of chromosomes, and in the position of the centromere are important factors in distinguishing individual chromosomes from each other.

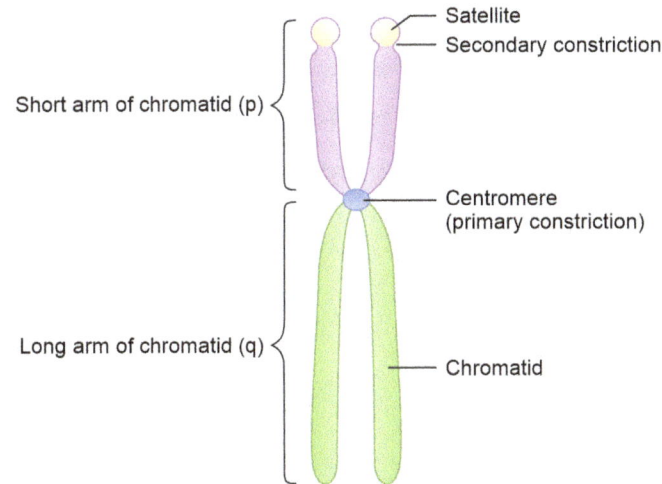

FIG. 2.4: Diagram to show the terms applied to some parts of a typical chromosome. Note that this chromosome is submetacentric.

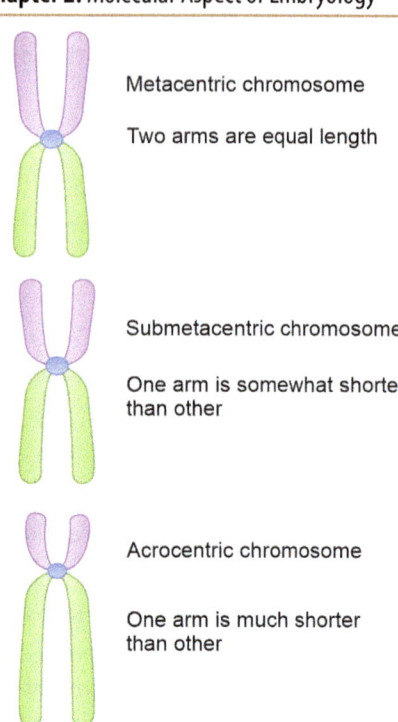

FIG. 2.5: Nomenclature used for different types of chromosomes, based on differences in lengths of the two arms of each chromatid.

- Additional help in identification is obtained by the presence in some chromosomes of *secondary constrictions*. Such constrictions lie near one end of the chromatid.
- The part of the chromatid 'distal' to the constriction may appear to be a rounded body almost separate from the rest of the chromatid: such regions are called *satellite bodies*. (Secondary constrictions are concerned with the formation of nucleoli and are, therefore, called *nucleolar organizing centers*).

- Identification of individual chromosomes is also obtained by the use of special staining procedures by which each chromatid can be seen to consist of a number of dark and light staining transverse bands.
- Chromosomes are distinguishable only during mitosis. In the interphase (between successive mitoses), the chromosomes elongate and assume the form of long threads. These threads are called *chromonemata* (Singular = *chromonema*).

Classification of Chromosomes

The Denver system of chromosome classification is a standardized method used to classify human chromosomes based on their size and centromere position. The chromosomes are grouped into seven categories, labeled A to G as shown in **Table 2.1**.

KARYOTYPING

It is a fundamental cytogenetic technique used to analyze the number, size, and shape of chromosomes in a cell. This diagnostic procedure is important in identifying chromosomal abnormalities that underlie various genetic disorders.

Procedure

Various steps in karyotype are:
- **Peripheral blood collection:** A sterile syringe collects 1–2 mL of blood through venipuncture, containing heparin to prevent clotting.
- **Blood culture procedure:**
  1. *Planting:* The heparinized blood is added to a test tube containing karyotyping medium (RPMI medium with calf/AB serum, L-glutamine, gentamicin, and PHA-M).
  2. *Incubation:* Kept at 37°C with periodic shaking for 72 hours to stimulate cell growth.

TABLE 2.1: Classification of chromosomes.

Group	Chromosomes	Size	Centromere position	Features
A	1, 2, 3	Largest	Metacentric	Large chromosomes with near-central centromeres
B	4, 5	Large	Submetacentric	Slightly smaller than group A; centromere off-center
C	6, 7, 8, 9, 10, 11, 12, X	Medium	Submetacentric	Medium-sized chromosomes with off-center centromeres; includes the X chromosome
D	13, 14, 15	Medium	Acrocentric	Medium-sized with centromeres near the end; contain satellite structures
E	16, 17, 18	Short	Metacentric/submetacentric	Short chromosomes with central or slightly off-center centromeres
F	19, 20	Short	Metacentric	Short chromosomes with near-central centromeres
G	21, 22, Y	Smallest	Acrocentric	Small chromosomes with centromeres near the end; includes the Y chromosome, which is smaller and has fewer genes

3. *Harvesting:* At 70 hours, colchicine is added to arrest cells at metaphase, the stage where chromosomes are most visible.
4. *Centrifugation:* Cells are spun at 1,500 rpm for 7 minutes to collect them at the bottom of the tube.
5. *Hypotonic treatment:* Cells are treated with hypotonic saline to swell and separate chromosomes.
6. *Fixation:* Cells are fixed using a solution of glacial acetic acid and methanol to preserve chromosome structure.
7. *Slide preparation:* Chromosomes are dropped onto slides to create spreads suitable for examination.
8. *Staining:* Slides are treated with trypsin and stained with Giemsa stain to highlight banding patterns.
9. *Microscopic examination:* Chromosomes are observed under a microscope to analyze their number, size, and structure.
10. *Photography:* Photomicrographs are taken to document and analyze the chromosome patterns for abnormalities.

During prenatal period, to detect the fetal chromosomal abnormalities, sample is collected from amniotic fluid.

Clinical Applications

- Karyotyping is crucial for diagnosing conditions such as Down syndrome (trisomy 21), Turner syndrome (monosomy X), Klinefelter syndrome (XXY), and many others.
- It plays a vital role in genetic counseling, prenatal diagnosis, and understanding the genetic basis of developmental disorders.

Karyotype

A karyotype (also know as *idiogram*) is a complete set of chromosomes in an individual or species, displayed in a systematic arrangement **(Figs. 2.6A and B)**. It is used to examine the number, size, shape, and overall structure of chromosomes.

LYON HYPOTHESIS AND SEX CHROMATIN

- **Chromatin:** Chromosomes during interphase. *Highly extended filaments* forming a diffuse network.
- **Euchromatin:** *Uncoiled portion* of chromosomes during interphase which is *genetically active*.
- **Heterochromatin:** *Coiled portion* of chromosomes in interphase (chromatin granules) which is *genetically inert*.

Lyon Hypothesis

- Dr Mary Lyon proposed that one of the two X chromosomes in a normal female is functional,

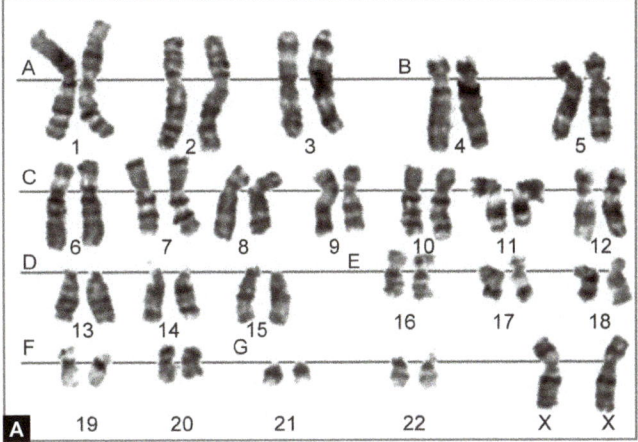
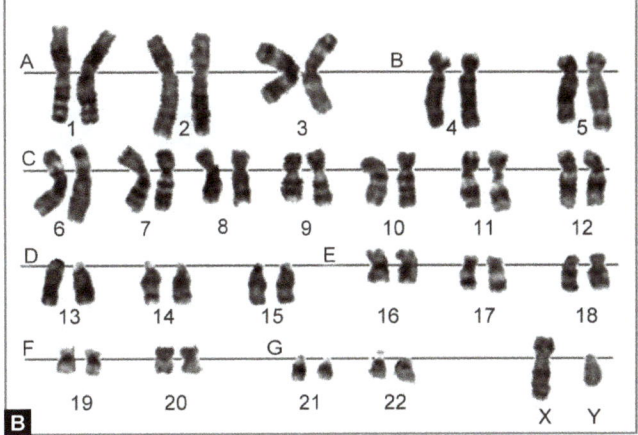

FIGS. 2.6A and B: Karyotype: (A) Normal female; (B) Normal male.

and the other is condensed and inactive in early development. This inactive X chromosome is called a *Barr body or sex chromatin*.
- The inactivated X chromosome can be either paternal or maternal in origin. Once inactivated, the same X chromosome remains inactive in all daughter cells. This process is called *Lyonization*.
- In normal males, there is no sex chromatin or Barr body because they have only one active X chromosome.
- X chromosome inactivation occurs around the 15th day of gestation.
- The number of Barr bodies is always one less than the total number of X chromosomes.

Sex Chromatin

- A small, dark-staining, condensed mass of inactivated X chromosome within the nucleus of a nondividing cell (interphase).
- Typically located just inside the nuclear membrane of the interphase nucleus.
- The inactive mammalian X chromosome is late-replicating, heterochromatic, and hypermethylated.
- The term sex chromatin comprises two structures—*Barr bodies and Drumstick/Davidson body.*

Barr Body

- Found in epithelial (oral, skin, vaginal, urethral, corneal) and other tissue cells (placenta, dental pulp, skin fibroblasts) and located at the periphery of the nucleus.
- **Sex differences:** Males 1–2%; Females 20–80%.
- **Measurement:** Approximately 1 µm.
- **Shapes:** Planoconvex, wedge-shaped, rectangular.
- **Maximum number per nucleus:** 0 or 1.

Drumstick (Davidson Body)

- Appears as a deeply stained body attached to the nucleus of polymorphonuclear leukocytes predominantly in neutrophils.
- **Incidence:** 2–3% or 6/500 cells in normal females.

CELL CYCLE AND CELL DIVISION

CELL CYCLE (FIG. 2.7)

The cell cycle is the series of stages a cell goes through to grow and divide. It ensures that cells reproduce accurately and maintain healthy tissue function. Each phase of the cell cycle is regulated to ensure cells divide correctly and maintain genetic integrity. This process is vital for growth, development, and tissue repair. Two main parts of the cell cycle are the cell growth and cell division. The phases of cell cycle are as follows:

Interphase: This is the preparation phase, where the cell grows and duplicates its DNA.
- **G1 Phase (Growth phase 1/Gap 1):** The cell grows and carries out normal functions. The duration of this phase is highly variable (2–100 hours). It checks for the necessary conditions to divide.

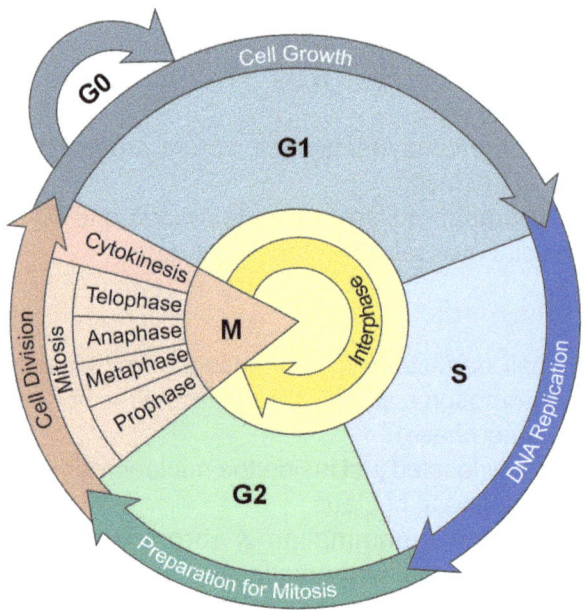

FIG. 2.7: Cell cycle.

- **S Phase (synthesis):** The cell replicates its DNA, so each new cell will have a complete set of chromosomes. Duration is 6–10 hours.
- **G2 Phase (Gap 2):** The cell continues to grow and prepares for division. It checks for any DNA errors and makes necessary repairs. Duration is 2 to 4 hours.

Mitotic (M) phase: This is the division phase, where the cell splits into two new cells.
1. **Mitosis:** The cell's chromosomes are separated into two identical sets. This phase has several steps: prophase, metaphase, anaphase, and telophase. Duration is 1–2 hours
2. **Cytokinesis:** The cell's cytoplasm divides, creating two separate daughter cells.

CELL DIVISION

Multiplication of cells takes place by division of pre-existing cells. Such multiplication constitutes an essential feature of embryonic development. Cell multiplication is equally necessary after the birth of the individual for growth and for replacement of dead cells. We have seen that chromosomes within the nuclei of cells carry genetic information that controls the development and functioning of various cells and tissues; and, therefore, of the body as a whole. When a cell divides, it is essential that the entire genetic information within it be passed on to both the daughter cells resulting from the division. In other words, the daughter cells must have chromosomes identical in number (and in genetic content) to those in the mother cell. This type of cell division is called *mitosis*.

A different kind of cell division called *meiosis* occurs during the formation of the gametes. This consists of two successive divisions called the *first* and *second meiotic divisions*. The cells resulting from these divisions (i.e., gametes) differ from other cells of the body in that:
- The number of chromosomes is reduced to half the normal number, and
- The genetic information in the various gametes produced is not identical.

MITOSIS

Many cells of the body have a limited span of functional activity, at the end of which they undergo division into two daughter cells. The daughter cells in turn have their own span of activity, followed by another division. The period during which the cell is actively dividing is the phase of mitosis. The period between two successive divisions is called the *interphase*.

Mitosis is conventionally divided into a number of stages called *prophase, metaphase, anaphase* and *telophase*.

* With the progress of telophase, the chromatin of the chromosome uncoils and elongates and the chromosome can no longer be identified as such. However, it is believed to retain its identity during the interphase (which follows telophase). This is shown diagrammatically in **Figure 2.8A**.
* During a specific period of the interphase, the DNA content of the chromosome is duplicated so that another chromatid identical to the original one is formed; the chromosome is now made up of two chromatids **(Fig. 2.8B)**.
* During *prophase*, the chromatin of the chromosome becomes gradually more and more coiled so that the chromosome becomes recognizable as a thread-like structure that gradually acquires a rod-like appearance **(Fig. 2.8C)**.
* Towards the end of prophase, the two chromatids constituting the chromosome become distinct **(Fig. 2.8D)** and the chromosome now has the typical structure.

While these changes are occurring in chromosomes, a number of other events are also taking place.
* The two centrioles separate and move to opposite poles of the cell. They produce a number of microtubules that pass from one centriole to the other and form a *spindle*. Meanwhile the nuclear membrane breaks down and nucleoli disappear **(Fig. 2.8D)**.
* With the formation of the spindle, chromosomes move to a position midway between the two centrioles (i.e., at the equator of the cell) where each chromosome becomes attached to microtubules of the spindle by its centromere. This stage is referred to as *metaphase* **(Fig. 2.8E)**.
* In the *anaphase*, the centromere of each chromosome splits longitudinally into two so that the chromatids now become independent chromosomes. At this stage, the cell can be said to contain 46 pairs of chromosomes. One chromosome of each such pair now moves along the spindle to either pole of the cell **(Fig. 2.8F)**.

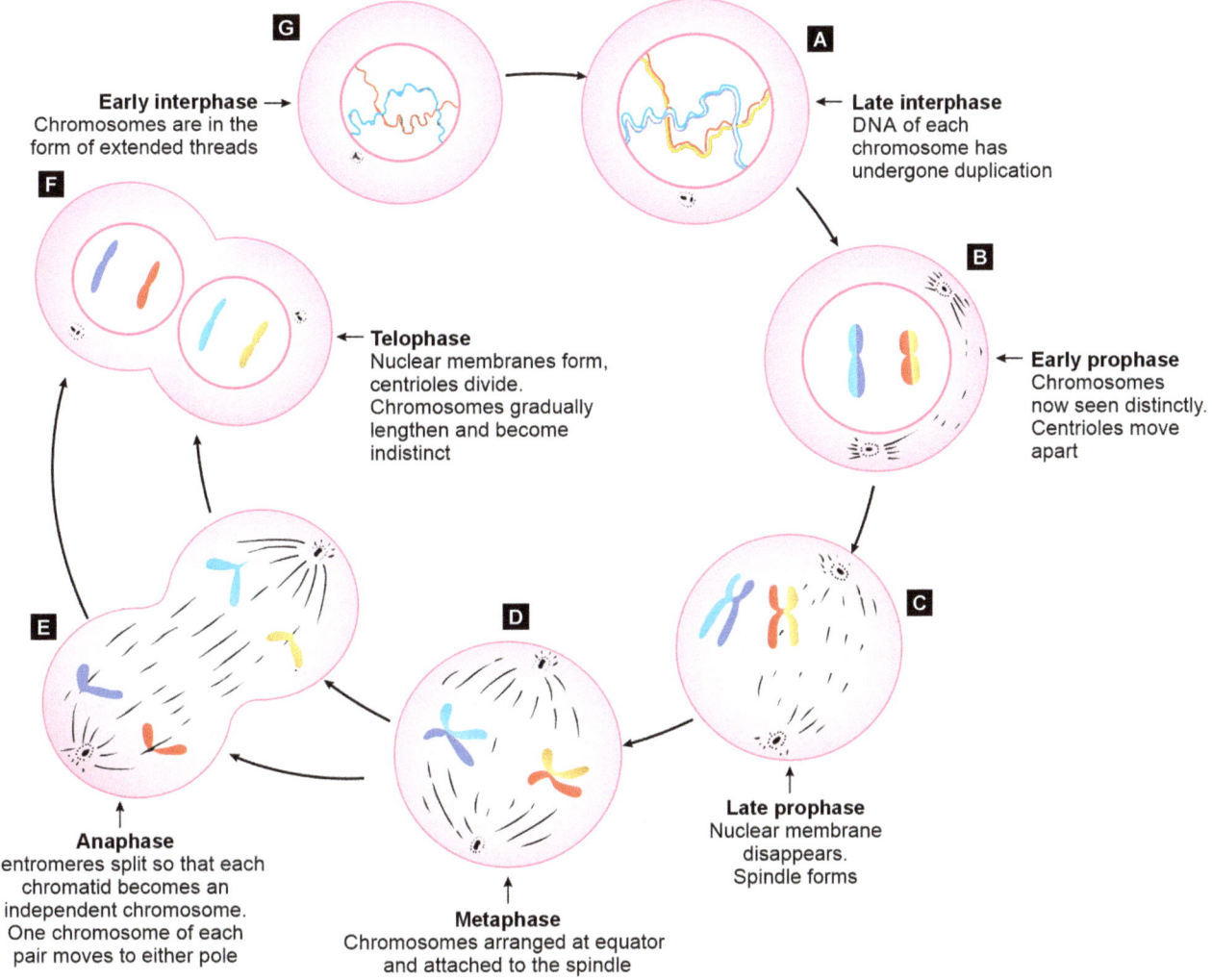

FIGS. 2.8A to G: Scheme to show the main steps of mitosis.

- ❖ This is followed by *telophase* in which the two daughter nuclei are formed by appearance of nuclear membranes. Chromosomes gradually elongate and become indistinct. Nucleoli reappear. The centriole is duplicated at this stage or in early interphase **(Fig. 2.8G)**.
- ❖ The division of the nucleus is accompanied by the division of the cytoplasm. In this process, the organelles are presumably duplicated and each daughter cell comes to have a full complement of them.

Clinical Importance

Mitosis
- **Growth and development:** Mitosis allows for the rapid cell division necessary for the growth and development of the embryo from a single fertilized egg to a multicellular organism.
- **Tissue repair and maintenance:** Mitosis is essential for the repair and maintenance of tissues, ensuring that damaged or old cells are replaced.
- **Genetic consistency:** Mitosis ensures that each daughter cell receives an identical set of chromosomes, maintaining genetic consistency throughout the developing organism.

MEIOSIS

As already stated, meiosis consists of two successive divisions called the first and second meiotic divisions.
- ❖ During the interphase preceding the first division, duplication of the DNA content of chromosomes takes place as in mitosis.
- ❖ As a result, another chromatid identical to the original one is formed. Thus, each chromosome is now made up of two chromatids.

First Meiotic Division

The *prophase* of the first meiotic division is prolonged and is usually divided into a number of stages as follows:

- **Leptotene:** The chromosomes become visible (as in mitosis). Although each chromosome consists of two chromatids, these cannot be distinguished at this stage **(Fig. 2.9A)**.
- **Zygotene:** We have seen that the 46 chromosomes in each cell consist of 23 pairs (the X and Y chromosomes of a male being taken as a pair). The two chromosomes of each pair come to lie parallel to each other, and are closely apposed. This *pairing* of chromosomes is also referred to as *synapsis* or conjugation. The two chromosomes together constitute a *bivalent* **(Fig. 2.9B)**.
- **Pachytene:** The two chromatids of each chromosome become distinct.
  The bivalent now has four chromatids in it and is called a *tetrad*. There are two central and two peripheral chromatids, one from each chromosome **(Fig. 2.9C)**. An important event now takes place. The two central chromatids (one belonging to each chromosome of the bivalent) become coiled over each other so that they cross at a number of points. This is called *crossing over*.
  For sake of simplicity only one such crossing is shown in **Figure 2.9D**. At the site where the chromatids cross, they become adherent; the points of adherence are called *chiasmata*.
- **Diplotene:** The two chromosomes of a bivalent now try to move apart. As they do so, the chromatids involved in crossing over 'break' at the points of crossing and the 'loose' pieces become attached to the opposite chromatid. This results in exchange of genetic material between these chromatids. A study of **Figure 2.9E** will show that each of the four chromatids of the tetrad now has a distinctive genetic content.

- ❖ The *metaphase* follows. As in mitosis the 46 chromosomes become attached to the spindle at the equator, the two chromosomes of a pair being close to each other **(Fig. 2.10A)**.
- ❖ The *anaphase* differs from that in mitosis in that *there is no splitting of the centromeres*. One entire chromosome of each pair moves to each pole of the spindle **(Fig. 2.10B)**. The resulting daughter cells, therefore, have 23 chromosomes, each made up of two chromatids **(Fig. 2.10C)**.
- ❖ The anaphase is followed by the *telophase* in which two daughter nuclei are formed. The division of the nucleus is followed by division of the cytoplasm.

Second Meiotic Division

- ❖ The first meiotic division is followed by a short *interphase*. This differs from the usual interphase in that *there is no duplication of DNA*. Such duplication is unnecessary as chromosomes of cells resulting from the first division already possess two chromatids each **(Fig. 2.10C)**.
- ❖ The second meiotic division is similar to mitosis. However, because of the crossing over that has occurred during the first division, the daughter cells are not identical in genetic content **(Fig. 2.11)**.

Clinical Importance

Meiosis
- **Genetic diversity:** Meiosis introduces genetic variation through processes like crossing over and independent assortment, which are crucial for the evolution and adaptation of species.
- **Formation of gametes:** Meiosis produces haploid gametes (sperm and eggs) with half the chromosome number of the parent cell, which is essential for sexual reproduction.
- **Prevention of polyploidy:** By reducing the chromosome number by half, meiosis ensures that upon fertilization, the resulting zygote has the correct diploid number of chromosomes, preventing polyploidy.

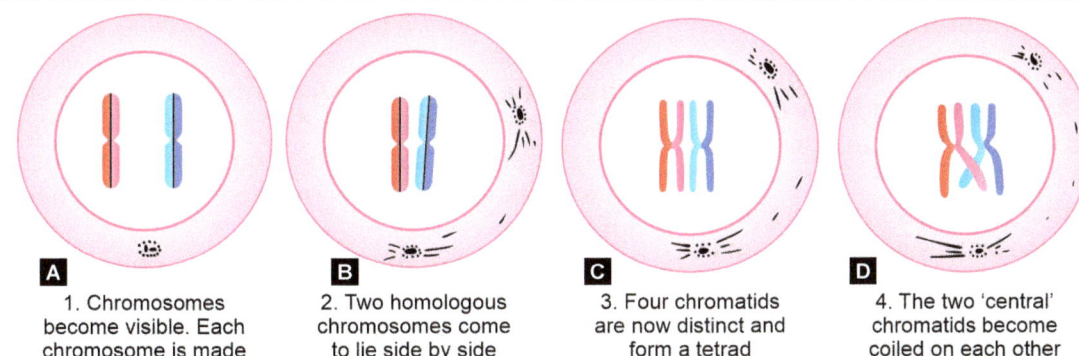

FIGS. 2.9A to E: Stages in the prophase of the first meiotic division.

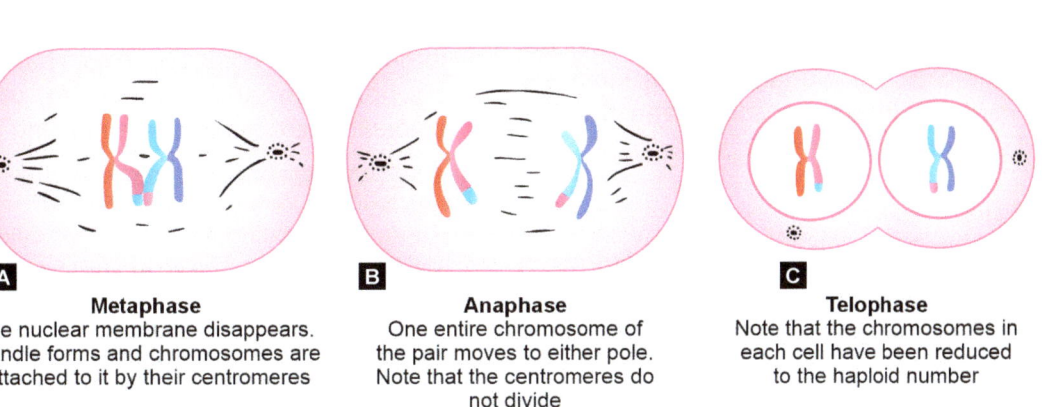

FIGS. 2.10A to C: Metaphase (A), anaphase (B), and telophase (C) of the first meiotic division.

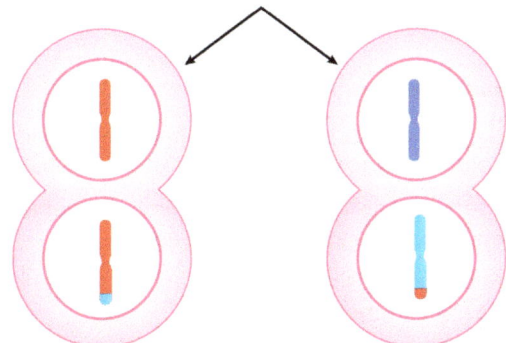

FIG. 2.11: Daughter cells resulting from the second meiotic division. These are not alike because of the crossing-over during the first meiotic division.

MOLECULAR CONTROL OF DEVELOPMENT OF EMBRYO

In Chapter 1, we have studied about the growth and differentiation and role of organizer in development of embryo. Certain regions of the embryo have the ability to influence the differentiation of neighboring regions. For example, the influence exerted by the optic vesicle on the overlying surface ectoderm to differentiate into lens vesicle. If the optic vesicle is removed, the lens vesicle fails to form.

The influence exerted by an area (optic vesicle) is called *induction* whereas the area exerting induction is called *organizer*. In interactions between tissues, one is *inducer*, and the other is *responder*. Capacity to respond to the inductor is called *competence*. The factors that influence the competence to respond are called *competence factors*.

Regulation of Gene Expression

Various processes and factors play an important role in correct expression of genes for the embryonic development. These are:

- **Signaling molecules:** These are present outside cells and have the effect on the neighboring cells. They bind to receptors and activate the transcription factors.
- **Transcription factors:** These are gene regulatory proteins present in nucleus and are responsible for gene expression.

Regulation of Growth and Differentiation

The interaction between inducer and responder as discussed is crucial for events of growth during development of zygote into multicellular organism. These interactions can be of two types:
1. **Epithelial-mesenchymal interaction:** Interaction between epithelial tissue and underlying mesenchymal tissue, e.g., development of liver and pancreas are due to interaction between endoderm of gut and adjacent mesoderm. Similarly, interaction between endoderm of ureteric bud and metanephric blastema of mesodermal origin form nephron.
2. **Epithelial-epithelial interaction:** Interaction between two different types of epithelial tissues, e.g., interaction between optic vesicle (neuroectodermal derivative) and lens vesicle (surface ectodermal derivative). Similarly, the formation of the inner ear structures involves interactions between the otic vesicle and surrounding epithelial cells.

Cell to Cell Signaling

Transmission of signals in the form of growth and differentiation factors, are transmitted from one cell to another by endocrine, paracrine, autocrine or juxtacrine interaction.
- **Autocrine signaling:** A cell produces signaling molecules that bind to receptors on its own surface. Example: Certain growth factors, such as TGF-β (transforming growth factor-beta), can act on the same cells that release them, promoting their own proliferation.
- **Paracrine signaling:** A cell produces signaling molecules that affect nearby target cells. *Example:* The secretion of sonic hedgehog (Shh) by notochord cells influences the differentiation of adjacent neural tube cells.
- **Juxtacrine signaling:** Direct cell-to-cell contact is required for signaling, involving membrane-bound signaling molecules and receptors. *Example:* The interaction between Delta ligand on one cell and Notch receptor on an adjacent cell is crucial for processes like lateral inhibition during neurogenesis.
- **Endocrine signaling:** Hormones are secreted into the bloodstream and affect distant target cells throughout the body. *Example:* Hormones like human chorionic gonadotropin (hCG) produced by the placenta are critical for maintaining pregnancy.

Sonic Hedgehog (Shh) Proteins
- These are signaling molecules that guide embryonic cell differentiation, also known as *master gene*.
- Crucial for the development of the central nervous system, eyes, lungs, limbs, and teeth.
- Mutations can cause holoprosencephaly, resulting in incomplete brain cleavage, cyclopia, cleft palate and other development abnormalities.

The various growth and differentiation factors and their functions are presented in **Table 2.2**.

TABLE 2.2: Important growth differentiation factors.

Growth differentiation factors	Role in embryology/organogenesis
Sonic hedgehog (Shh)	• Development of the central nervous system, eyes, limbs, teeth, and lungs • Limb and neural tube patterning, formation of the gastrointestinal tract
Fibroblast growth factors (FGFs)	Mesoderm differentiation, angiogenesis, axon growth, limb development, brain patterning, and formation of the inner ear and lungs
Bone morphogenetic proteins (BMPs 1 to 9)	Bone and cartilage formation, cell division, migration, apoptosis, kidney development, and neural tube closure
Transforming growth factor-beta (TGF-β)	Regulation of cell proliferation, differentiation, and extracellular matrix production, crucial for heart and lung development
Mullerian inhibiting factor (MIF)	Regression of paramesonephric duct, sexual differentiation
Wnt proteins	Patterning of limb development, development of midbrain, somites, differentiation of urogenital system, and organogenesis of kidneys and heart
Notch signaling	Neuronal differentiation, segmentation of somites, B and T lymphocytes differentiation and development of the cardiovascular system
Hedgehog (Hh) proteins	Limb and neural tube patterning, formation of the gastrointestinal tract
Nodal	Formation of primitive streak, mesoderm, left-right symmetry
Insulin-like growth factors (IGFs)	IGF-1 bone growth, IGF-2 fetal growth
Epidermal growth factor	Growth and proliferation of cells of ectodermal and mesodermal origin

Chapter 2: Molecular Aspect of Embryology

HIGHLIGHTS

- Characters of parents are transmitted to offspring through codes borne on strands of DNA. *Genes* are made of such strands of DNA. They are located on *chromosomes*.
- A typical cell contains 46 chromosomes (= *diploid number*).
- A gamete contains 23 chromosomes (= *haploid number*). The diploid number of chromosomes is restored as a result of fertilization.
- The parts of a chromosome are two *chromatids* joined by a *centromere*. Depending on the position of centromere the chromosomes are classified.
- **Karyotyping** is the process by which chromosomes can be classified individually.
- **Sex-chromatin** is the small, dark-staining, condensed mass of inactivated X-chromosome within the nucleus of nondividing cell, i.e., during interphase.
- Multiplication of cells takes place by *cell division*. The usual method of cell division, seen in most tissues, is called *mitosis*. Daughter cells resulting from a mitotic division are similar to the parent cell, and have the same number of chromosomes (46).
- A special kind of cell division takes place in the testis and ovary for formation of gametes. It is called *meiosis*. The gametes resulting from meiosis have the haploid number of chromosomes (23). The various gametes formed do not have the same genetic content.

TEST YOUR UNDERSTANDING

REVIEW QUESTIONS

1. Describe the structure of fully formed chromosome.
2. Discuss the procedure of karyotyping with its clinical applications.
3. What is Lyon hypothesis?
4. What are sex chromatins?
5. Classify chromosomes.
6. Discuss stages of mitosis.
7. Discuss stages of meiosis.
8. Discuss cell to cell interactions with examples.
9. What are cell to cell signaling? Discuss with examples.

MULTIPLE CHOICE QUESTIONS

1. Which of the following correctly describes the structure of a typical human chromosome?
   A. Composed of a single circular DNA molecule
   B. Contains two sister chromatids joined at a centromere
   C. Consists solely of RNA molecules
   D. Contains multiple origins of replication but no centromere

2. How does the process of crossing over during meiosis contribute to genetic diversity?
   A. By increasing the number of chromosomes in a cell
   B. By allowing exchange of genetic material between non-homologous chromosomes
   C. By allowing exchange of genetic material between homologous chromosomes
   D. By preventing mutations

3. What is the significance of nondisjunction during meiosis?
   A. It results in normal chromosomal separation
   B. It can lead to aneuploidy, such as trisomy or monosomy.
   C. It ensures genetic diversity
   D. It occurs during mitosis only

4. Which of the following best describes the role of sex chromatin (Barr body)?
   A. It indicates an extra Y chromosome
   B. It is found only in male cells
   C. It is involved in meiosis
   D. It represents an inactive X chromosome

5. During which phase of cell division are chromosomes most visible and suitable for karyotyping?
   A. Metaphase
   B. Interphase
   C. Anaphase
   D. Telophase

6. Which of the following statements about karyotyping is accurate?
   A. Karyotyping can only be performed on blood cells
   B. Karyotyping reveals the number and structure of chromosomes in a cell
   C. Karyotyping cannot detect chromosomal translocations
   D. Karyotyping is used to determine gene expression levels

7. A mutation in the gene coding for mullerian inhibiting factor (MIF) would most likely result in which of the following?
   A. Normal regression of the paramesonephric duct
   B. Defective sexual differentiation
   C. Abnormal kidney development
   D. Impaired limb formation

8. An experiment involves disrupting the Wnt signaling pathway in developing embryos. Which of the following developmental abnormalities would most likely be observed?
   A. Impaired midbrain development
   B. Defective limb patterning

C. Abnormal urogenital system differentiation
D. All of the above
9. A child presented with a congenital anomaly characterized by the failure of neural tube closure. Which growth differentiation factor is most likely implicated in this defect?
   A. Bone morphogenetic proteins (BMPs)
   B. Fibroblast growth factors (FGFs)
   C. Wnt proteins
   D. Insulin-like growth factors (IGFs)
10. A researcher removes the optic vesicle from a developing embryo and observes that the lens vesicle fails to form. This scenario best illustrates which of the following principles?
    A. Competence
    B. Differentiation
    C. Induction
    D. Segmentation

Answers:
1. B
2. C
3. B
4. D
5. A
6. B
7. B
8. D
9. A
10. C

Gametogenesis, Ovarian and Menstrual Cycle

CHAPTER 3

COMPETENCIES COVERED/LEARNING OUTCOMES

The student should be able to:

AN77.1	Describe the uterine changes occurring during the menstrual cycle.
AN77.2	Describe the synchrony between the ovarian and menstrual cycles.
AN77.3	Describe spermatogenesis and oogenesis along with diagrams.

Reproduction is the biological process by which new individuals are generated from existing organisms. It is essential for the continuation of species.

Central to this process are *gametes (germ cells)*—spermatozoa and ova—formed through gametogenesis. *Gametogenesis* involves the complex and highly regulated sequence of events leading to the production of these haploid cells, which carry half the genetic material necessary for the formation of a new individual.

Gametogenesis is different in males and females. *Spermatogenesis* is the process of forming sperm cells in the testes of males. *Oogenesis* is the process of forming egg cells in the ovaries of females.

In an individual, the formation of gametes takes place only during the *reproductive period* which begins at the age of puberty (10–14 years). In women it ends between the ages of 45 and 50 years, but in men it may continue till the age of 60 years or more.

This chapter explores the details of mechanisms of gametogenesis and highlights its importance in growth and development for the formation of the embryo and the subsequent stages of human development.

STRUCTURE OF A MATURE SPERMATOZOON

A spermatozoon is a highly specialized, free swimming, actively motile cell. The spermatozoon has a *head*, a *neck*, a *middle piece* and a *principal piece* or *tail* (**Figs. 3.1 and 3.2**). An *axial filament* passes through the middle piece and extends into the tail. The spermatozoon measures about 60 μm in length.

The Head

The head of the human spermatozoon is piriform in shape and measures 4 μm in length. It is derived from the nucleus, which consists of 23 highly condensed chromosomes. The head is covered by a cap-like structure

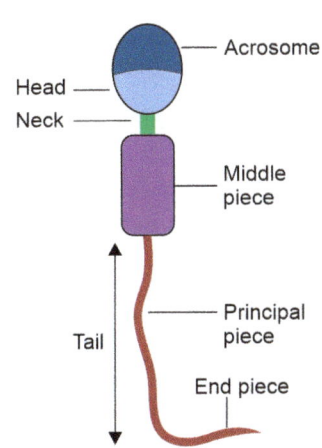

FIG. 3.1: Parts of a spermatozoon.

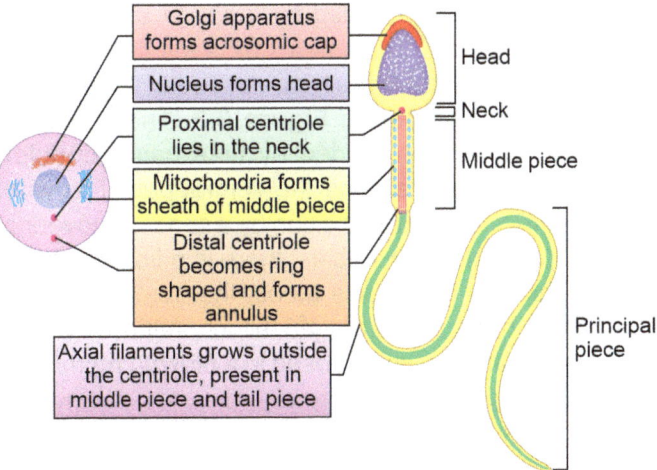

FIG. 3.2: Parts of a spermatozoon and their derivation. According to some authorities, the distal centriole forms the basal body, not the annulus.

called the *acrosome* (also called the *acrosomic cap* or *galea capitis*). The acrosome contains enzymes that help in penetration of the spermatozoon into the ovum during fertilization (*see* **Chapter 4**).

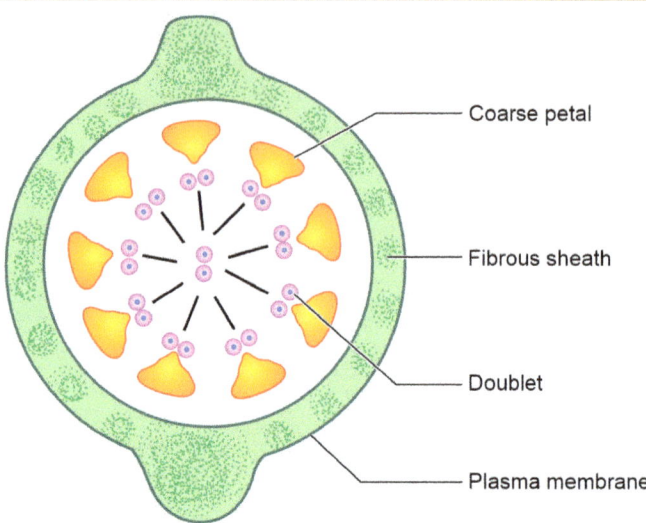

FIG. 3.3: Transverse section across the principal piece (tail) of a spermatozoon to show the arrangement of fibrils.

The Neck

The neck is narrow—it contains a funnel-shaped *basal body* and a spherical *centriole*. The basal body is also called the *connecting piece* because it helps to establish an intimate union between the head and the remainder of the spermatozoon.

The Axial Filament

The axial filament begins just behind the centriole. It passes through the middle piece and most of the tail. At the point where the middle piece joins the tail, the axial filament passes through a ring-like structure called the *annulus*. The part of the axial filament, which lies in the middle piece, is surrounded by a *spiral sheath* made up of mitochondria.

The axial filament is really composed of several fibrils arranged as illustrated in **Figure 3.3**. There is a pair of central fibrils, surrounded by nine pairs (doublets) arranged in a circle around the central pair. The whole system of fibrils is kept in position by a series of coverings. Immediately outside the fibrils, there is a fibrous sheath. In the region of the middle piece, the fibrous sheath is surrounded by spirally arranged mitochondria. Finally, the entire spermatozoon is enclosed in a plasma membrane.

> **Further Details**
> - The chromatin in the head of the spermatozoon is extremely condensed. This makes the head highly resistant to various physical stresses. The chemical basis for condensation is the replacement of histones by protamines.
> - The basal body is made up of nine segmented rod-like structures. On its proximal side (i.e., towards the head of the spermatozoon), the basal body has a convex articular surface which fits into a depression (implantation fossa) in the head.
> - In addition to the doublets, the axial filament contains nine coarser petal-shaped fibrils, one such fibril lying just outside each doublet.

SPERMATOGENESIS

It is the formation of male gametes involving a series of changes leading to the conversion of spermatogonia into spermatozoa, which begins at the age of puberty (12–16 years) and continues to old age.

- Spermatozoa are formed in the wall of the seminiferous tubules of the testes by the influence of primordial germ cells (PGC).
- The duration of spermatogenesis is around 64–74 days.
- The various cell-stages in spermatogenesis are *spermatocytosis, meiosis and spermiogenesis*.

Spermatocytosis

- It is a process of conversion of spermatogonia to primary spermatocytes through series of mitotic divisions. The PGCs give rise to spermatogonial stem cells.
- These stem cells form type A spermatogonia or germ cells which is the indicator of beginning of spermatogenesis.

Various processes in the formation of primary spermatocytes are:

- The *spermatogonia (type A)* or *germ cells* (44 + X + Y) divide mitotically, to give rise to more spermatogonia of type A, and also to spermatogonia of type B **(Fig. 3.4)**.
- The *spermatogonia (type B)* (44 + X + Y) enlarge, or undergo mitosis, to form *primary spermatocytes*.

Meiosis

It a process events of further division of primary spermatocytes to spermatids. Various events are **(Fig. 3.4)**:

- The *primary spermatocytes* (44 + X + Y) now divide so that each of them forms *two secondary spermatocytes*. This is the *first meiotic division*: it reduces the number of chromosomes to half.
- Each *secondary spermatocyte* has 22 + X or 22 + Y chromosomes. It divides to form *two spermatids*. This is the *second meiotic division* and this time there is no reduction in chromosome number.

Spermiogenesis

The process of metamorphosis by which a spermatid becomes a spermatozoon is called *spermiogenesis* (or *spermateleosis*) **(Figs. 3.2 and 3.5)**. This takes 24 days to complete. The spermatid is a more or less circular cell containing a nucleus, Golgi apparatus, centriole and mitochondria. All these components take part in forming the spermatozoon.

- The nucleus condenses and forms the head.
- The Golgi apparatus is transformed into the acrosomic cap that covers 2/3rd of nucleus.

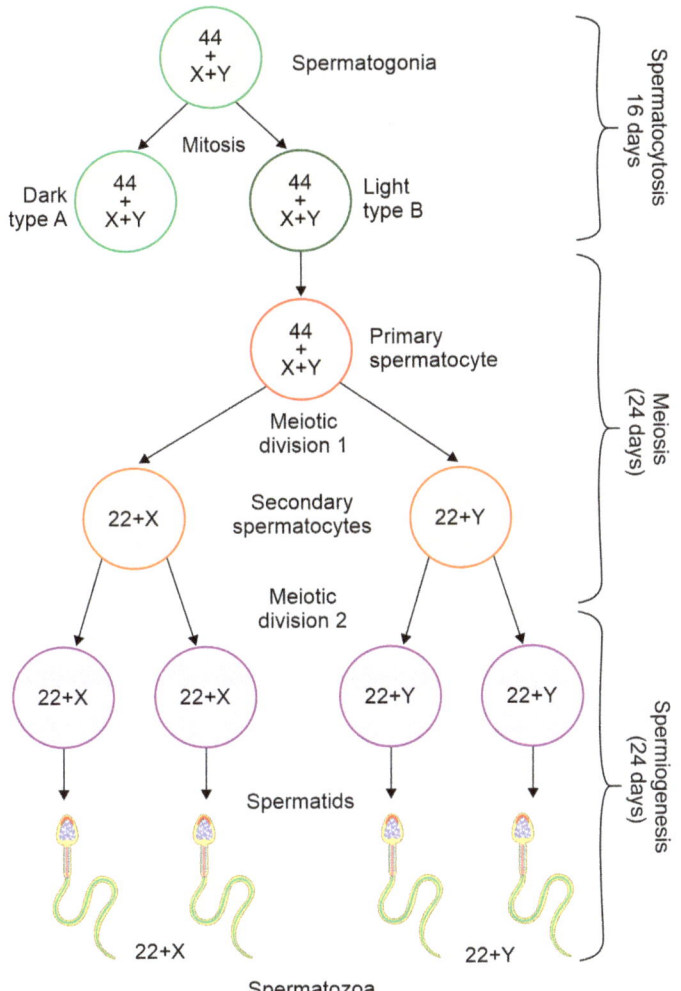

FIG. 3.4: Stages in spermatogenesis.
Note the number of chromosomes at each stage.

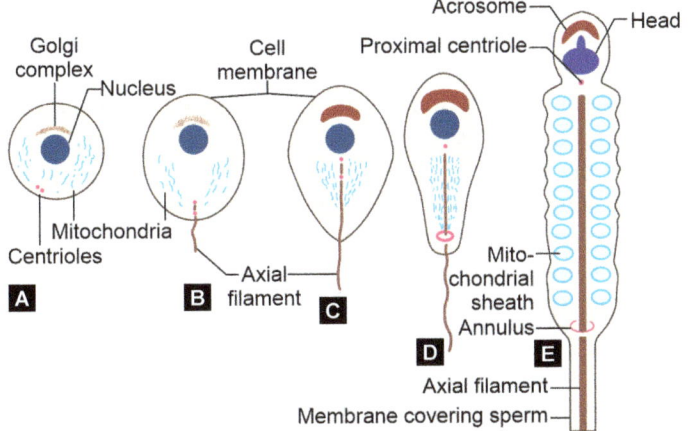

FIGS. 3.5A to E: Stages in spermiogenesis.
Also see **Figure 3.2**.

❖ The centriole divides into two parts that are at first close together—the axial filament appears to grow out of them. The proximal centriole becomes spherical and comes to lie in the neck. Distal centriole forms the distal end of middle piece, i.e., annulus.
❖ The part of the axial filament between the neck and the annulus, becomes surrounded by mitochondria (which forms spiral sheath), and together with them forms the middle piece.
❖ The remaining part of the axial filament elongates to form the principal piece or tail.
❖ Most of the cytoplasm of the spermatid is shed as residual bodies of Regnaud and are engulfed by Sertoli cells.
❖ Cell membrane persists as a covering for the spermatozoon. It becomes specialized for process of fertilization.

Maturation and Capacitation of Spermatozoa

❖ When first formed in seminiferous tubules, spermatozoa are immature. They are nonmotile and incapable of fertilizing an ovum.
❖ A current of fluid in seminiferous tubules carries spermatozoa from the testis to the epididymis. Here they are stored and duration of travel is 2–3 days.
❖ As spermatozoa pass through the epididymis they undergo a process of *maturation*. Changes take place in glycoproteins of the plasma membrane covering the sperm head.
❖ Spermatozoa acquire some motility after maturation, but become fully motile only after ejaculation when they get mixed with secretions of the prostate gland and seminal vesicles.
❖ Spermatozoa acquire the ability to fertilize an ovum only after they have been in the female genital tract for some time. This final step in their maturation is called *capacitation*.
❖ In the process of capacitation, the glycoprotein coat and seminal proteins lying over the surface of the spermatozoon are altered. Spermatozoa usually undergo capacitation in the uterus or uterine tube, under the influence of substances secreted by the female genital tract.
❖ When a spermatozoon comes in contact with the zona pellucida, changes take place in the membranes over the acrosome and enable release of lysosomal enzymes. This is called the *acrosome reaction.*
❖ Some enzymes help in digesting the zona pellucida and in penetration of the spermatozoa through it. Changes in the properties of the zona pellucida constitute the *zona reaction*.

Difference between Spermatogenesis and Spermiogenesis

❖ Spermatogenesis is the complete process of formation of a spermatozoon from a spermatogonium. It includes the first and second meiotic division and spermiogenesis.
❖ On the other hand, spermiogenesis is the process of transformation of a rounded spermatid into a spermatozoon.

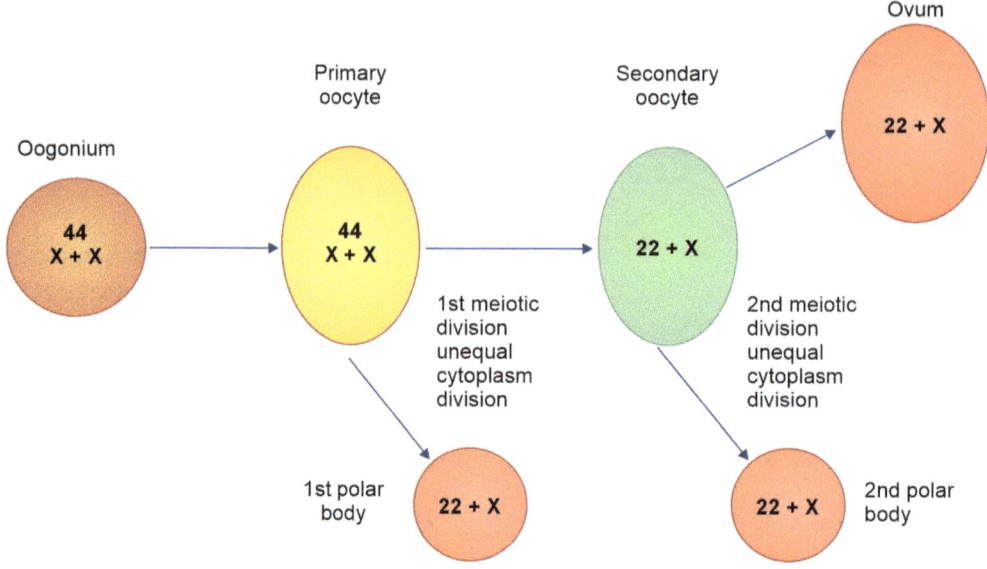

FIG. 3.6: Stages in oogenesis. Compare each stage with the corresponding one in **Figure 3.4**.

OOGENESIS

It is the process by which female gametes, or ova (eggs), are produced in the ovaries. It involves the differentiation and maturation of oogonia (precursor cells) into mature oocytes through a series of developmental stages.

- The oogenesis occurs in ovarian cortex.
- It starts at 10th week of IUL, stops at birth and restarts at puberty (11–13 years). It continues till menopause.
- Various processes involved are *mitosis, meiosis, growth and differentiation of follicles.* Oogenesis stages are described in **Figure 3.6**.
- All the oogonia to be used throughout the life of a woman are produced at a very early stage (possibly before birth) and do not multiply thereafter.

Differences between Spermatogenesis and Oogenesis

- One primary spermatocyte gives rise to four spermatozoa, one primary oocyte forms only one ovum.
- When the primary spermatocyte divides, its cytoplasm is equally distributed between the two secondary spermatocytes formed. However, when the primary oocyte divides, almost all its cytoplasm goes to the daughter cell, which forms the secondary oocyte. The other daughter cell (first polar body), receives half the chromosomes of the primary oocyte, but almost no cytoplasm. The first polar body is, therefore, formed merely to get rid of unwanted chromosomes.

Oogenesis at Different Stages of Life

- In the late fetal period, primary oogonia enlarge to form *primary oocytes*.
- At the time of birth, all primary oocytes are in the *prophase of first meiotic division*. Their number is about 40,000.
- The primary oocytes remain in prophase and do not complete their first meiotic division and enters *resting/ diplotene stage* until they begin to mature and are ready to ovulate at the start of puberty.
- The reproductive period of a female is between 12 to 50 years of age. With each menstrual cycle, a few primary oocytes (about 5 to 30) begin to mature and complete the first meiotic division shortly before ovulation.
- The first meiotic division of a primary oocyte produces two unequal daughter cells. Each daughter cell has the haploid number of chromosomes (23). The large cell, which receives most of the cytoplasm, is called the *secondary oocyte,* and the smaller cell is known as *the first polar body*.
- The secondary oocyte immediately enters the second meiotic cell division. *Ovulation takes* place while the oocyte is in metaphase. The secondary oocyte remains arrested in metaphase till fertilization occurs.
- The second meiotic division is completed only if fertilization occurs. This division results in two unequal daughter cells. The larger cell is called *ovum* while the smaller daughter cell is called the *second polar body*. The first polar body may also divide during the second meiotic division, resulting in formation of three polar bodies.
- If fertilization does not occur, the secondary oocyte fails to complete the second meiotic division and degenerates about 24 hours after ovulation.
- In each menstrual cycle, 5 to 30 primary oocytes start maturing, but only one of them reaches maturity and is ovulated. The remaining degenerate.
- During the entire reproductive life of a female, only around 400 ova are discharged (out of 40,000 primary oocytes available).

The reproductive period in a woman's life spans from *menarche* (onset of menses), around age 12, to *menopause*, typically around age 45, marked by the cessation of menstruation. The monthly flow of blood from the uterus during this period is referred to as *menstruation* (or menses). Menstruation, or menses, reflects cyclic changes within the uterus, known as the *menstrual cycle.*

Simultaneously, cyclic changes also take place in the ovaries known as the *ovarian cycle* resulting most important event of *ovulation*.

OVARIAN CYCLE

It is the cyclic changes in the ovaries during 28 days of reproductive cycle that result in the formation of single mature ovum.
- It includes follicular development, ovulation, and the formation and regression of the corpus luteum which are divided into three phases: preovulatory, ovulatory and postovulatory.
- These events are regulated by hormonal signals, primarily from the hypothalamus, pituitary gland, and ovaries themselves, which are part of hypothalamo-pituitary-ovarian axis.

Formation of Ovarian Follicles/Folliculogenesis

This is the first step of ovarian cycle which extends from 5th day to 14th day (ovulation).
- **Primordial follicles:** The oogonia are surrounded by other cells that form the stroma. Some cells of the stroma become flattened and surround an oocyte **(Fig. 3.7)**. These flattened cells ultimately form the ovarian follicle and are, therefore, called *follicular cells*. Follicles up to this stage of development are called *primordial follicles*.
- The further differentiation of primordial follicles is arrested till puberty.
- **Primary follicles:** At puberty the oocyte complete its first meiotic division, resulting in formation of *primary follicle* **(Fig. 3.8)**. Each primary follicle consists of primary oocyte surrounded by a layer of cuboidal or low columnar follicular cells.
- A homogeneous membrane, the *zona pellucida*, appears between the follicular cells and the oocyte **(Fig. 3.8)**.
- **Secondary follicle:** The follicular cells proliferate to form several layers. These constitute the *membrana granulosa* **(Fig. 3.9)**. The cells may now be called *granulosa cells*.
- **Preantral follicle:** Secretion of fluid by granulosa cells result in appearance of fluid filled spaces. This is called preantral follicle.

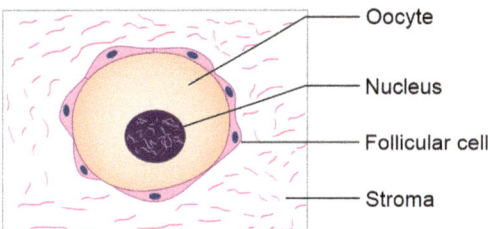
FIG. 3.7: Primordial follicle.

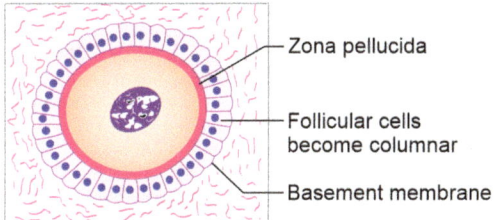
FIG. 3.8: Primary follicle.

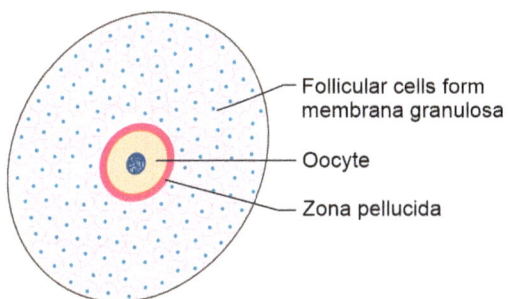
FIG. 3.9: Secondary follicle.

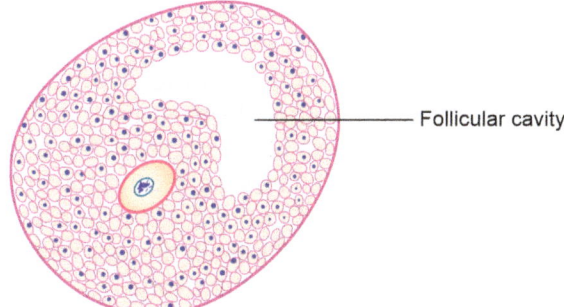
FIG. 3.10: Tertiary/antral follicle.

- **Antral/tertiary follicle:** These small fluid filled spaces joined to form bigger cavity called antrum **(Fig. 3.10)**.
- **Mature/Graafian follicle:** The cavity of the follicle rapidly increases in size. As a result, the wall of the follicle (formed by the granulosa cells) becomes relatively thin. The oocyte now lies eccentrically in the follicle, surrounded by some granulosa cells that are given the name *cumulus oophoricus* (or *cumulus ovaricus*). The cells that attach it to the wall of the follicle are given the name *discus proligerus* **(Fig. 3.11)**. The layer of cells immediately surrounding the oocyte and zona pellucida are called *corona radiata cells.*

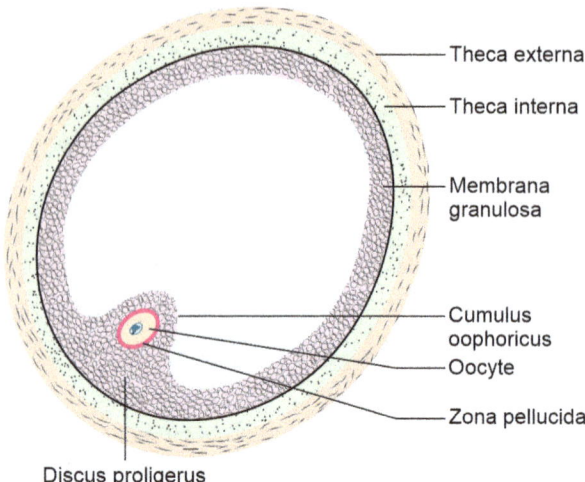

FIG. 3.11: Mature Graafian follicle.

- As the follicle expands, the stromal cells surrounding the membrana granulosa become condensed to form a covering called the *theca interna* (theca = cover). The cells of the theca interna later secrete a hormone called estrogen; and they are then called the cells of the *thecal gland* (Fig. 3.11).
- Outside the theca interna some fibrous tissue becomes condensed to form another covering for the follicle called the *theca externa* (Fig. 3.11). The ovarian follicle is now fully formed. Fully mature Graafian follicle is about 3–5 mm in size.

Ovulation

The shedding of the ovum from the ovary is called *ovulation*. The ovarian follicle is at first very small compared to the thickness of the cortex of the ovary.

- As it enlarges, it becomes so big that it not only reaches the surface of the ovary, but also forms a bulging in this situation. Ultimately, the follicle ruptures and the ovum is shed from the ovary.
- Just before ovulation the follicle may have a diameter of 15 mm. The stroma and theca on this side of the follicle become very thin. An avascular area *(stigma)* appears over the most convex point of the follicle. At the same time, the cells of the cumulus oophorus become loosened by accumulation of intercellular fluid between them.
- During the process of ovulation there is rupture of mature follicle and release of secondary oocyte in metaphase of 2nd meiotic division.
- The ovulated oocyte with its surrounding cells swims toward the fimbrial end of fallopian tube.
- In the ampulla of fallopian tube, one sperm penetrates the various barriers surrounding the secondary oocyte. This initiates resuming of meiosis II of secondary oocyte.

- ❖ **Stage of meiosis at ovulation:** Completion of meiosis I resulting in secondary oocyte and the first polar body.
- ❖ **Time of ovulation:** 14 days ± 1 day before the onset of next menstrual cycle.

The following factors may lead to ovulation:
- Ovulation occurs due to high concentration of luteinizing hormones (LH) in blood just before ovulation (*see* **Fig. 3.3**).
- A high concentration of LH leads to increase activity of the enzyme **collagenase,** which in turn digests the collagen fibers surrounding the follicle.
- Increase in concentration of **prostaglandins** causes contraction of smooth muscle in the wall of the ovary.
- The increased pressure of fluid in the follicular cavity is also a significant factor for ovulation to occur.
- However, the enzymatic digestion of the follicular wall seems to be the main factor responsible for ovulation.

Clinical Importance

Ovulation
- **Detection of time of ovulation:** Basal body temperature recording—it falls 0.3–0.5°C just before ovulation (follicular phase) and increases slightly thereafter (luteal phase). Time of ovulation can be determined by recording the morning temperature during mid-cycle. The rise in temperature after ovulation is due to the increase in the concentration of progesterone.
- **Endometrial biopsy:** To observe changes specific for ovulation under the influence of progesterone.
- **Observation of cervical mucus:** It is sticky and presents fern pattern.
- **Hormonal estimation:** Blood progesterone, estrogen, FSH, LH estimation during mid-cycle—increased LH and estrogen and decreased FSH at the time of ovulation and increased progesterone after ovulation.
- **Ultrasonography:** Process of ovulation can be recorded. Corpus luteum can be detected in ovary.
- **Uterine bleeding:** Intermenstrual occurs.
- **Vaginal smear:** Increased cornification of mucosa.
- **Mittelschmerz:** Mid-cycle pain.
- **Conditions affecting ovulation:**
  - *Age:* Anovulatory cycles are common before puberty, initial cycles after puberty, after menopause.
  - *Pregnancy*
  - *Lactation*
  - *Diseases*—nutritional, endocrine and emotional
  - *Environment*—extremes of temperature.

Structure of the Ovum

The ovum that is shed from the ovary is not fully mature. It is really a secondary oocyte that is undergoing division to shed off the second polar body (Fig. 3.6).

At this stage, the ovum has the appearance illustrated in **Figure 3.12**. Note that it is surrounded by the zona pellucida. Some cells of the corona radiata can be seen sticking to the outside of the zona pellucida. No nucleus is seen, as the nuclear membrane has dissolved for the

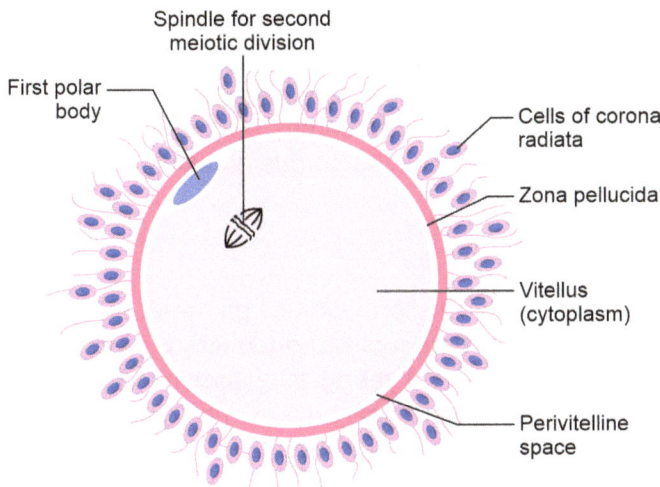

FIG. 3.12: Structure of ovum at the time of ovulation.

second meiotic division. A spindle is, however, present. Between the cell membrane (or *vitelline membrane*) and the zona pellucida, a distinct *perivitelline space* is seen. The first polar body lies in this space.

> **NOTE**
> The ovum is a very large cell and measures more than 100 μm in diameter. In contrast, most other cells of the body measure less than 10 μm (one μm is one thousandth of a millimeter).

Fate of the Ovum

Let us see what happens to the ovum that is shed from the ovary. You already know that the ovary is closely embraced by the fimbriated end of the uterine tube.
- Therefore, the ovum is easily carried into the tube partly by the follicular fluid discharged from the follicle and partly by the activity of ciliated cells lining the tube.
- The ovum slowly travels through the tube towards the uterus, taking three to four days to do so.
- If sexual intercourse takes place at about this time, the spermatozoa deposited in the vagina swim into the uterus and into the uterine tube.
- One of these spermatozoa may fertilize the ovum. If this happens, the fertilized ovum begins to develop into an embryo. It travels to the uterus and gets implanted in its wall. On the other hand, if the ovum (secondary oocyte) is not fertilized it dies in 12–24 hours. It passes through the uterus into the vagina and is discharged.

Corpus Luteum

The corpus luteum is an important structure. It mainly secretes a hormone progesterone, but secretes some estrogen also. The corpus luteum is derived from the ovarian follicle, after the latter has ruptured to shed the ovum, as follows **(Figs. 3.13A to D)**:
- When the follicle ruptures, its wall collapses and becomes folded.
- At this stage, the follicular cells are small and rounded. They now rapidly enlarge. As they increase in size, their walls press against those of neighboring cells so that the cells acquire a polyhedral shape. Their cytoplasm becomes filled with a yellow pigment called *lutein*. They are now called *luteal cells*. The presence of this yellow pigment gives the structure a yellow color and that is why it is called the corpus luteum (= yellow body). Some cells of the theca interna also enlarge and contribute to the corpus luteum.

The subsequent fate of the corpus luteum depends on whether the ovum is fertilized or not.
- If the ovum is not fertilized, the corpus luteum persists for about 14 days. During this period, it secretes progesterone. It remains relatively small and is called the *corpus luteum of menstruation*. At the end of its functional life, it degenerates and forms a mass of fibrous tissue called the *corpus albicans* (= white body) **(Fig. 3.14)**.
- If the ovum is fertilized and pregnancy results, the corpus luteum persists for three to four months. This

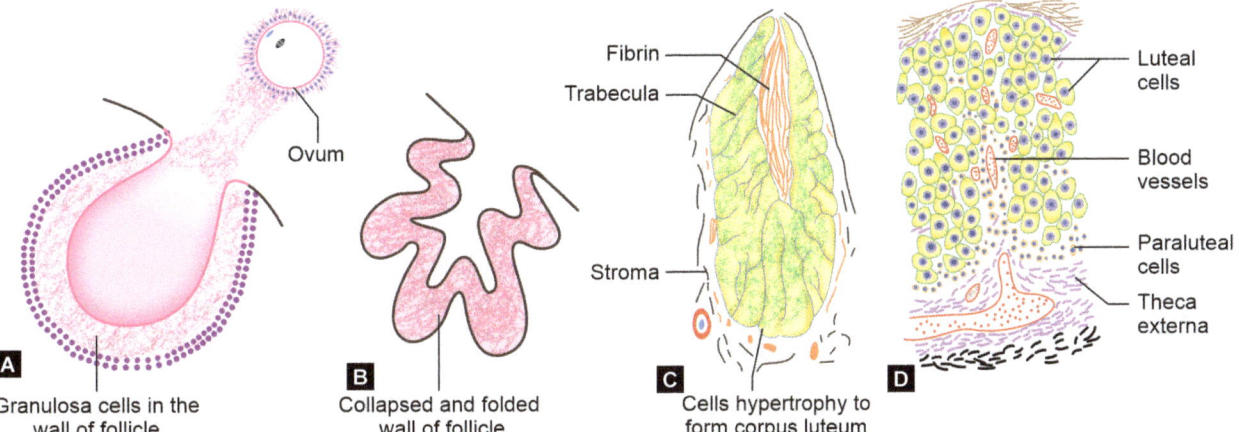

FIGS. 3.13A to D: Stages in the formation of corpus luteum and transformation of follicular cells to luteal cells.

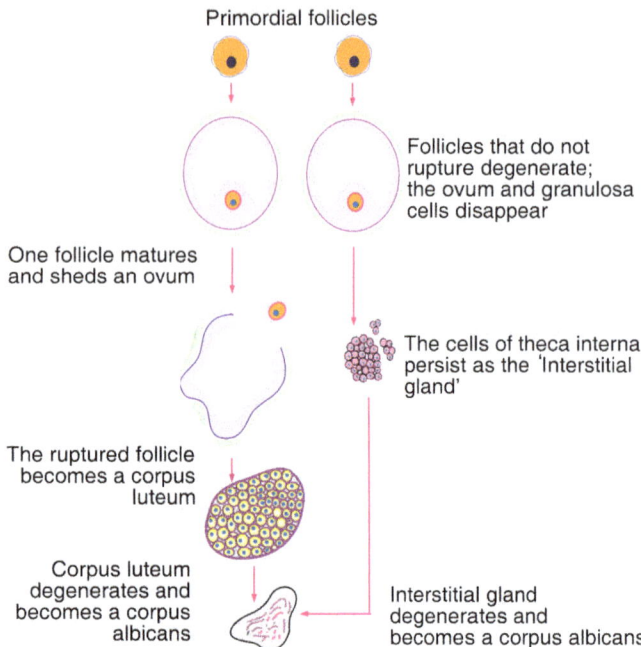

FIG. 3.14: Fate of ovarian follicles.

is larger than the corpus luteum of menstruation, and is called the *corpus luteum of pregnancy*.

The corpus luteum of pregnancy may occupy one-third to half the total volume of the ovary. The progesterone secreted by it is essential for the maintenance of pregnancy in the first few months. After the fourth month, the corpus luteum is no longer needed, as the placenta begins to secrete progesterone. Degeneration of the corpus luteum in the early months of pregnancy is prevented by human chorionic gonadotropin (hCG) secreted by the trophoblast cells of the developing embryo.

Clinical Importance

Corpus Lutem of Pregnancy
- The corpus luteum is essential for implantation of the blastocyst into the uterine endometrium and for continuation of pregnancy.
- Treatment with prostaglandins in early pregnancy either via intravenous, intramuscular or vaginal routes causes degeneration of the corpus luteum and abortion of the embryo/fetus.

Fate of Ovarian Follicles

In each ovarian cycle, one follicle reaches maturity, sheds an ovum, and becomes a corpus luteum. At the same time, several other follicles also begin to develop, but do not reach maturity **(Fig. 3.14)**. It is interesting to note that, contrary to what one might expect, these follicles do not persist into the next ovarian cycle, but undergo degeneration. The ovum and granulosa cells of each follicle disappear. The cells of the theca interna, however, proliferate to form the *interstitial glands*, also called the *corpora atretica* (singular = *corpus atreticum*). These glands are believed to secrete estrogens. After a period of activity, each gland becomes a mass of scar tissue indistinguishable from the corpus albicans formed from the corpus luteum.

Reproductive Period

In an individual, the formation of gametes takes place only during the reproductive period which begins at the age of puberty (10–14 years). In women it ends between the ages of 45 and 50 years, but in men it may continue till the age of 60 years or more.

Viability of Gametes

An ovum usually degenerates 24 hours after ovulation. However, at the most it may survive for two days. Similarly, sperms usually degenerate 48 hours after ejaculation, but may survive up to four days in female genital tract.

MENSTRUAL CYCLE

Definition: The menstrual cycle, also known as the uterine cycle, refers to the cyclic changes that occur in the endometrium every month **(Figs. 3.15 and 3.17)**. The onset of menstruation *(menarche)* takes place at about 10–12 years of age.
- The most evident feature is the monthly flow of menstrual blood which typically lasts 3–6 days.
- The cycle spans approximately 28 days, though it can vary from 21 to 40 days. It begins with the first day of bleeding in the current cycle and ends with the first day of bleeding in the subsequent cycle.
- The menstrual cycle prepares the endometrium to receive and support a fertilized ovum.

To understand the menstrual cycle, it is necessary to know the structure of the uterus. The wall of the uterus is made up of three layers.
1. The outermost layer or *perimetrium* is made up of peritoneum and the connective tissue.
2. The main thickness of the wall is made up of smooth muscle. This is the *myometrium*.
3. The innermost layer (corresponding to mucous membrane) is called the *endometrium*. It is this layer which undergoes changes during the menstrual cycle.

The constituents of the endometrium are as follows (Fig. 3.16):
- The epithelium lining the surface of the endometrium.
- The stroma fills the interval between surface epithelium and myometrium. It contains numerous simple tubular glands (uterine glands).
- The arteries that supply the endometrium tend to run vertically towards the surface. Some of these run spirally and supply the whole thickness of the

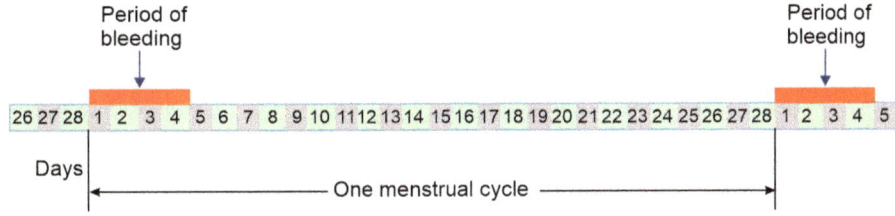

FIG. 3.15: Diagram illustrating the definition of a menstrual cycle.

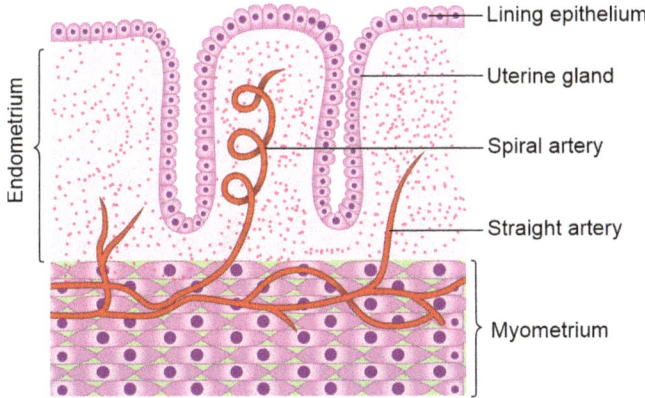

FIG. 3.16: Components of the uterine endometrium. These undergo changes during each menstrual cycle.

endometrium, while others that remain straight are confined to the basal part.

Phases of the Menstrual Cycle

The menstrual cycle is usually divided into the following phases, on the basis of changes taking place in the uterine endometrium **(Fig. 3.17)**:
1. *Postmenstrual*
2. *Proliferative*
3. *Secretory or premenstrual*
4. *Menstrual*

❖ The changes that occur during the postmenstrual phase and most of the proliferative phase happen under the influence of estrogen produced by the developing follicles in the ovary. This period is therefore called the *follicular phase* of the menstrual cycle, which makes up the first half of the cycle.

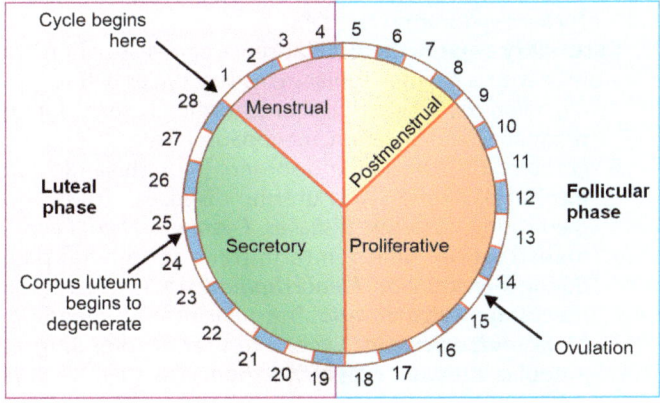

FIG. 3.17: Phases of the menstrual cycle.

❖ Following ovulation, the corpus luteum is formed and starts secreting progesterone. During the second half of the menstrual cycle, this hormone (along with estrogens) produces striking changes in the endometrium. As these changes take place under the influence of the corpus luteum, this half of the menstrual cycle is called the *luteal phase*.

❖ Just before the onset of the next bleeding, there is lowering of levels of both progesterone and estrogens, and it is believed that this 'withdrawal' leads to the onset of menstrual bleeding.

Endometrial Changes: Phase-wise

❖ **General changes:**
 – The endometrium progressively increases in thickness. In the postmenstrual phase, it is 0.5–1 mm thick; in the proliferative phase, it is 2–3 mm thick; and in the secretory phase its thickness reaches 5–7 mm.
 – The uterine glands grow in length. At first, they are straight, but gradually become convoluted acquiring 'saw-toothed' appearance when seen in longitudinal section.
 – *During the postmenstrual phase,* the cells of the stroma are uniformly distributed and are compactly arranged **(Figs. 3.16 and 3.18A)**.

❖ **Proliferative phase:** As the endometrium increases in thickness, the superficial part of the stroma remains compact, but the part surrounding the bodies of the uterine glands becomes spongy. The deepest part of the stroma also remains compact. The stroma can, therefore, be divided into the following three layers **(Fig. 3.18B)**:
 1. *Stratum compactum*
 2. *Stratum spongiosum*
 3. *Stratum basale*

The stratum compactum and spongiosum together are called *functional zone* as these layers are sloughed off during menstruation. The basal layer is retained and is the *regenerative zone* from which regeneration of endometrium occurs.
 – *During the secretory phase,* these layers become better defined. The endometrium becomes soft and edematous, because of the fluid secreted by the uterine glands **(Figs. 3.18C and D)**.

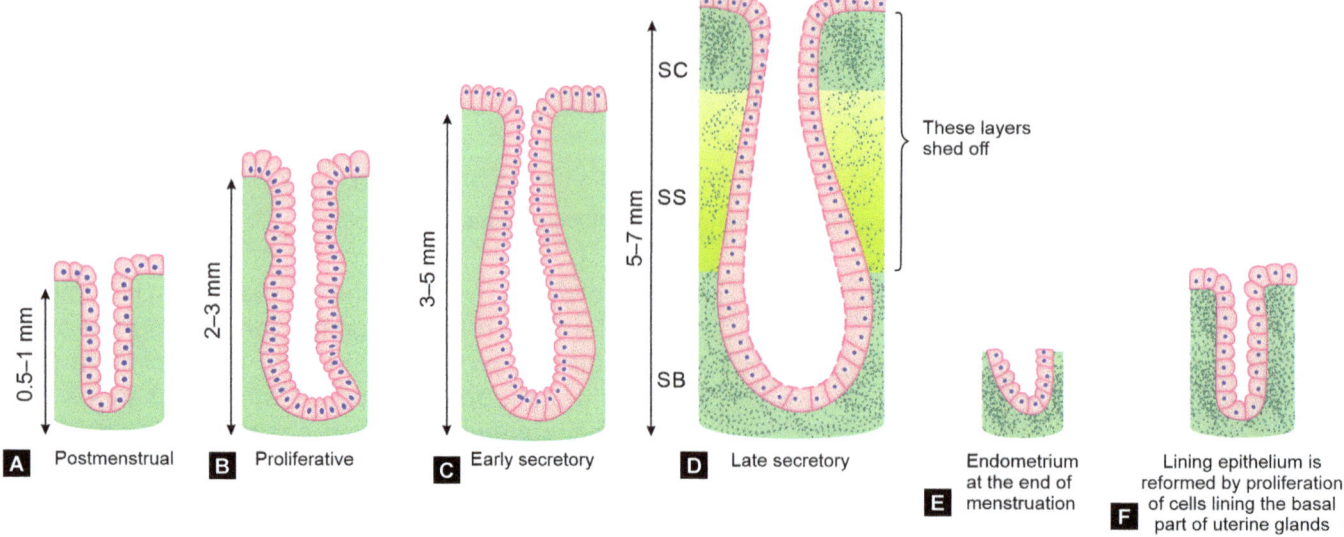

FIGS. 3.18A to F: Changes in uterine epithelium, glands and endometrium during menstrual cycle.
(SC: stratum compactum; SS: stratum spongiosum; SB: stratum basale)

- The arteries of the endometrium are small to begin with. They grow in length during the proliferative phase. During the secretory phase, the arteries supplying the superficial two-thirds of the endometrium become very tortuous and are called spiral arteries. The arteries to the basal third of the endometrium (which does not participate in the changes associated with the menstrual cycle) remain straight and short.
- Towards the end of the secretory phase the endometrium is thick, soft, and richly supplied with blood. The secretory activity of the uterine glands not only makes the endometrium soft, but also provides nutrition to the embryo. These changes are, therefore, an obvious preparation for providing a suitable environment for the fertilized ovum, when it reaches the uterus.
❖ **Menstrual phase:** In the absence of pregnancy, however, these measures are abortive—the superficial parts of the thickened endometrium (stratum compactum and stratum spongiosum) are shed off **(Fig. 3.18D)**, and this is accompanied by menstrual bleeding.
  - Menstrual bleeding causes the endometrium to be shed off bit by bit, and the blood along with shreds of endometrium flows out through the vagina. At the end of menstruation, the endometrium that remains is only 0.5 mm thick. It consists of the stratum basale along with the basal portions of the uterine glands **(Fig. 3.18E)**. The epithelium of these glands rapidly proliferates and reforms the lining epithelium **(Fig. 3.18F)**.
  - The endometrial changes associated with the menstrual cycle are confined to the body of the uterus. The cervical mucosa is not affected.

> **NOTE**
> Mechanism for onset of menstrual bleeding is as follows:
> - A few hours before the onset of menstrual bleeding, spiral arteries constrict, cutting off blood supply to the superficial endometrium.
> - Ischemia results, causing degeneration of the endometrium and damage to blood vessel walls.
> - As arteries relax, blood flows back into the endometrium, leaking from the damaged vessels.
> - This leaking blood leads to the gradual shedding of the endometrium during menstruation.

Clinical correlation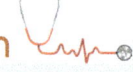

Disorders of Menstrual Cycle
Amenorrhea: Absence of menstrual cycle. Amenorrhea is of two types—primary and secondary with each having physiological and pathological causes.
1. **Primary amenorrhea:** It is absence of menstruation from the beginning and throughout the reproductive age of a woman.
   A. *Physiological:* Before puberty (12–14 years), delayed onset of menstruation (up to 18 years).
   B. *Pathological:* Menstruation does not start even after 18 years and is due to sex-chromosomal anomalies—Turner's syndrome (45, XO).
2. **Secondary amenorrhea:** It is absence of menstruation in a woman who is having regular menstrual cycles before.
   A. *Physiological:* Physiological amenorrhea is seen during pregnancy and lactation, menopause, stress.
   B. *Pathological:* Endocrine disorders (hypothalamic and pituitary); ovarian and uterine diseases, drugs and medication, systemic diseases. **Dysmenorrhea:** Painful menstruation. Sharp, intermittent abdominal pain during menstruation. **Menorrhagia:** Excessive menstrual bleeding. **Metrorrhagia:** Irregular uterine bleeding. **Menometrorrhagia:** Excessive uterine bleeding at irregular intervals. **Polymenorrhea:** Less than 21 days duration of menstrual cycles. **Oligomenorrhea:** More than 35 days duration of menstrual cycles.

Time of Ovulation

There are many methods of finding out the exact time of ovulation, but the one commonly used is the temperature method. *Temperature method:* In this technique, the woman's basal body temperature is recorded every morning.

The temperature is low during actual menstruation. Subsequently it rises. At about the middle of the cycle, there is a sudden fall in temperature followed by a rise. This rise is believed to indicate that ovulation has occurred **(Fig. 3.19)**. *Importance of determining the time of ovulation and "safe period"*

- **Where pregnancy is not desired:** After ovulation, the ovum is viable (i.e., it can be fertilized) for not more than 2 days. Spermatozoa introduced into the vagina die within 4 days. Therefore, fertilization can occur only if intercourse takes place during a period between 4 days before ovulation to 2 days after ovulation.
  The remaining days have been regarded as **safe period** as far as prevention of pregnancy is concerned. This forms the basis of the so-called **rhythm-method** of family planning.
- **Where pregnancy is desired:** Knowledge regarding the time of ovulation is also of importance in cases of sterility (difficulty in having children), where the couple can be advised to have intercourse during the days most favorable for conception.

Correlation between Ovarian and Uterine Cycles

The ovarian and uterine cycles run parallel to each other. Both are of 28 days duration **(Fig. 3.20)**. The uterine cycle is dependent on ovarian cycle. The uterine endometrium shows cyclic changes, which are dependent on the hormones secreted by developing ovarian follicles and corpus luteum of the ovary.

HORMONAL CONTROL OF OVARIAN AND UTERINE CYCLES

These cycles are under the control of various hormones, which can be briefly summarized as follows **(Fig. 3.21)**:

- The hypothalamus acts as a major center for the control of reproduction. It secretes the *gonadotropin-releasing hormones (GnRH),* which in turn controls the secretion of *gonadotrophic hormones* from the anterior pituitary gland (adenohypophysis).
- There are two gonadotropic hormones. They are the *follicle stimulating hormone (FSH)* and the *luteinizing hormone (LH).*
- In the first half of the menstrual cycle, the GnRH acts on the anterior pituitary to release FSH. The FSH acts on the ovary and stimulates the formation and maturation of ovarian follicles **(Fig. 3.21)**.
- The maturing ovarian follicles now start secreting estrogens. The repair and proliferation of endometrium takes place under the influence of estrogens. The endometrial stroma progressively thickens, the glands in it elongate and the spiral arteries begin to grow towards the surface epithelium.
- The level of estrogen rises to a peak about two days before ovulation. This leads to sudden increase in the level of LH secreted by the anterior pituitary

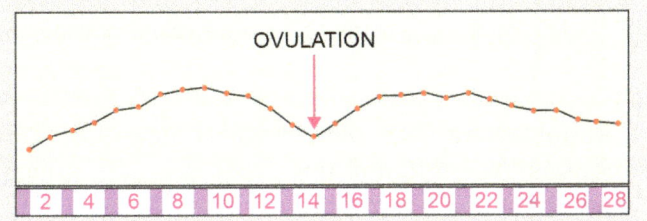

FIG. 3.19: Graph showing the morning temperature of a woman, on various days of the menstrual cycle. There is a fall in temperature at about the time of ovulation, followed by a rise.

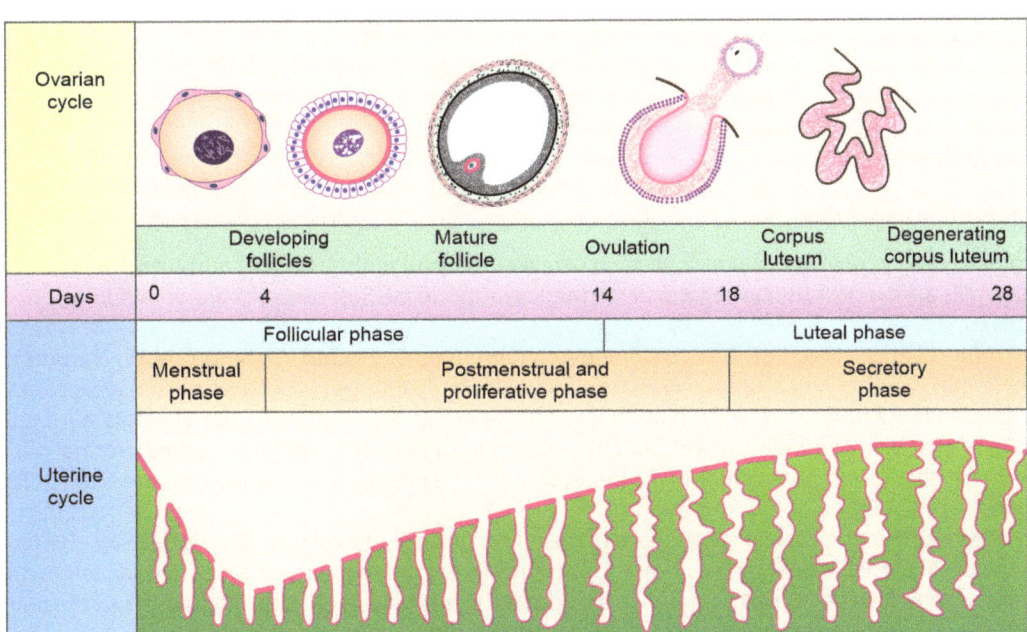

FIG. 3.20: Diagram showing correlation between ovarian and uterine cycles.

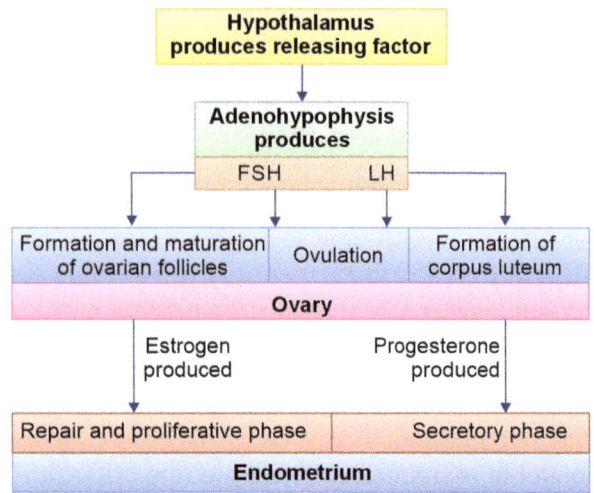

FIG. 3.21: Hormonal control of ovarian and uterine cycles. (FSH: follicle-stimulating hormone; LH: luteinizing hormone)

(LH surge) about 24–36 hours before ovulation **(Fig. 3.22)**. The LH surge leads to ovulation; and the Graafian follicle is transformed to the corpus luteum.

- The LH stimulates the secretion of progesterone by the corpus luteum. Though the secretion of progesterone predominates, some estrogen is also produced. The combined action of estrogen and progesterone stimulates the endometrial glands to secrete glycogen-rich mucoid material **(Fig. 3.21)**.
- If fertilization does not occur, the granulosa cells produce the protein *inhibin,* which acts on the anterior pituitary and inhibits the secretion of gonadotrophins. This leads to regression of the corpus luteum.
- Due to the regression of the corpus luteum there is a fall in the blood level of estrogen and progesterone. The withdrawal of these hormones causes the endometrium to regress. and triggers the onset of menstruation.
- If fertilization occurs, the corpus luteum does not regress. It continues to secrete progesterone and estrogen. The secretory phase of endometrium continues and menstruation does not occur.

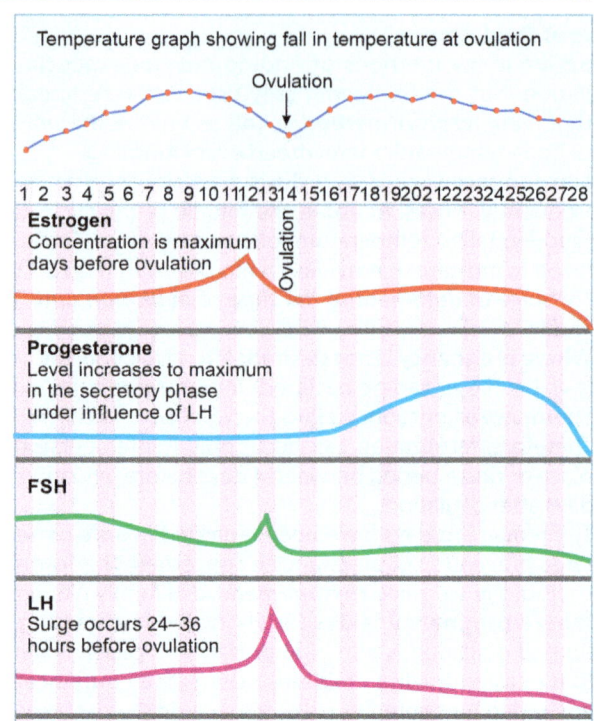

FIG. 3.22: Concentration of the hormones FSH, LH, estrogen and progesterone during a normal menstrual cycle. Ovulation occurs because of a LH surge just before ovulation.
(FSH: follicle-stimulating hormone; LH: luteinizing hormone)

Clinical correlation

Use of Hormones for Contraception

Ovulation in a woman (and by corollary, pregnancy) can be prevented by administration of contraceptive pills. The most important ingredients of such pills are progestins (in the form of synthetic compounds). Better results are obtained when a small amount of estrogen is also given.

In the most common variety of pill (distributed by government agencies in India), the progestin is **norethisterone acetate** (1 mg); and the estrogen is in the form of *estradiol* (50 μg). The pills are distributed in packets, each packet containing 28 pills out of which 21 pills contain these hormones, and 7 pills do not (for use in the last 7 days). The use of pills is started 5 days after onset of menstruation. They are taken continuously without any break as long as contraception is desired. Normal menstruation occurs during the 7 days in which pills without hormones are being taken. If the pills are taken regularly there is a regular menstrual cycle of 28 days duration.

Presence of progesterone in the preovulatory phase prevents occurrence of ovulation. This is because the progesterone in the pill prevents the secretion of FSH and LH by the pituitary. This interferes with the maturation of follicles, and ovulation.

Stoppage of pills reduces levels of these hormones in blood. It is this withdrawal that leads to menstrual bleeding. Such pills have almost 100% success in suppressing maturation of follicles and ovulation.

Chapter 3: Gametogenesis, Ovarian and Menstrual Cycle

HIGHLIGHTS

- Male gametes produced by the testis are called *spermatozoa*. The process is called *spermatogenesis*.
- Female gametes produced by the ovary are called *ova*. The process is called *oogenesis*. Spermatogenesis and oogenesis are together called *gametogenesis*.
- **Fertilization** takes place when one spermatozoon enters an ovum. The fused ovum and sperm form the *zygote*.
- A *spermatozoon* has a head, a neck, a middle piece and a principal piece or tail.
- Spermatozoa are derived from rounded *spermatids*. The process of conversion of a spermatid to a spermatozoon is called *spermiogenesis*.
- An *ovarian follicle* is a rounded structure that contains a developing ovum surrounded by follicular cells. The follicle has a cavity filled with fluid.
- Ovarian follicles have a cellular covering called the *theca interna*. The cells of the theca interna produce estrogens.
- The follicle gradually increases in size and finally bursts and expels the ovum. This process of shedding of the ovum is called *ovulation*.
- The *corpus luteum* is formed by enlargement and transformation of follicular cells, after-shedding of the ovum. The corpus luteum secretes progesterone, which is essential for maintenance of pregnancy.
- The term *menstrual cycle* is applied to cyclical changes that occur in the endometrium every month. The most obvious feature is a monthly flow of blood (*menstruation*).
- The menstrual cycle is divided into the following phases: *postmenstrual*, *proliferative*, *secretory*, *menstrual* (**Fig. 3.3**).
- The menstrual cycle is also divided into the *follicular phase* (in which changes are produced mainly by estrogens), and the *luteal phase* (in which effects of progesterone predominate). Both phases are of roughly equal duration.
- The *main changes in the endometrium* are (a) increase in thickness, (b) growth of uterine glands, (c) changes in epithelial cells lining the glands and (d) increase in thickness and fluid content of the endometrial stroma.
- Just before onset of menstruation, the blood supply to superficial parts of the endometrium is cut off. This part is *shed off* and there is *bleeding*.
- The menstrual cycle is *influenced by* estrogens, progesterone, follicle stimulating hormone (FSH) and luteinizing hormone (LH).

Summary

- Reproductive cycle in males (**Flowchart 3.1**).
- Reproductive cycle in females (**Flowchart 3.2**).
- Differences between sperm and ovum (**Table 3.1**).
- Differences between spermatogenesis and oogenesis (**Table 3.2**).

FLOWCHART 3.1: Reproductive cycle in male.

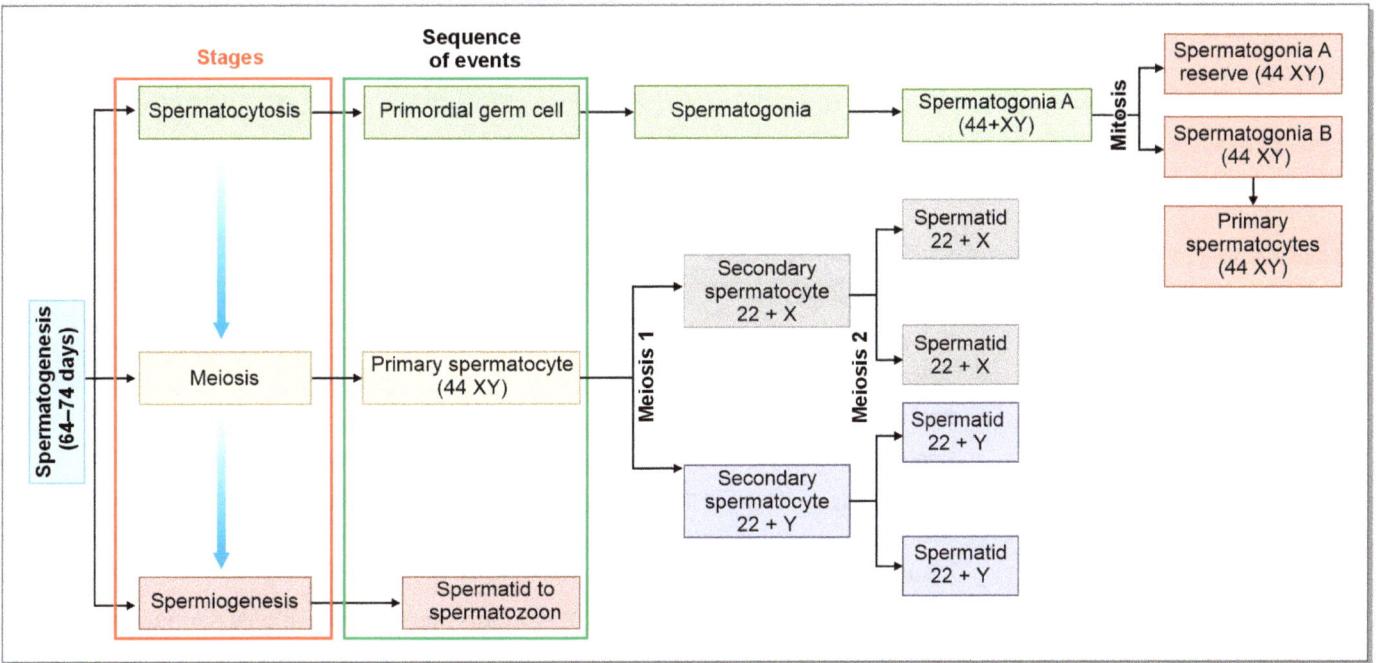

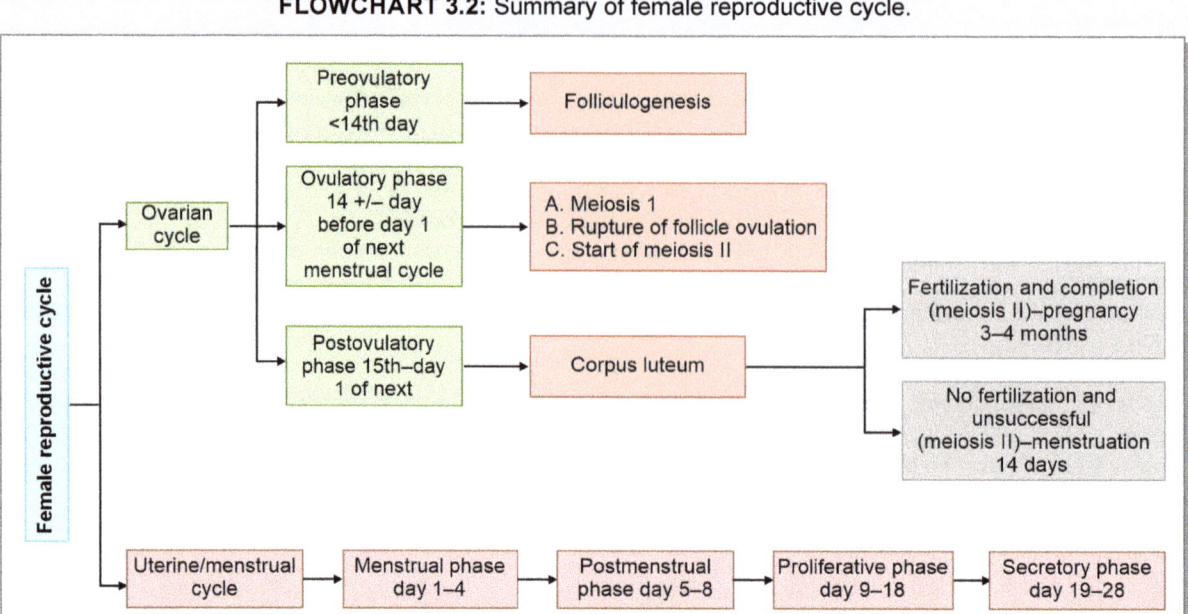

FLOWCHART 3.2: Summary of female reproductive cycle.

TABLE 3.1: Differences between spermatozoon and ovum.

Feature	Sperm (spermatozoon)	Ovum (oocyte)
Size	Smaller (approximately 60 μm long)	Larger (approximately 100–200 μm in diameter)
Shape	Head, midpiece, and tail (flagellum)	Round and large
Motility	Motile, due to flagellum	Nonmotile
Number produced	Millions per ejaculate	Typically, one per menstrual cycle
Lifespan	Survives 1–3 days in female reproductive tract	Survives 12–24 hours after ovulation
Origin	Produced in the testes	Produced in the ovaries
Chromosome	Haploid (23 chromosomes, either X or Y)	Haploid (23 chromosomes, always X)
Maturation process	Spermatogenesis	Oogenesis
Cell division	Continuous after puberty	Arrested in prophase I until puberty, then in metaphase II until fertilization
Mitochondria	Numerous in midpiece for energy	Fewer, dispersed in the cytoplasm
Acrosome	Present, contains enzymes to penetrate the ovum	Not present
Protective layers	Plasma membrane only	Surrounded by zona pellucida and corona radiata
Completion of meiosis	Completes meiosis after leaving the testis	Completes meiosis only upon fertilization

TABLE 3.2: Differences between spermatogenesis and oogenesis.

Feature	Spermatogenesis	Oogenesis
Definition	The process of sperm cell development	The process of ovum (egg cell) development
Location	Seminiferous tubules of the testes	Ovaries
Onset	Begins at puberty	Begins during fetal development
Duration	Continuous throughout life after puberty	Cyclical, typically 28 days
Primary germ cell	Spermatogonia	Oogonia
Mitosis	Spermatogonia undergo mitosis throughout life	Oogonia undergo mitosis only during fetal development

Feature	Spermatogenesis	Oogenesis
Meiosis I	Primary spermatocytes undergo meiosis I to form secondary spermatocytes	Primary oocytes begin meiosis I during fetal development and arrest in prophase I until puberty
Meiosis II	Secondary spermatocytes undergo meiosis II to form spermatids	Secondary oocytes begin meiosis II at ovulation and arrest in metaphase II until fertilization
Number of gametes produced	Four spermatids from each primary spermatocyte	One ovum and three polar bodies from each primary oocyte
Timing of gamete release	Continuous, millions produced daily	Monthly, one oocyte released per menstrual cycle
Hormonal regulation	Regulated by FSH and LH, testosterone	Regulated by FSH and LH, estrogen, progesterone
Cellular transformation	Spermatids undergo spermiogenesis to become mature spermatozoa	Oocytes undergo no significant transformation post-meiosis II
Support cells	Sertoli cells	Follicular cells (granulosa cells, theca cells)
End result	Motile spermatozoa	Nonmotile ovum

TEST YOUR UNDERSTANDING

REVIEW QUESTIONS

1. Draw the structure of spermatozoon.
2. Discuss the stages of spermatogenesis.
3. What are the differences between spermatogenesis and spermiogenesis?
4. What is gametogenesis? Enumerate differences between the spermatogenesis and oogenesis.
5. Discuss ovarian cycle.
6. Discuss oogenesis and ovulation.
7. Describe functions of corpus luteum.
8. Discuss hormonal regulation of ovarian and menstrual cycles.
9. Write a short note on menstrual disorders.

EXPLAIN WHY? (REASONING QUESTIONS)

1. Oogenesis results in only one viable ovum, whereas spermatogenesis results in four viable sperm cells.
2. Process of oogenesis begins before birth but is completed only upon fertilization.
3. The luteal phase of the ovarian cycle is critical for maintaining early pregnancy.
4. The endometrial lining is shed during menstruation in absence of sperm.

MULTIPLE CHOICE QUESTIONS

1. Galea capitis is:
   A. Acrosome of sperm
   B. Oocyte
   C. Gonads
   D. Head of sperm
2. Mittelschmerz refers to:
   A. Ovarian torsion
   B. Dysmenorrhea
   C. Mid-cycle pain
   D. Amenorrhea
3. Corpus luteum of pregnancy lasts for:
   A. 5–6 months
   B. 7–8 months
   C. 1–2 months
   D. 3–4 months
4. During which phase of the menstrual cycle does ovulation typically occur?
   A. Menstrual phase
   B. Follicular phase
   C. Luteal phase
   D. Proliferative phase
5. What is the primary hormone responsible for triggering ovulation during the menstrual cycle?
   A. Estrogen
   B. Progesterone
   C. Human chorionic gonadotropin (hCG)
   D. Luteinizing hormone (LH)
6. Which structure is formed from the ruptured follicle after ovulation and secretes progesterone?
   A. Corpus luteum

B. Corpus albicans
C. Corpus callosum
D. Corpus cavernosum

7. The viability of ovum released at ovulations is:
   A. 24–48 hours
   B. 12 hours
   C. 72–90 hours
   D. 6 hours

8. A female patient undergoing assisted reproductive technology (ART) has her oocytes retrieved for in vitro fertilization (IVF). At what stage of meiosis are the oocytes typically arrested at the time of retrieval?
   A. Prophase I
   B. Metaphase I
   C. Metaphase II
   D. Anaphase II

9. In a study of spermatogenesis, researchers discovered a mutation that leads to the production of non-functional sperm. The mutation affects a protein required for the condensation of chromatin during the later stages of spermatogenesis. Which stage is most likely disrupted by this mutation?
   A. Spermatogonia
   B. Primary spermatocytes
   C. Spermatids
   D. Sertoli cells

Answers: 1. A 2. C 3. D 4. D 5. D 6. A 7. A 8. C 9. C

CHAPTER 4

First Week of Development

COMPETENCIES COVERED/LEARNING OUTCOMES

The student should be able to:

AN77.4	Describe the stages and consequences of fertilization.
AN77.5	Enumerate and describe the anatomical principles underlying contraception.
AN77.6	Describe fertility and sterility, surrogate motherhood.
AN78.1	Describe cleavage and formation of blastocyst.
AN78.2	Describe the development of trophoblast.
AN78.3	Describe the process of implantation and common abnormal sites of implantation.
AN78.5	Describe decidual reaction; abortion and pregnancy test.

As discussed in Chapter 1 about the stages of human development, the germinal period is most crucial for human embryonic development. This stage spans from the first to the third week of development. It begins with fertilization and includes the initial cell divisions and differentiation of the germ layers.

We will discuss the embryonic development during the first week, second week and third week in detail in separate chapters.

OVERVIEW OF FIRST WEEK OF DEVELOPMENT

Ovum is released from ovary and in case of absence of spermatozoon in the uterine tube, it degenerates, and menstrual cycle goes on. But in case sperm penetrates the ovum, fertilization happens, and series of events takes place to form the zygote.

Human embryonic development starts from the stage of fertilization. During the first week of embryonic development, following series of events occur until the fertilized ovum is implanted in the uterus:

1. **Fertilization:** The process begins with the fertilization of the ovum by a sperm cell, forming a *zygote*. This typically occurs in the ampulla of the fallopian tube.
2. **Cleavage:** The zygote undergoes rapid mitotic divisions, known as *cleavage*, without increasing in size, resulting in a cluster of smaller cells called *blastomeres*.
3. **Morula formation:** By day 3–4 postfertilization, the cells compact into a solid ball known as the *morula*.
4. **Blastocyst formation:** Around day 5–6, the morula develops into a *blastocyst*, consisting of an inner cell mass *(embryoblast)* and an outer cell layer (the *trophoblast*, which will form the placenta).
5. **Implantation:** By the end of the first week, the blastocyst reaches the uterus and begins the process of implantation into the endometrial lining, which will provide it with the necessary nutrients for further development.

These stages are critical for establishing the foundation for all subsequent development and successful pregnancy.

Changes in ovum from maturation to fertilization are shown in **Figure 4.1**.

FERTILIZATION

Definition

Fertilization is the process of fusion of mature/highly differentiated male gamete (spermatozoon) and female gamete (ovum) to form the undifferentiated diploid mononucleated single cell, the zygote.

Human fertilization is a complex process and involves many steps. Male and female gametes must undergo several biological processes before fertilization occurs.

Site and time of fertilization is shown in **Figure 4.2**.

Stages of Fertilization

The process of fertilization takes place in three major steps which are:
1. Gametes approximation
2. Fusion of gametes with completion of meiosis II
3. Formation of zygote and results of fertilization

Gametes Approximation

* **Transport of spermatozoon:** After spermatozoa deposition, uterine contraction is stimulated by

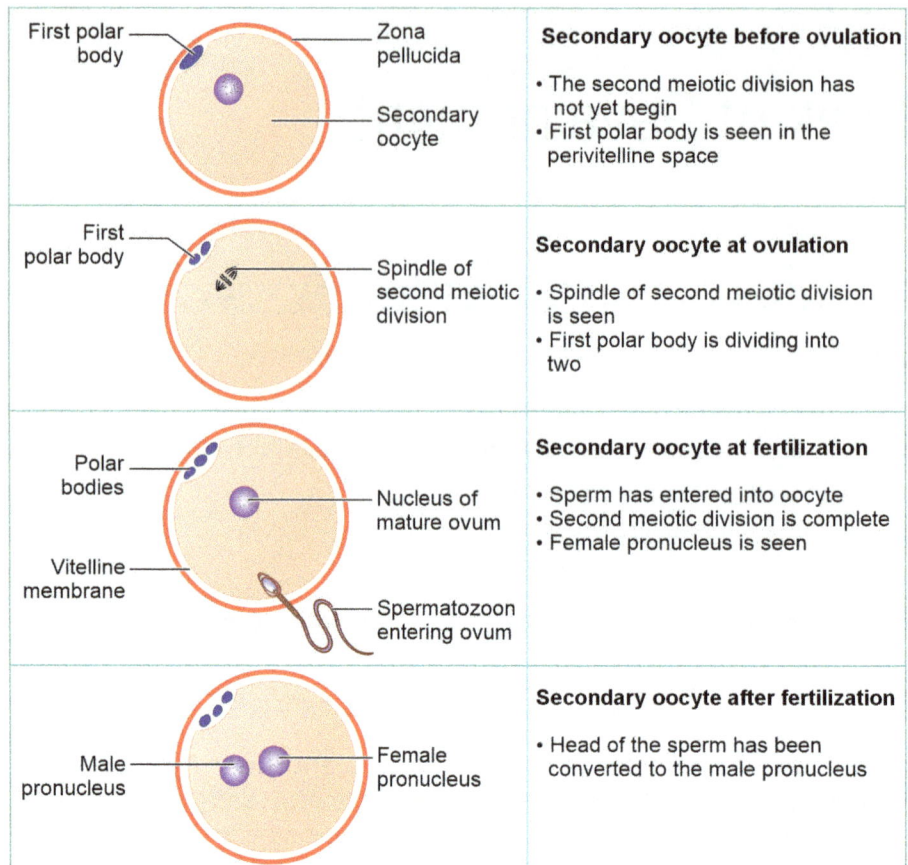

FIG. 4.1: Stages of maturation of ovum during different phases.

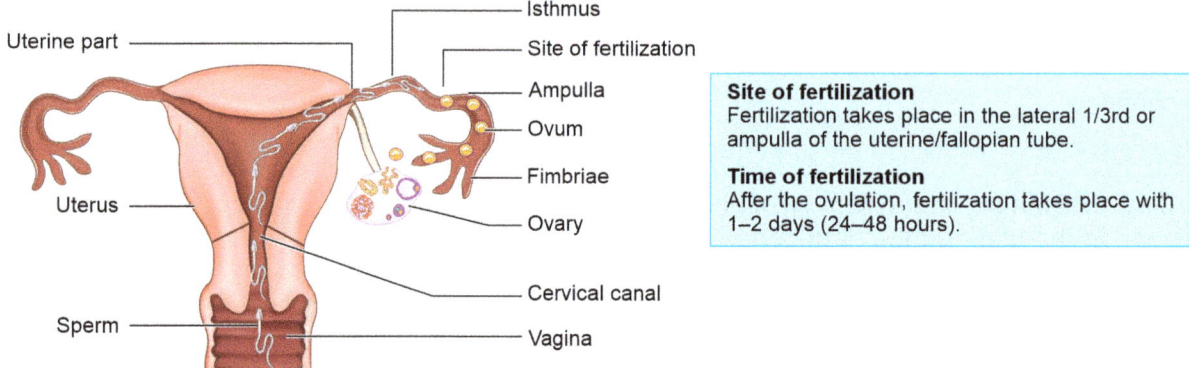

FIG. 4.2: Path taken by the sperm (red), and ovum (blue), site and time of fertilization.

Site of fertilization
Fertilization takes place in the lateral 1/3rd or ampulla of the uterine/fallopian tube.

Time of fertilization
After the ovulation, fertilization takes place with 1–2 days (24–48 hours).

prostaglandins in the semen and oxytocin released during the coital reflex. Most spermatozoa die within 24 to 48 hours after ejaculation and they are gradually reduced in number by constrictions at the cervix and uterine ostium. Approximately 200–500 million sperm are deposited in the female reproductive tract, but only about 300–500 reach the site of fertilization. The spermatozoa are attracted to the ovum by the method of chemotaxis, i.e., release of certain chemical by the follicular cells of ovum.

- **Transport of ovum:** In contrast to spermatozoa, the ciliary beats and rhythmic muscular contractions of the uterine tube are responsible for transcoelomic migration of ovum from the surface of ovary into the ampulla of uterine tube. The ovum released during ovulation remains viable for 24–48 hours. If fertilization does not occur, it degenerates.

Typically, both sperm and the oocyte reach the ampulla of the fallopian tube as shown in **Figure 4.2**.

- **Capacitation** is a series of physiological changes that spermatozoon undergoes to acquire the ability to fertilize an egg. This process occurs in the uterus or uterine tube. As already discussed in Chapter 2, capacitation is important for *acrosome reaction*.
- Specific proteins and signaling pathways are activated during capacitation, leading to changes in sperm motility patterns, known as *hyperactivation.*

- Hyperactivated sperm exhibit a more vigorous and erratic swimming pattern, which helps them navigate the female reproductive tract and penetrate the zona pellucida.

Fusion of Gametes

The ovum has three primary barriers that sperm must penetrate to achieve fertilization:
1. Corona radiata
2. Zona pellucida
3. Vitelline membrane

For spermatozoon to penetrate the ovum, four processes are involved as discussed below **(Figs. 4.3A to D)**.

- **Acrosome reaction:** During the acrosome reaction, enzymes such as hyaluronidase, acrosin and acid phosphatase are released from the acrosome, a cap-like structure covering the sperm head. These enzymes cause the disintegration of the covering of sperm head which comprises of nuclear envelope, acrosomal membrane and plasma membrane. It occurs when sperms come in contact with corona radiata of the oocyte.
- **Barriers disintegration:**
  - *Corona radiata:* Penetration of the first barrier relies on the release of hyaluronidase from the sperm's acrosome. Tubal mucosal enzymes and the movements of the sperm's tail also assist sperm in penetrating the corona radiata. The

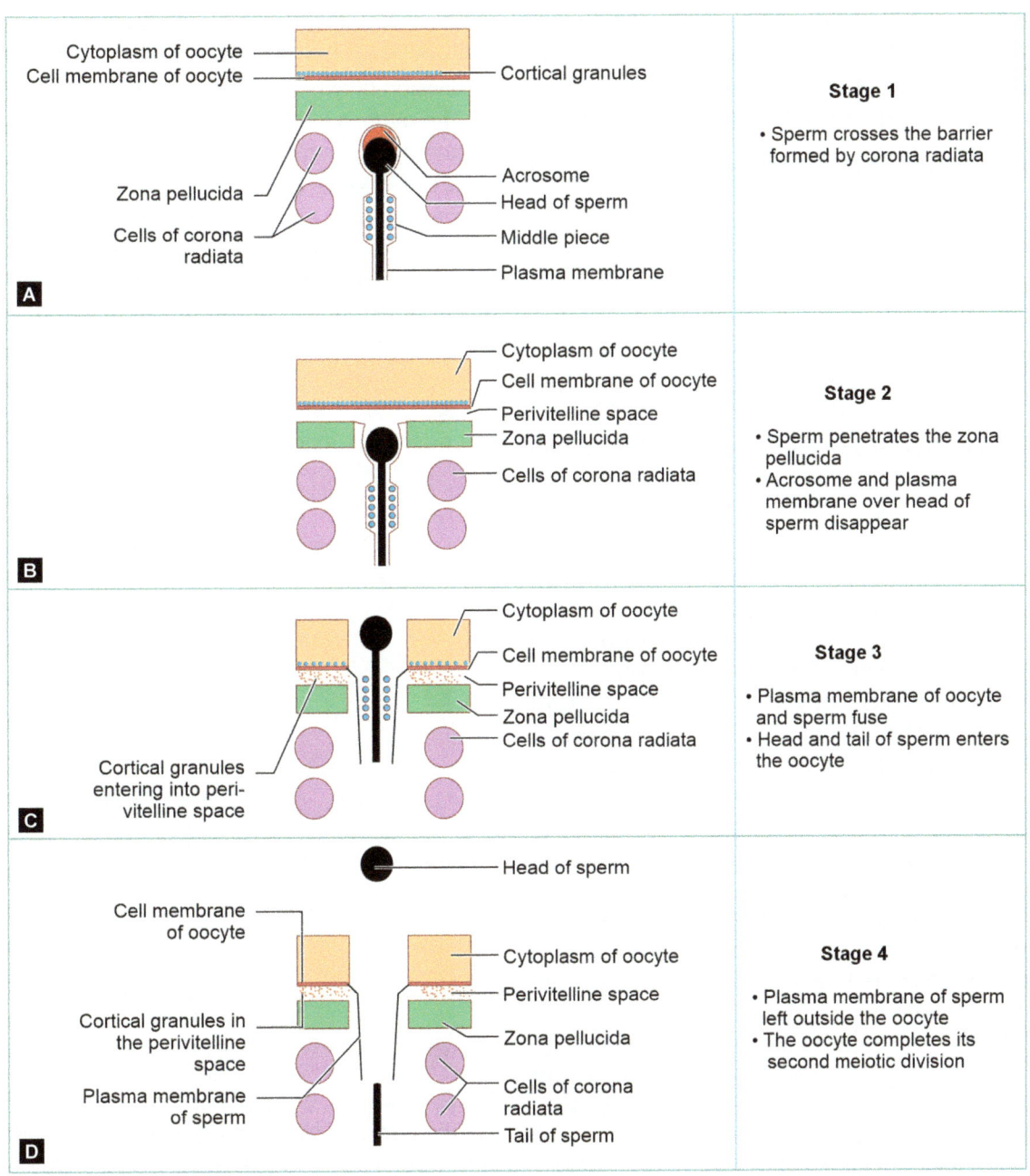

FIGS. 4.3A to D: Stages in penetration of a spermatozoon into an ovum.

hyaluronidase enzyme digests the cells of the corona radiata, enabling the sperm to enter the ovum.
- *Zona pellucida:* Glycoproteins on the sperm head bind to glycoproteins on the ovum's zona pellucida, specifically to Zp3 and Zp2 receptors. Acrosin then dissolves the zona pellucida around the sperm head. The zona pellucida is altered due to lysosomal enzymes released by the oocyte's plasma membrane, a process known as *the zona reaction*. Alterations in plasma membrane of oocyte and zona pellucida ensures that no other spermatozoon enters the oocyte, thus preventing *polyspermy*.
- *Vitelline membrane:* When a spermatozoon contacts the oocyte, their plasma membranes fuse together, likely at species-specific receptor sites. Fusion is initiated by the disintegrin peptide released from the sperm head, while integrin peptides are present in the vitelline membrane. This fusion process typically takes about 30 minutes.

> **NOTE**
> Upon the entry of a single sperm, a cascade of cellular processes known as the *cortical reaction* occurs. This reaction aims to create an impermeable zona pellucida, preventing *polyspermy*. Cortical granules are released and secrete serine proteases, peroxidases, and glycosaminoglycans. These enzymes work to cleave protein connections, removing receptors, and to harden the vitelline envelope. Additionally, they attract water into the perivitelline space, creating a gap to form the hyaline layer.

- ❖ **Calcium wave in oocyte:** Upon sperm entry into the oocyte, it triggers the release of calcium ions from intracellular stores within the oocyte, such as the endoplasmic reticulum. The calcium wave spreads throughout the oocyte in a wave-like fashion, signaling various cellular processes essential for fertilization, including the completion of meiosis, activation of the oocyte, and initiation of embryo development.
- ❖ **Fusion of nucleus:** Only the sperm head and midpiece enter the ovum, while the tail, plasma membrane and remaining parts are left outside. *The sperm's mitochondria, located in the midpiece, are typically degraded, ensuring that only maternal mitochondria are passed on to the offspring.* With nuclear fusion, following events occur:
  - The entry of the sperm into the ovum triggers the *completion of the second meiotic division* in the ovum, which had been arrested at metaphase II during ovulation.
  - This division results in the *formation of the female pronucleus* and the extrusion of the second polar body, which is a small cell containing excess genetic material.
  - After the sperm enters the ovum, its nuclear envelope disintegrates, and the chromatin decondenses resulting in *formation of the male pronucleus*.
  - The fusion of the male and female pronuclei forms a single diploid nucleus with 46 chromosomes resulting in *formation of zygote*, which contains complete set of genetic material.

> **NOTE**
> The first polar body may also divide during meiosis II, creating two smaller polar bodies. Therefore, the total number of polar bodies formed is typically three.

Formation of Zygote and Results of Fertilization

With fertilization of male and female gamete, zygote is formed. This undergoes cleavage to form the multicellular structures. From what we have discussed so far, the results of fertilization are as follows:
- ❖ Fertilization results in completion of second meiotic division of ovum and release of the second polar body.
- ❖ The ovum's nucleus becomes the female pronucleus, and the sperm's head becomes the male pronucleus (**Fig. 4.4A**). These pronuclei lose their nuclear membranes, and their 23 haploid chromosomes each combine resulting in fusion to form 23 pairs, totaling 46 diploid chromosomes (**Fig. 4.4B**).
- ❖ Determination of chromosomal sex takes place.
- ❖ The fertilized ovum (zygote) begins to divide into several cells (i.e., it undergoes cleavage). After fertilization and formation of 46 chromosomes, it undergoes mitotic division to form a two-cell embryo (**Fig. 4.4C**).

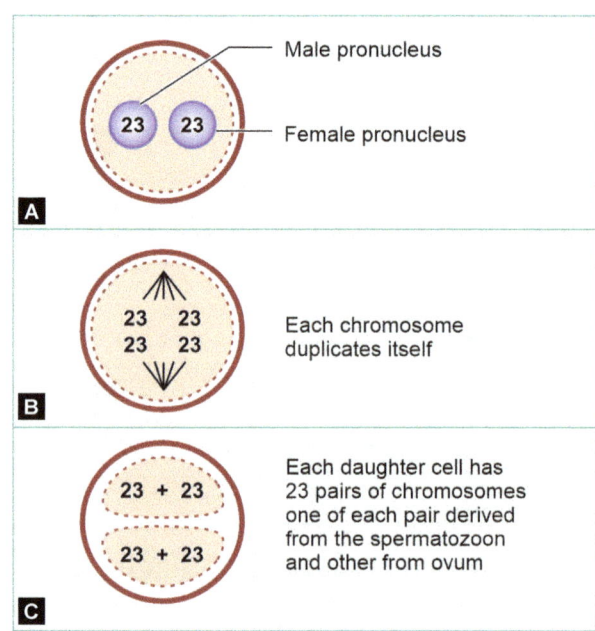

FIGS. 4.4A to C: Behavior of chromosomes during fertilization. The female pronucleus has 22 + X chromosomes. The male pronucleus may have 22 + X or 22 + Y chromosomes.

The important points to note at this stage are that:
- The two daughter cells are still surrounded by the zona pellucida **(Figs. 4.1 and 4.3)**
- Each daughter cell is much smaller than the ovum.
- With subsequent divisions, the cells become smaller and smaller until they acquire the size of most cells of the body.

Clinical Importance

- **Fertility:** The ability to conceive a child or become pregnant is called fertility.
- **Sterility:** Sterility refers to the absolute inability to conceive or induce conception after one year of regular, unprotected sexual intercourse. Unlike infertility, which implies a reduced ability to conceive, sterility indicates a complete lack of reproductive capacity.
- **Infertility:** Infertility is the inability to conceive a child after one year of regular, unprotected sexual intercourse. Unlike sterility, infertility suggests a reduced or impaired ability to achieve pregnancy, which may be due to factors affecting either partner, such as ovulatory disorders, sperm abnormalities, tubal blockage, or other reproductive system dysfunctions. Infertility can sometimes be treated or managed with medical interventions.
- **Surrogacy:** Surrogacy is a method of assisted reproduction where a woman, known as a surrogate, carries and delivers a child for another person or couple. This process can be beneficial for individuals who are unable to conceive or carry a pregnancy to term. There are two main types of surrogacy: traditional and gestational.

Further Information

Gestation and expected date of delivery: The gestation period, commonly referred to as pregnancy, lasts about 40 weeks from the first day of the last menstrual period (LMP) to childbirth. This period is divided into three trimesters and involves the development and growth of the fetus from a single cell to a fully formed baby.

Expected date of delivery (EDD): The EDD is typically calculated by adding 280 days (or 40 weeks) to the first day of the LMP. This method, known as Naegele's rule, assumes a regular 28-day menstrual cycle. The EDD is an estimate. Most of births occur within a two-week period before or after the EDD.

EDD = LMP + 280 days ± 7 days

Menstrual age (gestational age): Based on the first day of the last menstrual period (LMP).

Fertilization age (fetal developmental age): Typically, 14 days less than gestational age, starting from the day of fertilization.

TEST TUBE BABIES/IN VITRO FERTILIZATION (IVF)

The so-called test tube babies are produced by the technique of *in vitro fertilization* (*in vitro* = outside the body, as against *in vivo* = within the body). This technique is being increasingly used in couples who are not able to achieve fertilization due to many medical reasons and this form of fertilization is assisted reproductive technique (ART).

Gonadotropins are administered to the woman to stimulate growth of follicles in the ovary. Just before ovulation, the ovum is removed (using an aspirator) and is placed in a suitable medium. Spermatozoa are added to the medium. Fertilization and early development of the embryo take place in this medium. The process is carefully monitored, and when the embryo is at the 8-cell stage it is put inside the uterus. Successful implantation takes place in about 20% of such trials.

The reasons for using the technique can be as follows:
- The number of spermatozoa may be inadequate (usually about 2–5 mL of semen is ejaculated. Each milliliter contains about 100 million spermatozoa. If the count of spermatozoa is less than 20 million per mL, there may be difficulty in fertilization).
- There may be inadequate motility of spermatozoa.
- There may be obstruction of the uterine tube.
- There may be absence of ovulation.

SEX DETERMINATION

Ova contain 22 + **X** chromosomes. However, the spermatozoa are of two types. Half of them have 22 + **X** chromosomes and the other half of them have 22 + **Y** chromosomes. We speak of these as 'X-bearing', or 'Y-bearing', spermatozoa. An ovum can be fertilized by either type of spermatozoon. If the sperm is **X**-bearing, the zygote has 44 + **X** + **X** chromosomes and the offspring is a girl. If the sperm is **Y**-bearing the zygote has 44 + **X** + **Y** chromosomes and the offspring is a boy.

Thus, the sex of a child is determined at the time of fertilization. It will now be clear that one chromosome of each of the 23 pairs is derived from the mother and the other from the father.

CLEAVAGE

The two-cells formed as described above undergo a series of divisions **(Fig. 4.5A)**. One-cell divides first so that we have a '3-cell' stage of the embryo **(Fig. 4.5B)** followed by a '4-cell' stage **(Fig. 4.5C)**, a '5-cell' stage, etc. This process of subdivision of the ovum into smaller cells is called *cleavage*. The zygote undergoes its first mitotic division, resulting in two *blastomeres*. Continued mitotic divisions lead to 4, 8, and so on, blastomeres.

As cleavage proceeds the ovum comes to have 16 cells. It now looks like a mulberry and is called the *morula* **(Fig. 4.5D and Table 4.1)**. It is still surrounded by the zona pellucida. If we cut a section across the morula, we see that it consists of an *inner cell mass* that is completely surrounded by an outer layer of cells. The

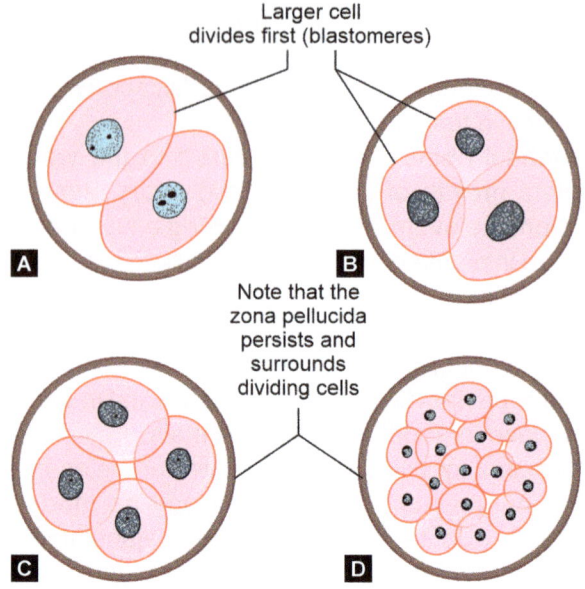

FIGS. 4.5A to D: Some stages in segmentation of the fertilized ovum: (A) Two-cell stage; (B) Three-cell stage; (C) Four-cell stage; (D) Morula.

TABLE 4.1: Relationship of cleavage stages and fertilization.

Cleavage stage	Time after fertilization when it can be observed
One-cell stage	<24 hours (not visible as it stays for a very short period)
Two-cells stage	24–36 hours
3–4 cells stage	36–48 hours
5–8 cells stage	48–72 hours
9–16 cells stage	72–96 hours

cells of the outer layer will later give rise to a structure called the *trophoblast* (Fig. 4.6A).

The inner cell mass gives rise to the embryo proper and is, therefore, also called the *embryoblast*. The cells of the trophoblast help to provide nutrition to the embryo.

During 32–64 cells stage and between 4th to 5th day, some fluid passes into the morula from the uterine cavity, and partially separates the cells of the inner cell mass from those of the trophoblast (Fig. 4.6B). As the amount of fluid increases, the morula acquires the shape of a cyst. The cells of the trophoblast become flattened, and the inner cell mass gets attached to the inner side of the trophoblast on one side only (Fig. 4.6C).

The morula has now become a *blastocyst*. The cavity of the blastocyst is the *blastocoele*. That side of the blastocyst to which the inner cell mass is attached is called the *embryonic or animal pole*, while the opposite side is the *abembryonic pole*.

The trophoblast divides into the one in contact with embryoblast known as *polar trophoblast* (30 cells) and the rest of it lining the wall of blastocyst is known as *mural trophoblast* (69 cells).

The zona pellucida starts thinning on the 4th day and disappears by the 5th day postfertilization, initiating the attachment of trophoblastic cells to the uterine epithelium for implantation on the 6th or 7th day. This is known as *hatching of blastocyst*.

> **NOTE**
>
> Cleavage plays a important role in maintaining the nucleus-to-cytoplasm (N/C) ratio by rapidly increasing the number of cells while the overall size of the embryo remains unchanged, ensuring proper distribution of cytoplasmic components among smaller cells.

Function of the Zona Pellucida

- **Prevents premature implantation:** It prevents the embryo from implanting into the epithelium of uterine tube and uppermost endometrium during its travel through the tube.
- **Glycoproteins (ZP1, ZP2, ZP3, ZP4):**
  - *ZP2:* Plays a crucial role in sperm binding, gamete recognition, penetration, and prevention of polyspermy.
  - *ZP Glycoproteins:* Induce the acrosomal reaction, allowing species-specific sperm penetration.
  - *Holds blastomeres together:* Maintains the integrity of the early embryo.
  - *Immunological barrier:* Lacks histocompatibility antigens, preventing maternal immune response against the genetically different embryo. After the disappearance of zona pellucida various

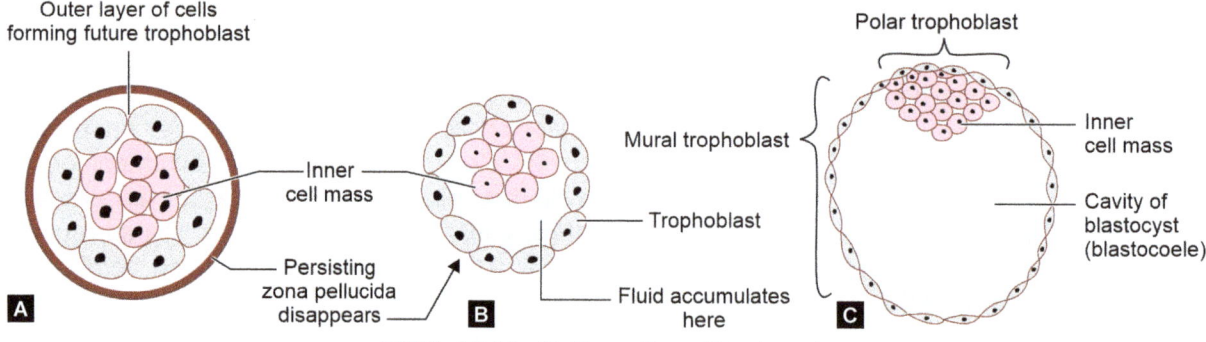

FIGS. 4.6A to C: Formation of blastocyst.

immunosuppressive cytokines and proteins are produced by the implanting embryo. This blocks the recognition of the embryo as a foreign tissue to the mother.
- *Disappears before implantation:* Allows the blastocyst to attach to the uterine endometrium for further development.

Clinical Importance

Contraceptive Methods
It is the use of various artificial methods or techniques to prevent pregnancy (contraception). The different contraceptive methods are:
- **Temporary**
  - *Physical/barrier technique*
    - *Male condom*—A sheath made of latex or polyurethane which is often used with a chemical spermicide to increase effectiveness by killing sperm.
    - *Female condom*—A pouch made of polyurethane or nitrile that is inserted into the vagina before intercourse.
    - *Others*—diaphragm, cervical cap, can be used with spermicide.
  - *Chemical method*—use of contraceptive pill, to prevent ovulation in the female.
    - *Use of intrauterine device*—intrauterine insertion of copper that prevents implantation of fertilized ovum.
- **Permanent/surgical method**—male/female sterilization (vasectomy/tubectomy). This is permanent method of sterilization.

IMPLANTATION

Definition and Implantation Period
Implantation is the process of attachment of a blastocyst to the uterine endometrium and its subsequent invasion, or embedding, into the uterine lining. This occurs between the 6th and 12th days following fertilization, i.e., it start late in first week and continues till mid of second week of development.

Process of Implantation
To understand the process of implantation, it is divided into two phases:
1. Events preliminary to fertilization
2. Stages of implantation.

Processes Preceding Implantation (Fig. 4.7)
By day 3 or 4, zygote is developed into the blastocyst as discusses previously.
- ❖ **Blastocyst formation:** The morula develops into a blastocyst, consisting of an inner cell mass and an outer trophoblast layer.
- ❖ **Zona pellucida thinning:** The zona pellucida begins to thin.
- ❖ **Zona pellucida disappearance:** The zona pellucida disappears, allowing the blastocyst to hatch.
- ❖ **Blastocyst hatching:** By day 5–6 the blastocyst hatches from the zona pellucida, enabling direct interaction with the uterine lining.

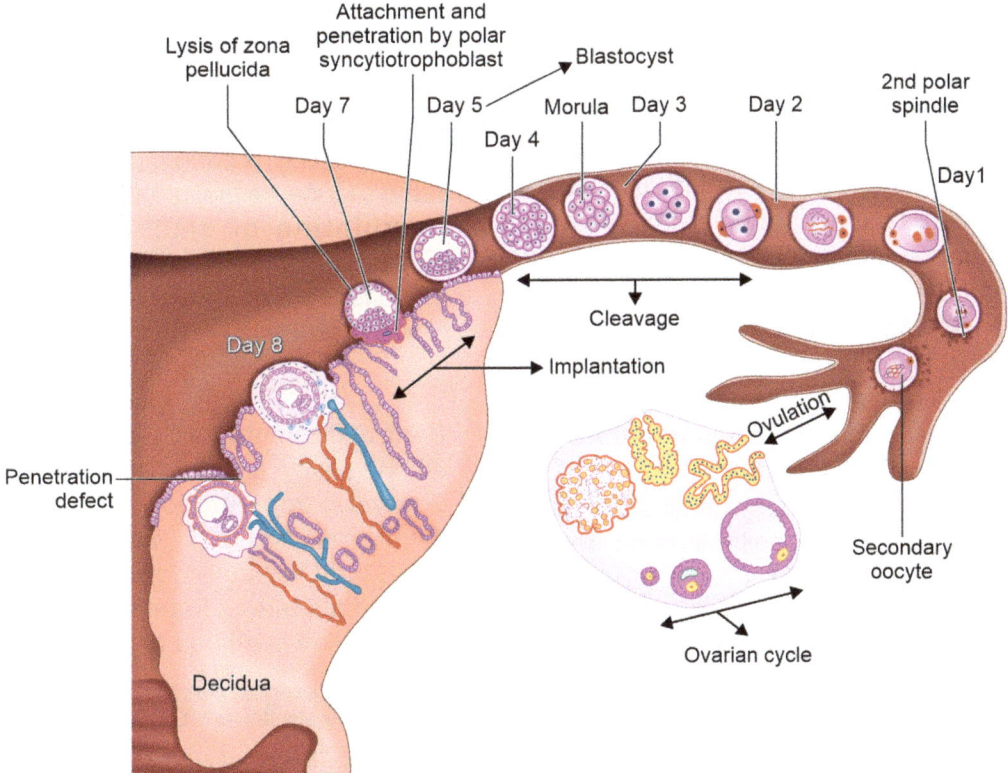

FIG. 4.7: Various processes before and during implantation—ovulation, fertilization, cleavage, blastocyst, trophoblast differentiation, decidual change, hatching of blastocyst, penetration defect.

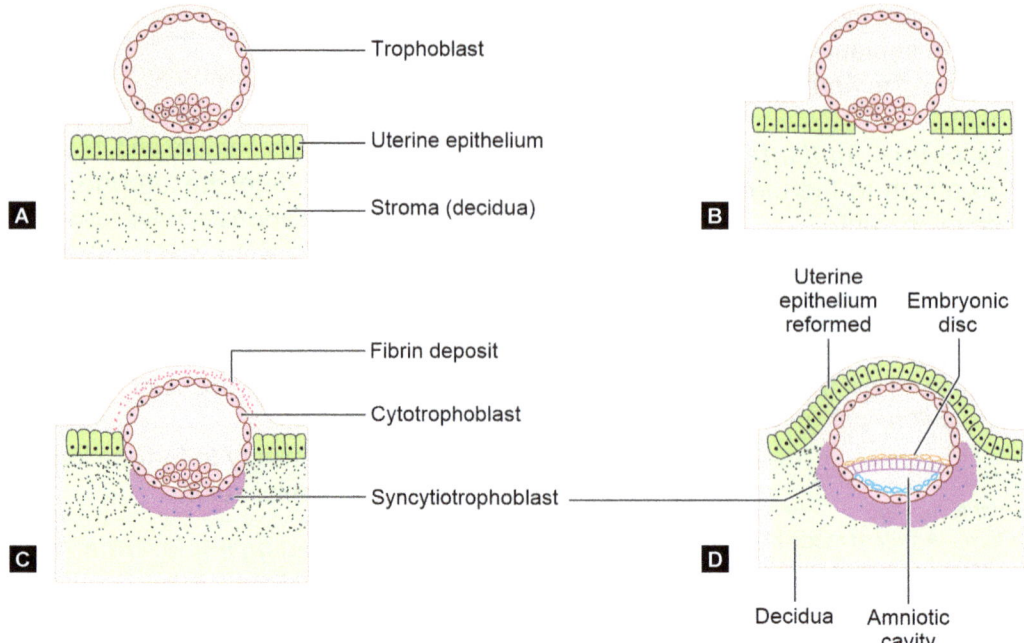

FIGS. 4.8A to D: Stages of implantation: (A) Hatching blastocyst; (B) Adhesion of blastocyst to uterine epithelium; (C) Penetration of blastocyst through uterine epithelium and erosion of endometrium; (D) Closure of penetration defect and differentiation of trophoblast and embryoblast.

Stages of implantation

- **Decidual reaction:** It refers to the changes in the endometrial stroma as the morula reaches the uterus during the secretory phase.
- **Hatching of blastocyst:** The zona pellucida thins and disappears by the 6th day, allowing the blastocyst to hatch. This thinning is due to action of enzyme trypsin **(Fig. 4.8D)**.
- **Adhesion of polar trophoblast to columnar uterine epithelium:** Trophoblastic cells which have tendency to stick, adhere to the uterine endometrium. On the 6th day postfertilization, zona pellucida disappears and it initiates the attachment of polar trophoblastic cells to the columnar uterine epithelium **(Figs. 4.8A and B)**.
- **Penetration of blastocyst through uterine epithelium:** The trophoblastic cells have got the penetrating/burrowing nature. The polar trophoblastic cells penetrate the uterine epithelium, creating a passage for the blastocyst **(Fig. 4.8C)**.
- **Erosion of the endometrium:** Proteolytic enzymes from trophoblast and uterine epithelium erode the endometrium, embedding the blastocyst deeper and deeper into the uterine mucosa till the whole of it comes to lie within the thickness of the endometrium.
- **Trophoblast differentiation:** By the 8th day, the trophoblast differentiates into cytotrophoblast (inner layer composed of mononucleated cells, divide actively) and syncytiotrophoblast layers (outer layer composed of multinucleated cells formed by fusion of cytotrophoblasts cells).

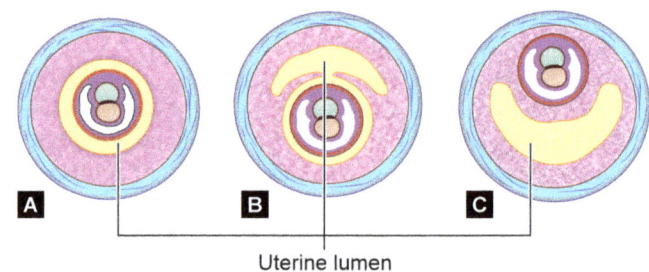

FIGS. 4.9A to C: Types of implantation: (A) Central; (B) Eccentric; (C) Interstitial.

- **Closure of penetration defect in uterine epithelium:** By the 9th day, a fibrin plug forms to close the defect in the uterine epithelium **(Fig. 4.8D)**.
- **Completion of embedding:** By 12th day of fertilization, the blastocyst is fully embedded and establishes a nutritive relationship with maternal blood vessels.

Types of Implantation (Figs. 4.9A to C)

1. **Central implantation:** Blastocyst is implanted in the uterine cavity, e.g., carnivores—cow.
2. **Eccentric implantation:** Blastocyst is implanted in the uterine crypt, e.g., mouse.
3. **Interstitial implantation:** Blastocyst is implanted in the endometrium of uterine wall. This is the type of implantation in guinea pig and human.

Clinical Importance

Normal and Abnormal Sites of Implantation
- **Normal site of implantation:** The upper part of body of uterus in midsagittal plane, in the posterior wall (55%) or in the anterior wall (45%) **(Fig. 4.10)**.

- **Abnormal sites of implantation (Fig. 4.10)**
  - Lower uterine segment: If the implantation is in the lower uterine segment, it is called placenta previa.
  - Extrauterine:
    - Tubal implantation: This is most common cause of abnormal implantation after uterine. The various parts of fallopian tube involved in order of frequency are: (1) Interstitial, (2) Ampulla, (3) Isthmic.
    - Abdominal implantation: It is rare. It can be primary (implantation in relation to mesentery) or secondary (re-implantation of ruptured tubal or ovarian pregnancy).
  - Ovarian implantation: It is rare and can cause teratoma.

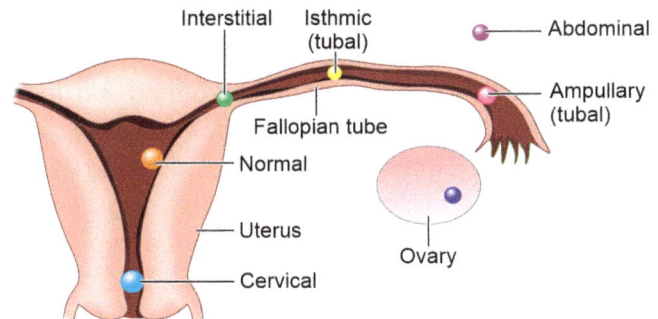

FIG. 4.10: Normal and abnormal sites of implantation: Normal site of implantation in the upper uterine segment; Abnormal sites of implantation are: tubal, interstitial, cervical, abdominal and ovary.

Clinical correlation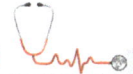

Placenta Previa

Introduction: Placenta previa occurs when the placenta implants low in the uterus, covering the cervix partially or completely, leading to complications like severe bleeding during pregnancy and delivery. It is one of the most common causes of antepartum hemorrhage.

Embryological basis
- **Implantation site:** Normally, the blastocyst implants in the upper uterus. In placenta previa, it implants near or over the cervix.
- **Trophoblast invasion:** Abnormal lower segment implantation affects trophoblastic invasion and the establishment of uteroplacental blood supply.
- **Chorionic villi formation:** Chorionic villi form in the lower uterine segment, resulting in a low placental position.
- Mechanisms leading to placenta previa are previous uterine scar, abnormal endometrial lining, and multiple gestations. Diagnosis is done by ultrasonography.

Clinical implications
Placenta previa increases risks of antepartum hemorrhage, preterm birth, and cesarean delivery. Early diagnosis via ultrasound is crucial for management and safe delivery planning.

Ectopic Pregnancy

- This results from abnormal sites of implantation, i.e., extrauterine pregnancies.
- Ectopic pregnancies do not progress and usually result in death of the embryo. Rarely does this embryo develop to full term.
- The most common ectopic pregnancy is tubal pregnancy with a 95% incidence. Tubal pregnancies are terminated by medical intervention. If it is permitted to progress, it can result in rupture of uterine tube with severe internal bleeding.
- Other types of ectopic pregnancies are abdominal, ovarian.

Clinical Importance

Abortion

Definition
The termination of pregnancy before the fetus is viable outside the womb, typically defined as before 20 weeks of gestation.

Types
- **Spontaneous abortion (miscarriage):** Natural loss of pregnancy due to various reasons including genetic abnormalities, infections, or maternal health issues.
- **Induced abortion:** Deliberate termination of pregnancy through medical or surgical means.

Causes
- **Genetic factors:** Chromosomal abnormalities in the fetus.
- **Maternal health:** Conditions such as anatomical alterations, diabetes, thyroid disorders, and infections.
- **Lifestyle factors:** Smoking, alcohol use, and exposure to harmful substances.

Symptoms
Vaginal bleeding, cramping, and pain in the lower abdomen.

Management
- **Medical management:** Use of medications such as misoprostol and mifepristone.
- **Surgical management:** Procedures like dilation and curettage (D and C) or vacuum aspiration.

Pregnancy Tests

Pregnancy tests are essential diagnostic tools used to confirm pregnancy by detecting specific hormones produced during early embryonic development.

Hormonal basis
- **Human chorionic gonadotropin (hCG):** hCG is the key hormone detected in pregnancy tests.
- Produced by the trophoblast cells of the developing embryo shortly after fertilization.
- Levels of hCG rise rapidly in the early weeks of pregnancy, doubling approximately every 48–72 hours.

Types of pregnancy tests
- **Urine pregnancy test:**
  - Most common and convenient method.
  - Can be performed at home or in a clinical setting.
  - Detects the presence of hCG in the urine.
  - Typically positive as early as 10–14 days after conception (around the time of the missed menstrual period).
- **Blood pregnancy test:**
  - Conducted in a clinical laboratory.
  - More sensitive and can detect lower levels of hCG compared to urine tests.
  - Can confirm pregnancy as early as 7–10 days after conception.

- **Two types:**
  1. **Qualitative hCG test:** Confirms the presence or absence of hCG.
  2. **Quantitative hCG test:** Measures the exact level of hCG in the blood, useful for tracking the progress of early pregnancy or diagnosing potential complications.

CHANGES IN THE ENDOMETRIUM OF THE UTERUS

After implantation, the endometrial features resembling the secretory phase are enhanced by human chorionic gonadotropin (hCG) secreted by syncytiotrophoblast cells. By the 17th or 18th day of the menstrual cycle, corresponding to the 5th day postfertilization and implantation, the uterine endometrium becomes markedly modified, edematous, and vascular, termed *decidua*.

Decidua

Definition

Decidua refers to the functional and specialized endometrial lining (stratum compactum) of the uterus during pregnancy after implantation, supporting the embryonic development.

Decidual Reaction

Under the influence of maternal progesterone and the hCG, stromal cells of the endometrium undergo decidualization, becoming enlarged, vacuolated and glycogen and lipid rich. These cells are called *decidual cells.* The intercellular substance increases, and it gives edematous appearance. The decidualized endometrium provides structural support and a nutrient-rich environment for embryonic development during early pregnancy. The decidual reaction is a defensive mechanism to protect the endometrium.

Types/Subdivisions of Decidua (Fig. 4.11)

- ❖ **Decidua basalis/serotina:** Found adjacent to the implanted blastocyst, forms the maternal part of the placenta. The maternal blood vessels (spiral arteries) proliferate in the region of decidua basalis and are filled with blood and dilate to form sinusoids. The decidua basalis is also referred to as the *decidual plate*, and is firmly united to the chorion.
- ❖ **Decidua capsularis/reflexa:** The part of endometrium that surrounds the conceptus, becoming compressed as the conceptus expands.
- ❖ **Decidua parietalis/vera:** The part of decidua that lines the remainder of the uterine cavity.

Fate of Decidua

As the conceptus enlarges during development, the decidua capsularis enlarges into the uterine cavity and finally fuses with decidua parietalis during 3rd month of pregnancy thus obliterating the uterine cavity. At the end of pregnancy, the decidua is shed off, along with the placenta and membranes. It is this shedding off which gives the decidua its name (c.f. deciduous trees).

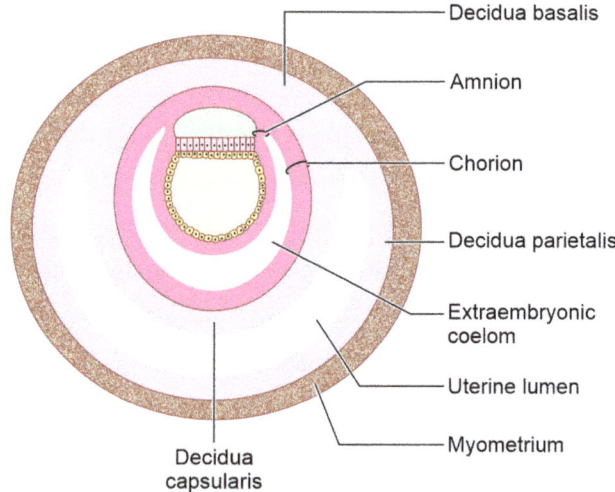

FIG. 4.11: Subdivisions of decidua—basalis, capsularis, parietalis.

Case Based Learning

Embryological Basis of Case of Infertility

Patient details: A 32-year-old woman married for 6 years, and regular menstrual cycles presented with her husband for consultation regarding infertility. They have been trying to conceive for the past 4 years without success and have not used any contraceptive methods. A detailed physical examination of both partners is conducted, and the following investigations are recommended to identify the cause of infertility.

- **Seminal analysis of the male:** It is done to assess the male's fertility potential by evaluating the quantity and quality of sperm. Key parameters include sperm count, motility, morphology, and pH of semen. Embryologically, spermatogenesis occurs in the seminiferous tubules of the testes, and any disruption in this process can lead to abnormalities in sperm parameters.
- **Transvaginal ultrasound for antral follicle count (AFC) of the female:** It is done to assess the number and size of antral follicles in the ovaries. Antral follicles are small fluid-filled sacs within the ovaries that contain immature eggs. The number of antral follicles

is a direct indicator of a woman's ovarian reserve and fertility potential. Each menstrual cycle, a cohort of antral follicles is recruited, but typically only one reaches maturity and ovulates.
- **Laparoscopy for tubal patency in the female:** The fallopian tubes play a crucial role in the transportation of the oocyte from the ovary to the uterus and in the process of fertilization. Any blockage or structural anomaly in the tubes can prevent the sperm from reaching the egg or the fertilized egg from reaching the uterus.
- **Blood test for anti-Müllerian hormone (AMH) levels in the female:** It is done to evaluate ovarian reserve and provide an estimate of the remaining egg supply, which can be critical in planning fertility treatment. AMH is produced by granulosa cells of preantral and small antral follicles. It reflects the size of the remaining egg supply or ovarian reserve. AMH levels provide insight into the functional status of the ovaries and their capacity to produce viable eggs.
- **Karyotyping of both partners:** Karyotyping examines the chromosomal composition of individuals. Chromosomal abnormalities, such as aneuploidies, translocations, or inversions, can lead to infertility, miscarriages, or congenital anomalies.

Case Findings and Recommendations
- **Seminal analysis:** Normal sperm count and morphology but reduced motility.
- **Transvaginal ultrasound (AFC):** An antral follicle count of 6, indicating a reduced ovarian reserve.
- **Laparoscopy:** No significant blockage.
- **AMH levels:** Low, suggesting diminished ovarian reserve.
- **Karyotyping:** Both partners have normal karyotypes.

Advice to the couple: Given the reduced sperm motility, low antral follicle count, and diminished ovarian reserve, the couple should be advised to consider assisted reproductive technologies (ART), such as in vitro fertilization (IVF). IVF can bypass the issues with sperm motility and reduced ovarian reserve by directly fertilizing the eggs in the laboratory and transferring the resulting embryos into the uterus. The couple should also be counseled about the potential for using intracytoplasmic sperm injection (ICSI) during IVF to enhance fertilization success given the sperm motility issue.

HIGHLIGHTS

- **Fertilization**
  - It is the process of fusion of male and female gametes resulting in the formation of single celled zygote.
  - It takes place in the ampulla of the uterine tube.
  - It involves the biological processes of completion of meiotic division of ovum, fusion of male and female pronuclei and initiation of mitotic cell division of zygote.
  - The process of fertilization has three stages and it involves four processes.
- **Cleavage**—the series of divisions the fertilized cell undergoes.
- **Morula**—the 16 cell stage of fertilized ovum. It has an inner cell mass (embryoblast) covered by an outer layer of cells (trophoblast).
- **Blastocyst**—reorganized cells of morula (blastomeres) into an inner cell mass (embryoblast) covered by an outer layer of cells (trophoblast). Fluid filled cavity (blastocyst) separates the two.
- **Polar bodies** are the byproducts of oocyte during the two meiotic divisions.
- **Parthenogenesis** is asexual reproduction without fertilization.
- **Contraception** is an artificial method or technique to prevent pregnancy.
- **In vitro fertilization (IVF)** is a form of artificial reproductive technique (ART).
- The process of attachment of developing embryo to the uterine endometrium is called **implantation**. The type of implantation in the human being is called interstitial implantation as the embryo gets buried in the substance of endometrium.
- **Decidua** is the functional stratum of uterine endometrium after the implantation of blastocyst.

 Summary

- Events taking place during the first week of germinal period is summarized in **Flowchart 4.1**.
- Process of implantation is summarized in **Flowchart 4.2**.

Chapter 4: First Week of Development

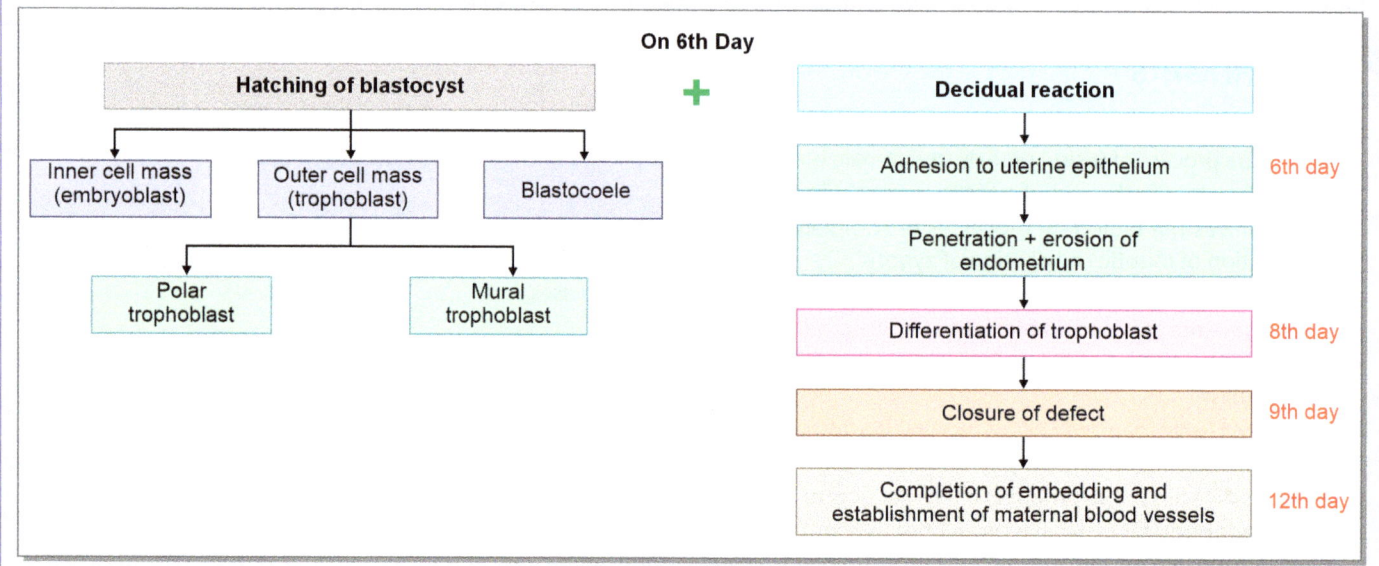

FLOWCHART 4.1: Events taking place during the first week of germinal period.

FLOWCHART 4.2: Process of implantation.

TEST YOUR UNDERSTANDING

REVIEW QUESTIONS

1. Define fertilization.
2. Describe the stages involved in fertilization.
3. What is capacitation?
4. What is acrosome reaction?
5. Explain in vitro fertilization.
6. Describe cleavage.
7. Write short notes on blastocyst.
8. Write short notes on morula.
9. Write short notes on implantation.
10. What are the abnormal sites of implantation?
11. Explain the decidual reaction.
12. What are the different types of decidua?

EXPLAIN WHY? (REASONING QUESTIONS)

1. Failure of capacitation can result in infertility.
2. Zona pellucida is crucial in preventing ectopic pregnancies.
3. Dysfunction of trophoblast cells can lead to placenta previa.
4. Cortical reaction is most important step to prevent polyspermy.
5. Fallopian tube is most common site for abnormal implantation.

MULTIPLE CHOICE QUESTIONS

1. The correct order of barriers through which the sperm has to pass through are:
   A. Zona pellucida, vitelline membrane, corona radiata
   B. Zona pellucida, corona radiata, vitelline membrane
   C. Vitelline membrane, corona radiata, zona pellucida
   D. Corona radiata, zona pellucida, vitelline membrane

2. Haploid nuclei that are fusing at fertilization are called:
   A. Centrioles
   B. Nucleoli
   C. Pronuclei
   D. None of the above

3. The first week of human development is characterized by the formation of all of the following, *except*:
   A. Inner cell mass
   B. Hypoblast
   C. Blastocyst
   D. Yolk sac

4. During a viva, examiner ask the medical student about the changes in uterus of pregnant woman to support embryo implantation. What term describes the changes in the endometrium to support implantation?
   A. Ovulation
   B. Menstruation
   C. Decidual reaction
   D. Fertilization

5. A 29-year-old woman experiences sharp lower abdominal pain and spotting. She is diagnosed with an ectopic pregnancy. Where does an ectopic pregnancy most commonly implant?
   A. Cervix
   B. Uterine cavity
   C. Fallopian tube
   D. Ovary

6. A couple is undergoing fertility treatment and asks about how long after fertilization does the zygote reach the blastocyst stage and prepare for implantation?
   A. 24 hours
   B. 2–3 days
   C. 4–5 days
   D. 6–7 days

7. Which of the following events marks the completion of the fertilization process and the formation of a zygote?
   A. Penetration of the zona pellucida by the sperm
   B. Fusion of the male and female pronuclei
   C. Release of the secondary oocyte from the ovary
   D. Capacitation of the sperm in the female reproductive tract

8. During fertilization, which enzyme released by the acrosome of the sperm allows it to penetrate the zona pellucida surrounding the oocyte?
   A. Trypsin
   B. Hyaluronidase
   C. Acrosin
   D. Lipase

9. What critical process occurring in the female reproductive tract enables sperm to acquire the ability to fertilize an oocyte?
   A. Acrosome reaction
   B. Capacitation
   C. Cortical reaction
   D. Zygote formation

Answers: 1. D   2. C   3. B   4. C   5. C
6. C   7. B   8. C   9. B

CHAPTER 5

Second Week of Development

> **COMPETENCIES COVERED/LEARNING OUTCOMES**
>
> The student should be able to:
>
> | AN78.2 | Describe the development of trophoblast. |
> |---|---|
> | AN78.4 | Describe the formation of extraembryonic mesoderm and coelom, bilaminar germ disc and prochordal plate. |

The process implantation that starts around the 6th or 7th day after fertilization, completes during the second week. From the second week of development, the various events take place which include the formation of the bilaminar embryonic disc, the establishment of extraembryonic structures such as the amnion, yolk sac, and primitive streak which are important for further embryonic and fetal development.

This period plays an important role in embryogenesis, characterized by rapid cellular proliferation and differentiation, setting the foundation for organogenesis and tissue specialization.

EVENTS OF SECOND WEEK OF DEVELOPMENT

For better understanding of the embryonic development during second week, it can be divided into three major headings depicting three changes that takes place in second week:

1. Changes in the embryoblast
2. Changes in the trophoblast
3. Changes in the uterine endometrium

As the blastocyst develops, it differentiates into tissues and organs of the embryo, as well as extraembryonic structures necessary for its support.

CHANGES IN THE EMBRYOBLAST

Formation of Bilaminar Germ Disc

As we have studied in chapter 4, the blastocyst is a spherical cyst-like structure which has an outer layer of trophoblasts and inner mass of cells known as embryoblast with cavity in between **(Fig. 5.1A)**. On 8th day after fertilization, embryoblast cells undergo differentiation to form two layers **(Fig. 5.1B)**:

- **Formation of hypoblast:** The inner cell mass cells towards the blastocyst cavity differentiate into flattened cells to form the *hypoblast, or primitive endoderm* and forms the yolk sac.

- **Formation of epiblast:** The remaining cells of the inner cell mass become columnar, forming the *epiblast or primitive ectoderm*.

  Together with the hypoblast, the epiblast, the embryo is now bilayer disc shaped and this refers to the *bilaminar germ disc*.

> **NOTE**
> - Hypoblast is the first germ layer to be formed.
> - Reorganization of cells of inner cell mass into hypoblast and epiblast occurs before completion of implantation of conceptus.

With this, there is further developmental changes that are as follows:

- **Formation of amniotic cavity:** A space appears between the epiblast and the trophoblast, forming the *amniotic cavity,* filled by amniotic fluid, or liquor amnii. The *amniogenic cells* (derived from trophoblast) line its roof, while the epiblast forms its floor **(Fig. 5.1C)**.

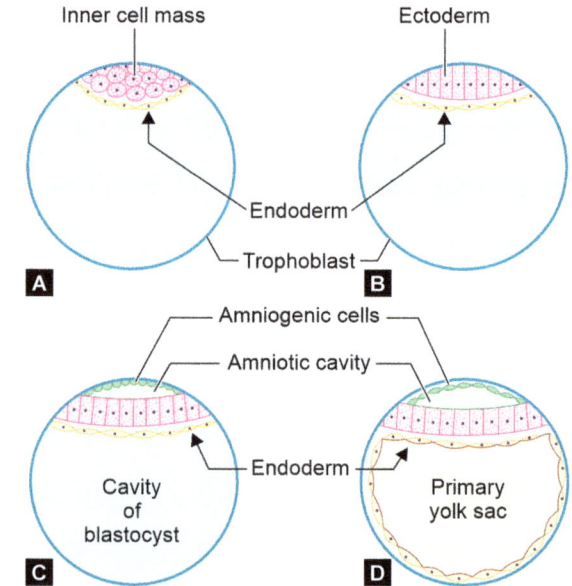

FIGS. 5.1A to D: Differentiation of endoderm and ectoderm, and the formation of the amniotic cavity and the yolk sac.

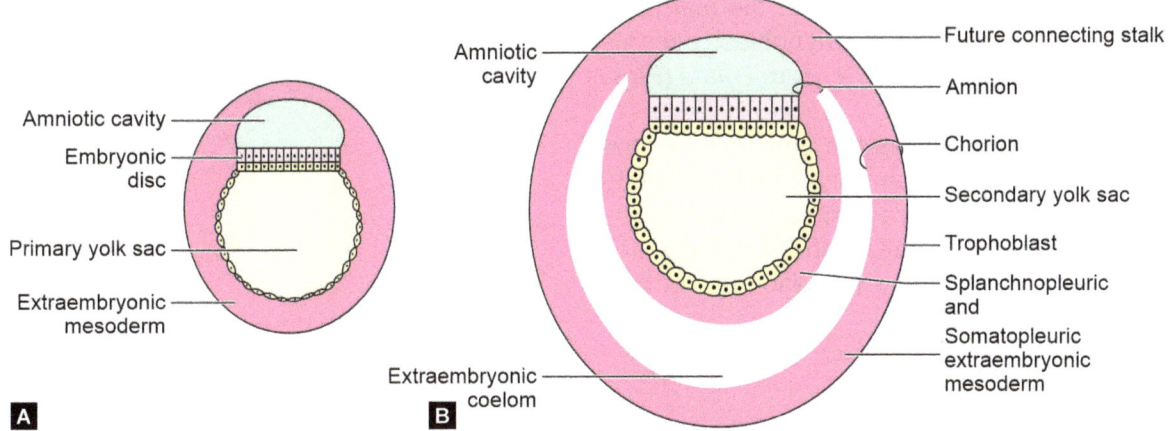

FIGS. 5.2A and B: Formation of extraembryonic mesoderm and extraembryonic coelom. Note carefully, the composition of the amnion, and of the chorion.

- **Formation of primary yolk sac:** On 9th day, flattened cells of hypoblast cells spread and line the blastocyst cavity, which is called *Heuser's membrane* and the now the blastocyst cavity formed is known as *primary yolk sac* lined by cells of endodermal origin (Fig. 5.1D).

Formation of Extraembryonic Mesoderm, Coelom and Connecting Stalk

- **Formation of extraembryonic mesoderm:** Trophoblast cells give rise to new cell mass forming a new layer called *extraembryonic mesoderm or primary mesoderm* between the trophoblast and the primary yolk sac endoderm, separating the amniotic cavity wall from the trophoblast (Fig. 5.2A).

> **NOTE**
>
> The cells of extraembryonic mesoderm lie outside the embryonic disc and don't give rise to any tissues of body during organogenesis

- **Formation of extraembryonic coelom and secondary yolk sac:** Within the extraembryonic mesoderm, a few small cavities appear which merge to form the *extraembryonic coelom (chorionic cavity)*, dividing the primary mesoderm into parietal and visceral layers. Due to this the primary yolk sac becomes smaller in size and is referred to as the *secondary yolk sac,* which is important for early blood formation and development of the gut and respiratory tract linings. This coelom splits the extraembryonic mesoderm into two layers, i.e., the part lining the inside of the trophoblast is called the *parietal or somatopleuric extraembryonic mesoderm* (it is also referred to *as the chorionic plate*). The part lining the outside of the yolk sac is called the *visceral or splanchnopleuric extraembryonic mesoderm.*

- **Formation of connecting stalk:** The extraembryonic coelom doesn't extend into the mesoderm that connects the amniotic cavity to the trophoblast. This part of the extraembryonic mesoderm forms *the connecting stalk,* which later becomes *umbilical cord* with development of blood vessels.

- **Formation of chorion and amnion:** Formation of extraembryonic coelom results in formation of two membranes: *The chorion*, formed from the parietal mesoderm and trophoblast, and *the amnion*, formed from the roof of amniogenic cells and visceral mesoderm. The chorion and amnion are the fetal membranes and they play an important role in childbirth (parturition) and we will refer to them again.

Formation of Prochordal Plate

By the time of development of above discussed structure, the embryo proper is a circular disc, composed of two layers, epiblast and hypoblast layers. There is no indication yet of a head or tail end of the embryonic disc (Figs. 5.3A and B).

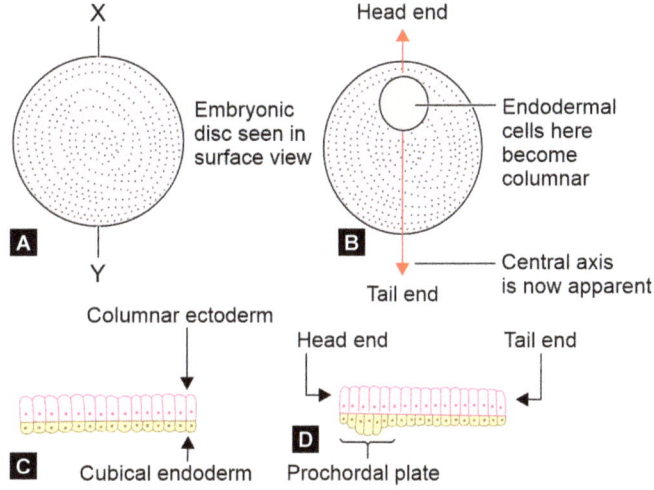

FIGS. 5.3A to D: Formation of prechordal plate.

On day 14, at one circular area near the margin of the disc, the cuboidal cells of the hypoblast become columnar. This area is called the *prochordal plate* (Figs. 5.3C and D).

The prochordal plate defines the embryo's *central axis (right and left halves)* and indicates the future *head and tail ends (cephalocaudal axis)*. At this site, epiblastic and hypoblastic cells adhere closely and remain connected even with the formation of the third germ layer in the next week.

Chorionic Cavity and Gestational Sac (Fig. 5.4)

The chorionic cavity is a fluid-filled space that forms within the chorion, one of the fetal membranes surrounding the embryo. It develops alongside the gestational sac, which encloses the embryo and its surrounding fluid, providing protection and nourishment during early pregnancy. Together, these structures play crucial roles in supporting embryonic development and establishing maternal-fetal circulation for nutrient and waste exchange.

CHANGES IN THE TROPHOBLAST

Trophoblast is the first embryonic membrane. When all the changes were happening in embryoblast, changes

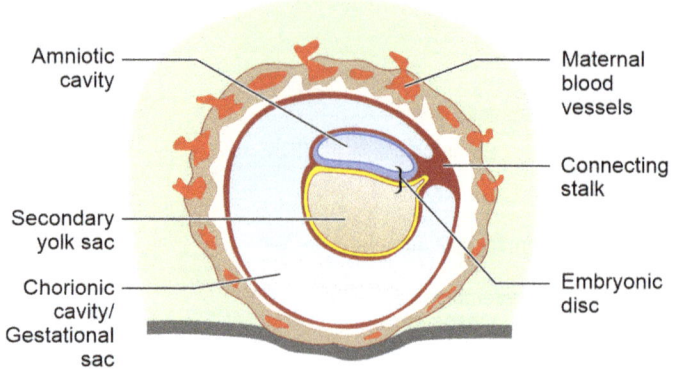

FIG. 5.4: Chorionic cavity in which embryo, amniotic sac and secondary yolk sac are suspended though connecting stalk.

in the trophoblast are occurring simultaneously. The trophoblast, which will form the human placenta, initially consists of a single layer but becomes bilaminar with the formation of blastocyst.

Differentiation of Two Layers of Trophoblast

This is essential for the formation of chorionic villi. On 8th day, as these cells multiply, two distinct layers are formed **(Figs. 5.5A to D)**:

1. **Syncytiotrophoblast:** The cells nearest to the decidua lose their boundaries, forming a continuous

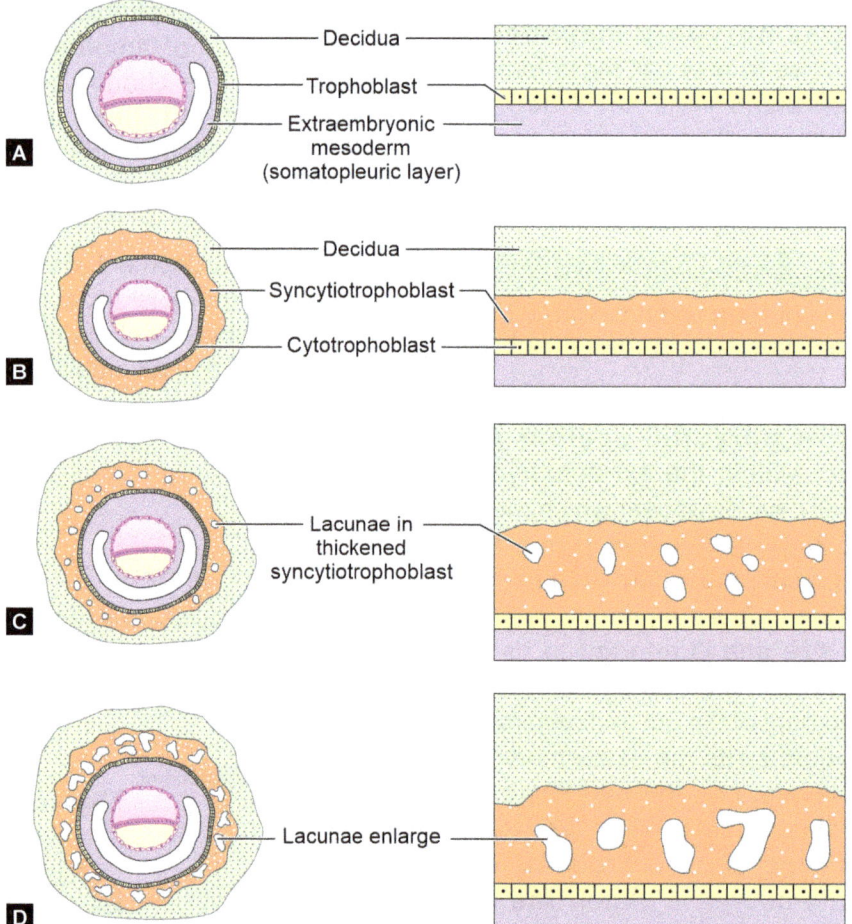

FIGS. 5.5A to D: Differentiation of trophoblast and early stages in the formation of chorionic villi. (A) Cytotrophoblast in contact with decidua; (B) Formation of syncytiotrophoblast; (C) Lacunae in syncytiotrophoblast; (D) Enlarging lacunae.

cytoplasmic sheet with many nuclei called a syncytium. This layer of the trophoblast is known as the *syncytiotrophoblast or plasmodiotrophoblast*.
2. **Cytotrophoblast:** Deep to the syncytium, the cells of the trophoblast retain their cell walls and form the inner second layer called the *cytotrophoblast or Langhans' layer*. This single layer of cuboidal cells with a clear outline rests on the extraembryonic mesoderm.

All these elements (syncytium, cytotrophoblast and mesoderm) take part in forming chorionic villi.

Formation of Chorion and Chorionic Villi

We should study chorionic villi formation during the placenta formation but since this process starts during the second week of development, it is explained here.

Chorion

Definition

The cellular, outermost extraembryonic membrane composed of trophoblast lined with extraembryonic somatopleuric mesoderm.

Formation

- The chorion forms from the extraembryonic somatic mesoderm and the two trophoblast layers (cytotrophoblast and syncytiotrophoblast).
- The extraembryonic coelom becomes the chorionic cavity, with the embryo, amniotic sac, and yolk sac suspended in it by the connecting stalk.
- Blood vessels develop in the extraembryonic mesoderm, becoming chorionic vessels.
- Chorionic villi develop from the chorion and cover the chorionic sac until the 8th week, becoming vascularized by allantoic vessels.

Chorionic Villi

The essential functional elements of the placenta are tiny finger-like processes called villi, which are surrounded by maternal blood. Inside the villi, capillaries circulate fetal blood. Exchanges between maternal and fetal blood occur through the villi walls. These villi form as offshoots from the trophoblast's surface. Since the trophoblast and underlying extraembryonic mesoderm make up the chorion, these structures are known as chorionic villi.

Types of Chorion Villi

The chorionic villi are first formed all over the trophoblast and grow into the surrounding decidua (**Figs. 5.6A and B**).
- **Chorion laeve:** The villi related to the decidua capsularis are transitory. After some time, they

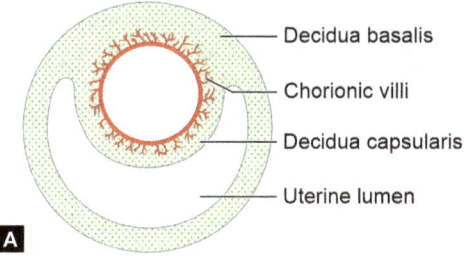

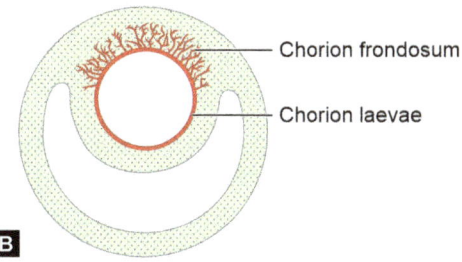

FIGS. 5.6A and B: Types of chorion: Chorion frondosum in relation to decidua basalis and chorion laeve in relation to decidua capsularis.

degenerate. This part of the chorion becomes smooth and is called the *chorion laevae* (**Fig. 5.6A**). It regresses in 3rd month of pregnancy.
- **Chorion frondosum:** In contrast, the villi that grow into the decidua basalis undergo considerable development. Along with the tissues of the decidua basalis, these villi form a disc-shaped mass which is called the *placenta* (**Fig. 5.6B**). The part of the chorion that helps to form the placenta is called the *chorion frondosum*.

Process of Chorionic Villus Formation

The following three stages in formation of chorionic villi are seen:
1. **Primary villi** consist of a central core of cytotrophoblast covered by a layer of syncytiotrophoblast. Adjoining villi are separated by an intervillous space.
2. **Secondary villi** show three layers—outer syncytiotrophoblast, an intermediate layer of cytotrophoblast, and an inner layer of extraembryonic mesoderm.
3. **Tertiary villi** are like secondary villi except that there are blood capillaries in the mesoderm.

The essential features of the formation of chorionic villi are as follows:
- As already discussed above, the trophoblast is at first made up of a single layer of cells (**Fig. 5.5A**). As these cells multiply, two distinct layers are formed i.e., syncytiotrophoblast and cytotrophoblast (**Fig. 5.5B**). The cytotrophoblast rests on extraembryonic mesoderm. All these elements (syncytium,

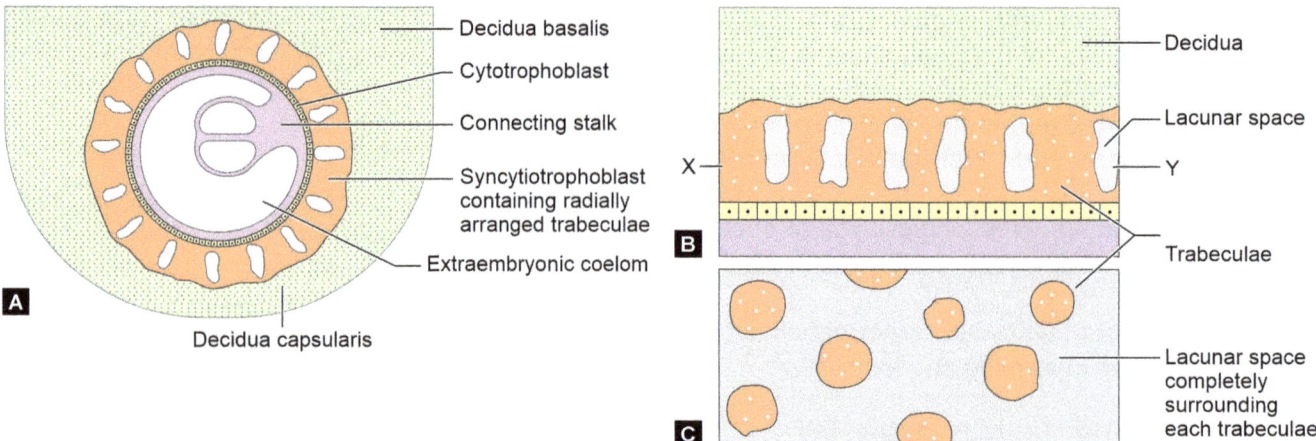

FIGS. 5.7A to C: (A) Radial arrangement of trabeculae and lacunae around the blastocyst; (B) Regularly arranged syncytial trabeculae; (C) Transverse section through trabeculae containing syncytiotrophoblast.

cytotrophoblast and mesoderm) take part in forming chorionic villi.

- The syncytiotrophoblast grows rapidly and becomes thick. Small cavities (called lacunae) appear in this layer **(Fig. 5.5C)**. Gradually, the lacunae increase in size. At first they are irregularly arranged **(Fig. 5.5D)**, but gradually, they come to lie radially **(Figs. 5.7A to C)** around the blastocyst. The lacunae are separated from one another by partitions of syncytium, which are called trabeculae. The lacunae gradually communicate with each other, so that eventually one large space is formed. Each trabeculus is now surrounded all around by this lacunar space **(Fig. 5.7C)**.
- The syncytiotrophoblast (in which these changes are occurring) grows into the endometrium. As the endometrium is eroded, some of its blood vessels are opened up, and blood from them fills the lacunar space **(Fig. 5.8A)**.
- Each trabeculus is, initially, made up entirely of syncytiotrophoblast **(Fig. 5.8B)**. Now the cells of the cytotrophoblast begin to multiply and grow into each trabeculus **(Fig. 5.8C)**. The trabeculus thus comes to have a central core of cytotrophoblast covered by an outer layer of syncytium. It is surrounded by maternal blood, filling the lacunar space. The trabeculus is now called *a primary villus* **(Fig. 5.8D)** and the lacunar space is now called *the intervillous space*.
- Extraembryonic mesoderm invades the center of each primary villus **(Fig. 5.9A)**. The villus now has a core of mesoderm **(Fig. 5.9B)** covered by cytotrophoblast and by syncytium. This structure is called *a secondary villus*.
- Soon thereafter, blood vessels can be seen in the mesoderm forming the core of each villus. With their appearance, the villus is fully formed and is called *a tertiary villus* **(Fig. 5.10)**. The blood vessels of

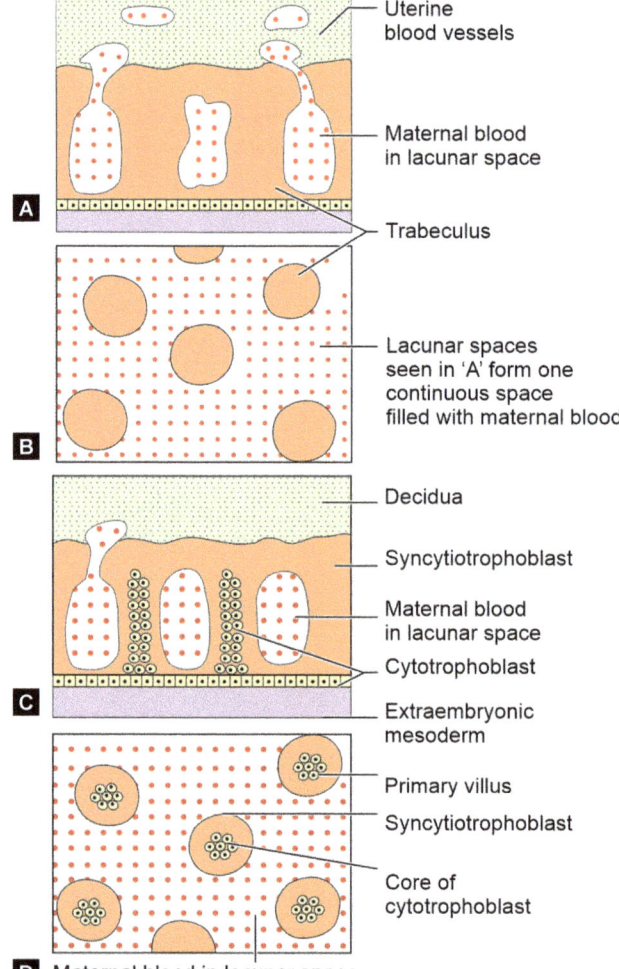

FIGS. 5.8A to D: (A) Uterine blood vessels in the decidua open into the lacunar space and fill with maternal blood and trabecular filled with syncytiotrophoblast; (B) Transverse section through trabeculae containing syncytiotrophoblast surrounded by lacunar spaces filled with maternal blood; (C) Primary villi with central cytotrophoblast cells surrounded by syncytiotrophoblast; (D) Transverse section of primary villi with central cytotrophoblast and peripheral syncytiotrophoblast in contact with maternal blood in intervillous space.

Chapter 5: Second Week of Development

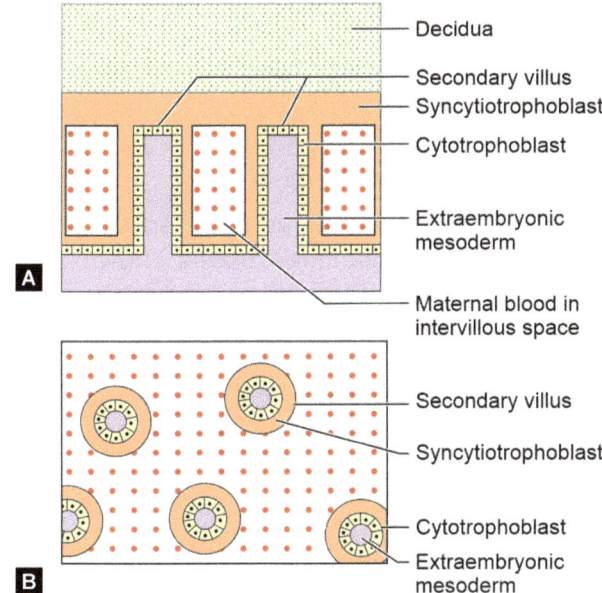

FIGS. 5.9A and B: (A) Secondary chorionic villi with central extraembryonic mesoderm, intermediate cytotrophoblast cells surrounded by syncytiotrophoblast; (B) Transverse section of secondary villi with central core of extraembryonic mesoderm, intermediate cytotrophoblast and peripheral syncytiotrophoblast in contact with maternal blood in intervillous space.

the villus establish connections with the circulatory system of the embryo. Fetal blood now circulates through the villi, while maternal blood circulates through the intervillous space.

❖ From **Figures 5.8C, 5.9A and 5.10A**, it is evident that the cytotrophoblast, that grows into the trabeculus (or villus) does not penetrate the entire thickness of syncytium and, therefore, does not come in contact with the decidua.

At a later stage, however, the cytotrophoblast emerges through the syncytium of each villus. The cells of the cytotrophoblast now spread out to form a layer that completely cuts off the syncytium from the decidua. This layer of cells is called the cytotrophoblastic shell **(Fig. 5.11)**. The cells of this shell multiply rapidly and the placenta increases in size.

Subdivisions of Villi (Fig. 5.12)

❖ Initially, villi attach to fetal extraembryonic mesoderm and maternal cytotrophoblastic shell, known as *anchoring villi.*
❖ Each anchoring villus includes a stem villus or *truncus chorii.*
❖ Stem villi branch into *rami chorii.*

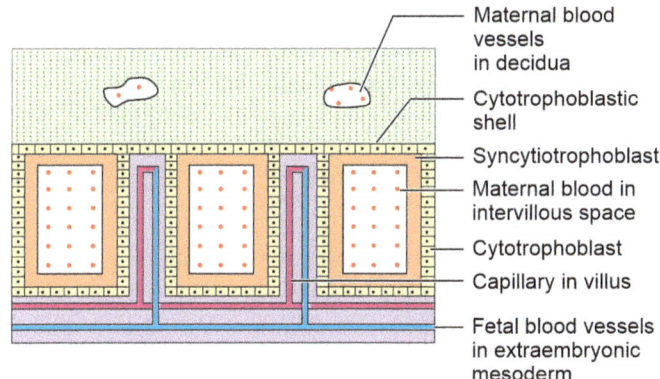

FIG. 5.11: Formation of cytotrophoblast shell.

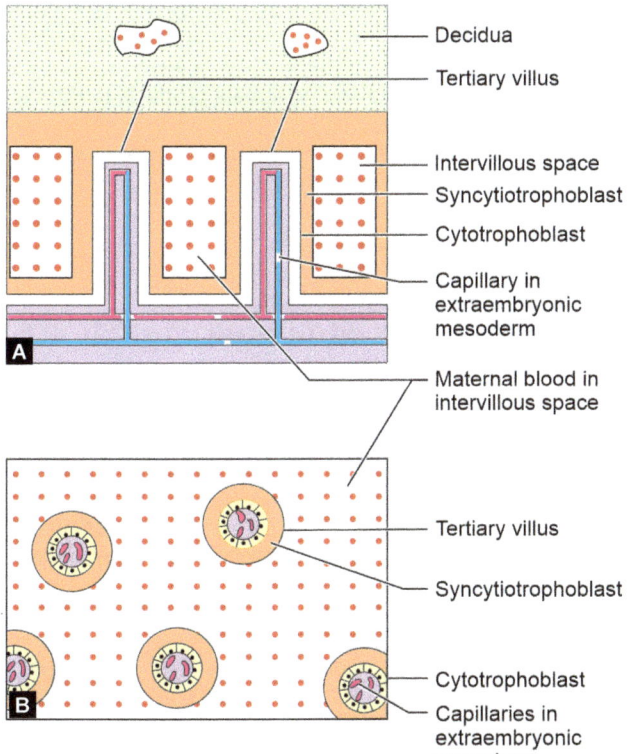

FIGS. 5.10A and B: (A) Tertiary chorionic villi with central core of extraembryonic mesoderm with capillaries, intermediate cytotrophoblast cells surrounded by syncytiotrophoblast; (B) Transverse section of tertiary villi with central extraembryonic mesoderm with capillaries, intermediate cytotrophoblast and peripheral syncytiotrophoblast in contact with maternal blood in intervillous space.

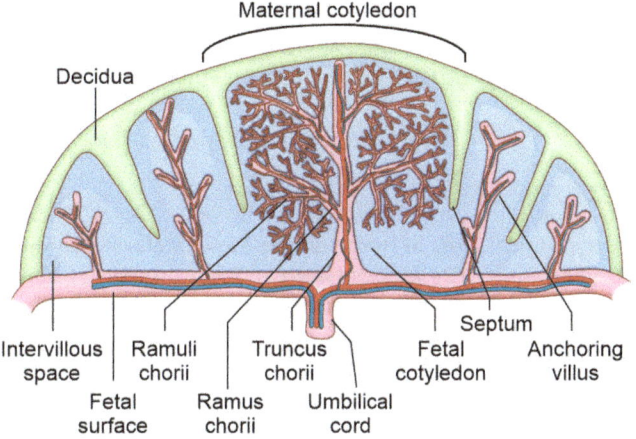

FIG. 5.12: Maternal and fetal cotyledons. Subdivisions of villus—truncus, ramus and ramuli chorii, and anchoring villi.

- ❖ Rami chorii further divide into finer branches called *ramuli chorii*, attaching to the cytotrophoblastic shell.
- ❖ Anchoring villi branch into *free/floating villi* in the intervillous space. Additional villi grow from the chorionic side of this space. Eventually, the intervillous space becomes nearly filled with villi, greatly enhancing surface area for maternal-fetal circulation exchange.
- ❖ The newly formed villi at first consist only of syncytiotrophoblast. They are subsequently invaded by cytotrophoblast, mesoderm, and blood vessels, and pass through the stages of primary, secondary and tertiary villi as described above.

> **NOTE**
> The primary and secondary villi appear during the second week of development. The tertiary villi are formed in third week of development. For a comprehensive view of chorionic villi, all are presented at one place.

Changes in the Endometrium of the Uterus

Decidual reaction and types of decidua are presented in Chapter 4, please refer.

Pre-organogenesis Period

The development of the embryo from fertilization until the formation of the bilaminar disc is known as the pre-organogenesis period because no organs are yet recognizable. This period encompasses the first 14 days of pregnancy. Teratogens acting during this time typically cause anomalies that result in the embryo's death, so such anomalies are rarely seen in full-term babies.

Clinical Importance

Hydatidiform Mole/Molar Pregnancy
- Abnormal form of pregnancy/conceptus where non-viable fertilized egg is implanted in the uterus and it fails to continue until term.
- The trophoblast develops and forms fetal membranes (placenta) but, the embryonic tissue is little or absent.
- In this condition, the embryo dies but there is abnormal growth of trophoblast. Cystic swellings resembling a bunch of grapes that develop from the degenerating and avascular villi.
- **Types:** There are two types of hydatidiform mole:
    1. *Complete mole*: It is caused by a single sperm or two sperms combining with an oocyte having no female pronucleus. Hence, no embryo is seen.
    2. *Partial mole*: A normal oocyte combines with one or two sperm which then reduplicates resulting triploid or tetraploid genotypes. In this condition, a part of embryo is seen.
- **Diagnosis is by:**
    - Ultrasound that shows *snowstorm* appearance of uterine cavity.
    - Appearance of vesicles in urine. No fetal movements and fetal heart sounds.
    - High levels of human chorionic gonadotropin (hCG) after two months of pregnancy suggests hydatidiform mole.
- Moles can undergo malignant change and form choriocarcinoma. The chances of developing choriocarcinoma are 10–15% for complete moles.
- **Treatment:** Evacuating the contents of uterus by uterine suction immediately after diagnosis to avoid the risk of choriocarcinoma.

Immunological Rejection of Conceptus by the Mother
- The antigens expressed by the fetus and placenta are different from that of the mother. But they are not rejected by the maternal immune system during pregnancy.
- Implantation of an embryo brings changes in the DNA packaging of chemokine genes of the stromal cells of decidua. This permanently deactivates, or "silences," the expression of chemokine genes and recruitment of T cells to the site of implantation.

Case Based Learning

Embryological Basis of Hydatidiform Mole (Molar Pregnancy)
Patient details: A 28-year-old woman, G1P0, presents at 10 weeks gestation with vaginal bleeding and severe nausea. She reports that this pregnancy was a long-awaited event for her and her husband. On examination, her uterus is larger than expected for gestational age. There is no fetal heartbeat on Doppler ultrasound.
Diagnostic Evaluation
- **Ultrasound:** Characteristic "snowstorm" appearance with the absence of a viable fetus.
- **β-hCG levels:** Elevated β-hCG levels disproportionate to gestational age.
- **Histopathology:** Examination of products of conception reveals hydropic villi with trophoblastic proliferation.

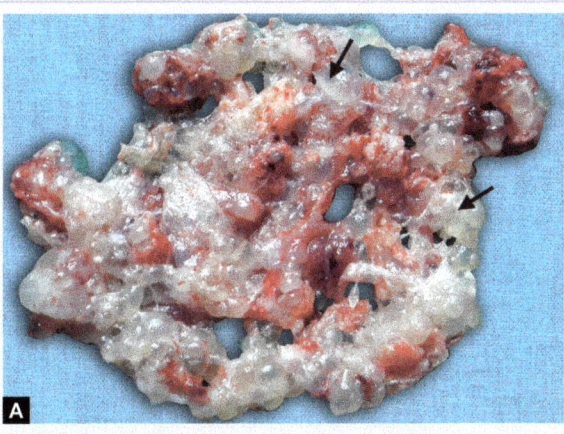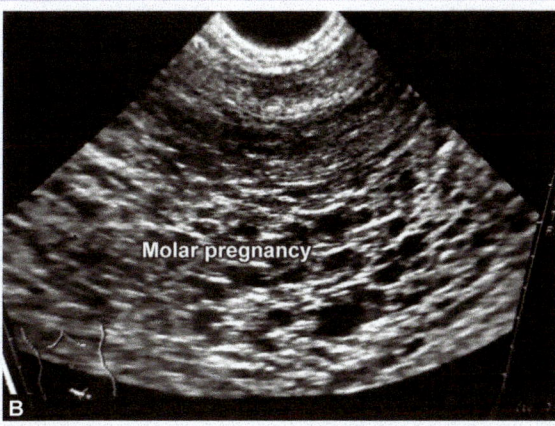

FIGS. 5.13A and B: (A) Showing grape-like vesicles of varying sizes. These are the tissues of molar pregnancy (see the arrows); (B) An ultrasonogram showing snowstorm appearance of a molar pregnancy.
(Reproduced with permission from Dr Hiralal Konar. Source: Chapter 42. In: Konar H, Textbook of Obstetrics, Jaypee Brothers Medical Publishers Pvt Ltd, 2023).

Embryological Basis

Hydatidiform mole (HM) arises from abnormal fertilization events that lead to trophoblastic proliferation and aberrant placental development. Complete HM results from fertilization of an empty ovum (lacking maternal genetic material) by a single sperm that duplicates its own genetic material (paternal origin). Partial HM arises from fertilization of a normal ovum by two sperm (paternal origin). This abnormal genetic constitution results in partial development of fetal tissue alongside abnormal trophoblastic proliferation.

In both the cases, trophoblasts proliferate and invade the uterine wall more aggressively than in normal pregnancies. The abnormal trophoblastic proliferation leads to the formation of characteristic vesicular structures within the placenta, seen as the "snowstorm" appearanc e on ultrasound.

Management

Evacuation of molar tissue through dilation and curettage (D&C) is done, followed by regular monitoring of β-hCG levels to ensure resolution. Patients are advised on contraception to prevent pregnancy temporarily, while persistent gestational trophoblastic disease may require chemotherapy or surgery. Regular follow-up with clinical and laboratory assessments is advised to detect any recurrence or complications.

HIGHLIGHTS

- The cells of the inner cell mass rearranged to form an embryonic disc having two layers *(bilaminar germ disc)*. These layers are the epiblast and the *hypoblast*.
- A cavity appears on the ectodermal side of the disc. This is the *amniotic cavity*. Another cavity appears on the endodermal side. This is the *yolk sac*.
- At first, the walls of the amniotic cavity and yolk sac are in contact with trophoblast. They are soon separated from the latter by *extraembryonic mesoderm*.
- A cavity, the *extraembryonic coelom* appears and splits the extraembryonic mesoderm into a *somatopleuric layer* (in contact with trophoblast) and a *splanchnopleuric layer* (in contact with yolk sac).
- The trophoblast and underlying somatopleuric mesoderm form a membrane called the *chorion*. The cells forming the wall of the amniotic cavity form the *amnion*.
- The amniotic cavity is now attached to trophoblast by a part of extraembryonic mesoderm into which the extraembryonic coelom has not extended. This mesoderm forms the *connecting stalk*.
- Embryonic disc from the ectodermal aspect near one edge developes rounded area called the *prochordal plate*. Here ectoderm and endoderm are not separated by mesoderm.
- The prochordal plate defines the embryo's *central axis (right and left halves)* and indicates the future *head and tail ends (cephalocaudal axis)*.
- The trophoblast differentiates into two layers: *the syncytiotrophoblast*, forming a multinucleated continuous layer, and *the cytotrophoblast*, maintaining distinct cell boundaries.
- **Chorion** is the cellular, outermost extraembryonic membrane composed of trophoblast lined with extraembryonic somatopleuric mesoderm.
- *Chorionic villi* develop from the chorion and cover the entire chorionic sac until the beginning of 8th week. It is of two types—primary and secondary.
- **Tertiary villi** are like secondary villi except that there are fetal blood capillaries in the mesoderm.

Summary

- Events taking place during the second week of germinal period (**Flowchart 5.1**).

FLOWCHART 5.1: Second week of development—events.

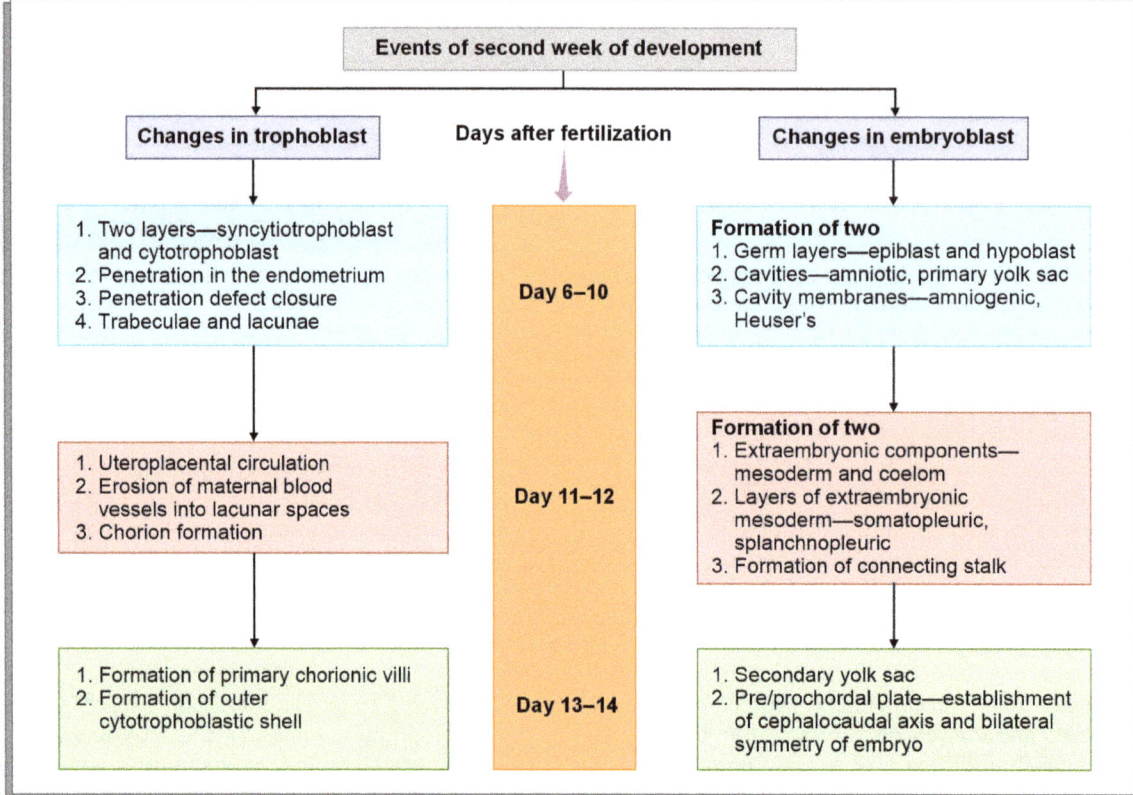

Week of 2's

1. Embryoblast/Inner cell mass differentiates into two germ layers
   – Hypoblast
   – Epiblast
2. Appearance of two cavities
   – Amniotic
   – Yolk sac—primary and secondary
3. Two layers of trophoblast
   – Cytotrophoblast
   – Syncytiotrophoblast
4. Formation extraembryonic components
   – Extraembryonic mesoderm
   – Extraembryonic coelom
5. Division of extraembryonic mesoderm into two layers
   – Somatopleuric
   – Splanchnopleuric
6. Two cavity membrane
   – Amniogenic membrane
   – Haueser's membrane
7. Two fetal membranes
   – Amnion
   – Chorion
8. Two ends of embryo—axis differentiation by prochordal plate
   – Cephalic
   – Caudal axis
9. Formation of two types of villi
   – Primary
   – Secondary

TEST YOUR UNDERSTANDING

REVIEW QUESTIONS

1. Describe the differentiation of the embryoblast during the second week of development.
2. What roles do the syncytiotrophoblast and cytotrophoblast play in development?
3. Explain the formation of chorionic villi.
4. Discuss the formation of amniotic cavity and its significance.
5. What is the role of the hypoblast in early embryonic development?
6. Describe the changes that occur in the trophoblast during the second week of human development.
7. What is the significance of lacunae formation in the syncytiotrophoblast?
8. What is the function of human chorionic gonadotropin (hCG) secreted by the syncytiotrophoblast?

Chapter 5: Second Week of Development

MULTIPLE CHOICE QUESTIONS

1. Which is called as primitive ectodermal layer?
   A. Epiblast
   B. Hypoblast
   C. Blastocele
   D. Trophoblast

2. Which villi is attached to the extraembryonic mesoderm of fetus and cytotrophoblastic shell of maternal side?
   A. Rami chorri
   B. Stem villus
   C. Anchoring villi
   D. Floating villi

3. "Snowstorm appearance" of uterine cavity in USG is suggestive of:
   A. Choriocarcinoma
   B. Ectopic pregnancy
   C. Hydatidiform mole
   D. Twin pregnancy

4. Trophoblast and somatopleuric mesoderm forms:
   A. Amnion
   B. Yolk sac
   C. Primitive streak
   D. Chorion

5. Endodermal layer of GIT is formed from:
   A. Hypoblast
   B. Epiblast
   C. Yolk sac
   D. Neural crest cells

6. During the second week of human embryonic development, which of the following structures undergoes differentiation to form the bilaminar embryonic disc?
   A. Morula
   B. Blastocyst
   C. Trophoblast
   D. Chorionic villi

7. In the second week of human embryonic development, what structure plays a crucial role in forming the placenta and facilitates nutrient exchange between the embryo and mother?
   A. Amniotic cavity
   B. Syncytiotrophoblast
   C. Bilaminar germ disc
   D. Chorionic villi

8. A 28-year-old pregnant woman at 6 weeks gestation complains of nausea and vomiting (morning sickness). On ultrasound, a yolk sac is noted within the gestational sac. Which embryonic structure is primarily responsible for the production of hormones that maintain the early pregnancy and contribute to her symptoms?
   A. Syncytiotrophoblast
   B. Epiblast
   C. Hypoblast
   D. Cytotrophoblast

9. What is the fate of the cytotrophoblast cells during the second week of human embryonic development?
   A. They differentiate into the epiblast and hypoblast layers.
   B. They form the amniotic cavity.
   C. They contribute to the formation of the yolk sac.
   D. They form the inner layer of the chorionic villi.

10. A 35-year-old woman presents for her first prenatal visit at 8 weeks gestation. Ultrasound reveals a developing embryo with visible heart motion. Which embryonic structure is primarily responsible for the formation of the fetal blood vessels that will eventually connect to the placenta?
    A. Epiblast
    B. Hypoblast
    C. Extraembryonic mesoderm
    D. Chorionic villi

Answers:
1. A   2. C   3. C   4. D   5. C
6. B   7. D   8. A   9. D   10. C

CHAPTER 6

Third Week of Development

COMPETENCIES COVERED/LEARNING OUTCOMES

The student should be able to:

AN78.4	Describe the formation of prochordal plate.
AN79.1	Describe the formation and fate of the primitive streak.
AN79.2	Describe formation and fate of notochord.
AN79.3	Describe the process of neurulation.
AN79.4	Describe the development of somites and intraembryonic coelom.
AN79.5	Explain embryological basis of congenital malformations, nucleus pulposus, sacrococcygeal teratomas, neural tube defects.

With the start of 3rd week, the bilaminar germ disc undergo further differentiation and give rise to *trilaminar germ disc*, which is made up of three layers—the ectoderm (outer), endoderm (inner) and mesoderm (middle). During the third week of development the embryo proper acquires the form of a three-layered disc. This is called the *embryonic disc* (also called embryonic area, embryonic shield, or germ disc).

All tissues of the body are derived from one or more of these three germ layers. Much of the student's study of embryology concerns itself with learning from which of these germ layers particular tissues and organs develop.

OVERVIEW OF THIRD WEEK OF DEVELOPMENT

The embryonic development during third week can be studied into following headings:
1. Changes in the germ disc/embryonic area
2. Changes in the trophoblast

The major events encompassing the third week are formation of primitive streak, gastrulation notochord, neuralization and formation of intraembryonic mesoderm.

CHANGES IN THE GERM DISC OR EMBRYONIC AREA

These topics can be examined under the following subheadings:
- **Changes in the shape of the embryonic disc:** The disc undergoes morphological alterations, establishing three distinct axes.
- **Changes in the ectodermal layer of the disc:** The ectoderm differentiates into three functional zones.

Changes in the Shape of Embryonic Disc

- During the 2nd and 3rd week of development there is changes in the shape of embryonic disc. At the beginning of 3rd week of development the disc is *circular in shape*. At about 15th/16th day it becomes *oval in shape*. Around 18th day of development it becomes *pear shaped* with broad cephalic and narrow caudal ends. The connecting stalk is attached to the caudal end **(Figs. 6.1A to C)**.

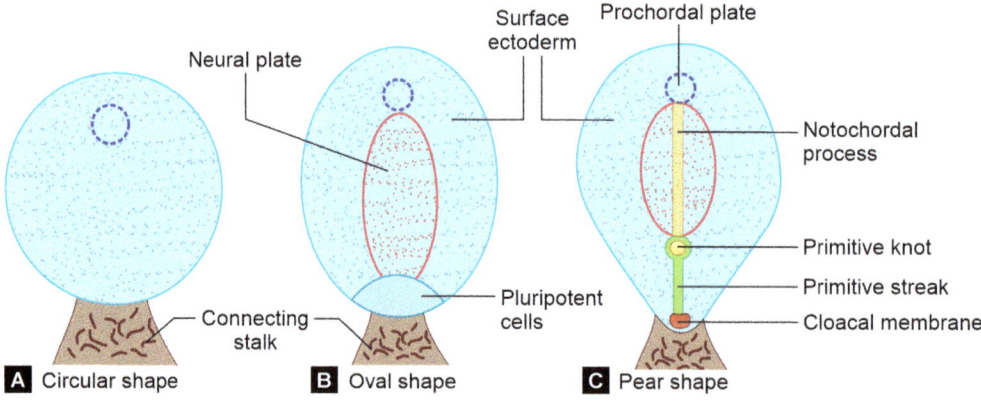

FIGS. 6.1A to C: Changes in the shape of embryonic disc from circular (A) to oval (B) and then pear shape (C).

- The three axes of embryo, the *cephalocaudal, dorsoventral and right left axes* are established with the appearance of prochordal plate and migration of connecting stalk.

Changes in the Ectodermal Layer of Disc

The ectodermal layer of bilaminar germ disc differentiates into three functional zones. They are:
1. **Surface ectoderm:** The cell along the cephalic margin and sides of embryonic disc. From this develops the *epidermis of skin*.
2. **Neuroectoderm:** The cells of surface ectoderm lying dorsal to the notochord. These cells form the neural plate or neuroectoderm. This gives rise to *central nervous system*.
3. **Pluripotent cells:** The cells of epiblast at the caudal end of bilaminar embryonic disc are pluripotent (Figs. 6.1A to C). These cells form the *primitive streak* and *primitive node* which in turn form the three germ layers, the notochord and the primordial germ cells.

FORMATION OF PRIMITIVE STREAK

- It is a transient structure that forms in the blastula during the early stages of embryonic development.
- On 15th day of gestation, soon after the formation of prochordal plate there is active proliferation, migration, and invagination of the pluripotent epiblast cells lying on the dorsal aspect of the caudal end of the embryonic disc.
- These proliferating cells form an elevation that bulges into the amniotic cavity called the *primitive streak* **(Figs. 6.2A and B).**
- These cells lying along the central axis between epiblast and hypoblast form a narrow median groove and raised lateral margins, the *primitive streak* **(Figs. 6.1A to C)** from which *notochord* and the *3rd germ layer (intraembryonic mesoderm)* are formed during the early part of 3rd week resulting in trilaminar germ disc.
- The primitive streak is at first a rounded or oval swelling, but with the elongation of the embryonic disc it becomes a linear structure lying in the central axis of the disc. With the formation of prochordal plate and primitive streak, the shape of embryonic disc changes from circular to oval **(Figs. 6.1 and 6.3)**.
- The primitive streak gradually elongates, along the central axis of the embryonic disc. The disc becomes pear-shaped **(Fig. 6.4)**.
- **Primitive streak is the primary organizer** as it induces formation of notochord and intraembryonic mesoderm. *Formation of notochord and intraembryonic mesoderm determines the craniocaudal axis and right and left sides of embryo.*

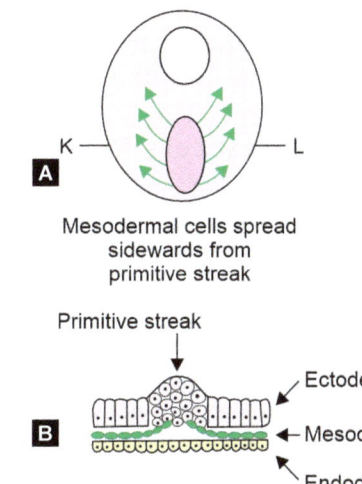

FIGS. 6.3A and B: Formation of intraembryonic mesoderm. 'B' is a section along axis KL in 'A'.

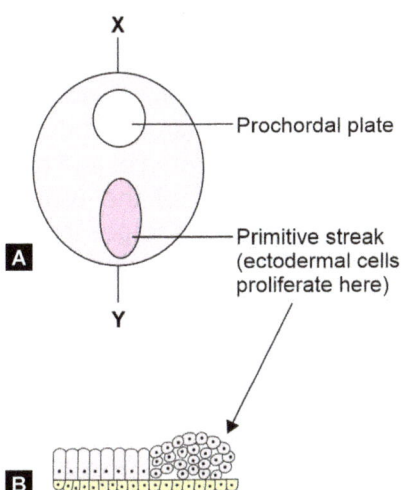

FIGS. 6.2A and B: Appearance of primitive streak. 'B' is a section along axis XY shown in 'A'.

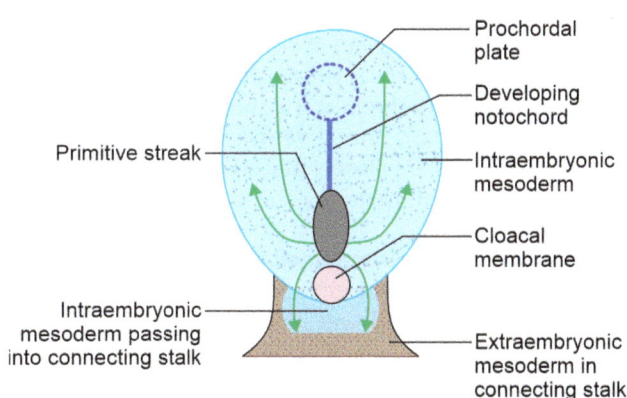

FIG. 6.4: Spread of intraembryonic mesoderm. Note that the mesoderm comes to lie between ectoderm and endoderm in all parts of the embryonic disc except at the: (1) prochordal plate, (2) cloacal membrane and (3) region of the notochord.

Importance and Fate of Primitive Streak

❖ Formation of primitive streak acts as the initiation of *gastrulation*.
❖ It also establishes the *fundamental axes* and bilateral symmetry of developing embryo.
❖ Primitive streak regresses at the end of 3rd week with complete disappearance by 26th day, hence it is a transient structure.

GASTRULATION

Gastrulation is defined as the process during early embryonic development that *transforms the bilaminar embryonic disc into a trilaminar disc,* forming three germ layers: ectoderm, mesoderm, and endoderm from pluripotent epiblast.

Trilaminar Germ Disc

❖ The cells of epiblast invade the hypoblast and eventually replace the hypoblast forming the *definitive endoderm*.
❖ Other cells migrate between the epiblast and the definitive endoderm to form the *intraembryonic mesoderm*.
❖ The remaining epiblast cells form the definitive *ectoderm*.
❖ Thus the epiblast, through the process of gastrulation, is the source of all the germ layers which will give rise to all the tissues and organs of the embryo.

Molecular Regulation of Primitive Streak

Migration of primitive streak cells and their specification to form various derivatives are controlled by various factors, i.e., Nodal, WNT, FGF8 and Chordin.

Clinical correlation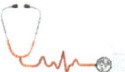

Teratogenesis Associated with Gastrulation
- **Teratogenic effects on primitive streak:** The embryo is highly sensitive to teratogens during 15th to 18th day (3rd week/gastrulation period) of development as the primitive streak and its derivatives will be affected.
- **Holoprosencephaly:** In this condition, the forebrain is small and the two lateral ventricles fuse into a single cavity. The eyes are closely placed (hypertelorism). High doses of alcohol intake by the mother can cause this condition.
- **Caudal dysgenesis (sirenomelia):** Deficiency of mesoderm in the caudal part of the embryo that normally contributes for the formation of lower limbs, urogenital system and lumbosacral vertebrae will result in abnormalities in these structures. The child is born with a fused lower limbs and presents renal, genital and vertebral anomalies including imperforate anus. This condition is more common in mother with diabetes.

- **Sacrococcygeal teratoma:** Persistence of pluripotent cells of primitive streak at the caudal end of embryonic disc after 4th week of gestation gives rise to a large tumor called *sacrococcygeal teratoma*. Sacrococcygeal teratoma (SCT) is a type of tumor that arises at the base of the coccyx (tailbone) and is the most common germ cell tumor in neonates. These teratomas, as they retain the potential to differentiate into various tissue types, including ectoderm, mesoderm, and endoderm. SCTs can contain a mix of tissues such as hair, muscle, and bone, reflecting their pluripotent origin. It can cause obstruction during labor and is usually malignant. It has to be removed within 6 months after birth.
- **Chordoma:** Malignant tumor arising from remnants of notochord. It can be seen at cranial or caudal end of notochord.

Connecting Stalk

❖ When the embryonic disc is first formed, it is suspended (along with amniotic cavity and yolk sac) from the trophoblast by the connecting stalk **(Fig. 6.5)**.
❖ The connecting stalk is the unsplit part of extraembryonic mesoderm.
❖ To begin with, the connecting stalk is very broad compared to the size of the embryo.
❖ Due to the enlargement and elongation of embryonic disc, the connecting stalk becomes relatively small, and its attachment becomes confined to the region of the tail end of the embryonic disc.
❖ Some amount of intraembryonic mesoderm arising from the primitive streak passes backward into the connecting stalk **(Figs. 6.4 and 6.5)**.
❖ As it does so, it leaves a bilaminar area caudal to the primitive streak (ectoderm and endoderm are in contact without intervening mesoderm). This region forms the *cloacal membrane* **(Fig. 6.4)**.

FORMATION OF NOTOCHORD

With the formation of prochordal plate the cephalocaudal axis of the embryo is established. With the formation of notochord the ventrodorsal axis will be established. The notochord is a midline structure that develops in the region lying between the cranial end of the primitive streak and the caudal end of the prochordal plate **(Figs. 6.1 and 6.4)**. The various stages through which the notochord passes during its development are as follows:

❖ The cranial end of the primitive streak becomes thickened and elevated. This thickened part of the streak is called the *primitive knot, primitive node or Hensen's node* **(Fig. 6.6A)**.
❖ Primitive node is known as the 'organizer' as it regulates important processes, such as laterality (right and left side determination) and formation of the notochord.

Chapter 6: Third Week of Development

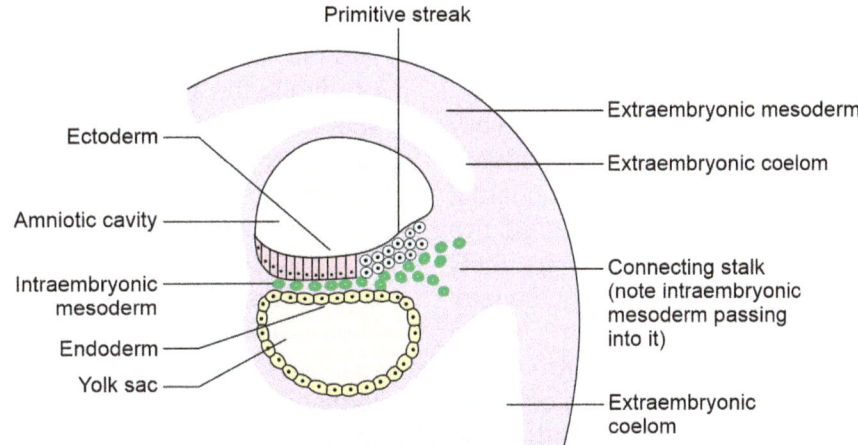

FIG. 6.5: Diagram showing the attachment of the connecting stalk to the caudal end of the embryonic disc. Note the cells of the intraembryonic mesoderm passing into the connecting stalk.

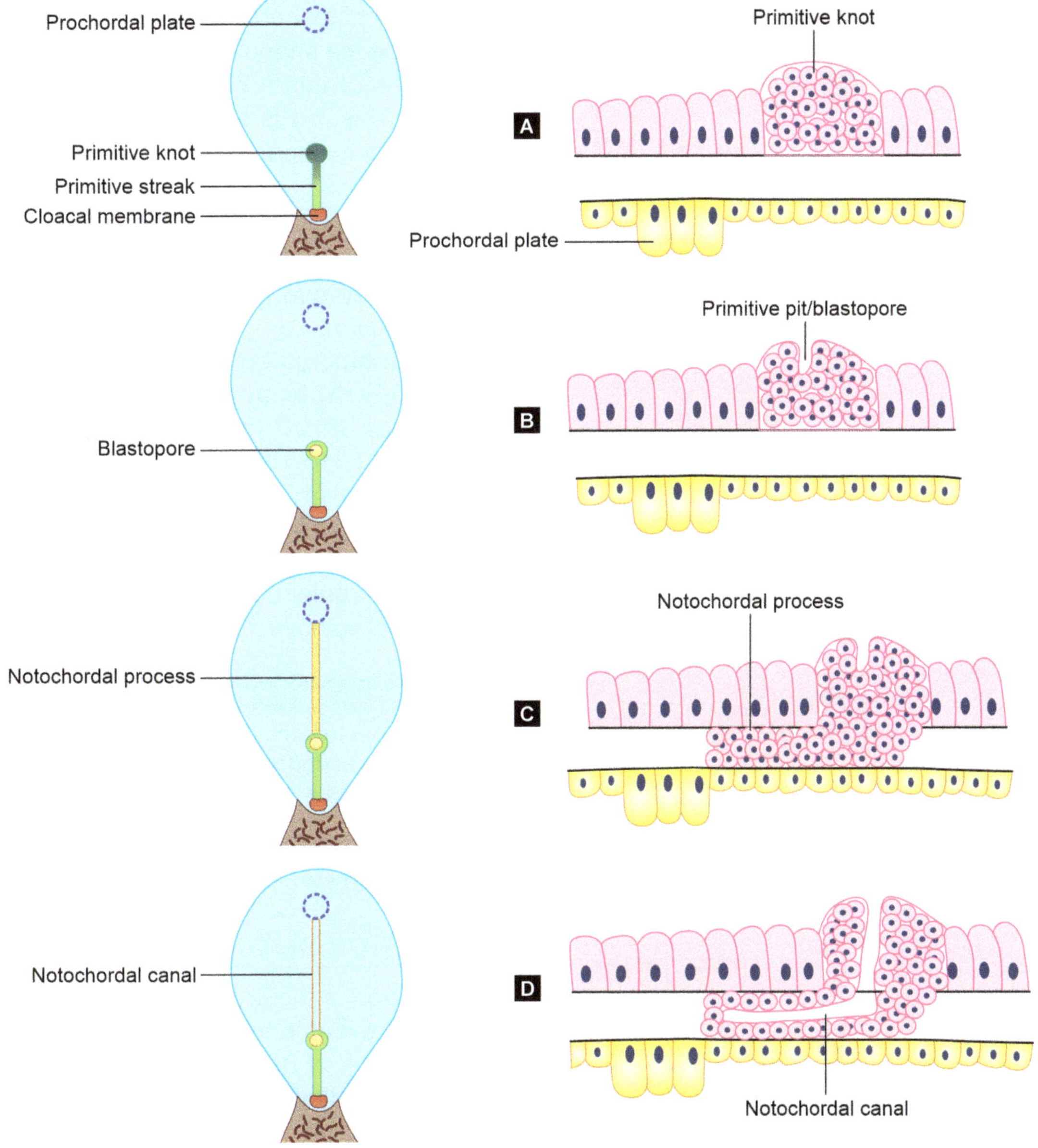

FIGS. 6.6A to D: Embryonic disc and its longitudinal section showing formation of (A) primitive knot; (B) blastopore; (C) notochordal process and (D) notochordal canal. Note that the notochordal process is deep to ectoderm and that its position is shown diagrammatically.

- A depression appears in the center of the primitive knot. This depression is called the *blastopore/primitive pit* **(Fig. 6.6B)**.
- Cells in the primitive knot multiply and pass cranially in the midline, between the ectoderm and endoderm, reaching up to the caudal margin of the prochordal plate. These cells form a solid cord called the *notochordal process or head process* **(Figs. 6.6C and 6.7A)**. The cells of this process undergo several stages of rearrangement **(Fig. 6.1)** ending in the formation of a solid rod called the notochord.
- The cavity of blastopore, extends into the notochordal process, and converts it into a tube called the *notochordal canal or neurenteric canal* **(Figs. 6.6D and 6.7B)**.
- The cells forming the floor of notochordal canal become intercalated in (i.e., become mixed up with) the cells of the endoderm **(Fig. 6.7C)**. The cells forming the floor of the notochordal canal now separate the canal from the cavity of the yolk sac.
- The floor of the notochordal canal begins to break down. At first, there are small openings formed in it, but gradually the whole canal comes to communicate with the yolk sac **(Fig. 6.7D)**. The notochordal canal also communicates with the amniotic cavity through the blastopore. Thus, *at this stage, the amniotic cavity and the yolk sac are in communication with each other.* This communication facilitates nutrition by diffusion to the ectodermal surface of germ disc. The germ disc starts *differentiating into the neural ectoderm, neural plate and neural tube.* As the blood vascular system was not formed nutrition is provided through this communication to the rapidly developing nervous system.
- Gradually the walls of the canal become flattened so that instead of a rounded canal there will be a flat plate of cells called the *notochordal plate* **(Fig. 6.7E)**.
- However, this process of flattening is soon reversed and the notochordal plate again becomes curved, to assume the shape of a tube **(Fig. 6.7F)**. Proliferation of cells of this tube converts it into a solid rod of cells. This rod is the *definitive notochord*. It gets completely separated from the endoderm.

Importance and Fate of Notochord

- It forms the central axis of embryonic disc.
- It induces overlying ectoderm for the process of *neurulation*.
- As the embryo enlarges, the notochord elongates considerably and lies in the midline, in the position to be later occupied by the vertebral column. However, the *notochord does not give rise to the vertebral column*. Most of it disappears, but parts of it persist in the region of each intervertebral disc as the *nucleus pulposus* and its cranial continuation the *apical ligament of dens of axis vertebra*.

Pluripotent Ectodermal Cells

Pluripotent ectodermal cells form the following:
- Definitive endoderm
- Intraembryonic mesoderm
- Definitive ectoderm
- Notochord
- Primordial germ cells (PGC)

FORMATION OF THE NEURAL TUBE

Neurulation is the process of formation of neural tube. The initial event in the process of neurulation begins in the 3rd week of development. The notochord induces the differentiation of adjacent ectoderm to thicken. This thickening forms the neural plate that passes through the various events of neurulation which are as follows **(Figs. 6.8A and B)**:

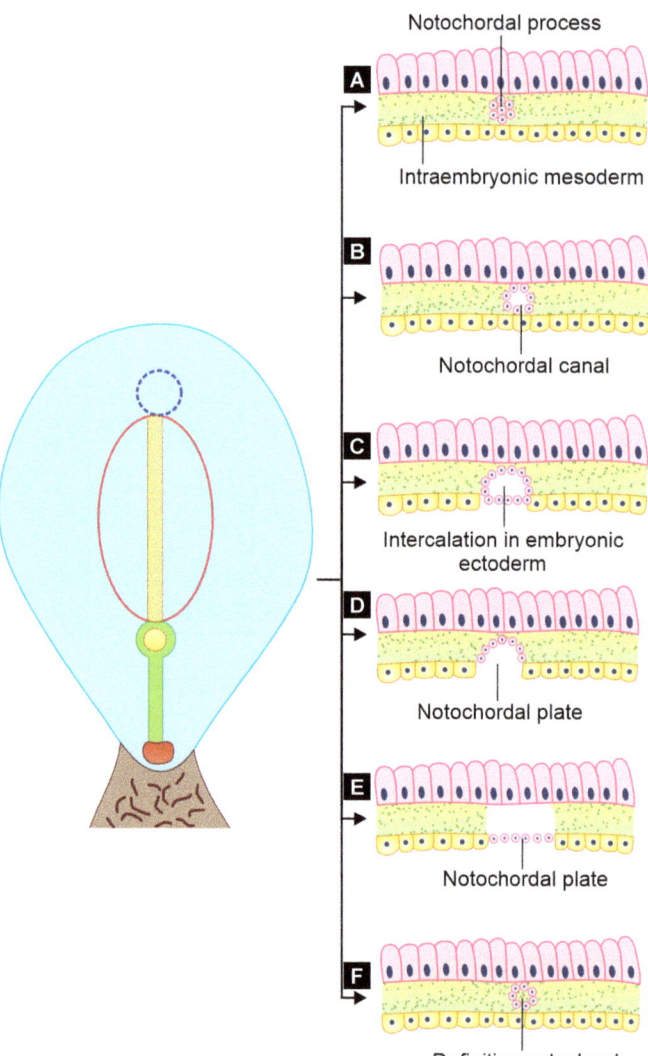

FIGS. 6.7A to F: Transverse sections through the embryonic disc to illustrate stages in the formation of the notochord.

Chapter 6: Third Week of Development

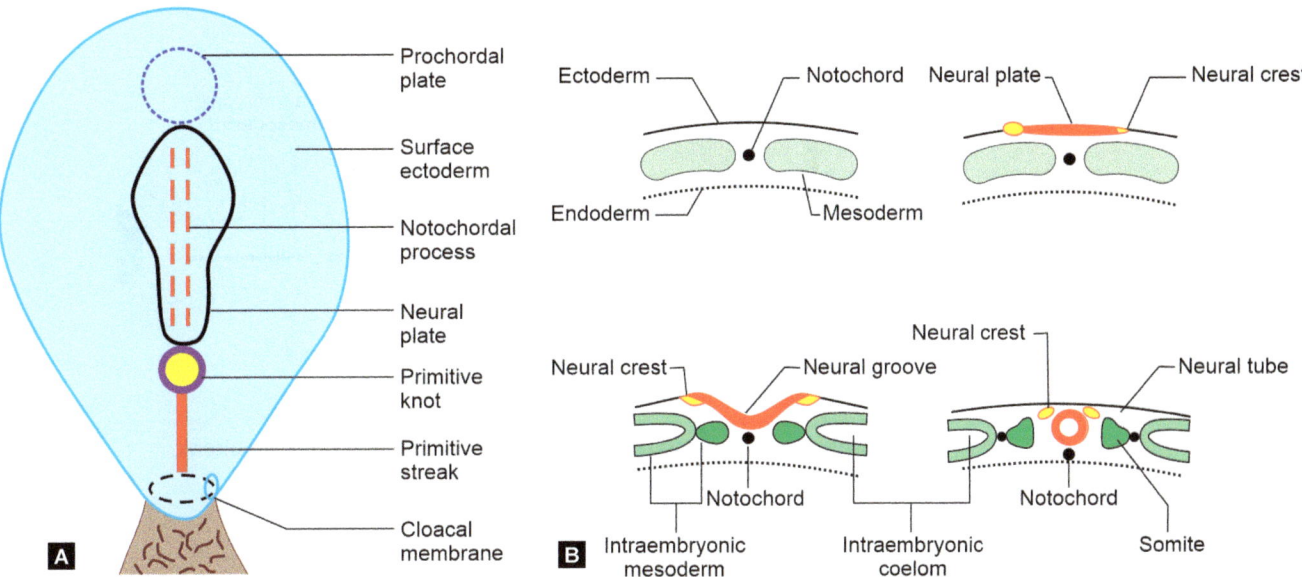

FIGS. 6.8A and B: Formation of neural tube. (A) Neural plate as seen in longitudinal section; (B) Various processes of formation of neural tube in transverse section

- Neurulation is induced by signaling molecules from the notochord and prechordal plate.
- The ectoderm above the notochord thickens to form the *neural plate*. This region is termed the *neuroectoderm*.
- The neural plate elongates and broadens in a cranial-to-caudal direction from prechordal plate to primitive knot.
- The lateral edges of the neural plate elevate to form *neural folds* with proliferation of paraxial mesoderm on both sides leading to formation of the *neural groove* in center.
- Neural folds move towards the midline and begin to fuse forming a cylindrical *neural tube*. Fusion starts in the cervical region and proceeds bidirectionally (cranially and caudally).
- The neural tube communicates with amniotic sac with two openings: cranial and caudal neuropore. These get closed by day 25 and day 27 respectively. The neural tube separates from the overlying ectoderm.
- The neural tube differentiates into the central nervous system. Cranial part of the neural tube forms the brain while caudal part of the neural tube forms the spinal cord.
- Some cells at the crest of the neural folds detach during fusion and forms *neural crest cells*.
- These neural crest cells migrate and differentiate into various cell types, including peripheral nerves, melanocytes, and facial cartilage.

FORMATION OF INTRAEMBRYONIC MESODERM (THIRD GERM LAYER)

The cells that proliferate in the region of the primitive streak pass sideways, pushing themselves between the epiblast and hypoblast **(Figs. 6.3A and B)**. These cells form the *intraembryonic mesoderm (or secondary mesoderm)*.

- **Extensions of intraembryonic mesoderm:**
  - The intraembryonic mesoderm spreads throughout the disc except in three regions: prechordal plate, notochord and cloacal membrane, where ectoderm and endoderm remains in contact.
  - In later development, the ectoderm and endoderm mostly persist as a lining epithelium. On the other hand, the *bulk of the tissues of the body are formed predominantly from mesoderm*.
  - Cranial to the prochordal plate, the mesoderm of the two sides meet in the midline **(Figs. 6.4 and 6.9)**.
  - At the edges of the embryonic disc, the intraembryonic mesoderm is continuous with the extraembryonic mesoderm **(Figs. 6.10 to 6.12)**.

Regions that Remain Bilaminar

- **Buccopharyngeal membrane:**
  - As there is no mesoderm in the prochordal plate, this region remains relatively thin, and later forms the buccopharyngeal membrane (future oral cavity).
  - The rupture of this membrane **(4th week of gestation)** establishes communication between primitive mouth and pharynx.
- **Cloacal membrane:**
  - At the caudal end of embryonic disc between primitive streak and connecting stalk the germ disc is bilaminar. It is called cloacal membrane. Later it is divided into anal membrane (future anal opening) and urogenital membrane (future urinary and genital openings).

64 Chapter 6: Third Week of Development

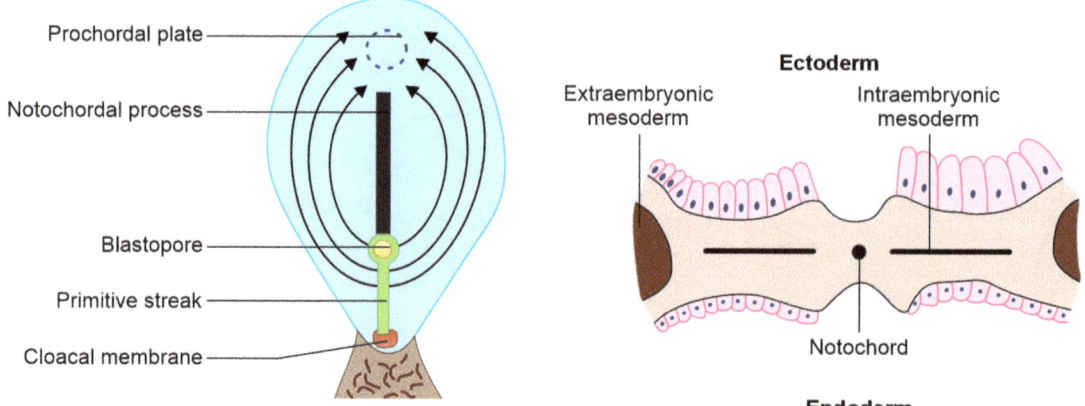

FIG. 6.9: Proliferating intraembryonic mesoderm from primitive node and primitive streak.

- The rupture of these membranes **(6th week of gestation)** establishes the communication of urinary, genital and digestive systems with the outside.
- In the midline caudal to the prochordal plate, as this place is occupied by the notochord.

Subdivisions of Intraembryonic Mesoderm

The intraembryonic mesoderm is further subdivided into three longitudinal parts **(Figs. 6.10 to 6.12)**:
1. Mesoderm, on either side of the notochord, becomes thick and is called the *paraxial mesoderm*.
2. More laterally, the mesoderm forms a thinner layer called the *lateral plate mesoderm*.
3. Between these two, there is a longitudinal strip called the *intermediate mesoderm*.

Paraxial Mesoderm

At first, the cells of the paraxial mesoderm are homogenously arranged. Later, the mesoderm gets segmented.
- The segments are of two categories—somitomeres and somites **(Figs. 6.11 and 6.12)**.
- **Somitomeres** lie in the region of the head. They are rounded structures. There are seven of them. They form the mesoderm and muscles of the head and jaw.
- **Somites** are cubical and more distinctly segmented. The most cranial somites are formed in the occipital region. New somites are progressively formed caudal to them.
- Ultimately there are about 44 pairs of somites (4 occipital, 8 cervical, 12 thoracic, 5 lumbar, 5 sacral and 8–10 coccygeal).

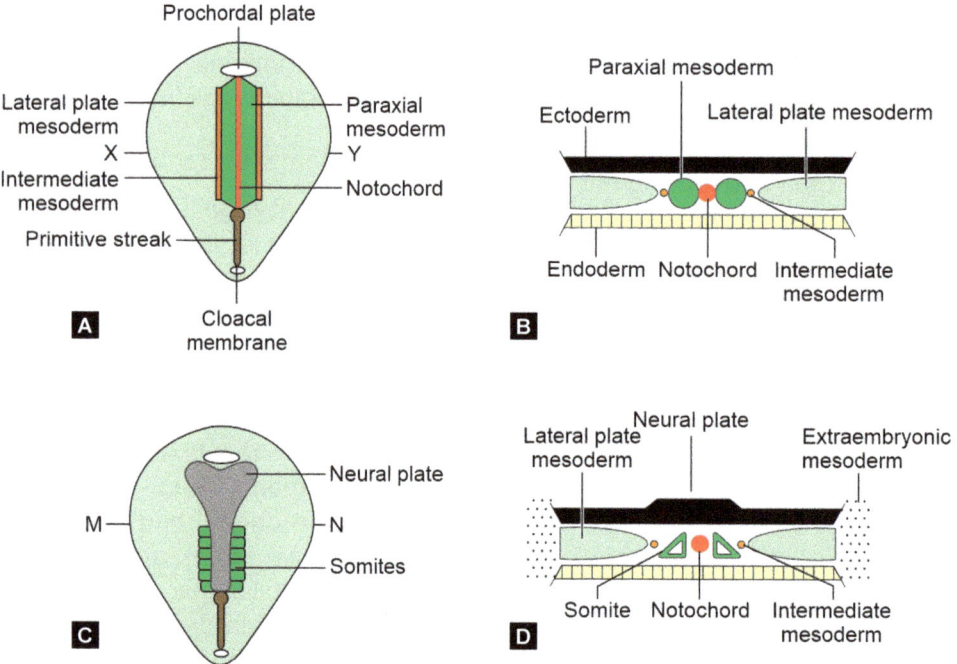

FIGS. 6.10A to D: Subdivisions of intraembryonic mesoderm.

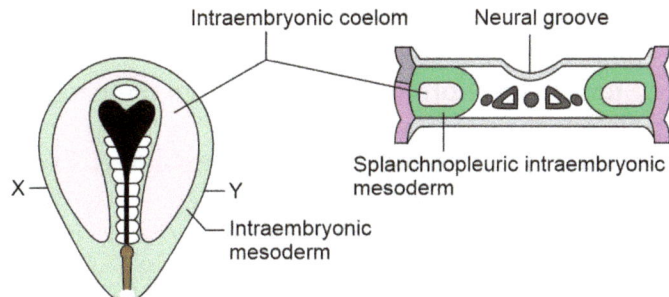

FIG. 6.11: Formation of intraembryonic coelom and its subdivisions.

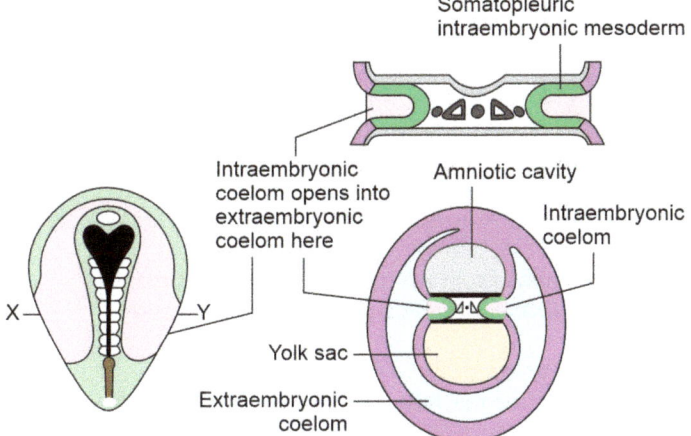

FIG. 6.12: Communication between intraembryonic coelom and extraembryonic coelom. Structures in the midline of germ disc before folding.

❖ Occipital somites form muscles of the tongue. Somites form the axial skeleton, skeletal muscle and part of skin.
❖ In the head region, cranial to somites, somitomeres give origin to some mesenchyme.
Formation of intraembryonic mesoderm and especially the somites establishes right and left axes of the embryo. Somitomere derived structures are mentioned in chapter on pharyngeal arches. The fate of somites is described in chapter on skeletal and muscular system.

Lateral Plate Mesoderm—Formation of Intraembryonic Coelom

❖ While the paraxial mesoderm is undergoing segmentation, to form the somites, changes are also occurring in the lateral plate mesoderm.
❖ Small cavities appear in it. These coalesce (come together) to form one large cavity called the *intraembryonic coelom*.
❖ The cavity has the shape of a horseshoe (**Fig. 6.11**). There are two halves of the cavity (one on either side of the midline) which are joined together cranial to the prochordal plate. At first, this is a closed cavity (**Fig. 6.11**) but soon it comes to communicate with the extra-embryonic coelom (**Fig. 6.12**).

❖ With the formation of the intraembryonic coelom, the lateral plate mesoderm splits into:
  – *Somatopleuric or parietal layer* of intraembryonic mesoderm that is in contact with ectoderm.
  – *Splanchnopleuric or visceral layer* of intraembryonic mesoderm that is in contact with endoderm (**Figs. 6.11 and 6.12**).
❖ The intraembryonic coelom gives rise to pericardial, pleural, and peritoneal cavities.
❖ The heart is formed in the splanchnopleuric mesoderm forming the floor of the pericardial part of the coelom (**Figs. 6.11 to 6.13**). This is, therefore, called the *cardiogenic area* (also called *cardiogenic plate, heart-forming plate*).
❖ Cranial to the cardiogenic area (i.e., at the cranial edge of the embryonic disc) the somatopleuric and splanchnopleuric mesoderm are continuous with each other. The mesoderm here does not get split, as the intraembryonic coelom has not extended into it. This unsplit part of intraembryonic mesoderm forms a structure called the *septum transversum* (**Figs. 6.11 to 6.13**).

Intermediate Mesoderm

The urinary and genital systems are derived from the intermediate mesoderm. *This will be discussed in detail in the chapters of urinary and genital systems.*

Extent of Components of Intraembryonic Mesoderm

❖ Paraxial mesoderm extends along the entire length of the embryo including its limbs as it contributes for the segmental muscles and dermis, but bones of axial skeleton only.
❖ Intermediate mesoderm though extends initially along the entire trunk of the embryo, its functional components are present only in the lower part of trunk region as it contributes for urinary and genital systems. The details will be discussed in the chapter on development of urinary and genital system.

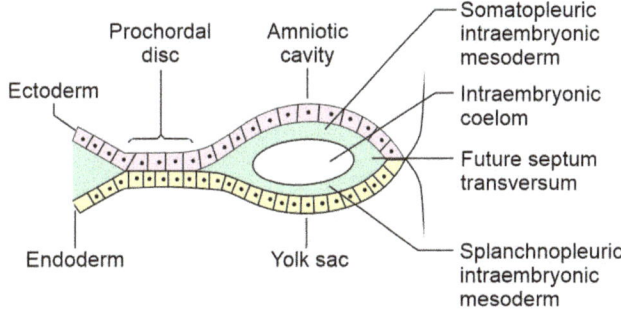

FIG. 6.13: Midline section through cranial end of the embryonic disc to show the relationship of the pericardial cavity to other structures.

- Lateral plate mesoderm is present in relation to the trunk region and it contributes for the development of heart and major blood vessels of the body and the coelomic cavities.

CHANGES IN THE TROPHOBLAST

- Mesodermal cells penetrate the core of the primary villi forming *secondary villi*.
- Blood vessels develop in the mesoderm by the end of the third week forming *tertiary villi*.
- The entire trophoblast becomes surrounded by a outer *cytotrophoblastic shell*.
- **Stem or anchoring villi** extend from the chorionic plate to the decidua basalis.
- Lateral branches of the stem villi are called *free or terminal villi*.
- The *chorionic cavity* becomes larger.
- The embryo is attached to its trophoblastic shell by a narrow *connecting stalk*, which later develops into the umbilical cord.

HIGHLIGHTS

- The two most important during this week are the *formation of third germ layer and establishment of body axes of the embryo.*
- **Primitive streak** is formed on the 15th day and is a transient structure formed from the cells of epiblast along the central axis of embryo as an elevation at the caudal end of the embryonic disc.
- Cells multiplying in the primitive streak move into the interval between ectoderm and endoderm and form the *mesoderm (third germ layer)*.
- **Gastrulation** is the process of formation of three germ layers by translocation of cells of inner cell mass of embryoblast.
- Caudal to the primitive streak we see a round area called the *cloacal membrane*. It is made up only of epiblast and hypoblast.
- The cranial end of the primitive streak enlarges to form the *primitive node or Hensen's node*.
- Cells of the primitive knot multiply and pass cranially to form a rod-like structure reaching up to the prochordal plate. This is the *notochordal process*.
- The notochordal process undergoes changes that convert it first into a canal and then into a plate and finally back into a rod-like structure. This is the notochord. Most of the notochord disappears. Remnants remain as the nucleus pulposus of each intervertebral disc and *apical ligament of dens of axis vertebra*.
- **Intraembryonic mesoderm** shows three subdivisions. The mesoderm next to the middle line is called the *paraxial mesoderm*. The mesoderm in the lateral part of the embryonic disc is called the *lateral plate mesoderm*. A cavity called the intraembryonic coelom appears in it and splits the mesoderm into a *somatopleuric layer* (in contact with ectoderm) and a *splanchnopleuric layer* (in contact with endoderm). A strip of mesoderm between the lateral plate mesoderm and the paraxial mesoderm is called the *intermediate mesoderm*.
- The intraembryonic coelom later forms the pericardial, pleural, and peritoneal cavities.

Summary

- Events taking place during the third week of germinal period (**Flowchart 6.1**).

FLOWCHART 6.1: Third week of development—events.

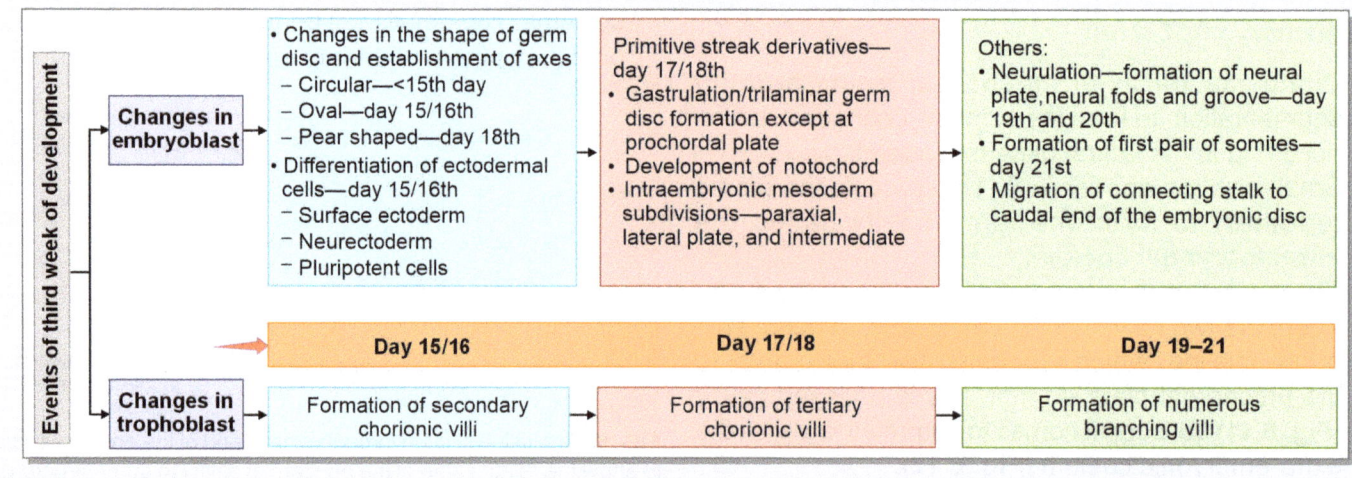

Chapter 6: Third Week of Development

TEST YOUR UNDERSTANDING

REVIEW QUESTIONS

1. Define gastrulation. Write steps of formation of three germ layers.
2. Write a note on primitive streak and its fate.
3. Describe formation of notochord.
4. Discuss the process of formation of neural tube.
5. What are the three subdivisions of intraembryonic mesoderm?
6. Give the embryological basis of teratomas.

EXPLAIN WHY? (REASONING QUESTIONS)

1. Process of gastrulation is crucial for proper embryonic development.
2. Intraembryonic mesoderm is essential for the formation of the musculoskeletal and cardiovascular systems.
3. Presence of sacrococcygeal teratomas can be traced back to primitive streak remnants.
4. Defects in ectoderm differentiation can cause neurodevelopmental disorders.
5. Notochord doesn't form vertebral column.

MULTIPLE CHOICE QUESTIONS

1. Apical ligament of dens is a remnant of:
   A. Primitive streak
   B. Neural plate
   C. Notochord
   D. Primitive node

2. Bilateral symmetry is established by:
   A. Hypoblast
   B. Epiblast
   C. Mesoderm
   D. Primitive streak

3. Genitourinary system develops from:
   A. Lateral plate mesoderm
   B. Intermediate mesoderm
   C. Paraxial mesoderm
   D. Extraembryonic mesoderm

4. Which gestational age shows oval shaped embryonic disc?
   A. 18th day
   B. 20th day
   C. 12th day
   D. 15th/16th day

5. A 28-year-old pregnant woman is found to have a fetus with an open neural tube defect. At what stage of development did the defect most likely occur, and which process was primarily involved?
   A. Second week, formation of the bilaminar disc
   B. First week, implantation
   C. Third week, neurulation
   D. Fifth week, organogenesis

6. During a routine ultrasound, a fetus is found to have a sacrococcygeal teratoma. This tumor arises from remnants of which embryonic structure, and at which developmental stage does this occur?
   A. Notochord, during neurulation
   B. Primitive streak, during gastrulation
   C. Neural crest cells, during neural tube closure
   D. Somites, during segmentation

7. A newborn presents with vertebral anomalies. During which event of the third week of development might these anomalies have originated, and which structure is primarily involved?
   A. Gastrulation, involving the ectoderm
   B. Formation of the notochord, involving the mesoderm
   C. Neural tube closure, involving the ectoderm
   D. Somite differentiation, involving the mesoderm

8. A pregnant woman is exposed to a teratogenic agent at the end of the third week of gestation. Which of the following structures is most likely to be affected, potentially leading to major congenital anomalies?
   A. Amniotic cavity
   B. Bilaminar germ disc
   C. Trilaminar germ disc
   D. Chorionic cavity

Answers: 1. C 2. D 3. B 4. D 5. C 6. B 7. B 8. C

CHAPTER 7

Embryonic Period (Fourth to Eighth Week) of Development

COMPETENCIES COVERED/LEARNING OUTCOMES

The student should be able to:

AN79.4	Describe the development of somites and intraembryonic coelom.
AN79.6	Diagnosis of pregnancy in first trimester.
AN80.1	Describe formation, functions and fate of—chorion; amnion; yolk sac; allantois and decidua.
AN80.2	Describe the formation and structure of umbilical cord.

❖ Period from *fourth to eighth week* is called *embryonic period*. During fourth week there is differentiation of three germ layers and folding of the embryonic disc to form the species specific shape of embryo.

❖ The important observable feature during the fourth week of development is the appearance of mesodermal *somites* on each side of the midline.

❖ During the second month, the primordia of organs are formed from the various germ layers. Hence, it is also known as *period of organogenesis*.

❖ **Functional subdivision of germ layer derivatives:** The ectodermal derivatives are means for protection as the epidermis of skin and its accessory structure, nervous system are developed from it. The endodermal derivatives are meant for nutrition and the digestive and respiratory systems develop from it. The mesodermal derivatives are the musculoskeletal, cardiovascular, urogenital systems and the serous cavities.

GROWTH OF THE EMBRYO AND ITS AGE DETERMINATION

After its formation, the embryonic disc undergoes folding. This folding leads to major changes in body form (during the 4th–8th weeks of fetal life). The embryo acquires the external features of a human being. All organ systems are formed. At the end of the embryonic period, the embryo can be recognized as human even though its size in crown-rump length (CRL) is only about 30 mm.

Estimation of the Age of an Embryo

This is important for understanding the age of the embryo, i.e., gestational sac in the early stages and the effect of teratogens during this period.

For understanding the age of the embryo during embryonic period it is divided into the three stages. They are

1. **Presomite:** 15th–20th day of development. Embryos younger than 20 days are called *presomite embryos* and their age is reckoned in days. The following structures develop during this period:
   - Primitive streak
   - Notochord
   - Intraembryonic mesoderm

2. **Somite:** 20th–30th day of development. These are series of mesodermal segments. The somites begin to be seen in embryos of about 21 days old. There are 44 pairs of somites that are derived from paraxial mesoderm. Once the somites appear, the age is described in terms of the number of somites present, e.g., one-somite stage, four- somite stage, etc. When the embryo is about 30 days old, it is large enough to be measured. The age of embryo is estimated between 20th to 30th day depending on the presence of number of somites as shown in **Table 7.1 and Figure 7.1**. During this period about 3/4 pairs of somites are formed on each day.

3. **Post-somite:** 31st–55th day. The length and weight of fetus is measured by transabdominal ultrasound. During this period, the growth of embryo is expressed by two measurements. However, the measurement of the length of an aborted embryo is not as simple as it sounds, as the embryo is bent on itself and cannot be straightened without fear of damage to it. Hence, instead of measuring its full length we measure what is called the crown-rump (CR) length.
   - *Crown-rump length* (CRL): It is the sitting height measured from the vertex of the skull to the midpoint between the apices of the buttocks. Various other measurements are also used. For example (with the use of ultrasound), we can measure the dimensions of some parts of the fetus (e.g., head, foot length).

Chapter 7: Embryonic Period (Fourth to Eighth Week) of Development

TABLE 7.1: Number of somites correlated with age of embryo and appearance of structures.

Age of embryo in days	No. of somite pairs	Structures that develop during the period
20	1–4	Formation of neural plate, neural folds and neural groove
21	4–8	Fusion of endocardial heart tubes
22	8–12	• Otic placode appears • Optic sulcus appears
23	12–16	Formation of lens and otic placodes
24	16–20	1st and 2nd pair of pharyngeal arches appear
25	20–24	• Closure of anterior neuropore • 3rd–5th pair of pharyngeal arches appear
26	24–28	• Upper limb bud appear • Primitive streak disappear
27	28–32	Closure of posterior neuropore
28	32–36	Lower limb bud appears
29	36–40	Limb buds become paddle-shaped
30	40–44	Face development begins

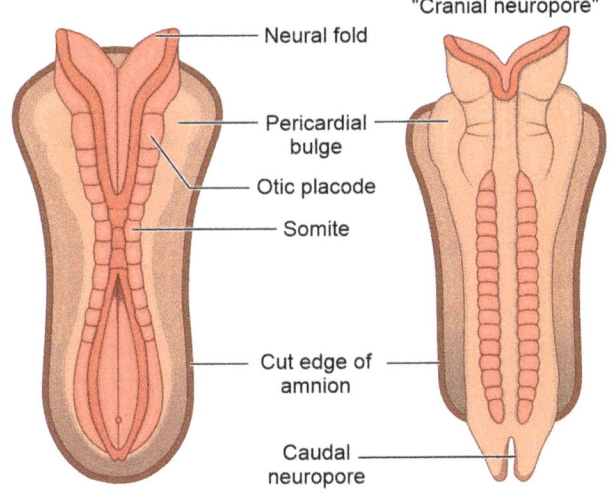

FIG. 7.1: Somite embryo—formation of neural folds and closure of neuropores.

- *Crown-heel length* (CHL): It is the standing height measured from the vertex of the skull to the heel.

Clinical correlation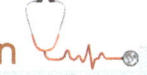

- Gestational sac is the first structure that an obstetrician looks during an early ultrasound in a married woman who comes with a history of missed periods or amenorrhea.
- When gestational sac is seen in transvaginal ultrasound between 3–5 weeks of gestation, it is positive sign of pregnancy.
- Between 5–7 weeks gestation a fetal pole or fetal heart beat can be detected. The fetal pole is the first visible sign of embryo which presents a curve with embryo's head at one end and the tail at the other end.
- Sometimes gestational sac is seen, but it is empty without evidence of an embryo by 6 weeks of gestation.
- The gestational sac increases at the rate of 1 mm per day during the first trimester.
- The yolk sac will be visible from 5th week of gestation and its mean diameter is about 6 mm at 10 weeks of gestation.

EMBRYONIC PERIOD

The changes during the embryonic period can be studied under the following headings:
- Folding of embryo
- Derivatives of ectoderm
- Derivatives of mesoderm
- Derivatives of endoderm

FOLDING OF EMBRYO

The changes that now take place will be best understood by a careful study of **Figures 7.2A to E.**
- There is progressive increase in the size of the embryonic disc due to rapid growth of cells of central part of embryonic disc and rapid growth of somites. The growth at the peripheral parts of disc is slow. This results in formation of a head fold, a tail fold and two lateral folds at the end of 3rd week of development.
- This causes conversion of flat pear-shaped germ disc into a *cylindrical embryo* **(Fig. 7.2A)**.
- The head and tail ends of the disc (X, Y), however, remain relatively close together. Hence, the increased length of the disc causes it to bulge upwards into the amniotic cavity **(Figs. 7.2B and C)**.
- With further enlargement, the edges of embryonic disc become folded on itself in the median and in the transverse planes. The folding in the median plane form ventrally directed *head fold* and *tail fold* **(Figs. 7.2D and E)**. The folding in the transverse plane forms ventrally directed *lateral folds*.
- Cephalocaudal folding is due to rapid, longitudinal growth of central nervous system. Lateral foldings are due to rapid growth of somites that convert the embryo into a tubular structure.

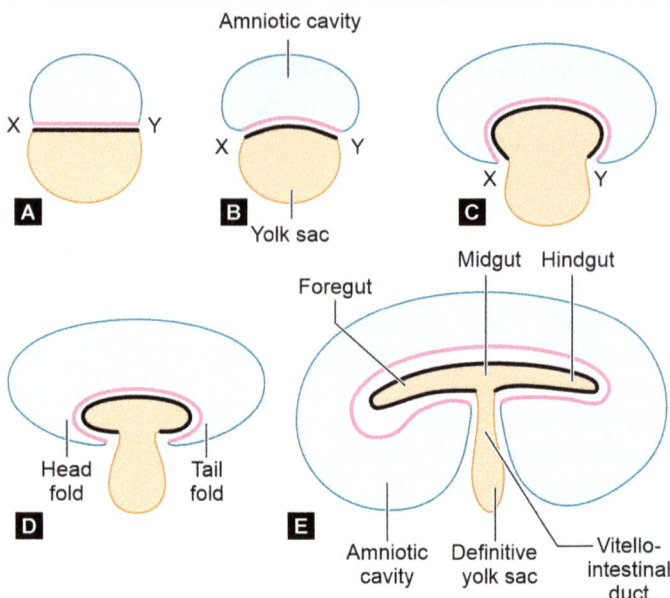

FIGS. 7.2A to E: Formation of head and tail folds and establishment of the gut.

❖ These are not three separate folds but occur simultaneously and merge into one another. The notochord, neural tube and somites stiffen the dorsal axis of the embryo making it more foldable.
❖ With the formation of the head and tail folds, parts of the yolk sac become enclosed within the embryo. In this way, a tube lined by endoderm is formed in the embryo. This is the *primitive gut*, from which most of the gastrointestinal tract is derived **(Figs. 7.2B to E)**. At first, the gut is in wide communication with the yolk sac. The part of the gut cranial to this communication and in the head fold is called the *foregut*; the part caudal to the communication and in the tail fold is called the *hindgut*; while the intervening part is called the *midgut* that is formed due to the formation of lateral folds that converge ventrally **(Fig. 7.2E)**. The communication with the yolk sac becomes progressively narrower. As a result of these changes, the yolk sac becomes small and inconspicuous, and is now termed the *definitive yolk sac* (also called the *umbilical vesicle*). The narrow channel connecting it to the gut is called the *vitellointestinal duct* (also called *vitelline duct; yolk stalk* or *omphalomesenteric duct*). This duct becomes elongated and eventually disappears.
❖ As the head and tail folds are forming, similar folds are also formed on each side in transverse or horizontal plane. These are the *lateral folds*. As a result, the embryo comes to be enclosed all around by ectoderm except in the region through which the *vitellointestinal duct (omphalomesenteric duct)* passes. Here, there is a circular aperture which may now be called the *umbilical opening* **(Fig. 7.2E)**.
❖ The folding facilitates growth and expansion of amniotic cavity that comes to surround the embryo on all sides. In this way, the embryo now floats in the amniotic fluid, which fills the cavity.
❖ Convergence of folds on ventral surface forms tubular investment of amnion for connecting stalk. This causes obliteration of extraembryonic coelom. Now, the amnion forms a covering for the umbilical cord.
❖ The events resulting from various folds are presented in **Table 7.2**.

TABLE 7.2: Events resulting from various embryonic folds.

Head fold	Tail fold	Lateral folds
Formation of *foregut*	Formation of *hindgut*	Encloses the part of yolk sac that becomes *midgut*
Opening of *stomodeum* into the amniotic cavity	Invagination of ectoderm to form ectodermal *cloaca*	Convergence of lateral folds with head and tail folds at the primitive umbilical ring forms the amnio-ectodermal junction
Pericardial cavity and cardiogenic mesoderm lies ventral to the foregut	Ventral shifting of connecting stalk	The intraembryonic coelom surrounds the gut tube. The communication between the intra- and extraembryonic coeloms becomes constricted and eventually obliterated
Transverse mesoderm between the pericardial cavity and the yolk sac—**septum transversum**	Ventral shifting of allantoic diverticulum	Splanchnopleuric intraembryonic mesoderm invests the ventrolateral surfaces of the primitive gut. It is reflected dorsolaterally as a bilaminar fold, the dorsal *mesentery of the gut*
Amniotic cavity—extends ventral to the cranial end of the embryo	**Amniotic cavity**—extension ventral to the caudal end of the embryo	The intraembryonic coelom becomes well defined and forms the peritoneal cavity. The intermediate mesoderm projects into it from the dorsal aspect, on either side of dorsal mesentery
Yolk sac is constricted from cranial end	Constriction of yolk sac from the caudal end	The part of yolk sac lying outside the embryonic folds becomes the umbilical vesicle. The temporary communication between the umbilical vesicle and the midgut is the vitellointestinal duct that traverses through the umbilical cord

Formation of Umbilical Cord

With the formation of extraembryonic coelom, the embryo (along with the amniotic cavity and yolk sac) remains attached to the trophoblast only by extraembryonic mesoderm into which the coelom does not extend **(Fig. 7.3A to F)**. This extraembryonic mesoderm forms the *connecting stalk*.

The trophoblast, and the tissues of the uterus, together form an important organ, the *placenta*. The importance of the connecting stalk is obvious when we see that this is the only connecting link between the embryo and the placenta.

- As the embryo grows, the area of attachment of the connecting stalk to it becomes relatively smaller. Gradually, this attachment is seen only near the caudal end of the embryonic disc **(Figs. 7.3D and E)**.
- With the formation of the tail fold, the attachment of the connecting stalk moves (with the tail end of the embryonic disc) to the ventral aspect of the embryo. It is now attached in the region of the umbilical opening **(Fig. 7.3F)**.
- By now, blood vessels have developed in the embryo, and also in the placenta. These sets of blood vessels are in communication by means of arteries and veins passing through the connecting stalk. At first, there are two arteries and two veins in the connecting stalk, but later the right vein disappears (the left vein is 'left').

It is clear from **Figure 7.3F** that, at this stage, the amnion has a circular attachment to the margins of the umbilical opening and forms a wide tube in which the following lie:

- Vitellointestinal duct and remnants of the yolk sac.
- Mesoderm (extraembryonic) of the connecting stalk. This mesoderm gets converted into a gelatinous substance called Wharton's jelly. It protects blood vessels in the umbilical cord.
- Blood vessels that pass from the embryo to placenta.
- A small part of the extraembryonic coelom.

This tube of amnion, and the structures within it, constitutes the *umbilical cord* **(Fig. 7.4)**. This cord progressively increases in length to allow free movement of the embryo within the amniotic cavity.

Allantoic Diverticulum

- Before the formation of the tail fold (during 3rd week), a small tubular endodermal diverticulum called the *allantoic diverticulum* arises from the yolk sac near the caudal end of the embryonic disc **(Fig. 7.4E)**.
- This diverticulum grows into the extraembryonic mesoderm of the connecting stalk.
- After the formation of the tail fold, part of this diverticulum is absorbed into the hindgut (that forms the urinary bladder). It now passes from the ventral side of the hindgut into the connecting stalk **(Fig. 7.4F)**.
- During second month, the extraembryonic part of allantoic diverticulum degenerates.
- It distends and acts as a reservoir for the urinary system in lower vertebrates. In the human embryo part of it is absorbed into the primitive urinary bladder (3rd month) and the remaining intraembryonic part

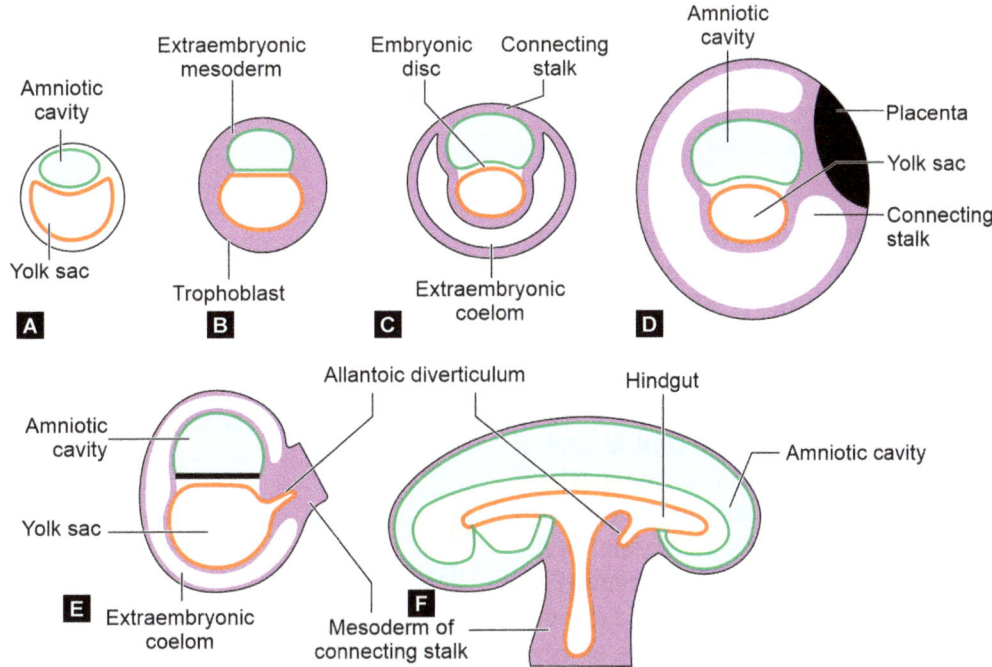

FIGS. 7.3A to F: Stages in the establishment of the umbilical cord, allantoic diverticulum and its relationship to the connecting stalk.

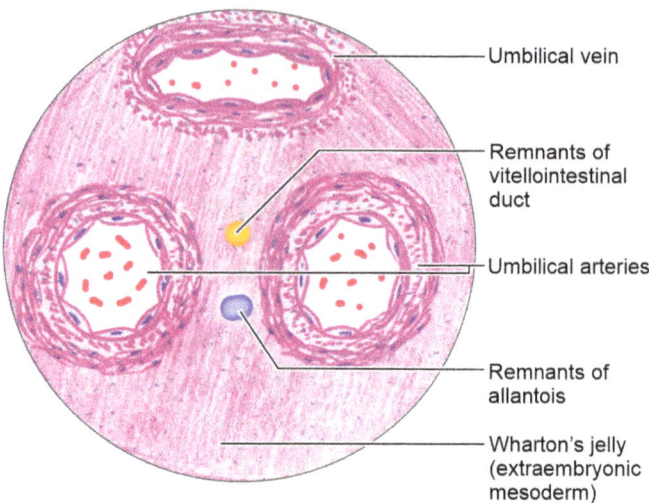

FIG. 7.4: Section through umbilical cord.

extends from the urinary bladder to umbilical cord as a thick tube called *urachus*. After birth the urachus forms the *median umbilical ligament* (extends from apex of urinary bladder to umbilicus).

❖ The blood vessels develop in allantois during 3rd–5th months that later become the *umbilical vessels*.

Effect of Head and Tail Folds on Positions of Other Structures

Just before the formation of the head and tail folds, the structures in the embryonic disc are oriented, as shown in **Figures 7.5 and 7.6** and in **Table 7.2**. A median (midline) section across the disc, at this stage, is shown in **Figure 7.5A**. From the *cranial to the caudal end*, the structures seen in the midline are the:

❖ Septum transversum
❖ Developing pericardial cavity and the heart
❖ Prochordal plate
❖ Neural plate
❖ Primitive streak
❖ Cloacal membrane

Note that the primitive streak is now inconspicuous. After folding, the relative positions of these structures change to that shown in **Figures 7.5B and C**. The important points to note here are as follows (**Fig. 7.7 and Table 7.2**):

❖ With the formation of head fold, the developing *pericardial cavity* comes to lie on the ventral side of the embryo, ventral to the foregut. The *heart*, which was developing in the splanchnopleuric mesoderm (cardiogenic plate) in the floor of the pericardial cavity (**Fig. 7.5A**), now lies in the roof of the cavity (**Fig. 7.5B**). The pericardium enlarges rapidly, and forms a conspicuous bulging on the ventral side of the embryo (**Fig. 7.5C**).

❖ The *septum transversum*, which was the most cranial structure in the embryonic disc, now lies caudal to the heart (**Fig. 7.5B**). At a later stage of development, the diaphragm and liver develop in relation to the septum transversum.

❖ The region of the *prochordal plate* now forms the buccopharyngeal or oral membrane, which closes the foregut cranially. When this membrane breaks down (during 4th week), the foregut communicates with the exterior and now the amniotic fluid can enter the gut.

❖ The most cranial structure of the embryo is now the enlarged cranial part of the neural tube, which later forms the brain (**Fig. 7.5B**). This enlarges enormously (**Fig. 7.5C**). There are now two big bulgings on the ventral aspect of the embryo. Cranially, there is the

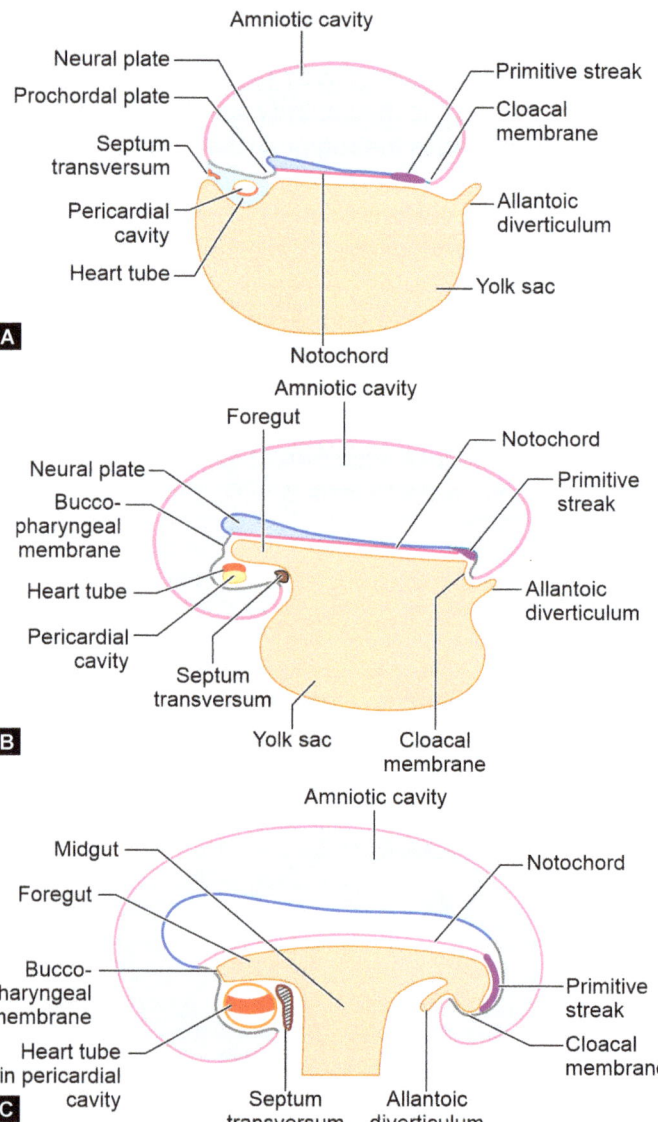

FIGS. 7.5A to C: A to C are embryonic disc-related structures before (A), during (B) and after (C) formation of head and tail folds. Note the changing relationships of septum transversum, pericardium, buccopharyngeal membrane, cloacal membrane and allantois.

Chapter 7: Embryonic Period (Fourth to Eighth Week) of Development

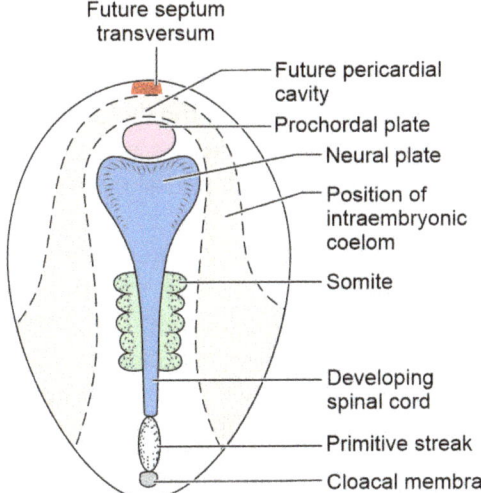

FIG. 7.6: Embryonic disc showing structures from cranial to caudal end.

developing brain, and a little below it there is the bulging pericardium **(Fig. 7.5C)**. In between these two, there is a depression called the *stomatodeum or stomodeum*, the floor of which is formed by the buccopharyngeal membrane.

❖ Towards the tail end of the embryo, the primitive streak is now an inconspicuous structure that gradually disappears. The distal end of the hindgut is closed by the *cloacal membrane*. At first, this is directed caudally **(Fig. 7.5B)**, but later it comes to face ventrally **(Fig. 7.5C)**.

We have traced the development of the embryo to a stage when the rudiments of the nervous system, the heart and the gut have been formed. *We are now in a position to trace the development of individual organ systems in detail in the chapters of Nervous System, Cardiovascular System and Alimentary System.*

DERIVATIVES OF GERM LAYERS

Ectoderm

Surface Ectoderm

Derivatives of surface ectoderm are:

❖ **Buccopharyngeal membrane:** With the formation of head fold the surface ectoderm lines a surface depression, *the stomodeum or primitive oral cavity.*

❖ **Cloacal membrane:** With the formation of tail fold the surface ectoderm lines *the proctodeum or ectodermal cloaca*. The cloacal membrane lines the proctodeum. Later, the cloacal membrane is divided into anal and urogenital membranes.

❖ **Protective covering:** These are epidermis, hairs, nails, sebaceous and sweat glands. *Details will be described in the chapter on Development of Skin and its Appendages.*

❖ **Special sense organs:** Olfactory pit, optic and lens vesicles, otic vesicle, branchial clefts, Rathke's pouch, mammary gland, pituitary gland. *Details will be described in the chapters on Development of Eye, Ear, Pharyngeal Arches, Mammary Gland and Endocrine Glands.*

❖ **Others:** Parts of mouth, salivary glands, nasal cavity and paranasal air sinuses. *Details will be discussed in the chapters on Development of Alimentary System and Respiratory System.*

Neuroectoderm and Neural Crest Cells

❖ During third week of development, the surface ectoderm overlying the developing notochord thickens to form the *neural plate* or *neuroectoderm* which takes part in formation of CNS and PNS.

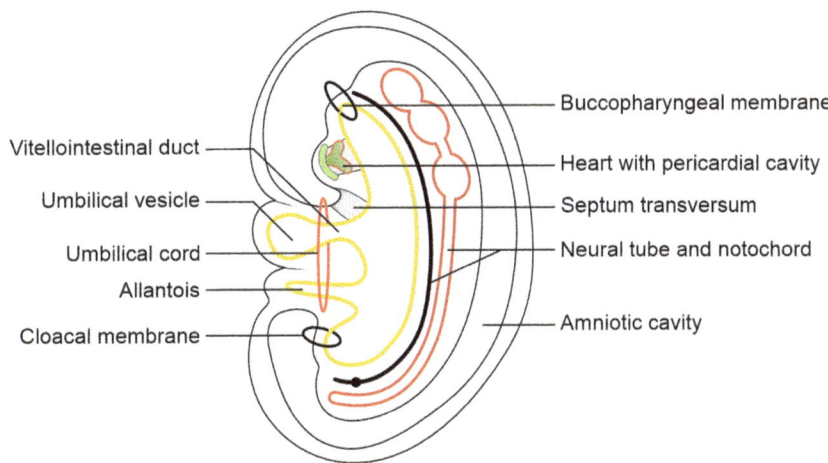

FIG. 7.7: Arrangement of embryonic structures after the formation of head and tail folds in a sagittal section.

Intraembryonic Mesoderm

Paraxial Mesoderm

- The developing otic capsules (membranous labyrinth) divide the paraxial mesoderm into preotic and postotic parts. The preotic part is unsegmented whereas the postotic part shows 40± 44 pairs of segments called *somites*.
- The somites appear from day 20 to day 30 in craniocaudal sequence.
- The somites are triangular in shape. Each somite differentiates into three parts:
  1. *Dermatome*: It forms segmental dermis of the skin.
  2. *Sclerotome*: It helps to form the vertebral column and ribs.
  3. *Myotome*: It forms skeletal muscle.
- Each dermatome and myotome has a segmental nerve supply which is retained no matter where the cells migrate.

  The somites will be discussed in detail in the Chapter 10.

Intermediate Mesoderm

- It temporarily connects paraxial mesoderm with lateral plate mesoderm.
- It contributes for the development of kidneys, gonads and the duct system of urinary and genital systems.

  The intermediate mesoderm will be discussed in detail in the chapters on Urinary and Genital Systems.

Lateral Plate Mesoderm

- It is the unsegmented part of intraembryonic mesoderm which also forms intraembryonic coelom.
- The pleural, pericardial and peritoneal cavities develop from the intraembryonic coelom.
- The two layers of mesoderm:
  1. *Somatopleuric layer:* It forms the parietal layer for the coelomic cavities, dermis and subcutaneous tissues of the body wall and skeletal elements of limbs.
  2. *Splanchnopleuric layer:* The layer in contact with endoderm is called splanchnopleuric intraembryonic mesoderm and it contributes for the visceral layer of coelomic cavities, musculature and connective tissue of gastrointestinal and respiratory tracts and the heart.
- The *septum transversum*, part of the intraembryonic mesoderm, forms the diaphragm and separates the pericardial cavity from the rest of the intraembryonic coelom.

Endoderm

With the formation of head fold and tail fold the endodermal yolk sac gets incorporated into the embryo to form the primitive.

- The *gastrointestinal tract* is the main organ system derived from the endodermal germ layer.
- *Further development* gives rise to, (a) epithelial lining of the respiratory tract, (b) the parenchyma of the thyroid, parathyroid, liver and pancreas, (c) reticular stroma of the tonsils and thymus, (d) epithelial lining of urinary bladder and urethra, (e) epithelial lining of the tympanic cavity and auditory tube.

HIGHLIGHTS

- The *embryonic disc* undergoes folding at the cranial and caudal ends. These are the *head and tail folds*. *Lateral folds* also appear. As a result of these folds, the endoderm is converted into a tube, *the primitive gut*. It is divisible into *foregut*, *midgut* and *hindgut*.
- After formation of the head fold the gut is closed cranially by the prochordal plate, which is now called the *buccopharyngeal membrane*. Caudally, the gut is closed by the *cloacal membrane*.
- The *umbilical cord* develops from the connecting stalk. It contains the right and left umbilical arteries, the left umbilical vein, and remnants of the vitellointestinal duct and yolk sac.
- The *allantoic diverticulum* arises from the yolk sac before the formation of the primitive gut. After formation of the tail fold, it is seen as a diverticulum of the hindgut.
- The *pericardial cavity* is derived from part of the *intraembryonic coelom* that lies cranial to the prochordal plate. The developing heart lies ventral to the cavity. After formation of the head fold the pericardial cavity lies ventral to the foregut; and the developing heart is dorsal to the pericardial cavity.
- The *septum transversum* is made of *intraembryonic mesoderm* that lies cranial to the pericardial cavity. After formation of the head fold, it lies caudal to the pericardium and heart. The liver and the diaphragm develop in relation to the septum transversum.

Chapter 7: Embryonic Period (Fourth to Eighth Week) of Development

Summary

- Derivatives of three germ layers **(Table 7.3)**

TABLE 7.3: Structured that are derived from three germ layers.

Ectoderm	Mesoderm	Endoderm
• Epidermis of skin • Hair, nails • Epithelium of all orifices • Lens of eye • Central nervous system (CNS) • Peripheral nervous system (PNS) • Neural crest cells (sensory neurons, melanocytes, adrenal medulla) • Sensory epithelium • Enamel of teeth • Subcutaneous glands (sweat, sebaceous) • Mammary glands • Pituitary gland	• Muscles (skeletal, smooth, cardiac) • Bones, cartilage • Connective tissue (tendons, ligaments) • Blood and lymphatic vessels • Blood cells • Heart • Kidneys, ureter • Gonads (testes, ovaries) • Uterus and vagina • Dermis of skin • Adrenal cortex • Pericardium, pleura, peritoneum	Epithelial lining of: • Digestive tract including liver and pancreas • Respiratory tract • Urinary bladder • Urethra • Pharyngotympanic tube • Tympanic cavity • Tonsils **Glands** • Thyroid gland • Parathyroid glands • Thymus

TEST YOUR UNDERSTANDING

REVIEW QUESTIONS

1. Write a short note on folding of embryo.
2. Enumerate the derivatives of three germ layers.
3. Discuss the development of connecting stalk.
4. Discuss formation of blood vessels.
5. Discuss significance of allantois diverticulum.
6. Discuss the effects of folding on embryo.

EXPLAIN WHY? (REASONING QUESTIONS)

1. Proper embryonic folding is crucial organogenesis.
2. Improper segmentation of somites can lead to musculoskeletal abnormalities.

MULTIPLE CHOICE QUESTIONS

1. What is umbilical vesicle?
   A. Primitive gut tube
   B. Vitillointestinal duct
   C. Definitive yolk sac
   D. Amniotic cavity
2. Degeneration of extraembryonic part of allantoic diverticulum occurs at:
   A. 7th month
   B. 2nd month
   C. 5th month
   D. 3rd month
3. Lower limb buds start to appear at:
   A. 15 days
   B. 10 days
   C. 28 days
   D. 35 days
4. During the 4th week of development, the embryonic folding process is crucial for:
   A. Forming the amniotic cavity
   B. Establishing the basic body plan of the embryo
   C. Differentiating the three germ layers
   D. Initiating placental development
5. Which of the following is a derivative of the ectoderm?
   A. Kidneys
   B. Liver
   C. Nervous system
   D. Heart
6. The mesodermal germ layer gives rise to which of the following structures?
   A. Epidermis of the skin
   B. Lungs
   C. Skeletal muscles
   D. Intestinal lining

Chapter 7: Embryonic Period (Fourth to Eighth Week) of Development

7. What is the significance of the connecting stalk during the embryonic period?
   A. It forms the central nervous system
   B. It links the embryo to the placenta
   C. It differentiates into the gut tube
   D. It forms the amniotic cavity

8. A newborn is found to have an imperforate anus, where the anal opening is absent. This condition is likely due to an issue in the development of which germ layer derivative?
   A. Ectoderm
   B. Mesoderm
   C. Endoderm
   D. Neural crest cells

9. An infant is diagnosed with congenital diaphragmatic hernia, where abdominal organs herniate into the chest cavity. This anomaly suggests a developmental defect in which structure formed during embryonic folding?
   A. Neural tube
   B. Septum transversum
   C. Primitive streak
   D. Notochord

10. A patient has a congenital heart defect. During embryonic development, which germ layer primarily contributes to the formation of the heart?
    A. Ectoderm
    B. Mesoderm
    C. Endoderm
    D. Trophoblast

Answers: 1. C   2. B   3. C   4. B   5. C
           6. C   7. B   8. C   9. B   10. B

Fetal Period of Development, Prenatal Diagnosis and Teratology

CHAPTER 8

COMPETENCIES COVERED/LEARNING OUTCOMES

The student should be able to:

AN79.6	Describe the diagnosis of pregnancy in first trimester and role of teratogens, alpha-fetoproteins.
AN80.6	Explain embryological basis of estimation of fetal age.
AN81.1	Describe various methods of prenatal diagnosis.
AN81.2	Describe indications, process and disadvantages of amniocentesis.
AN81.3	Describe indications, process and disadvantages of chorion villus biopsy.

At the beginning of *fetal period (9th week to 3rd month)* the embryo has developed into a recognizable human being and the primordia of all organ system have formed. From 9th week onwards the embryo is called *fetus*.

During the fetal period, development is mainly directed towards the rapid growth in body size and towards differentiation of tissues, organs and organ systems **(Fig. 8.1)**. The growth of the head is slow as compared to that of the rest of body. At the beginning of third month, the head is half the crown-rump (CR) length, while at birth, it is about one fourth of CR length. Fetal weight gain is very rapid in the last month of pregnancy.

FETAL PERIOD

- Extends from the beginning of the *3rd month to the end of pregnancy.*
- Characterized by *maturation of tissues and organs* and rapid growth of the body.
- The length of the fetus is indicated as the *crown-rump length* or *crown-heel length*.
- The *first half* of this period is characterized by a *rapid growth in length*, the *second half*, a *rapid increase in weight.*
- It is associated with complete development of the placenta, umbilical cord and fetal membranes.
- The *length of pregnancy* is considered to be *40 weeks* after the onset of the last menstrual period or *38 weeks* after fertilization.
- **In the 3rd month:**
  - Fetal head forms about 1/2 the CR length.
  - Face assumes a human form.
  - Upper extremity exceeds in length the lower one.
  - External genitalia become apparent, sex differentiation is possible to ascertain.
  - Intestinal loop in the *physiological hernia* is withdrawn into the abdominal cavity.
  - Primary ossification centers are present in the long bones and the skull.
- **In the 4th and 5th months:**
  - The fetus lengthens rapidly, the weight of the fetus increasing little.

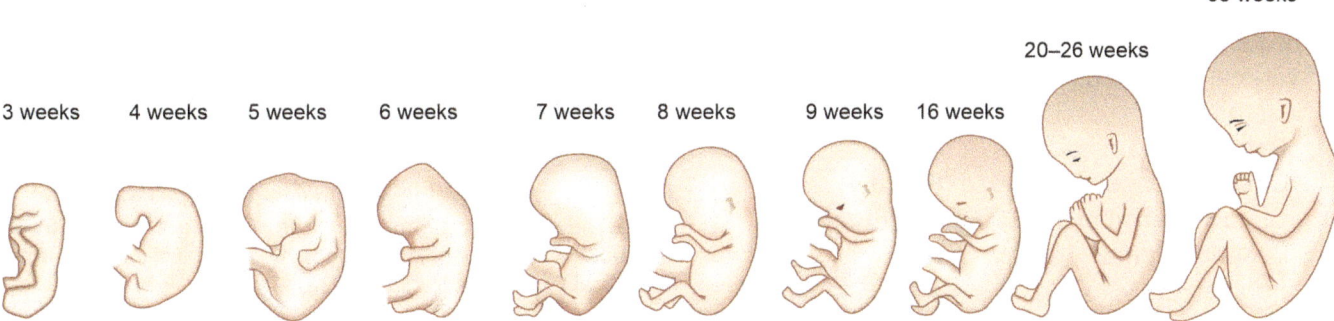

FIG. 8.1: Changes in external appearance and body proportions at different gestational ages.

- The head measures about 1/3 the CR length.
- The fetus is covered with fine hair, called *lanugo hair*.
- Eyebrows and head hair are also visible.
- During the 5th month movements of the fetus can be felt by the mother, known as *"quickening"*.

❖ **2nd half of pregnancy:**
  - Weight increases considerably.
  - Fetal head is reduced to 1/4 of the CR length.
  - Lower extremity exceeds in length the upper extremity.
  - In the *6th month* the skin of the fetus is reddish and has a *wrinkled appearance*.
  - By the end of the *7th month* the fetus is capable of an independent existence, pulmonary respiration being established, therefore called *viable age of the fetus*. According to MTP Act of India 1971, fetus is viable at the age of 24 weeks.
  - During the last 2 months the fetus assumes a well rounded contour and is covered by *vernix caseosa*.

❖ **Full-term fetus:**
  - Weight is around 2500–3,000 g and crown-heel length (CHL) is around 50 cm, the head having the largest circumference of all parts of the body.
  - Sexual characteristics are pronounced, the testes have completely descended into the scrotum.
  - An ossific center appears at the lower end of the femur.
  - The umbilical cord is attached near the center of the anterior abdominal wall.

DETERMINING THE AGE OF A LIVING FETUS

The ability to find out the age of a living fetus is very important clinically. The age of such a fetus can be determined by making measurements using ultrasound examination. Various structures are visible on USG **(Fig. 8.2)**

❖ Between 7 and 14 weeks, the CRL length can be measured **(Fig. 8.3)**. This is the most common and accurate method of fetal age estimation during early pregnancy.

❖ Estimation of fetal age in the second and third trimesters of pregnancy is based on the measurements of various body parts.
  These are:
  - Biparietal diameter
  - Circumference of the head **(Fig. 8.4)**
  - Circumference of the abdomen **(Fig. 8.5)**
  - Length of femur
  - Foot length

Estimation of fetal age facilitates management of pregnancy. The various congenital anomalies that can be identified include neural tube defects like anencephaly **(Fig. 8.6)**, encephalocele spina bifida, abdominal wall

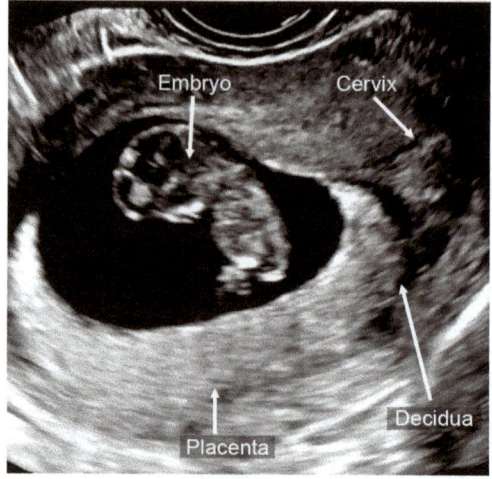

FIG. 8.2: Developing embryo with placenta and decidua. (Reproduced with permission from Dr Hiralal Konar. Source: Chapter 42. In: Konar H, Textbook of Obstetrics, Jaypee Brothers Medical Publishers Pvt Ltd, 2023).

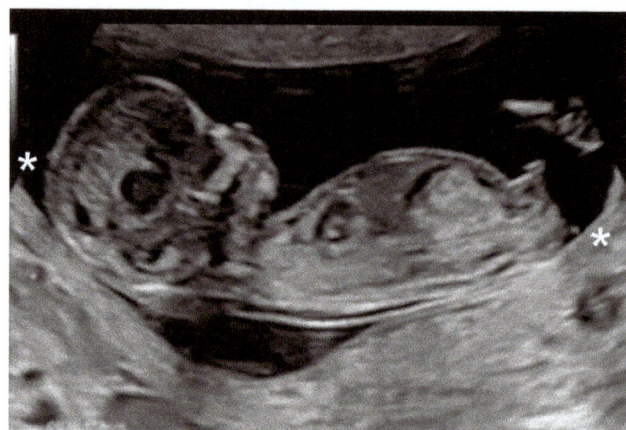

FIG. 8.3: USG showing measurement of crown-rump length (CRL).
(Reproduced with permission from Dr Hiralal Konar. Source: Chapter 42. In: Konar H, Textbook of Obstetrics, Jaypee Brothers Medical Publishers Pvt Ltd, 2023).

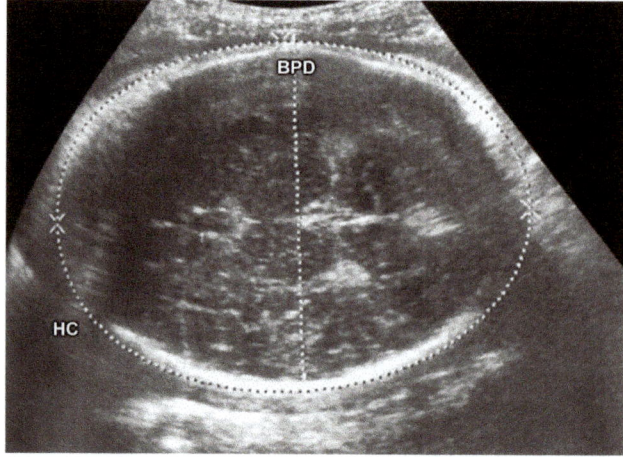

FIG. 8.4: Ultrasound image of fetal head.
(Reproduced with permission from Dr Hiralal Konar. Source: Chapter 42. In: Konar H, Textbook of Obstetrics, Jaypee Brothers Medical Publishers Pvt Ltd, 2023).

Chapter 8: Fetal Period of Development, Prenatal Diagnosis and Teratology

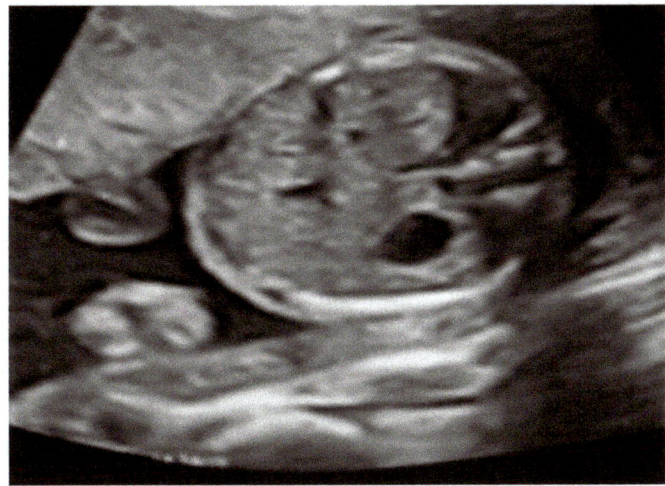

FIG. 8.5: Ultrasound image of fetal abdomen (24 weeks). (Reproduced with permission from Dr Hiralal Konar. Source: Chapter 42. In: Konar H, Textbook of Obstetrics, Jaypee Brothers Medical Publishers Pvt Ltd, 2023).

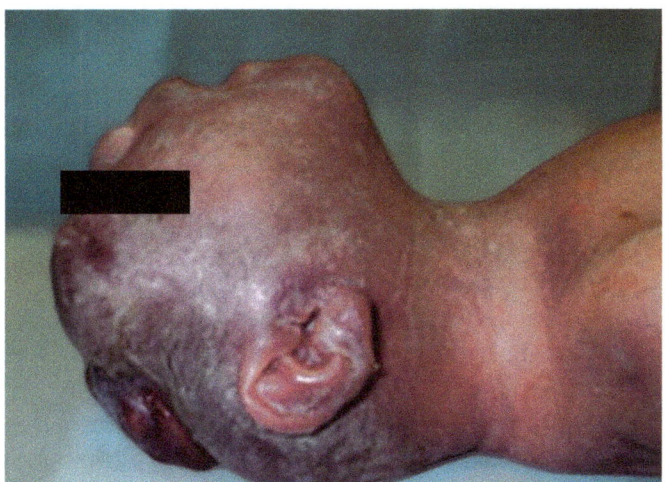

FIG. 8.6: Anencephalic aborted fetus.

defects like omphalocele, facial defects, cleft lip and palate, etc.

TERATOLOGY AND BIRTH DEFECTS

Teratology is the branch of science that studies the causes, mechanisms, and patterns of abnormal development, particularly focusing on birth defects and congenital malformations.

It examines how various environmental, genetic, and maternal factors influence the development of the fetus, leading to structural or functional anomalies.

Embryological Importance

- The study of teratology is important in embryology, as many birth defects originate during the different periods of embryonic and fetal development.
- During the *first trimester*, the embryo undergoes rapid cell division, differentiation, and organogenesis, making this period *highly susceptible* to teratogenic influences.
- Disruptions in these processes can lead to congenital abnormalities, which are often classified based on the affected embryonic tissues and the timing of exposure to teratogens.

Various Theories of Teratogenicity

- **Genotype of the embryo and maternal genome:** The genetic makeup of the embryo and the mother significantly influence susceptibility to teratogens. Some genetic mutations may predispose the embryo to defects.
- **Timing of exposure:** The most critical period for teratogenic effects is during organogenesis, typically between the *3rd and 8th weeks of gestation*.
- **Dose and duration:** The severity of birth defects often correlates with the dose and duration of exposure to the teratogen. Higher doses and prolonged exposure increase the risk of significant anomalies.
- **Specificity:** Different teratogens affect specific tissues or organs, leading to predictable patterns of malformations.
- **Mechanism of action:** Teratogens act through various mechanisms, such as disrupting cell proliferation, apoptosis, differentiation, or interfering with genetic and molecular signaling pathways.

Manifestations of abnormal development are death, *malformation, growth retardation*, and *functional disorders*.

Types of Birth Defects

- **Congenital malformations and structural birth defects:** These involve abnormalities in the structure of body parts resulting from abnormal development during the embryonic period, such as cleft lip and palate, heart defects, spina bifida, and limb deformities.
- **Functional birth defects:** These affect how a body part or system works, such as metabolic disorders, intellectual disabilities, and sensory impairments.
- **Deformations:** These are caused by mechanical forces altering the shape of a part of the fetus, such as clubfoot due to intrauterine constraint.
- **Disruptions:** These result from the destruction of previously normal fetal tissue, such as limb defects caused by amniotic band syndrome.
- **Dysplasias:** These involve abnormal organization of cells in tissues, leading to structural anomalies and impaired function. Examples include skeletal dysplasias like achondroplasia and thanatophoric dysplasia.

Causes of Birth Defects

Genetic Factors

- **Chromosomal abnormalities:** This can be due to chromosomal number abnormalities involving autosomes such as Down syndrome (Trisomy 21) and Edward syndrome (Trisomy 18) or involving sex chromosomes such as Turner syndrome (45 XO) and Klinefelter syndrome (47 XXY).
  These can also be due to structural defects in chromosomes like Cat's cry syndrome (Chr 5) and Prader Willi syndrome (Chr 15).
- **Single gene mutations:** Inherited conditions like cystic fibrosis, sickle cell anemia, Marfan syndrome, and Tay-Sachs disease.
- **Multifactorial inheritance:** Conditions resulting from the interaction of multiple genes and environmental factors, such as neural tube defects, talipes, cleft lip/palate, and congenital heart disease.

Environmental Factors

- **Teratogenic drugs:** Medications like thalidomide, isotretinoin, and certain anticonvulsants can cause severe birth defects.
- **Infections:** Maternal infections such as rubella, cytomegalovirus, toxoplasmosis, syphilis, and zika virus can lead to congenital anomalies.
- **Chemical exposures:** Exposure to environmental chemicals like lead, organic mercury, and pesticides can harm fetal development.
- **Radiation:** High levels of ionizing radiation can cause mutations and structural defects in the developing fetus.
- **Maternal conditions:** Conditions like diabetes, obesity, and malnutrition can influence fetal development and increase the risk of birth defects.
- **Alcohol and substance abuse:** Alcohol consumption during pregnancy can lead to fetal alcohol spectrum disorders (FASD), and drug abuse can cause various developmental issues.

PRENATAL DIAGNOSIS OF FETUS

Prenatal diagnosis involves testing the fetus for genetic, chromosomal, and structural abnormalities before birth. These techniques help detect congenital anomalies and guide clinical management and counseling for prospective parents.

Various methods include:
- Ultrasound imaging
- Amniocentesis
- Chorionic villus sampling (CVS)
- Fetal MRI
- Maternal screening
- Alpha fetoprotein assay
- Fetoscopy
- Percutaneous umbilical cord blood sampling (PUCBS)/cordocentesis

Ultrasound Imaging

- Ultrasound imaging is a noninvasive and widely used technique in prenatal diagnosis to visualize the fetus, placenta, and amniotic fluid.
- It uses high-frequency sound waves to create images of the developing fetus, allowing for the assessment of fetal growth, development, and well-being.
- *Soft markers* are minor ultrasound findings that may be associated with an increased risk of chromosomal abnormalities or other conditions. Common soft markers include:
  - *Nuchal translucency/nuchal test:* Down syndrome
  - *Shortened femur or humerus:* Down syndrome

Amniocentesis

Amniocentesis is the invasive procedure to collect amniotic fluid in which puncture of the amniotic fluid sac is done.

Indications

- **Genetic and chromosomal testing:**
  - Advanced maternal age (over 35 years)
  - Family history of genetic disorders (e.g., Down syndrome, cystic fibrosis)
  - Abnormal results from initial screening tests [e.g., noninvasive prenatal testing (NIPT) ultrasound]
- **Assessment of fetal health:**
  - Detection of neural tube defects (e.g., spina bifida)
  - Evaluation of fetal lung maturity (in later pregnancy)
  - Diagnosis of fetal infections (e.g., cytomegalovirus)
  - Investigation of Rh incompatibility and fetal anemia
- **Evaluation of pregnancy complications:**
  - Polyhydramnios or oligohydramnios (abnormal amniotic fluid levels)
  - Monitoring in pregnancies with multiple gestations

Procedure

- Explain the procedure, risks, and benefits to the patient. Perform an ultrasound to determine the position of the fetus and the placenta.
- **Anesthesia:** Local anesthesia may be applied to numb the abdominal area.
- **Needle insertion:** A long, thin needle is inserted through the abdominal wall and uterus into the amniotic sac under continuous ultrasound guidance **(Fig. 8.7)**.

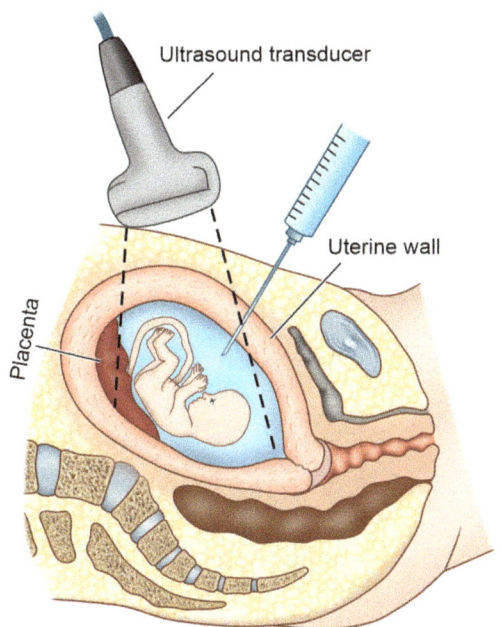

FIG. 8.7: Amniocentesis under USG guidance.

- **Fluid aspiration:** A small amount of amniotic fluid (about 20 mL) is withdrawn into a syringe.

Disadvantages or Complications

- There is a small risk of miscarriage, estimated to be about 1 in 300 to 1 in 500 procedures.
- The procedure can introduce an infection into the amniotic sac or cause uterine infections, though this is rare.
- Leakage of amniotic fluid can occur from the puncture site, which may lead to complications if it does not resolve on its own.
- There is a slight risk of needle injury to the fetus, though this is minimized by using ultrasound guidance during the procedure.

Chorionic Villus Sampling

In this procedure, a biopsy of chorionic villi is taken either by an abdominal route or by a cervical route. The procedure is performed between 10 and 12 weeks of gestation. The biopsies are used for detecting chromosomal abnormalities, inborn errors of metabolism or X-linked disorders *(refer Chapter 9 for details)*.

Alpha Fetoprotein Assay

- Alpha fetoprotein (AFP) is normally produced in the liver and in the gut of a fetus in the second trimester of pregnancy. It reaches amniotic fluid and maternal serum through the placenta.
- Its concentration increases when the fetus is suffering from congenital malformations, such as omphalocele, bladder exstrophy and intestinal atresia.
- However, its concentration decreases in a few chromosomal anomalies, such as Down's syndrome, and trisomy 18.

Fetoscopy

Fetoscopy is a minimally invasive diagnostic procedure that allows direct visualization of the fetus, amniotic cavity, umbilical cord, and placenta using a fetoscope, a specialized endoscope. This procedure is usually performed during 17th to 20th weeks of gestation.

Maternal Screening

Various screening of maternal serum is done in different stages of pregnancy. The biochemical markers tested are:
- **Pregnancy:** Associated plasma protein-A (PAPP-A)
- Free beta-human chorionic gonadotropin (β-hCG)
- α-fetoprotein (AFP)
- Unconjugated estriol
- Inhibin-A

Fetus MRI

It can be performed to get further information about conditions that have been detected in ultrasonographic images especially for fetal brain and spine. MRI is safe and provides high soft tissue contrast and resolution.

Percutaneous Umbilical Cord Blood Sampling (PUCBS/Cordocentesis)

In this procedure, fetal blood is drawn from the umbilical vein for diagnosis of many genetic conditions. The same procedure is also used for blood transfusion into the fetus or for injection of drugs. It should not be done earlier than 17th week.

FETAL THERAPY

Fetal therapy refers to a range of medical interventions performed on the developing fetus in utero to treat or manage congenital abnormalities, genetic disorders, or other medical conditions that can affect fetal development and postnatal health. Advancements in prenatal diagnostics and surgical techniques have made it possible to intervene before birth, improving outcomes for certain conditions.

Pharmacologic Therapy

Administering medications to the fetus, either through the mother or directly to the fetus. It is used in treating fetal arrhythmias, infections, or metabolic disorders. *Examples:* Digoxin for fetal tachycardia and antibiotics for fetal infections.

Fetal Surgery

Performing surgical procedures on the fetus while in utero to correct structural anomalies. *Examples:* Myelomeningocele repair for spina bifida and removal of fetal tumors (e.g., sacrococcygeal teratoma).

Intrauterine Blood Transfusion

Transfusing blood to the fetus through the umbilical vein like treating fetal anemia due to conditions like Rh incompatibility or parvovirus B19 infection.

Stem Cell Transplantation

Transplanting stem cells into the fetus to treat genetic or hematologic disorders. *Examples:* Stem cell transplantation for conditions like severe combined immunodeficiency (SCID).

Other Uses

- Gene therapy
- Amnioreduction and amnioinfusion. *Example:* Twin-to-twin transfusion syndrome.

HIGHLIGHTS

- **Fetal period:** Extends from 3rd month to term.
- **Estimation of fetal age:** It is estimated by measuring by the biparietal diameter, circumference of the abdomen, length of femur and foot length.
- **Control of fetal growth:** The various factors that control fetal growth are maternal (nutrition, hormones), placental (hormones) and fetal (genetic, endocrine).
- **Teratogenesis:** It is the study of congenital malformations. The various causes for congenital malformations are the hereditary, environmental and physical factors.
- **Prenatal diagnosis of fetal diseases and malformations:** It is by radiological imaging of fetus, biochemical and genetic analysis of amniotic fluid, chorionic villus and fetal blood like *amniocentesis, chorionic villus sampling, fetal MRI, cordocentesis, etc.*
- **Fetal therapies:** These are medical and surgical line of treatment options for treating a fetal condition or correcting an anomaly.

Summary

- Environmental teratogens are shown in **Table 8.1**

TABLE 8.1: Environmental teratogens and their associated birth defects.

Teratogen	Associated birth defects
Drugs and medications (absolute contraindication)	
Thalidomide	Limb defects (phocomelia), heart defects, ear and eye anomalies
Isotretinoin	Craniofacial defects, cardiovascular anomalies, CNS malformations
Antiepileptic drugs	Neural tube defects, craniofacial anomalies, cardiac defects
Warfarin	Nasal hypoplasia, stippled epiphyses, CNS abnormalities
ACE inhibitors	Renal dysgenesis, oligohydramnios, skull hypoplasia
Tetracycline	Discoloration of teeth, inhibition of bone growth
Methotrexate	Neural tube defects, limb abnormalities, craniofacial defects
Lithium	Ebstein's anomaly (tricuspid valve defect)
Misoprostol	Limb defects, cranial nerve palsy, skull defects
Alcohol	Fetal alcohol spectrum disorders (FASD), growth retardation, neurodevelopmental disorders
Cocaine	Placental abruption, preterm birth, low birth weight, congenital malformations

Teratogen	Associated birth defects
Infections	
Rubella	Congenital rubella syndrome, heart defects, cataracts, deafness
Cytomegalovirus (CMV)	Microcephaly, cerebral calcifications, hepatosplenomegaly
Zika virus	Microcephaly, brain defects, eye abnormalities
Toxoplasmosis	Hydrocephalus, intracranial calcifications, chorioretinitis
Chemicals and environmental exposures	
Lead	Neurodevelopmental disorders, cognitive impairments
Mercury	Neurological damage, cerebral palsy, cognitive impairments
Pesticides	Neural tube defects, limb defects, cognitive impairments
Radiation	Microcephaly, intellectual disabilities, growth retardation
Maternal conditions	
Diabetes	Cardiac defects, neural tube defects, macrosomia
Obesity	Neural tube defects, cardiac anomalies
Nutritional deficiencies	Neural tube defects (folic acid deficiency), growth retardation

TEST YOUR UNDERSTANDING

REVIEW QUESTIONS

1. Discuss the methods for determining the age of the fetus.
2. Name the factors that influence fetal growth.
3. Describe various theories of teratogenesis.
4. Write a short note on amniocentesis.
5. Discuss various prenatal diagnostic tests.
6. Discuss environmental teratogens.

EXPLAIN WHY? (REASONING QUESTIONS)

1. Teratogens more likely to cause major structural birth defects during the embryonic period compared to the fetal period.
2. Biochemical markers and ultrasound imaging used together in prenatal screening for neural tube defects.
3. Medications that cross the placental barrier pose a higher risk.

MULTIPLE CHOICE QUESTIONS

1. Which period is considered as "critical period of development"?
   A. Bilaminar germ disc formation
   B. Trilaminar germ disc formation
   C. Period of organogenesis
   D. Neural tube formation

2. Study of congenital malformations is called as:
   A. Perinatology
   B. Neonatology
   C. Teratology
   D. Genetics

3. A pregnant woman presents for her first prenatal visit. She is unsure of her last menstrual period (LMP) but reports feeling fetal movements for the past two weeks. Which method would be most accurate for estimating fetal age?
   A. Fundal height measurement
   B. Ultrasonography
   C. Maternal serum alpha-fetoprotein (AFP) levels
   D. Fetal heart rate monitoring

4. A pregnant woman is concerned about potential teratogenic effects of medications she has been taking. Which of the following factors primarily determines the extent of teratogenic risk?
   A. Maternal age
   B. Gestational age
   C. Genetic predisposition
   D. Drug dosage and timing of exposure

5. A newborn presents with characteristic facial anomalies, cardiac defects, and intellectual disability. Which teratogen is most likely responsible for these findings?
   A. Alcohol
   B. Thalidomide
   C. Retinoic acid
   D. Warfarin

6. A pregnant woman with a history of poorly controlled diabetes is at increased risk of which type of birth defect in her offspring?
   A. Neural tube defects
   B. Cardiac anomalies

   C. Cleft lip and palate
   D. Limb reduction defects

7. A pregnant woman is found to have elevated maternal serum alpha-fetoprotein (AFP) levels. Which prenatal diagnostic test would be most appropriate to confirm the presence of a neural tube defect in the fetus?
   A. Chorionic villus sampling (CVS)
   B. Amniocentesis
   C. Fetal ultrasound
   D. Maternal serum human chorionic gonadotropin (hCG) levels

8. A pregnant woman is diagnosed with severe fetal hydrops. What fetal therapy would be most appropriate to manage this condition?
   A. Intrauterine blood transfusion
   B. Maternal corticosteroid administration
   C. Maternal dietary modification
   D. Fetal surgery for amniotic band release

9. Which method is most commonly used to estimate fetal age during prenatal care?
   A. Maternal weight gain
   B. Maternal age
   C. Ultrasonography
   D. Fetal heart rate monitoring

10. Which parameter is commonly used in ultrasonography (USG) for estimating fetal age during pregnancy?
    A. Crown-rump length
    B. Fundal height measurement
    C. Maternal serum alpha-fetoprotein levels
    D. Fetal heart rate monitoring

Answers: 1. C   2. C   3. B   4. D   5. B   6. B   7. B   8. A   9. C   10. A

CHAPTER 9

Fetal Membranes, Placenta and Twinning

COMPETENCIES COVERED/LEARNING OUTCOMES

The student should be able to:

AN80.1	Describe formation, functions and fate of chorion: amnion; yolk sac; allantois and decidua.
AN80.2	Describe formation and structure of umbilical cord.
AN80.3	Describe formation of placenta, its physiological functions, fetomaternal circulation and placental barrier.
AN80.4	Describe embryological basis of twinning in monozygotic and dizygotic twins.
AN80.5	Describe role of placental hormones in uterine growth and parturition.
AN80.7	Describe various types of umbilical cord attachments.

Before studying the organogenesis in detail, we must study fetal membranes and placenta. The development of *fetal membranes* and *the placenta* is important for the nourishment and growth of the embryo and fetus. These structures facilitate the exchange of nutrients, gases, and waste between the mother and fetus, while also providing essential hormonal support to maintain pregnancy.

In this chapter, we will discuss the formation and functions of the amnion, chorion, yolk sac, and allantois, and discuss the processes involved in placental development along with the types of twinning, its embryological basis, and the clinical implications.

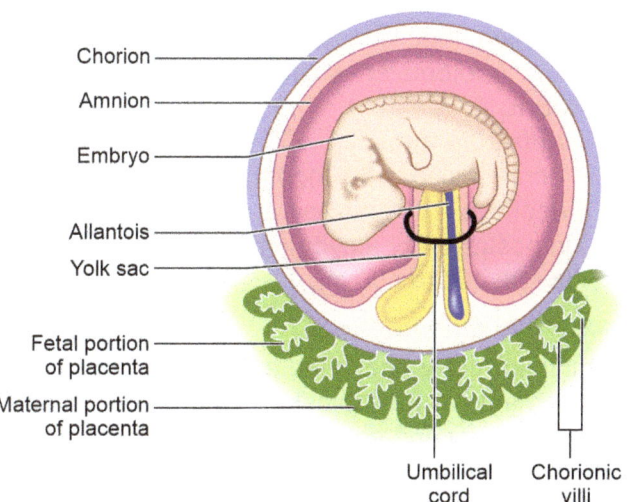

FIG. 9.1: Extraembryonic membranes.

FETAL/EXTRAEMBRYONIC MEMBRANES

Fetal membranes, also known as extraembryonic membranes, are structures that develop from the zygote but do not form part of the embryo itself.

* **Structures:** The structures that constitute the fetal membranes are **(Fig. 9.1)**:
  - Placenta formed by trophoblast and *chorion*.
  - *Amnion* or ectodermal vesicle filled with amniotic fluid covering the embryo/fetus.
  - *Yolk sac* (primary, secondary and tertiary)
  - *Allantois* or allantoenteric diverticulum
  - Connecting or body stalk and *umbilical cord*
* **Functions:** These are concerned with protection, and nutrition
  - Protection of embryo
  - Respiration through placenta
  - Excretion
  - Nutrition through amniotic fluid and umbilical cord

Clinical Importance

Prenatal diagnostic test like chorionic villus sampling and amniocentesis are performed through these structures.

Amnion and Amniotic Fluid

It is the fetal membrane that covers the embryo and forms the amniotic sac that is filled with *amniotic fluid*. It appears in the 2nd week of development.

Formation and Expansion of Amniotic Cavity

* The amniotic cavity is lined by extensions of ectodermal cells from the inner cell mass and amniogenic cells from the trophoblast (*refer* to **Figs. 5.1C and D**).

- The amniogenic cells line the roof and lateral walls of the amniotic sac, while the floor is formed by ectodermal cells.
- During the late embryonic period (around 8th week), the amniotic cavity expands due to the accumulation of fluid.
- This expansion gradually surrounds the entire embryo. It also ensheaths the umbilical cord and covers the fetal surface of the placenta.
- The amniotic cavity grows at the expense of extra-embryonic coelom, which gets obliterated and results in fusion between chorion and amnion.

NOTE

Animals that contain the amnion are called amniotes, e.g., reptiles, birds, mammals.

Amniotic Fluid

- It is a clear, watery fluid (98%) and contains 2% solids (inorganic salts, urea, proteins, sugars).
- **Source:** Fetal/maternal/both
  - Amnion, fetal kidney, fetal lung, placenta
  - Amnio-fetomaternal exchange
- **Amount:**
  - *10th–20th week:* 25–400 mL
  - Increases up to 6th month, then decreases. At 28 weeks, it is 800 mL and at term it is 1,000 mL and in postmaturity (beyond 40 weeks of gestation) it is reduced to 400 mL.

Functions of Amniotic Fluid

- Amniotic fluid supports the embryo or fetus, allowing movement for musculoskeletal growth, protecting against injury and adhesion to the amnion.
- By full term, amniotic fluid volume reaches about 1 liter.
- Water exchanges occur every 3 hours between amniotic fluid and maternal blood.
- Starting around the 5th month, the fetus swallows amniotic fluid, which transfers nutrients to maternal blood via the placenta.
- Once fetal kidneys function, urine, mostly water, passes into the amniotic fluid, with placental help removing metabolic wastes.

Clinical correlation

Abnormal Production of Amniotic Fluid
- **Polyhydramnios**—more than 2 L of amniotic fluid will be present. In some cases, this is associated with atresia of the esophagus or CNS defects, which prevents swallowing of amniotic fluid by the fetus.
- **Oligohydramnios**—scanty amniotic fluid. It is sometimes associated with renal agenesis, as no urine is added to the amniotic fluid.

Both conditions can cause abnormalities in the fetus. They can also cause difficulties during childbirth.

Amniocentesis
It is a technique to collect amniotic fluid. The fluid is collected either through cervix or anterior abdominal wall. This procedure is usually done during 15–20 weeks of pregnancy. There is risk of fetal injury or preterm delivery in performing this procedure. *Refer* Chapter 8 for more details.

Amniotic Bands
Tears in the amnion can lead to the formation of amniotic bands, which may encircle fetal limbs, causing constrictions and potential amputations. This condition, resulting from infections or toxins affecting the fetus or fetal membranes, can also lead to craniofacial malformations and other abnormalities.

Chorion

We have already discussed about chorion in chapter 5 during the second week of development.

Yolk Sac

The yolk sac is an extraembryonic membrane that forms during early embryonic development. It is also referred to as an umbilical vesicle.

Formation of Yolk Sac

- **Primary yolk sac:** It appears during the 2nd week of development. The cavity of blastocyst is converted to form *primary yolk sac* and is lined by flattened cells derived from trophoblast/endoderm **(Flowchart 9.1)**.
- **Secondary yolk sac:** During the 2nd week of development with appearance of extraembryonic coelom the primary yolk sac reduces in size and becomes the secondary yolk sac. The extension of secondary yolk sac into the connecting stalk is known as *allantoic diverticulum*.
- **Definitive/tertiary yolk sac:** During the 4th week of development, with the folding of embryo to form primitive gut, most of the yolk sac is taken up by body. The remaining part of secondary yolk sac in the extraembryonic mesoderm is known as the *tertiary or definitive yolk sac* and is in communication with the midgut by an elongated part called the *vitellointestinal duct*.

Functions

Functions of the yolk sac are:
- Transfer of nutrients to the developing embryo before the placental circulation is established.
- Early hematopoiesis till the development of liver.
- Formation of primitive gut.
- Source of primordial germ cells that later migrates to developing gonads to form gametes.

Chapter 9: Fetal Membranes, Placenta and Twinning

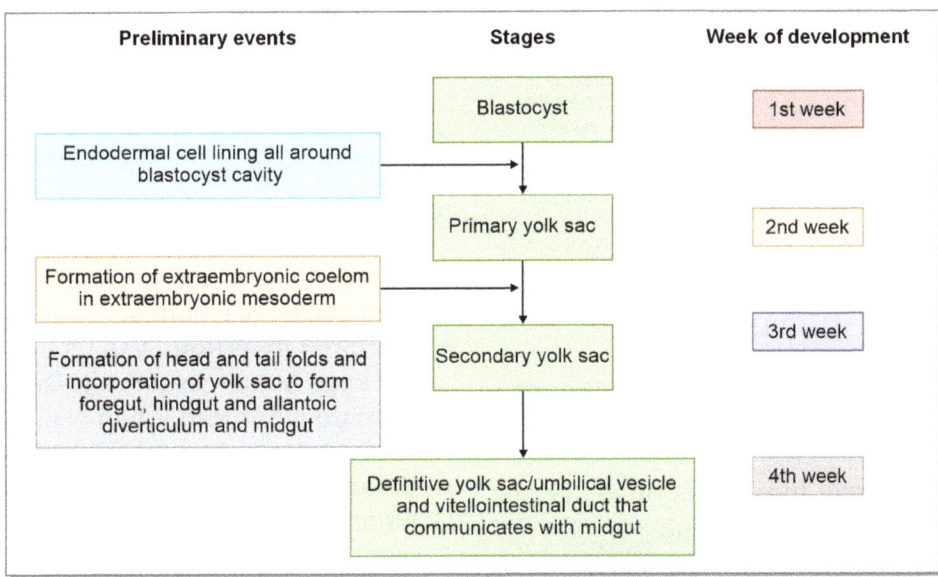

FLOWCHART 9.1: Formation and fate of yolk sac.

Clinical correlation

- **Meckel's diverticulum:** The vitellointestinal duct disappears by 6th week of development. If it persists, it results in a condition called *Meckel's diverticulum* that will be discussed in detail in development of digestive system.
- **Allantois/allantoenteric diverticulum:** By 16th day small diverticulum arises from caudal wall of yolk sac and extends into connecting stalk which later forms *fetal umbilical arteries and veins.* In adults it represents median umbilical ligament.
- In ultrasound examination, yolk sac can be seen within gestational sac between 5th and 6th week of gestation. The size of yolk sac increases up to 10th week and then gradually regresses and disappears between 14th to 20th week.
- It is the first component to be visualized on USG with gestational sac for the confirmation of pregnancy **(Fig. 9.2)**.

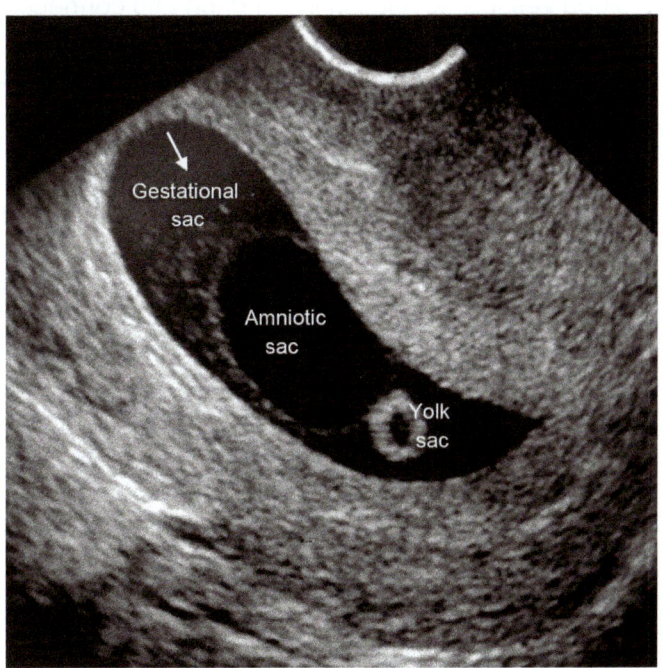

FIG 9.2: Yolk sac with gestational and amniotic sac. (Reproduced with permission from Dr Hiralal Konar. Source: Chapter 42. In: Konar H, Textbook of Obstetrics, Jaypee Brothers Medical Publishers Pvt Ltd, 2023).

Umbilical Cord

Introduction

The umbilical cord is a vital structure that connects the developing fetus to the placenta, allowing for the exchange of nutrients, gases, and waste products.
- It is one of the fetal membranes which develops from extraembryonic mesoderm and caudal extension of yolk sac and contains its remnants.
- Umbilical cord is tubular in structure and is covered by amniotic membrane.
- It contains blood vessels, yolk sac remnants and embryonic connective tissue.
- One end of it is attached to the anterior abdominal wall of fetus and the other end is fixed to the center of fetal surface of placenta.
- It is 50–55 cm in length and 2 cm in breadth at full term.

Function

The umbilical vessels transport oxygen and nutrients from the placenta to the developing fetus and eliminate carbon dioxide from fetal circulation into the placenta.

Formation of Umbilical Cord

- As discussed in Chapter 5, the unsplit area of extraembryonic mesoderm forms the connecting stalk (*refer* **Fig. 5.5**).
- With the establishment of cephalocaudal axis of the embryo, the connecting stalk moves toward the caudal end of the embryo. Allantoic diverticulum

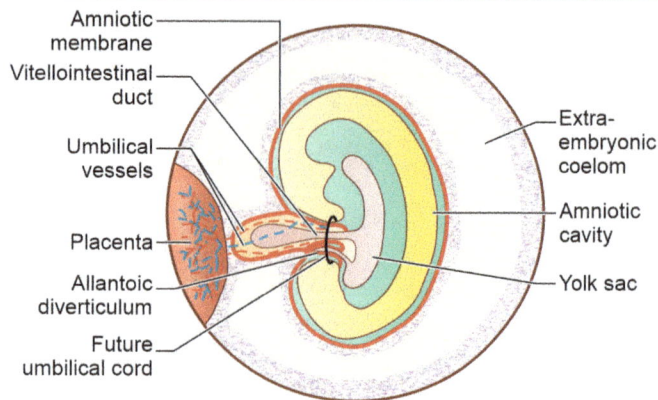

FIG. 9.3: Developing embryo with incorporation of yolk sac into the head and tail folds and its communication with the extraembryonic part of yolk sac.

extends into the primary mesoderm of connecting stalk during 3rd week of development.
- During 3rd week of development, extraembryonic blood vessels develop in the chorion and connecting stalk and are known as *umbilical vessels.*
- During the 4th week of development because of folding of embryo, the connecting stalk with its constituent allantoic diverticulum moves to the ventral surface of the developing embryo. With the incorporation of yolk sac into the head and tail folds of the embryo, contributing for the foregut and hind gut respectively the midgut between the two is in communication with the extraembryonic part of yolk sac and this is known as vitellointestinal duct **(Fig. 9.3)**. Because of the formation of embryonic folds, the amniotic membrane forms a tubular investment enclosing the connecting stalk along with allantoic diverticulum, vitellointestinal duct and umbilical vessels forming the umbilical cord.

Components

Components of umbilical cord vary with gestational age of the fetus. They are:
- **Vitellointestinal duct:** It is the communication between the midgut and extraembryonic part of yolk sac. In late fetal life, it disappears.
- **Umbilical arteries:** Two arteries (right and left) from the internal iliac arteries transport deoxygenated blood from the fetus to the placenta.
- **Umbilical veins:** Initially, two veins are present. Later right vein disappears and only the left vein remains, carrying oxygenated blood from the placenta to the fetus.
- **Wharton's jelly:** It is primary or intraembryonic mesodermal cells of connecting stalk that undergoes mucoid degeneration to cushions the umbilical vessels.
- **Allantoic diverticulum:** A ventral projection from the hindgut into connecting stalk, with the proximal part forming the bladder apex and the distal part becoming the urachus.
- **Vitellointestinal duct:** Connects the midgut to the yolk sac and disappears in late fetal life.

Types of Umbilical Cord Attachment to Placenta

- **Central insertion:** When attaches centrally to the middle of the placenta, normal **(Fig. 9.4A)**.
- **Paracental/eccentric:** When attaches 2 cms away from center. It is normal.
- **Marginal insertion:** The umbilical cord attaches to the edge or margin of the placenta **(Fig. 9.4B)**.
- **Furcate insertion:** When blood vessels of umbilical cord divides before reaching placenta **(Fig. 9.4C)**.
- **Velamentous insertion:** It inserts into the fetal membranes rather than directly into the placental mass **(Fig. 9.4D)**.
- **Battledore or battledoor insertion:** It attaches at or near the margin of the placenta, appearing flat and ribbon-like.

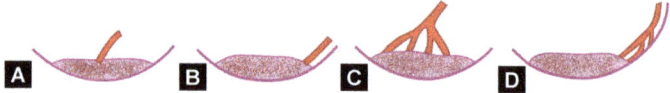

FIGS. 9.4A to D: Variations in attachment of umbilical cord to placenta: (A) Normal, (B) Marginal, (C) Furcate, (D) Velamentous insertion.

Clinical correlation

- **Physiological hernia:** The coelomic cavity surrounds the vitellointestinal duct at the fetal end of the umbilical cord until the 10th week of development. During this time, a U-shaped midgut loop herniates into the extraembryonic coelom known as physiological hernia.
- **Cord length:**
  - If the cord is long, it can encircle the neck of fetus causing *strangulation* or it can cause *cord prolapse* during childbirth which may cause *hypoxia of fetus* due to compression of cord.
  - Short cord can cause forceful placental separation during childbirth.
- **Single umbilical artery:** Instead of normal two umbilical arteries a single umbilical artery will be present. Usually, the left umbilical artery is absent. Its incidence is 1% and is associated with fetal anomalies.
- **Cord blood therapies:** Cord blood is the source of stem cells that are used for various disorders:
  - Hematopoietic stem cells
  - Cardiovascular diseases—myocardial infarction
  - Genetic diseases
  - Brain injury
  - Type I diabetes

PLACENTA

The placenta is a fetomaternal, highly vascular organ connecting the embryo/fetus to the uterine wall, facilitating physiological exchange between fetal and maternal tissues. It is a circular, disc-shaped structure weighing about 500 grams, with two surfaces and two structural components.

The two surfaces are:
1. **Maternal surface:** It is irregular and is divided into 15 ± 20 small lobules called maternal cotyledons.
2. **Fetal surface:** It is smooth and covered with amnion. Umbilical cord is attached at or near the center of this surface.

It has structural components of fetal and maternal origin:
- Maternal component is developed by *decidua basalis* or *decidual plate*.
- Fetal component is developed from *chorion frondosum* or *chorionic plate.*

Normal Attachment of Placenta

The normal attachment of placenta is in the upper uterine segment **(Fig. 9.5)**.

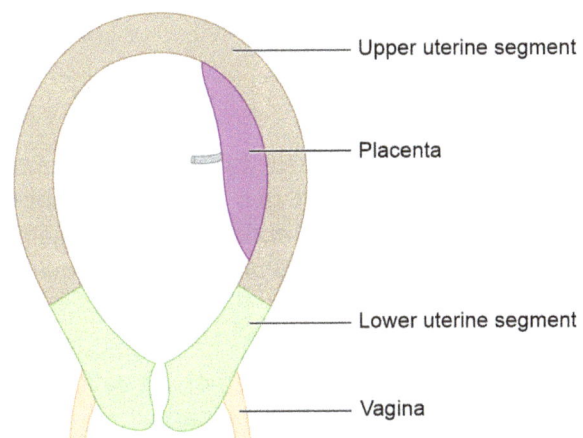

FIG. 9.5: Normal attachment of placenta—upper uterine segment.

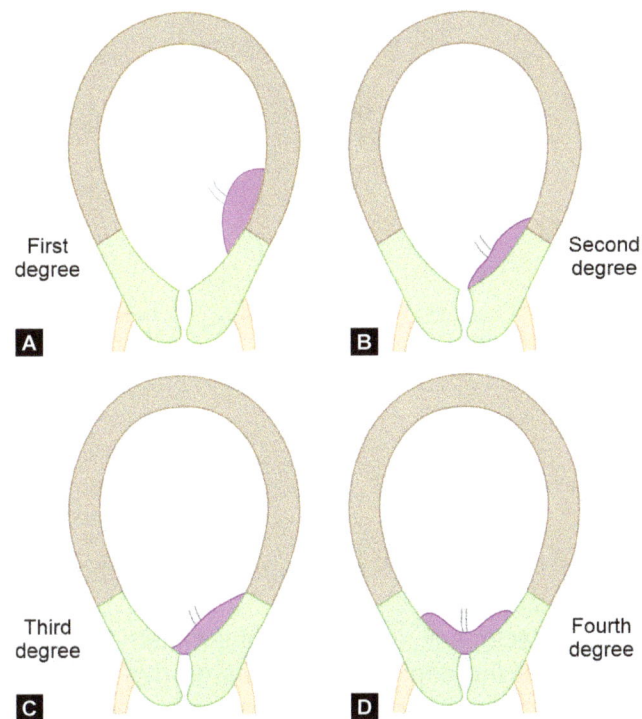

FIGS. 9.6A to D: Different degrees of placenta previa.

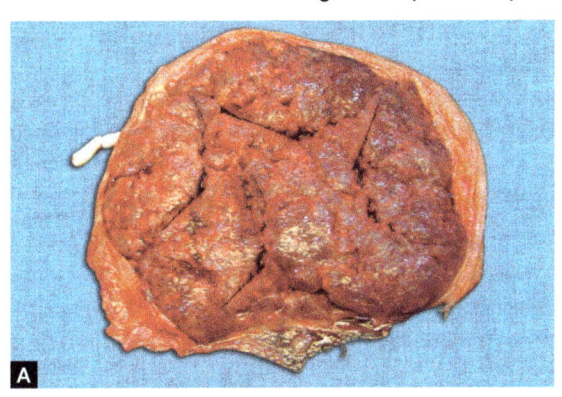

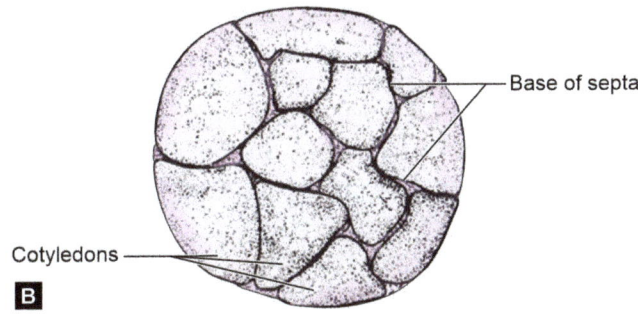

FIGS. 9.7A and B: Placenta: (A) Maternal surface; (B) After shedding, viewed from the maternal aspect.
(Reproduced with permission from Dr Hiralal Konar. Source: Chapter 42. In: Konar H, Textbook of Obstetrics, Jaypee Brothers Medical Publishers Pvt Ltd, 2023).

Maternal Surface

The maternal surface is rough and irregular **(Figs. 9.7A and B)**. It is subdivided into a number of lobes called *maternal cotyledons*.
- Septa that grow into the intervillous space from the maternal side **(Fig. 9.8)** divide this surface into 15–20 rough and irregular maternal cotyledons.

Clinical correlation

Placenta Previa
- The attachment of placenta may extend partially or completely into the lower uterine segment. This condition is called placenta previa. This is due to the implantation of the blastocyst close to the internal os.
- **Degrees of placenta previa (Figs. 9.6A to D):**
  - *First degree:* Attachment of placenta does not extend to internal os.
  - *Second degree:* Attachment of placenta extends up to internal os, but does not cover it.
  - *Third degree:* Placental edge covers the internal os. With the dilatation of internal os at the time of childbirth, the placenta will not occlude the internal os.
  - *Fourth degree:* Placenta completely covers the internal os even when the internal os is completely dilated. This can cause severe bleeding during pregnancy or during parturition.

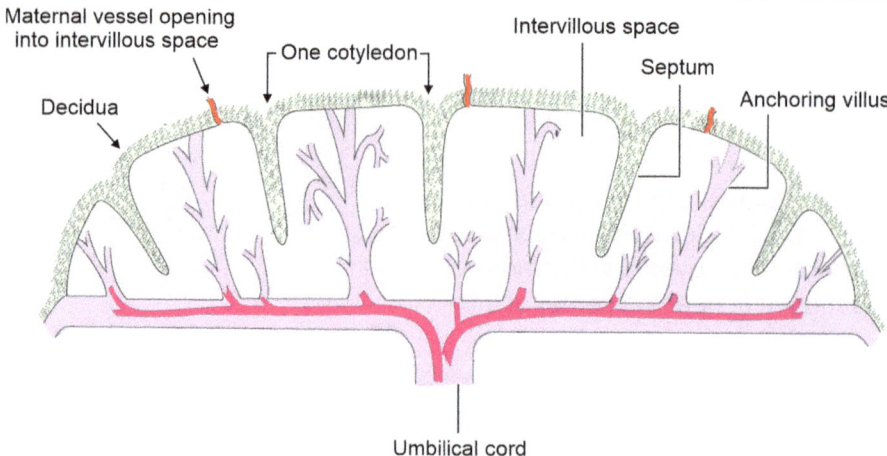

FIG. 9.8: Structure of a fully formed placenta. Each lobe (labeled cotyledon) contains a number of anchoring villus, but only one is shown here for the sake of simplicity.

- Each maternal cotyledon contains 2–4 anchoring villi and their branches.
- If the placenta is viewed from the maternal side, the bases of the septa are seen as grooves while the cotyledons appear as convex areas bounded by the grooves.

Fetal Surface

This surface is smooth and is covered by amnion (Fig. 9.9). The umbilical cord is attached close to the center and umbilical vessels radiate from the umbilical cord beneath the amnion.

- From the chorionic plate 40–60 extensions (fetal cotyledons) arise and extend toward the decidua basalis. Each *fetal cotyledon* (Fig. 9.10A) consists of a stem villus/truncus chorii that show ramifications into number of branches (ramus chorii), each further subdivides (ramuli chorii), such as the branches of a tree.
- Their terminal ramifications look, such as fingers and are called chorionic villi. The villi that are attached to decidua basalis are called *anchoring villi*. Others float in the maternal blood that flows in between the villi and are called *floating villi* (Fig. 9.10B).

Measurements of Placenta at Full Term

At full term (9 months after onset of pregnancy), the placenta has:
- **Diameter:** 6–8 inches
- **Thickness:** 3 cm
- **Weight:** About 500 g

Placental margin presents as fetal membrane contributed from inside outward by decidua capsularis and parietalis, chorion laeve and amnion. After the birth of the child, the placenta is shed off along with the decidua.

Structure of Placenta (Fig. 9.11)

Before going to the placental barrier, let us first see the structure of placenta. It has three parts:
1. **Maternal side—basal plate**
   - Stratum spongiosum of decidua basalis containing maternal blood vessels
   - Outer layer of syncytiotrophoblast (Nitabuch's layer)
   - Outer shell of cytotrophoblast
   - Inner layer of syncytiotrophoblast (Rohr's fibrinoid stria)
2. **Fetal side—chorionic plate**
   - Covered by amnion
   - Primary mesoderm with fetal blood vessels
   - Cytotrophoblast
   - Syncytiotrophoblast
3. **Between basal plate and chorionic plate**
   - *Intervillous space*
     - Volume—140 mL
     - Maternal blood passing through intervillous space—500 mL/minute
     - Volume of fetal blood flowing through fetal villi—400 mL/minute
   - Stem villi—primary, secondary, tertiary

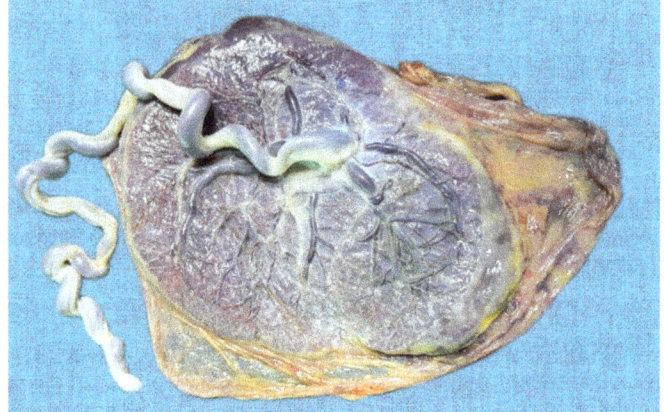

FIG. 9.9: Fetal surface.
(Reproduced with permission from Dr Hiralal Konar. Source: Chapter 42. In: Konar H, Textbook of Obstetrics, Jaypee Brothers Medical Publishers Pvt Ltd, 2023).

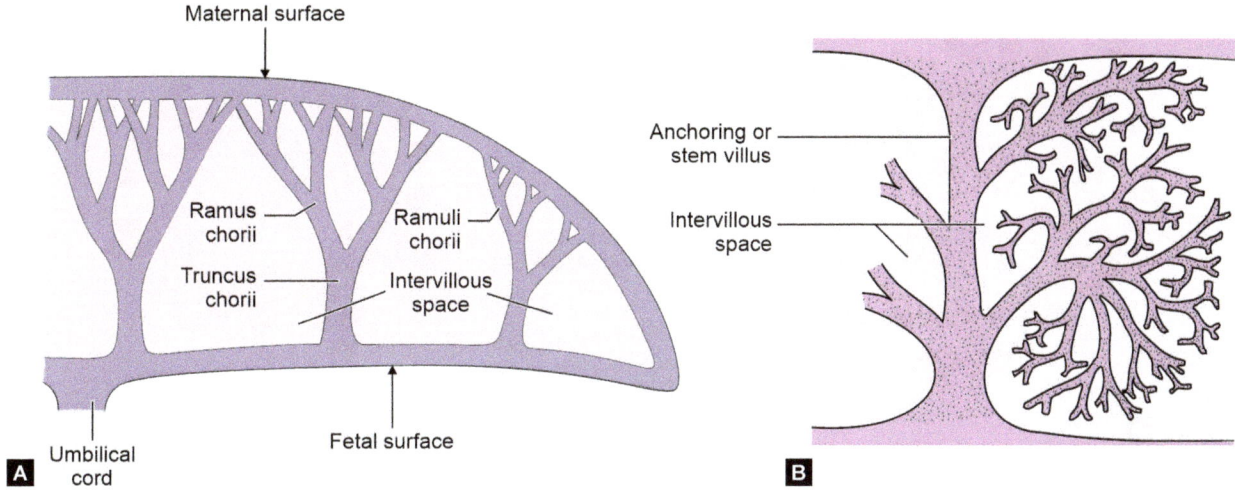

FIGS. 9.10A and B: (A) Arrangement of anchoring villi and intervillous space within the placenta. Note the subdivision of each anchoring villus; (B) Free villi arising from an anchoring villus.

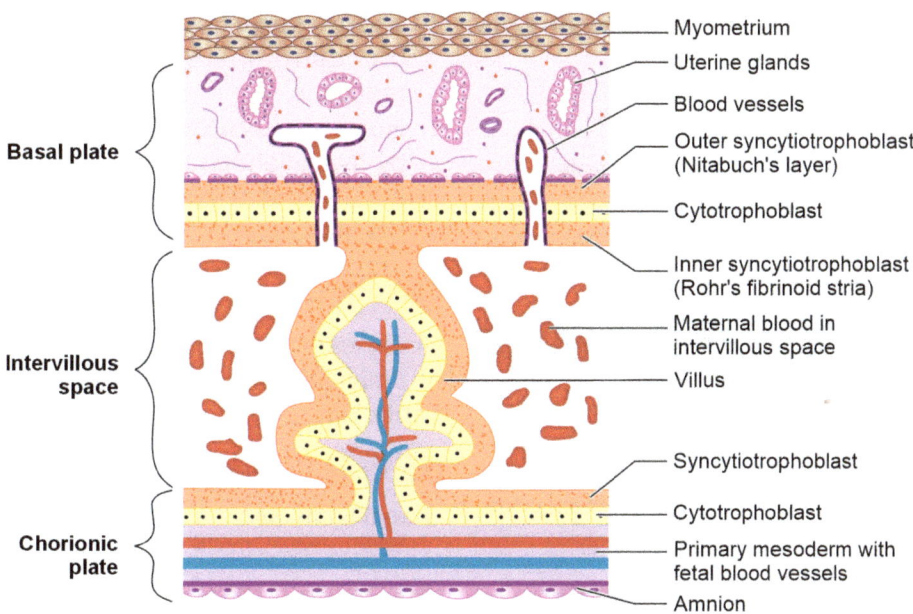

FIG. 9.11: Structural components of placental barrier or membrane.

Fetomaternal Circulation

- Fetomaternal circulation refers to the complex vascular exchange system between the mother and the fetus, facilitated by the placenta.
- This system ensures the transfer of oxygen, nutrients, and waste products between maternal and fetal blood without direct mixing.
- The fetal blood circulates through blood vessels within the chorionic villi of the placenta, while maternal blood flows through the intervillous spaces surrounding these villi.

Placental Membrane or Barrier

In the placenta, maternal blood circulates through the intervillous space, and fetal blood circulates through vessels in the villi. They flow side-by-side in opposite directions without mixing, separated by a membrane formed by layers of the villus wall.

The *placental membrane or barrier*, between fetal blood in the chorionic villi and maternal blood in the intervillous space, facilitates the exchange of oxygen, nutrients, and waste.

- In early pregnancy (until 20 weeks), the placental barrier is thick and consists of **(Fig. 9.12A)**:
  - Endothelium and basement membrane of fetal blood vessels
  - Surrounding mesoderm (connective tissue)
  - Cytotrophoblast and its basement membrane
  - Syncytiotrophoblast
- In the later part of pregnancy, due to increased nutrient demand, the efficiency of the membrane

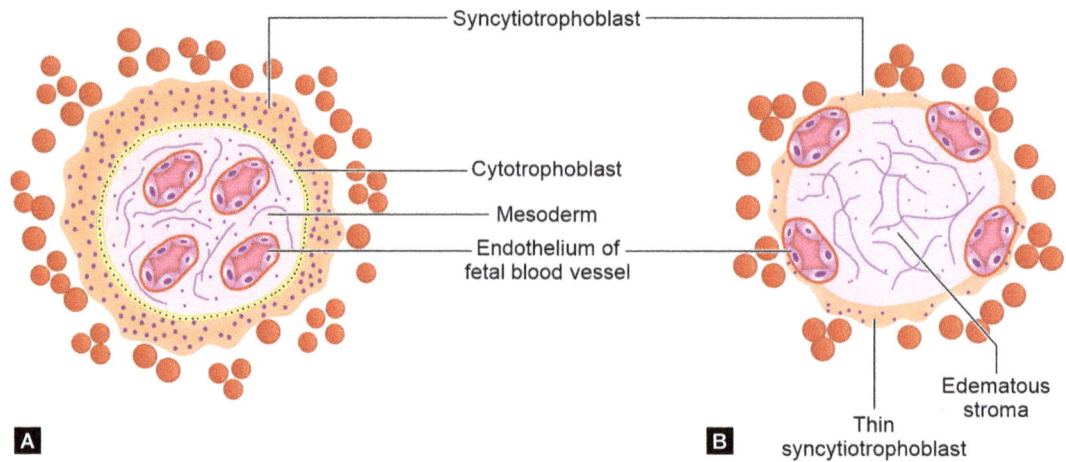

FIGS. 9.12A and B: Diagram of placental barrier: (A) In early part of pregnancy and (B) In later part of pregnancy.

is increased due to the reduction in its thickness **(Fig. 9.12B)** by:
- Disappearance of cytotrophoblast and its basement membrane
- Thinning of syncytiotrophoblast
- Edematous stroma
- Peripheral migration of fetal blood vessels

So, in later pregnancy, membrane/barrier presents endothelium of fetal capillaries resting on basement membrane and syncytiotrophoblast only.

> **NOTE**
> - The placental membrane area ranges from 4 m² to 14 m², similar to the adult intestinal tract, with numerous microvilli on the syncytiotrophoblast surface enhancing absorption.
> - Initially 0.025 mm thick, the membrane thins to 0.002 mm but becomes less efficient toward the end of pregnancy due to fibrinoid deposits.

Functions of Placenta

It has several functions that facilitate growth of the fetus:
- **Nutrient and oxygen transport:** Transports oxygen, water, electrolytes, and nutrients from maternal to fetal blood, maintaining fetal nutrition. A full-term fetus takes up about 25 mL of oxygen per minute.
- **Waste elimination:** Removes carbon dioxide, urea, and other waste products from fetal blood to maternal blood.
- **Immunity transfer:** Maternal antibodies (IgG) pass to the fetus, providing immunity against certain infections like polio, diphtheria and measles.
- **Barrier function:** Blocks many bacteria and other harmful substances, but some viruses and bacteria can pass through.
- **Drug transfer:** Drugs taken by the mother can enter fetal circulation and cause congenital malformations. Maternal hormone cannot cross placenta but synthetic hormones can cross and affect the fetus.
- **Blood separation:** Keeps maternal and fetal bloodstreams separate, preventing antigenic reactions.
- **Hormone synthesis:** Produces hormones mainly by syncytiotrophoblast like progesterone, estrogen, hCG, HPL and relaxin that are essential for pregnancy maintenance and maternal physiological changes.

Classification or Types of Placenta

Classification of placenta according to shape, attachment of umbilical cord and umbilical arteries are shown in **Table 9.1**.

TABLE 9.1: Classification of placenta.

Based on shape	- **Discoid**—round or disc like - **Bidiscoidal**—it consists of two discs - Oval - Triangular - Irregular - **Lobed**—it divides into lobes - **Diffuse/placenta membranacea**—chorionic villi persists all-round the blastocyst
According to distribution of umbilical arteries	- **Disperse type**—umbilical arteries show dichotomous branching and show progressive reduction in size - **Magistral type**—arteries present uniform caliber up to the periphery of placenta - **Furcate**—blood vessels divide before reaching the placenta
Phylogenetic classification	According to tissues from maternal and fetal parts of placenta contributing for placental barrier into epitheliochorial, syndesmochorial, endotheliochorial and hemochorial.

Clinical correlation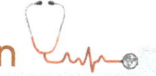

Congenital abnormalities: The various congenital abnormalities of placenta resulting from different factors are tabulated in **Table 9.2**.

Placental hormones:

- **Human chorionic gonadotropin (hCG)** produced by the placenta and is similar in its actions to the LH of the hypophysis cerebri. Gonadotropins are excreted through maternal urine where their presence is used as a test to detect a pregnancy in its early stages.
- **Human chorionic somatomammotropin (hCS)** has an anti-insulin effect on the mother. This leads to increased plasma levels of glucose and amino acids in the maternal circulation. In this way, it increases availability of these materials for the fetus. It also enhances glucose utilization by the fetus.
- **Progesterone** maintains pregnancy by inhibiting uterine contractions and supporting endometrial lining for implantation and fetal development.
- **Estrogen** stimulates uterine growth and preparation of myometrium for sensitization by oxytocin for parturition.
- **Relaxin** relaxes pelvic ligaments and joints to prepare for childbirth for vaginal delivery.

Chorionic villus biopsy: It is a prenatal diagnostic test involving the extraction of placental tissue. It is performed between the 10th and 12th weeks of pregnancy.

- **Types:**
  - Transcervical— a catheter is inserted through the cervix into the placenta.
  - Transabdominal—a needle is inserted through the abdomen and uterus into the placenta.
- **Indications:** To detect genetic or chromosomal abnormalities during 1st trimester:
  - Family history or sibling with abnormalities
  - Maternal >35 years at due date
  - Sex-linked genetic disease
  - Previous ultrasound with questionable abnormality
- **Risk involved with the procedure:**
  - Cramping, bleeding, or leaking of amniotic fluid
  - Infection
  - Miscarriage or preterm labor
  - Limb defects in infants if done before 9 weeks (rare)
  - Women with twins or other multiples will need sampling from each placenta
- **Limitations:** CVS does not provide information on neural tube defects, such as spina bifida, so need follow up blood tests between 16 to 18 weeks of their pregnancy to screen for neural tube defects.

TABLE 9.2: Congenital abnormalities of placenta.

Anomaly	Description
Adherence anomalies	• **Placenta accreta:** Abnormal adherence to the uterine wall due to defective decidua basalis. • **Placenta increta:** Penetration into the myometrium. • **Placenta percreta:** Penetration through the myometrium to the serosa.
Shape anomalies	• **Bilobed or multilobed:** Placenta with multiple lobes. • **Placenta succenturiate:** Accessory placental lobe connected by blood vessels **(Fig. 9.13)**. • **Placenta circumvallate:** Folded edge with fetal membranes attaching beyond the edge. • **Placenta fenestrate:** Placenta exhibits small fenestrations or windows within its structure.
Site anomalies	• **Placenta previa:** Implantation near or over the cervical os, obstructing delivery. • **Placenta accreta spectrum:** Placental attachment abnormalities associated with prior uterine surgery or scarring.

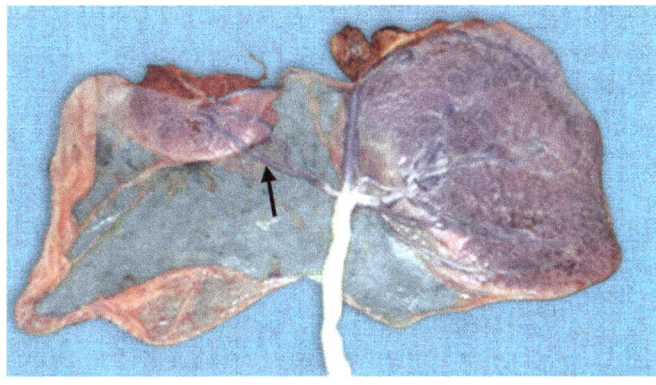

FIG. 9.13: Placenta succenturiate.
(Reproduced with permission from Dr Hiralal Konar. Source: Chapter 42. In: Konar H, Textbook of Obstetrics, Jaypee Brothers Medical Publishers Pvt Ltd, 2023).

MUTUAL RELATIONSHIP OF AMNIOTIC CAVITY, EXTRAEMBRYONIC COELOM AND UTERINE CAVITY

We have so far considered the fetal membranes (amnion and chorion), and the placenta, mainly in relation to the fetus. Let us now see their relationships to the uterine cavity. These are important, as they help us to understand some aspects of the process of childbirth.

❖ In **Figure 9.14**, we see three cavities, namely (1) the uterine cavity, (2) the extraembryonic coelom

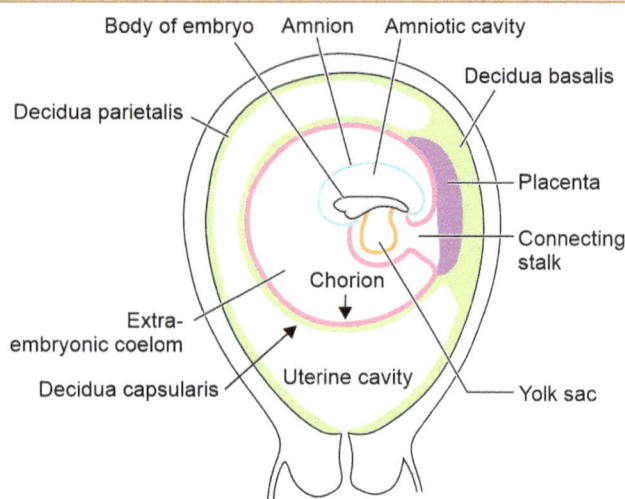

FIG. 9.14: Relationship of amniotic cavity, extraembryonic coelom and uterine cavity.

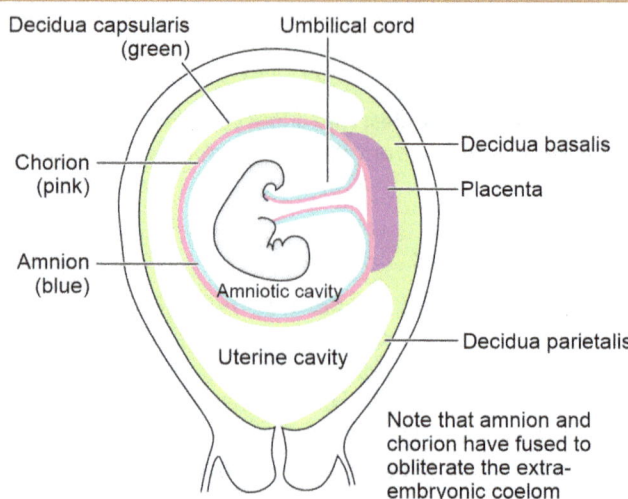

FIG. 9.15: Relationship of amniotic cavity and uterine cavity after obliteration of the extraembryonic coelom.

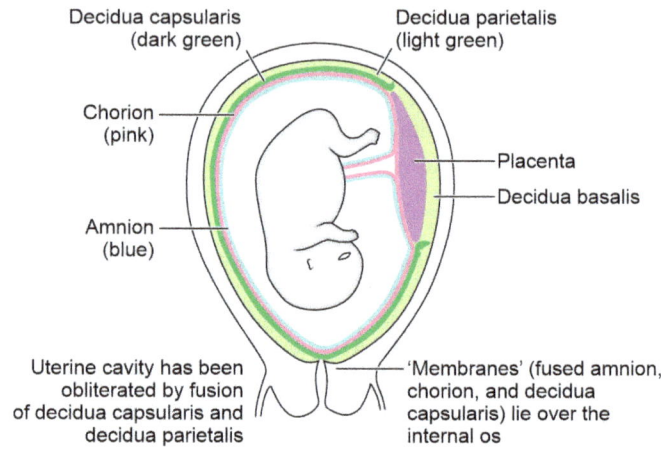

FIG. 9.16: Amniotic cavity after obliteration of the extraembryonic coelom and uterine cavity.

and (3) the amniotic cavity. The outer wall of the extraembryonic coelom is formed by chorion and the inner wall by amnion. As the amniotic cavity enlarges, the extraembryonic coelom becomes smaller and smaller. It is eventually obliterated by fusion of amnion and chorion. The fused chorion and amnion form the *amniochorionic membrane*.

- As seen in **Figure 9.15**, the wall of the amniotic cavity is now formed by: (1) amnion, (2) chorion and (3) decidua capsularis, all three being fused to one another.
- Further expansion of the amniotic cavity occurs at the expense of the uterine cavity. Gradually, the decidua capsularis fuses with the decidua parietalis, and the uterine cavity is also obliterated **(Fig. 9.16)**.
- Further expansion of the amniotic cavity is by enlargement of the uterus is accompanied by an increase in the amount of amniotic fluid. At the time of parturition (childbirth), the fused amnion and chorion (amniochorionic membrane) (along with the greatly thinned out decidua capsularis), constitute what are called *the membranes*.
- As the uterine muscle contracts, increased pressure in the amniotic fluid causes these membranes to bulge into the cervical canal. This bulging helps to dilate this canal. The bulging membranes can be felt through the vagina and are referred to as the *bag of waters*.
- Ultimately the membranes rupture. Amniotic fluid flows out into the vagina. After the child is delivered, the placenta and the membranes, along with all parts of the decidua, separate from the wall of the uterus and are expelled from it.

MULTIPLE BIRTHS AND TWINNING

If more than one fetus is carried to term in a single pregnancy. When a mother gives birth to two infants at the same time, they are called twins, three (triplets), four (quadruplets) or even more infants are sometimes born simultaneously.

Types of Twinning

Twins can be produced in two ways **(Flowchart 9.2)**:

Dizygotic Twins (Polyovular)

- Two ova may be shed simultaneously from the ovary. Each of them may be fertilized and may develop in the usual manner. This results in twins that are called *dizygotic or fraternal twins*.
- As each of them develops from a separate ovum, they have independent genetic constitutions. These twins, therefore, need not be of the same sex, nor do they resemble each other any more than children of the same parents that are born separately. Each fetus has its own chorionic and amniotic sacs *(bichorial, biamniotic)*. Dizygotic twinning is more

common in human beings than monozygotic twinning **(Fig. 9.17A)**.

Monozygotic Twins (Monoovulatory)

- Twins can also arise from a single fertilized ovum. These are called *monozygotic or identical or maternal or paternal twins*.
- The genetic constitution of the two twins is exactly the same. Hence, they are of the same sex and exactly alike in appearance.

Monozygotic twins are produced in one of the following ways:

- **Early blastomere separation:**
  - The cells formed in the first few divisions of the zygote are totipotent, i.e., each cell is capable of developing into a complete embryo. The two cells formed by the first division may separate and develop independently.
  - In such a case, the fetuses will have separate chorionic and amniotic sacs (bichorial, biamniotic) as in dizygotic twins.
  - The percentage incidence is 25–30% and can result up to 3rd day after fertilization as separation takes place after the first cellular division **(Fig. 9.17B)**.
- **Duplication of inner cell mass:**
  - The embryo may develop normally up to the stage of the morula. However, when the blastocyst is formed, two inner cell masses form within it and each develops into a complete fetus. In this case,

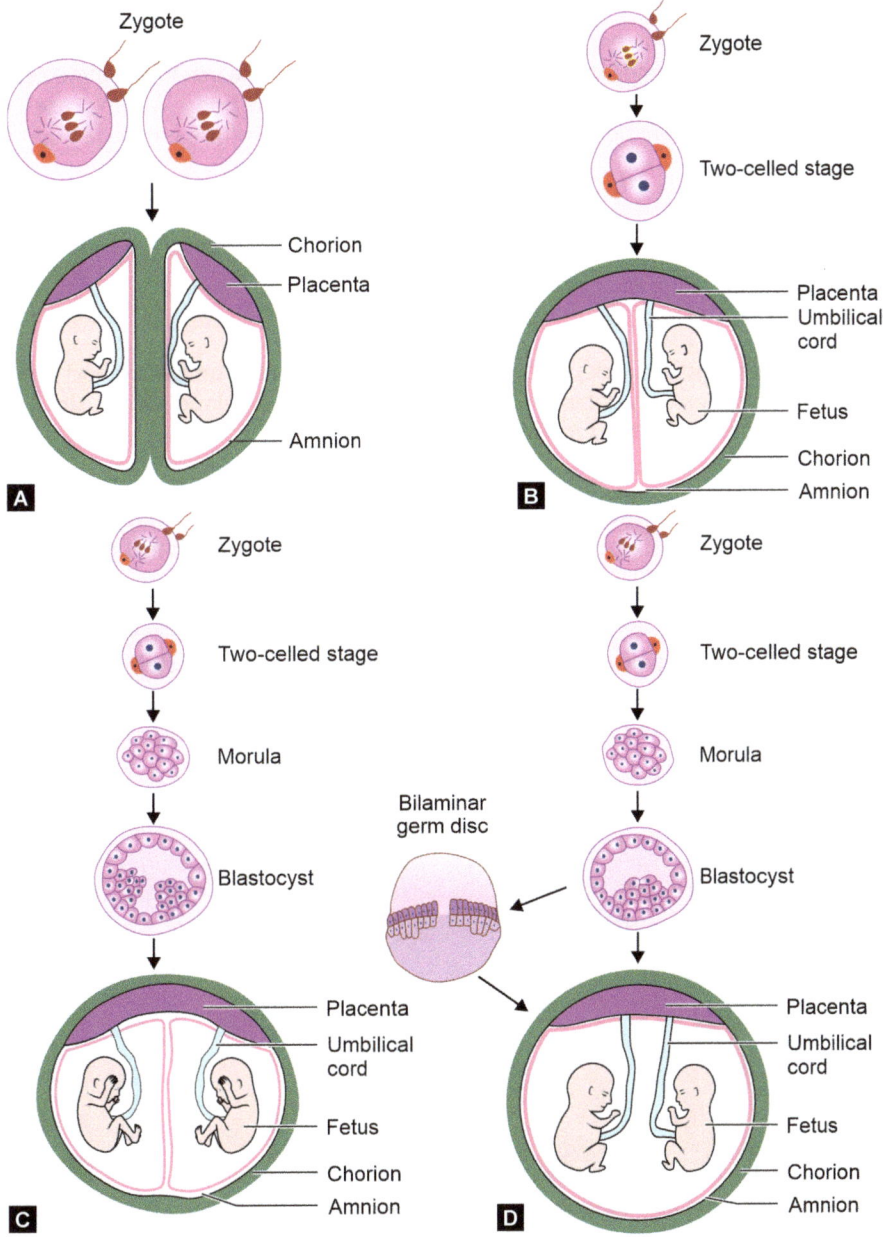

FIGS. 9.17A to D: Twinning: (A) Dizygotic twins resulting from fertilization of two different ova—bichorial, biamniotic; (B to D) Monozygotic twins: (B) Bichorial, biamniotic; (C) Monochorial, biamniotic; (D) Monochorial, monoamniotic.

the two fetuses have a common chorionic sac but each lies in an independent amniotic cavity *(monochorial, biamniotic)*.
- The percentage incidence is 70–75%. Separation takes place a little later in the development but before the blastocyst has defined the roles of each cell, i.e., between 4th and 7th day after fertilization **(Fig. 9.17C)**.

❖ **Duplication of embryonic disc:**
  - The inner cell mass may split into two; or two embryonic axes may be established in one inner cell mass. By this we mean that two separate embryonic discs are formed within it, each with its own prochordal plate and primitive streak. In this case, the two fetuses share a common chorion as well as a common amniotic cavity *(monochorial, monoamniotic)*.
  - The percentage incidence is 1 ± 2%. Separation takes place at the stage when the amniotic bag is already being formed, i.e., between 8th and 12th day after fertilization **(Fig. 9.17D)**.

Clinical correlation

Hazards of Monochorionic Monoamniotic Twinning

Incomplete duplication of disc (Figs. 9.18A to D)

This results in the formation of conjoined twins or double monsters or **Siamese twins**. Incomplete separation of monozygotic twins results in the birth of two infants that are joined together in some part of the body. In some cases, it is possible to separate them by operation, but most of them are born dead. Depending on the degree of incomplete separation or fusion, different types of conjoined twins result:
- **Craniopagus**—twins united at head
- **Thoracopagus**—twins showing fusion of thorax
- **Pygopagus**—fusion at sacral region
- **Cephalothoracopagus**—fusion of thorax and head

Acephalic, acardiac fetus

Sometimes the two twins do not undergo equal development, possibly as a result of unequal blood supply. The underdeveloped fetus may possess no heart of its own and may depend upon the other fetus for its blood supply. Unequal division of embryonic axis/unequal blood supply are responsible for this type of anomaly.

Parasitic twins

Sometimes the second conceptus may be represented as a mass attached to other fetus, or may be embedded within its body. This results from cessation of development of one embryo/fetus which is called parasitic as it is incompletely developed and is wholly dependent on the complete embryo/fetus for its growth and development.

Fetus papyraceous **(Fig. 19.19)**

Fetus papyraceous is a condition where one twin dies in utero, typically in the second trimester, and is compressed by the surviving twin, resulting in a flattened, parchment-like appearance.

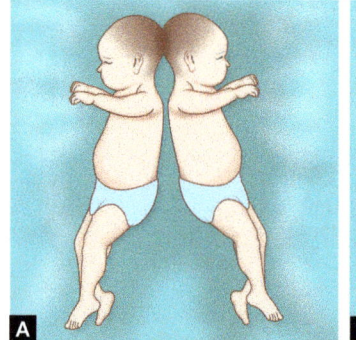 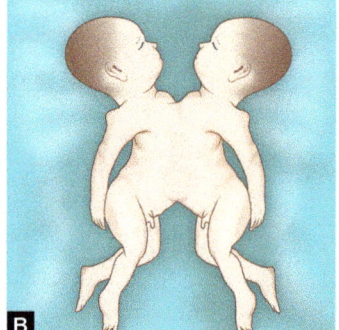 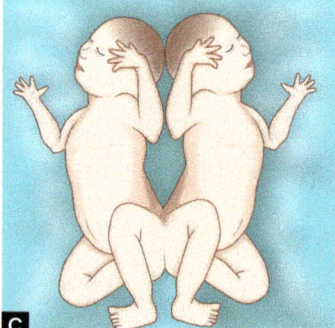 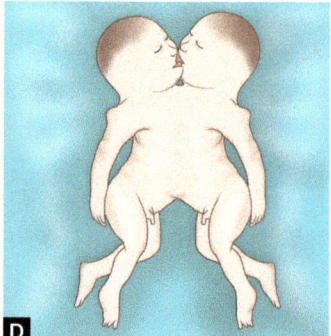

FIGS. 9.18A to D: Conjoined twins: (A) Craniopagus; (B) Thoracopagus; (C) Pygopagus; (D) Cephalothoracopagus—fusion of thorax and head.

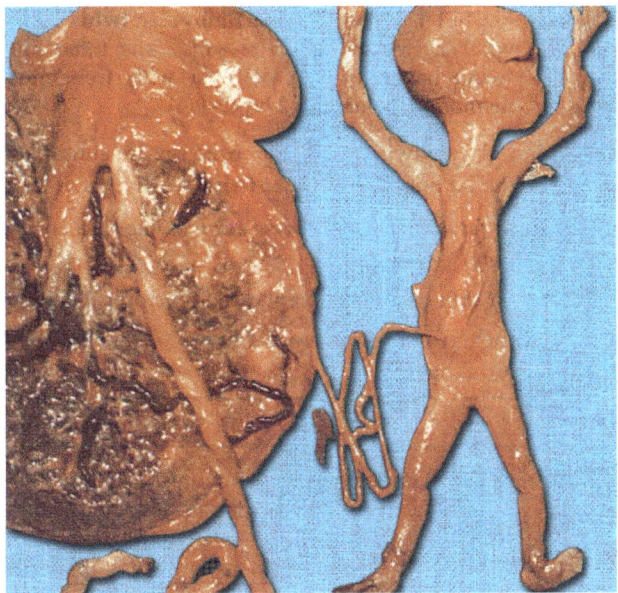

FIG. 19.19: Fetus papyraceous or compressus.
(Reproduced with permission from Dr Hiralal Konar. Source: Chapter 42. In: Konar H, Textbook of Obstetrics, Jaypee Brothers Medical Publishers Pvt Ltd, 2023).

HIGHLIGHTS

- Tissues or structures that develop from the zygote, but do not form part of embryo proper are *fetal membranes.*
- Fetal membranes include *chorion, amnion, yolk sac, allantois and connecting stalk.*
- **Amnion** is the fetal membrane that covers the embryo and forms the amniotic sac which is filled by *amniotic fluid.*
- **Chorion** is the outermost fetal membrane covering the embryo and helps in the formation of chorionic villi and placenta.
- **A yolk sac** is an extraembryonic membrane that forms during early embryonic development. It is of three types: *primary, secondary and tertiary.*
- **Umbilical cord** is tubular in structure and is covered by amniotic membrane. It contains blood vessels, yolk sac remnants and embryonic connective tissue.
- The *placenta* is formed partly from embryonic structures and partly from decidua. Placenta is responsible for transport of nutrients and oxygen to the fetus and for removal of waste products.
- The essential elements of the placenta are *chorionic villi.*
- The placenta is normally attached to the upper part of body of the uterus. A placenta attached lower down is called *placenta previa.* It can cause problems during childbirth.
- The embryo is surrounded by three large cavities. These are: (1) the *amniotic cavity*, (2) the *extraembryonic coelom* and (3) the *uterine cavity.* Enlargement of the amniotic cavity obliterates the extraembryonic coelom, leading to fusion of amnion and chorion. Further enlargement of amniotic cavity obliterates the uterine cavity. Fused amnion and chorion (called membranes) bulge into the cervical canal (during childbirth) and help to dilate it.
- If more than one fetus is carried to term in a single pregnancy, then it is referred to as *multiple births or pregnancy.*
- Twinning can be two types: *Dizygotic twins (polyovular)* and *monozygotic twins (monoovulatory).* Dizygotic twinning is more common in human beings than monozygotic twinning. The genetic constitution of the two twins is exactly the same in monozygotic twins.

Summary

- Twinning types and basis **(Flowchart 9.2).**
- Formation of placenta **(Flowchart 9.3).**
- Substances that can/not cross placental barrier **(Table 9.3).**
- Differences between monozygotic and dizygotic twins **(Table 9.4).**

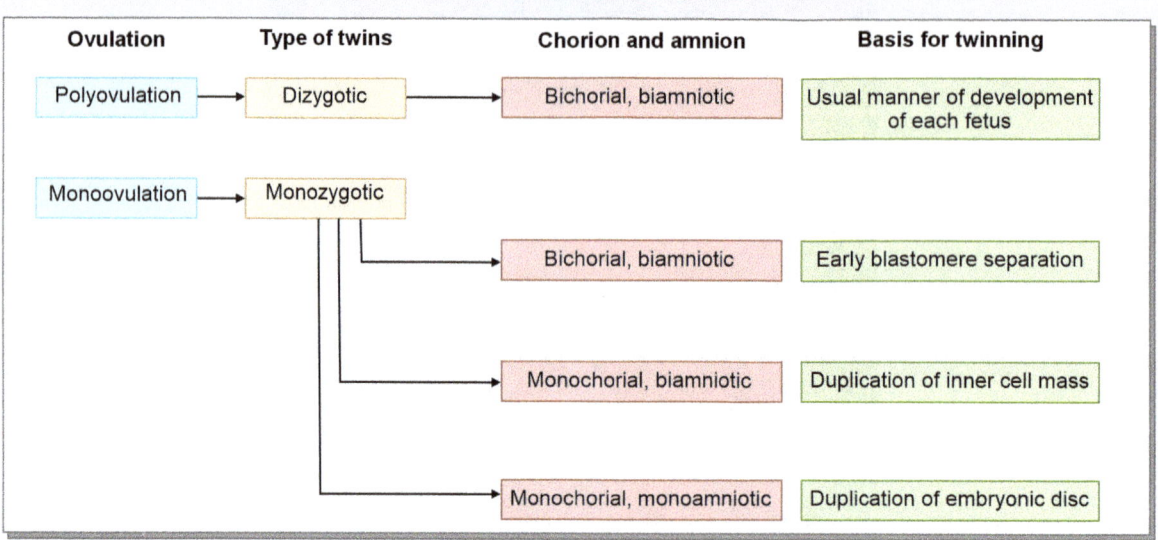

FLOWCHART 9.2: Twinning—types and basis.

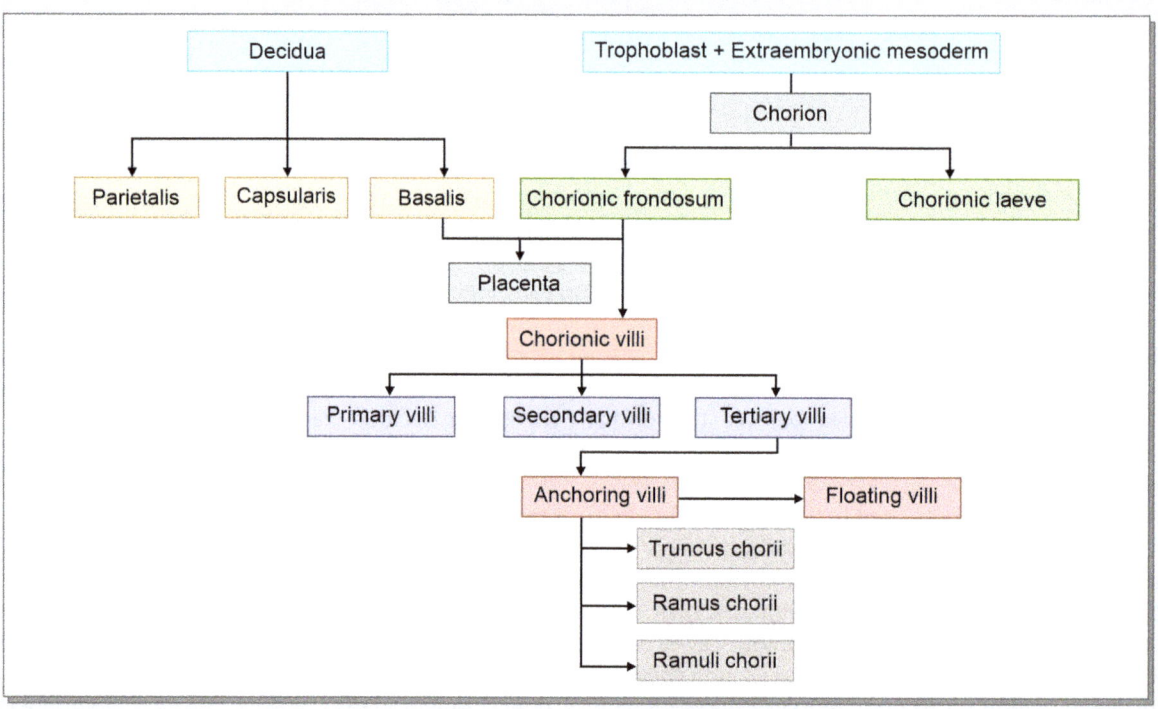

FLOWCHART 9.2: Development of placenta.

TABLE 9.3: Substances crossing placental barrier.

Substances that cross the placental barrier	Harmful substances that can cross the placental barrier	Substances that do not cross the placental barrier
Oxygen (O_2), water and electrolytes	Alcohol, nicotine, carbon monoxide, cocaine	Large protein molecules, maternal cholesterol, lipoproteins and triglycerides
Nutrients (glucose, amino acids, fatty acids, vitamins)	*Toxoplasmosis gondii, Treponema pallidum*	Heparin
Waste products (carbon dioxide, urea, bilirubin)	Category X drugs (e.g., opioids, phenytoin, oral contraceptives) and Category D drugs (e.g., tetracycline, phenobarbital, amikacin, streptomycin, diazepam, alprazolam)	Most bacteria

Substances that cross the placental barrier	Harmful substances that can cross the placental barrier	Substances that do not cross the placental barrier
Hormones (thyroxine, cortisol), α-fetoprotein	Rubella virus vaccine and anti-D antibodies	IgM, IgA, IgE, IgD antibodies
Antibodies (IgG)	Some viruses (e.g., rubella, CMV, HSV2)	Blood cells and maternal hormones

TABLE 9.4: Differences between monozygotic twins and dizygotic twins.

Feature	Monozygotic twins	Dizygotic twins
Origin	Single fertilized egg splits into two embryos	Two separate eggs fertilized by two separate sperm
Genetic similarity	Identical genetic material (identical twins)	Genetically similar as ordinary siblings (fraternal twins)
Number of placentas	Usually one (shared placenta)	Usually two (separate placentas)
Number of amniotic sacs	Can have one or two (monoamniotic or diamniotic)	Always two (diamniotic)
Sex	Always the same sex	Can be the same or different sex
Incidence	About 3–4 per 1,000 births worldwide	Varies by region, more common (about 12 per 1,000 births)
Factors influencing occurrence	Generally random, no significant hereditary influence	Hereditary factors, maternal age, and fertility treatments increase likelihood
Complications	Higher risk of complications such as twin-to-twin transfusion syndrome (TTTS)	Lower risk of complications compared to monozygotic twins

TIMETABLE OF SOME EVENTS MENTIONED IN THIS CHAPTER

Structure	Age
Chorion	7–10 days
Amnion	2 weeks

Structure	Age
Yolk sac	2–3 weeks
Allantois	3 weeks
Placenta	4 weeks
Maternal-fetal circulation	8–10 weeks

TEST YOUR UNDERSTANDING

REVIEW QUESTIONS

1. Describe the structure and function of the chorion.
2. Explain the roles of the amnion and amniotic fluid.
3. Discuss the formation and functions of the placenta.
4. Compare and contrast monozygotic and dizygotic twinning.
5. What are the primary functions of the yolk sac?
6. Describe the process of twinning and its variations.
7. Write a note on amniocentesis.
8. Write a note on chorionic villus sampling.
9. Describe the importance of placental barriers.

EXPLAIN WHY? (REASONING QUESTIONS)

1. Abnormalities in placental development impact development.
2. Assessment of amniotic fluid volume during prenatal examination is important.
3. Pregnant woman is restricted to take any medication with doctor consultation.
4. Placental hormones influence pregnancy outcomes.
5. Determination of placental location is significant in prenatal imaging.
6. Monitoring fetal growth discordance in monochorionic twins is crucial during prenatal care

MULTIPLE CHOICE QUESTIONS

1. The umbilical vesicle develops from:
   A. Ectoderm
   B. Endoderm
   C. Mesoderm
   D. Ectoderm and mesoderm
2. Fetal component of placenta is called as:
   A. Chorionic leave
   B. Chorionic frondosum
   C. Decidual plate
   D. Chorion
3. During late pregnancy, placental efficiency is increased due to all, *except*:
   A. Disappearance of cytotrophoblast
   B. Thining of syncytiotrophoblast
   C. Endothelium of fetal blood vessels
   D. Peripheral migration of fetal blood vessels
4. Attachment of placenta to lower uterine segment is termed as:
   A. Abruptio placentae
   B. Placenta previa
   C. Disperse placenta
   D. Circumvallate placenta
5. Nitabuch's layer is:
   A. Cytotrophoblast
   B. Extraembryonic mesoderm
   C. Outer layer of syncytiotrophoblast
   D. Inner layer of syncytiotrophoblast
6. A 30-year-old pregnant woman is undergoing a routine ultrasound at 20 weeks of gestation. The ultrasound reveals a monochorionic diamniotic twin pregnancy. Which of the following complications is most closely associated with this type of twin pregnancy?
   A. Twin-to-twin transfusion syndrome (TTTS)
   B. Vanishing twin syndrome
   C. Down syndrome
   D. Preeclampsia
7. A 25-year-old primigravida is found to have oligohydramnios during her third trimester. Which of the following fetal conditions is most likely to be associated with oligohydramnios?
   A. Fetal renal agenesis
   B. Fetal anencephaly
   C. Fetal macrosomia
   D. Fetal polyhydramnios
8. A 35-year-old woman is pregnant with dizygotic twins. She asks about the genetic risks for her twins. Which of the following statements is true regarding dizygotic twins?
   A. They share the same placenta and amniotic sac
   B. They have a higher risk of congenital anomalies compared to monozygotic twins
   C. They have different genetic makeup, similar to regular siblings
   D. They are always of the same sex

Answers: 1. B 2. B 3. C 4. B 5. C
         6. A 7. A 8. C

Basic Tissues of the Body

CHAPTER 10

COMPETENCIES COVERED/LEARNING OUTCOMES

The student should be able to:
There are no specific competencies given. We should study these for the correlation and comprehensive understanding.

AN65.1 and AN65.2	Epithelial tissue.	AN70.1	Exocrine glands.
AN66.1 and AN66.2	Connective tissue.	AN71.1 and AN71.2	Bone and cartilage.
AN67.1, AN67.2 and AN67.3	Muscular tissue.	AN26.6	Explain the concept of bones that ossify in membrane.
AN68.1, AN68.2 and AN68.3	Nervous tissue.		

During the embryonic period, differentiation of germ layers with organogenesis mark the initiation of complete development of human being. The three germ layers differentiates into many components of the body and body parts from surface epithelium to organs and mesenchyme.

The human body is made up of many types of tissue. These are known as *basic tissues of the body*. They are as follows:

- **Epithelial tissue:** Epithelium consists of cells arranged in the form of continuous sheets. Epithelia line the external and internal surfaces of the body and of body cavities. These also include glands and mesenchyme.
- **Connective tissue:** Connective tissue proper includes loose connective tissue, dense connective tissue and adipose tissue. Blood, cartilage and bone are special connective tissues.
- **Muscular tissue:** This is of three types: striated, cardiac and smooth muscles.
- **Nervous tissue:** This tissue consists of neurons (nerve cells), nerve cell processes (axons and dendrites) and cells of neuroglia.

In the present chapter we shall study the formation of these basic tissues, which will help us understanding the formation of organs in further chapters.

EPITHELIA

An epithelium may be derived from ectoderm, endoderm or mesoderm. In general, ectoderm gives rise to epithelia covering the external surfaces of the body; and some surfaces near the exterior. Endoderm gives origin to the epithelium of most of the gut; and of structures arising as diverticula from the gut (e.g., the liver and pancreas). Mesoderm gives origin to the epithelial lining of the greater part of the urogenital tract.

Some Epithelia Derived from Ectoderm

- Epithelium of skin, hair follicles, sweat glands, sebaceous glands, and mammary glands.
- Epithelium over cornea and conjunctiva, external acoustic meatus and outer surface of tympanic membrane.
- Epithelium of some parts of the mouth, lower part of anal canal, terminal part of male urethra, parts of female external genitalia.

Some Epithelia Derived from Endoderm

- Epithelium of the entire gut except part of the mouth and anal canal (lined by ectoderm).
- Epithelium of auditory tube and middle ear.
- Epithelium of respiratory tract.
- Epithelium over part of urinary bladder, urethra and vagina.

Some Epithelia Derived from Mesoderm

- Tubules of kidneys, ureter, trigone of urinary bladder.
- Uterine tubes, uterus, part of vagina.
- Testis and its duct system.
- Endothelium lining the heart, blood vessels and lymphatics.
- Mesothelium lining the pericardial, peritoneal and pleural cavities; and cavities of joints.

Glands

Almost all glands, both exocrine and endocrine, *develop as diverticula from epithelial surfaces* **(Fig. 10.1A)**:

* **Exocrine glands:** The gland may be derived from elements formed by branching of one diverticulum (e.g., parotid) or may be formed from several diverticula (e.g., lacrimal gland, prostate). The opening of the duct (or ducts) is usually situated at the site of the original outgrowth.
* **Endocrine glands:** The diverticula are generally solid to begin with **(Figs. 10.1A and B)** and are canalized later **(Fig. 10.1C)**. The proximal parts of the diverticula form the duct system. The distal parts of the diverticula form the secretory elements **(Fig. 10.1C)**.
  - In the case of endocrine glands (e.g., thyroid, anterior part of hypophysis cerebri) the gland loses all contact with the epithelial surface from which it takes origin **(Figs. 10.1D and E)**.
  - Depending on the epithelium from which they take origin, glands may be *ectodermal* (e.g., sweat glands, mammary glands), *endodermal* (e.g., pancreas, liver), *mesodermal* (e.g., adrenal cortex), or of *mixed origin* (e.g., prostate).

Mesenchyme

* A small proportion of mesodermal cells give rise to epithelia. The remaining cells, that make up the bulk of mesoderm, get converted into a loose tissue called *mesenchyme* **(Fig. 10.2)**.
* Mesenchymal cells have the ability to form many different kinds of cells that in turn give rise to various tissues **(Fig. 10.3)**. *Chondroblasts* arising from mesenchymal cells form cartilage, *osteoblasts* form bone, *myoblasts* form muscle, while *lymphoblasts* and *hemocytoblasts* form various cells of blood. Mesenchymal cells also give rise to *endothelial cells* from which blood vessels and the primitive heart tubes are formed.
* However, after all these tissues have been formed many mesenchymal cells are still left and they give rise to cells of various types of connective tissue.

CONNECTIVE TISSUE

As the name suggests, connective tissue serves as a connecting system binding, supporting and strengthening all other body tissues together. Connective tissue consists of three components, i.e., *cells, fibers and ground substance*. The fibers and ground substance are synthesized by the cells of the connective tissue.

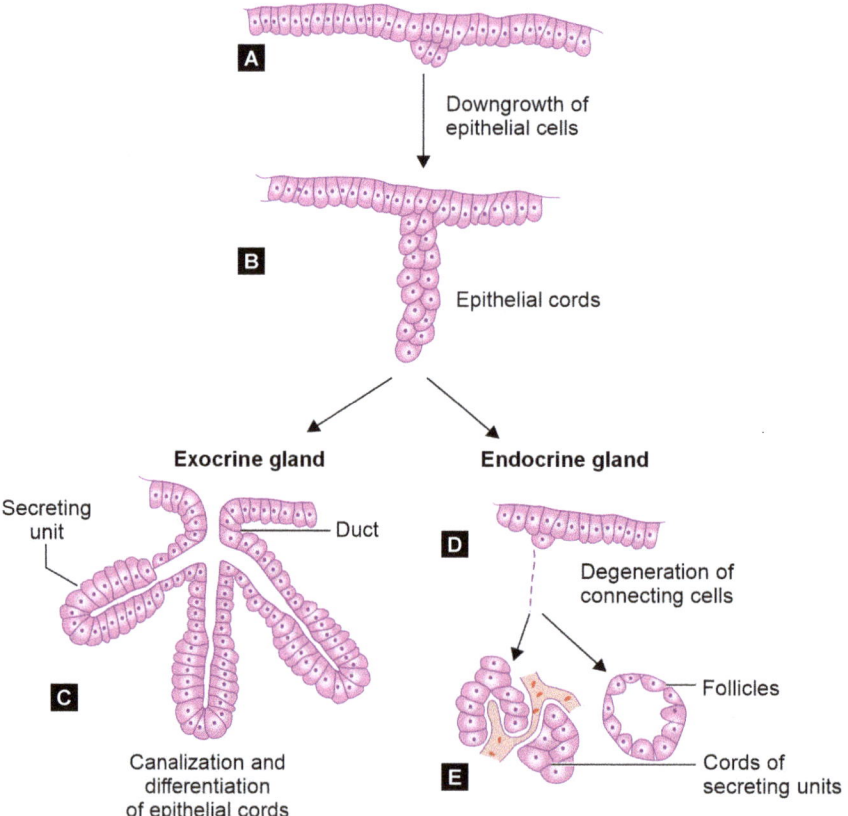

FIGS. 10.1A to E: Stages in the development of a typical gland.

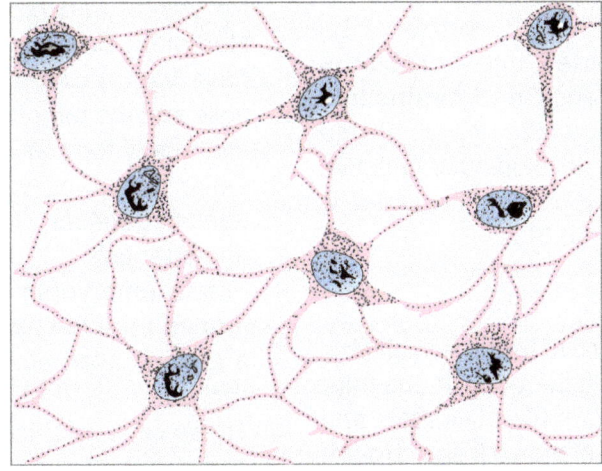

FIG. 10.2: Mesenchymal cells. Note the delicate cytoplasmic processes joining the cells to one another.

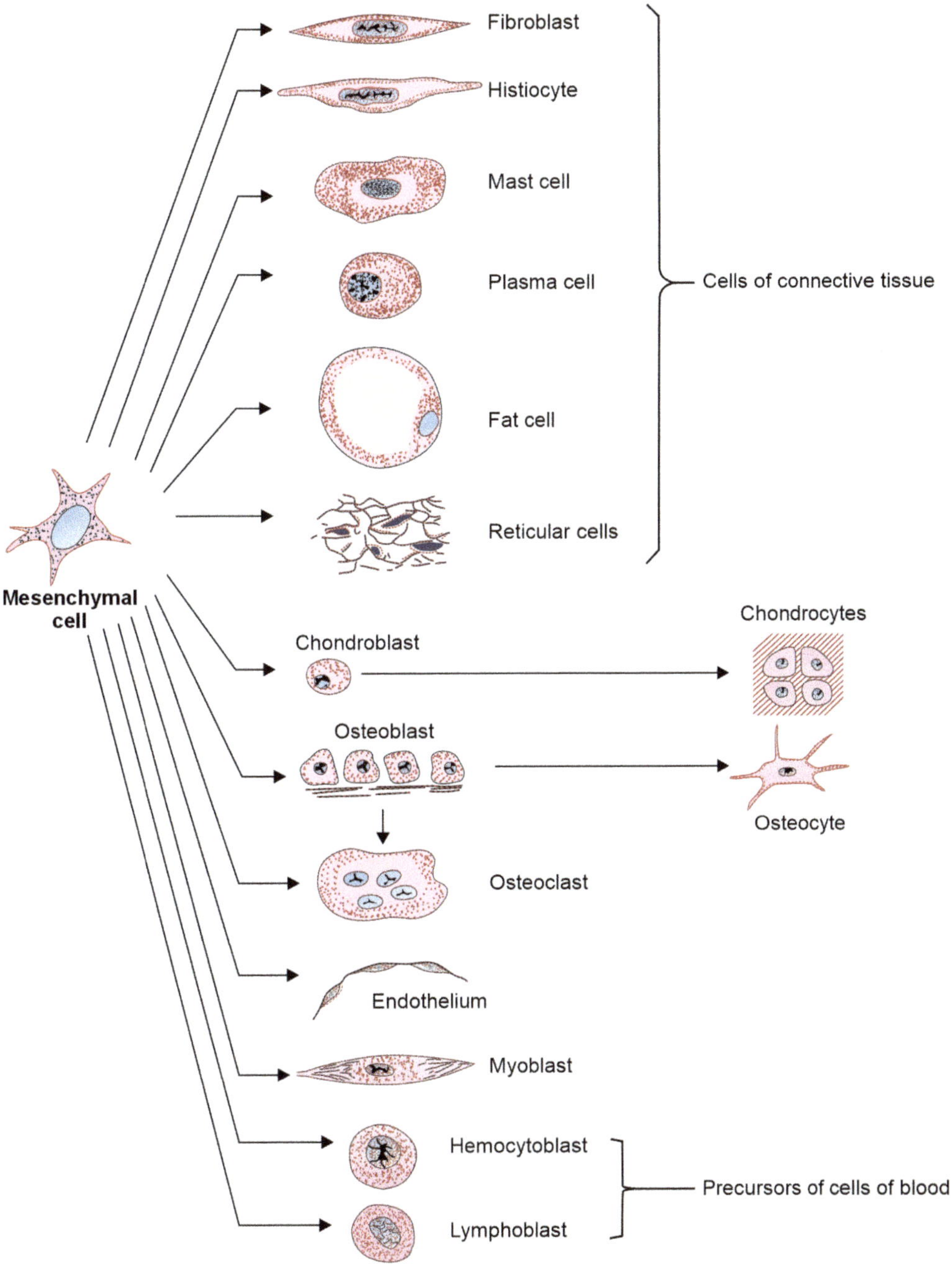

FIG. 10.3: Derivatives of mesenchymal cells.

Formation of Loose Connective Tissue

Mesenchymal cells get converted into fibroblasts that secrete the ground substance and synthesize the *collagen, reticular and elastic fibers*. Some mesenchymal cells present in the developing connective tissue also get converted into *histiocytes, mast cells, plasma cells and fat cells* (Fig. 10.3).

Formation of Blood

Blood is a specialized fluid connective tissue, which acts as a major transport system within the body. In the third week of embryonic life, formation of blood vessels and blood cells is first seen in the wall of the yolk sac, around the allantoic diverticulum and in the connecting stalk. In these situations, clusters of mesodermal cells aggregate to form *blood islands* (Fig. 10.4A).

- *Blood vessels* form in two ways, *vasculogenesis* and *angiogenesis*.
- In vasculogenesis vessels arise from blood islands. In angiogenesis new vessels sprout from existing ones.
- Blood islands first appear in the *mesoderm surrounding the yolk sac*, slightly later in the lateral plate mesoderm and other regions.
- The blood islands arise from mesodermal cells that form *hemangioblasts*, a common precursor for vessel and blood cell formation (Fig. 10.4B). Hemangioblasts in the center of the blood islands form *hemopoietic stem cells*, precursor for blood cells and the peripheral cells into *angioblasts*, which eventually form *endothelial cells* (Fig. 10.4C).
- Once the primary vascular bed is established by vasculogenesis, additional vessels are formed by angiogenesis.
- In late embryonic life, hemopoietic stem cells are formed from the mesoderm surrounding the aorta in a region called *aorta-gonad-mesonephros (AGM) region*.
- These cells colonize the *liver*, the major hemopoietic organ in the fetus until 6 months.
- Later stem cells from the liver colonize the *bone marrow*, the definitive blood forming region. At the time of the birth, blood formation is mainly in the bone marrow.
- All these are mediated mainly by *fibroblast growth factor (FGF)* and *vascular endothelial growth factor (VEGF)*.
- In bone marrow, totipotent haemal stem cells give rise to pleuripotent lymphoid stem cells and pleuripotent haemal stem cells (Fig. 10.5). These stem cells form *colony forming units (CFU)*.
- Cells of one particular colony forming unit are committed to differentiate only into one line of blood cells, i.e., erythrocytes, megakaryocyte, granulocytes, monocytes, macrophages and lymphocytes (Fig. 10.5).
- In the case of erythrocytes, stem cells divide so rapidly that they seem to burst. They are therefore called *burst forming units (BFU)*. Their daughter cells then form colony forming units.

It is to note that the precursors of the various types of blood cells are generally regarded as being of mesodermal in origin. However, blood forming cells differentiating in relation to the wall of the yolk sac and probably in the liver, may be endodermal in origin.

Formation of Cartilage

Cartilage is also formed from mesenchyme. At a site where cartilage is to be formed, mesenchymal cells become closely packed. This is called a *mesenchymal condensation*.

- The mesenchymal cells then become rounded and get converted into cartilage forming cells or *chondroblasts* (Fig. 10.3).
- Under the influence of chondroblasts, the *intercellular substance* of cartilage is laid down.
- Some chondroblasts get imprisoned within the substance of this developing cartilage and are called *chondrocytes*.

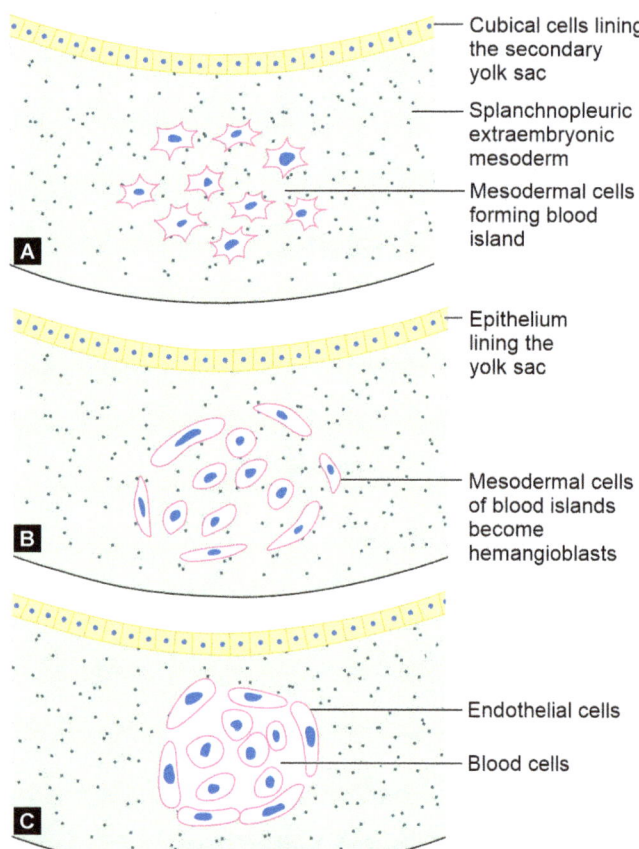

FIGS. 10.4A to C: Formation of blood cells and blood vessel from a blood island.

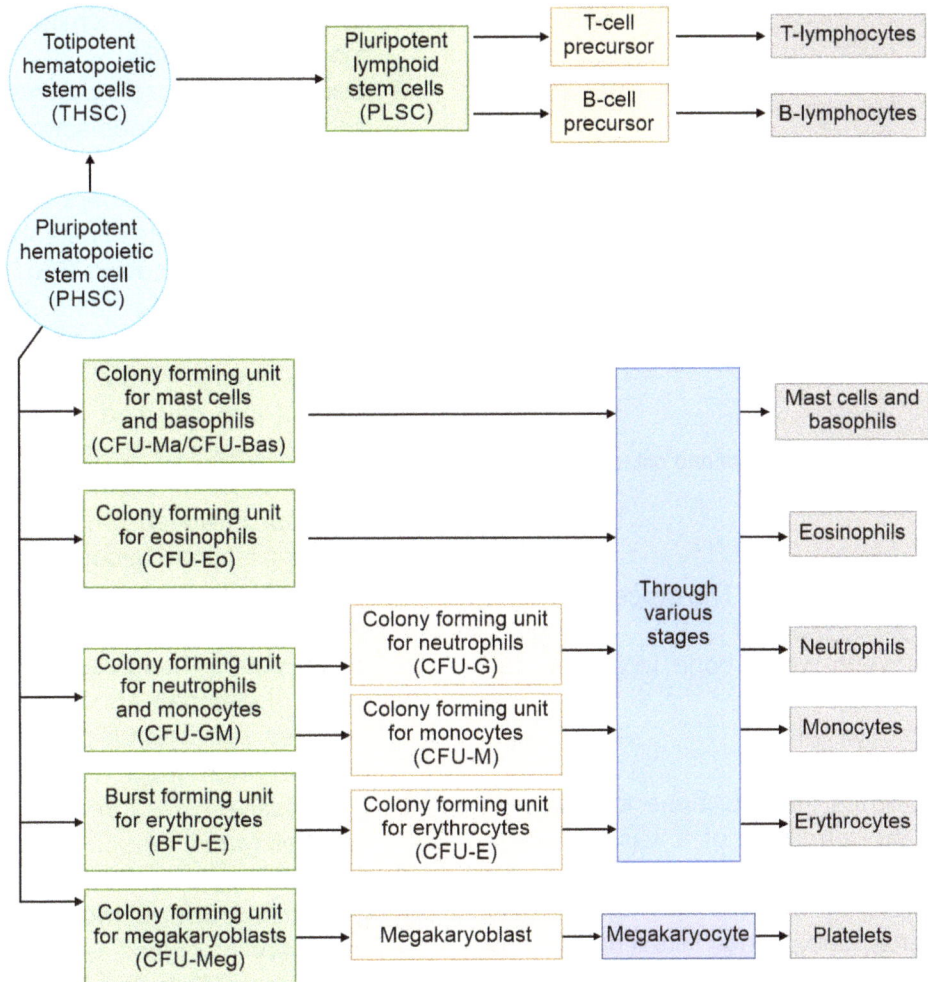

FIG. 10.5: Scheme showing the terms applied to precursors of various blood cells (CFU: colony forming unit; BFU: burst forming unit). Note the other abbreviations used for other precursor cells.

- Some fibers also develop in the intercellular substance. In *hyaline cartilage*, collagen fibers are present, but are not seen easily. In *fibrocartilage*, collagen fibers are numerous and very obvious. In some situations, the intercellular substance is permeated by elastic fibers, forming *elastic cartilage*.
- Mesenchymal cells surrounding the surface of the developing cartilage form a fibrous membrane, the *perichondrium*.

Bone

To understand the formation of bone, it is necessary for students to know its normal structure. This can be read up from the author's *Textbook of Human Histology*. Some features are shown in **Figure 10.6**.

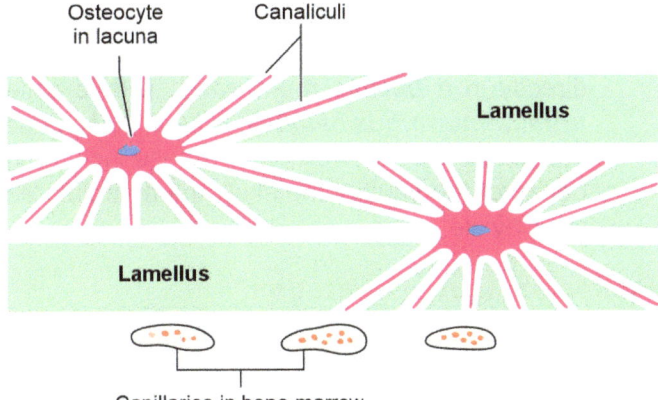

FIG. 10.6: Bone structure: The unit of bone structure is called *lamellus*, which stack upon each other (lamellae) to increase thickness. Between adjoining lamellae, there are spaces called *lacunae*. Osteocytes placed amongst lacunae of bone.

Cells of Bone

Three main types of cells are present in bone:
1. Osteocytes are cells that are seen in mature bone.
2. Osteoblasts are bone forming cells. These cells are, therefore, seen wherever bone is being laid down. They have abundant basophilic cytoplasm and are arranged in regular rows, looking very much like an epithelial lining **(Fig. 10.7)**.
- Osteoclasts are, on the other hand, responsible for bone removal. They are large multinucleated cells and are seen in regions where bone is being absorbed **(Fig. 10.7)**.

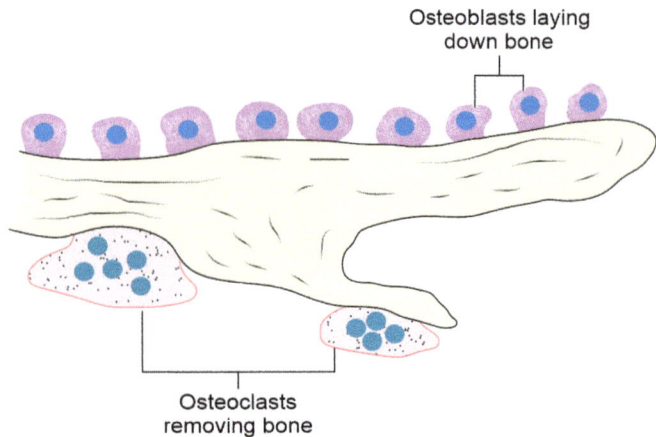

FIG. 10.7: Relationship of osteoblasts and osteoclasts to developing bone.

Formation of Bone

All bone is of *mesodermal origin*. The process of bone formation is called *ossification*.

There are two ways in which bone formation can occur. These are:
1. Intramembranous ossification
2. Endochondral ossification
    - In most parts of the embryo, bone formation is preceded by the formation of a *cartilaginous model* that closely resembles the bone to be formed. This cartilage is subsequently replaced by (not converted into) bone. This kind of bone formation is called *endochondral ossification*. Bones formed in this way are, therefore, called *cartilage bones*.
    - In some situations (e.g., the vault of the skull), formation of bone is not preceded by formation of a cartilaginous model. Instead, bone is laid down directly in a *fibrous membrane*. This is called *intramembranous ossification* and these bones are called *membrane bones*. These include the bones of the vault of the skull, the mandible and the clavicle.

Intramembranous Ossification

❖ It is direct conversion of mesenchymal tissue into bone.
❖ The various steps involved in this type of bone formation are:
  1. *Mesenchymal condensation:* Star-shaped mesenchymal cells of loose connective tissue aggregate in the area where bone is to be formed and are converted to spindle-shaped cells thus forming a condensed mesenchymal tissue model **(Fig. 10.8A)**.
  2. *Conversion into a fibrous membrane:* Spindle-shaped mesenchymal cells differentiate into fibroblasts which lay down collagen fibers converting the mesenchymal model into a fibrous model **(Fig. 10.8B)**.
  3. *Osteoblast and osteoid formation:* Fibroblasts get converted into osteoblasts and start laying down the early bone matrix, i.e., *osteoid* (uncalcified bone). It contains fibers and ground substance which are products of osteoblasts. This forms the *center of ossification* **(Fig. 10.8C)**.
  4. *Mineralization of osteoid:* Secretion of alkaline phosphatase by osteoblasts and deposition of hydroxyapatite crystals of calcium converts the osteoid into calcified bone matrix. Mineralized osteoid is seen as a *spicule of bone* **(Fig. 10.8D)**.
  5. *Conversion of osteoblast to osteocyte and formation of woven bone:* The osteoblasts trapped in matrix lacunae become osteocytes. Processes of osteoblasts traverse through mineralized canals of calcified matrix (tunnels) called *canaliculi*. The collagen fiber bundles run in different directions giving the appearance of a *woven bone*. The spicules are irregularly arranged with spaces between them **(Fig. 10.8E)**.
  6. *Progressive bone formation:* Fusion of adjacent spicules forms the bone model **(Fig. 10.8F)**.
  7. *Remodeling into lamellar bone:* Woven bone gets transformed into lamellar bone due to resorption by osteoclasts and bone deposition by osteoblasts. This results in formation of mature *compact or spongy bone*.

Endochondral Ossification

The essential steps in the formation of bone by endochondral ossification are:
1. **Mesenchymal condensation:** At the site where the bone is to be formed, the mesenchymal cells become closely packed to form a mesenchymal condensation **(Figs. 10.9A and B)**.
2. **Cartilaginous model:** Some mesenchymal cells become chondroblasts and lay down hyaline cartilage **(Fig. 10.9C)**. Mesenchymal cells on the surface of the cartilage form a membrane called the *perichondrium*. This membrane is vascular and contains osteogenic cells.
3. **Cartilage cell hypertrophy:** The cells of the cartilage are at first small and irregularly arranged. However, in the area where bone formation is to begin, the cells enlarge considerably **(Fig. 10.9D)**.
4. **Calcification of intercellular matrix:** The intercellular substance between the enlarged cartilage cells becomes calcified, under the influence of an enzyme called *alkaline phosphatase*, which is secreted by the cartilage cells. The nutrition to the

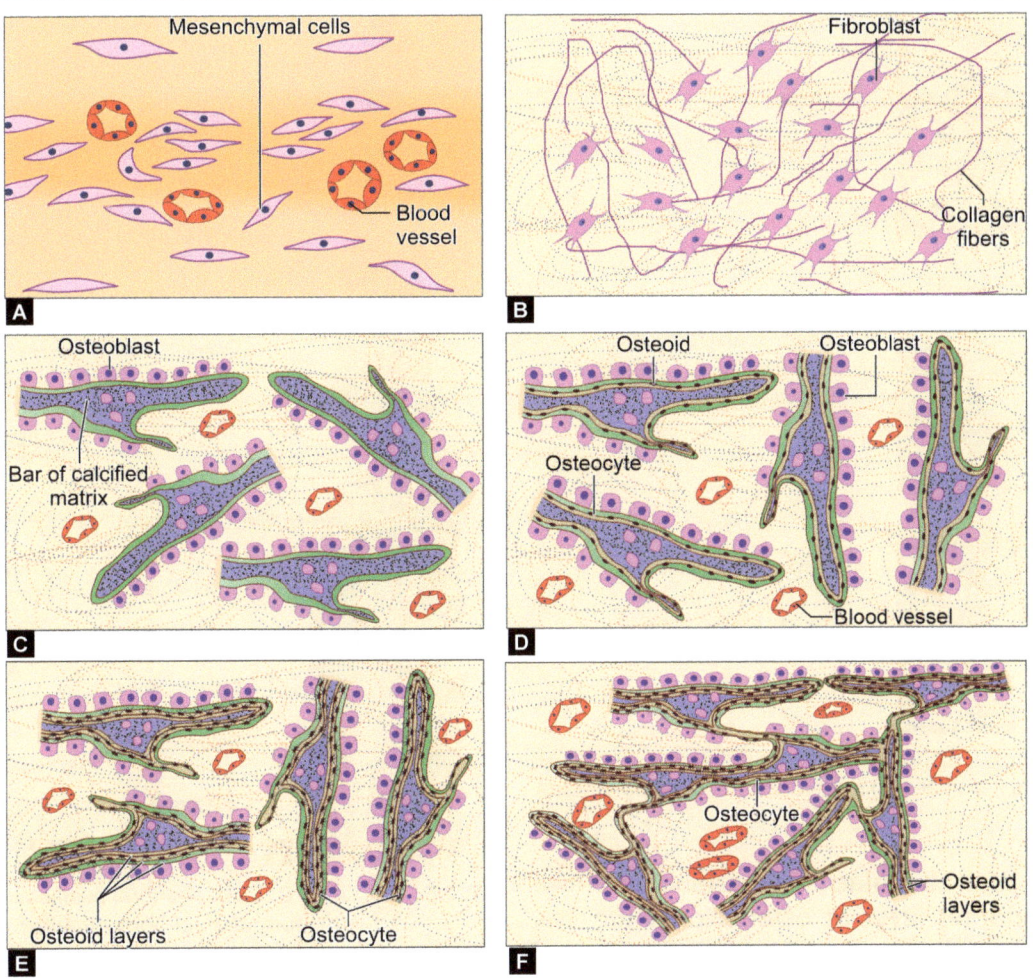

FIGS. 10.8A to F: Stages in intramembranous ossification.

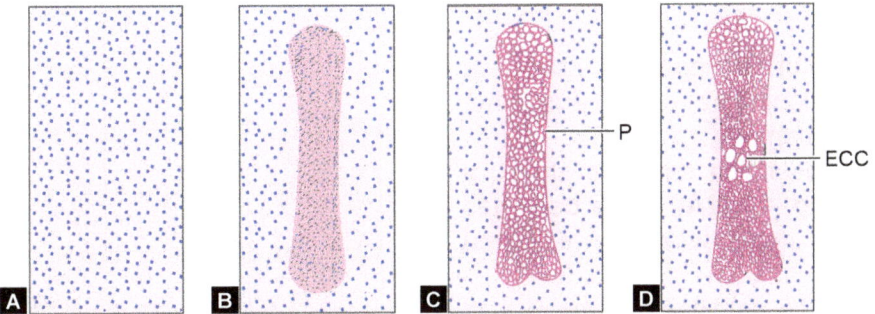

FIGS. 10.9A to D: Endochondral ossification. (A and B) Mesenchymal condensation; (C) Cartilaginous model with perichondrium (P); (D) Enlarged cartilage cells (ECC) at the site of bone formation.

cells is thus cut off and they die, leaving behind empty spaces called *primary areolae* (Figs. 10.10A and B).

5. **Vascularization of cartilaginous matrix:** Some blood vessels of the perichondrium (which may be called *periosteum* as soon as bone is formed) now invade the calcified cartilaginous matrix. They are accompanied by osteogenic cells. This mass of vessels and cells is called the *periosteal bud*. It eats away much of the calcified matrix forming the walls of the primary areolae, and thus creates large cavities called *secondary areolae* (Fig. 10.10C).

6. **Osteoid and lamella formation:** The walls of the secondary areolae are formed by thin layers of calcified matrix that have not been dissolved. The osteogenic cells become osteoblasts and arrange themselves along the surfaces of these bars, or plates, of calcified cartilaginous matrix (Fig. 10.11A). These osteoblasts now lay down a layer of ossein fibrils embedded in a gelatinous intercellular matrix (Fig. 10.11B). This material is called *osteoid*. It is calcified and a *lamellus* of bone is formed (Fig. 10.11C).

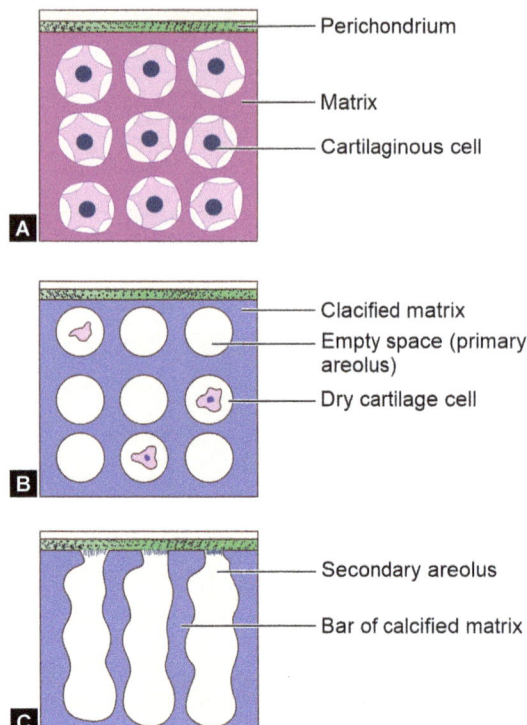

FIGS. 10.10A to C: Endochondral ossification. (A and B) Formation of primary areolae; (C) Formation of secondary areolae.

7. **Formation of trabeculae:** The osteoblasts now lay down another layer of osteoid over the first lamellus. This is also calcified. Thus, two lamellae of bone are formed. Some osteoblasts that get caught between the lamellae form *osteocytes*. As more lamellae are laid down, bony trabeculae are formed **(Fig. 10.11D)**.
   - The calcified matrix of cartilage only acts as a support for the developing trabeculae and is not itself converted into bone.
   - At this stage, the ossifying cartilage shows a central area **(1 in Fig. 10.12A)** where bone has been formed. As we move away from this area we see:
     - A region where the cartilaginous matrix has been calcified and surrounds dead, and dying, cartilage cells **(2 in Fig. 10.12A)**.
     - A zone of hypertrophied cartilage cells, in an uncalcified matrix **(3 in Fig. 10.12A)**.
     - A normal cartilage **(4 in Fig. 10.12A)** in which there is considerable mitotic activity.
   ❖ If we see the same cartilage a little later **(Fig. 10.12B)**, we find that ossification has now extended into zone 2, and simultaneously the matrix in zone 3 has become calcified. The deeper cells of zone 4 have meanwhile hypertrophied, while the more superficial ones have multiplied to form zone 5.

In this way, formation of new cartilage keeps pace with the loss due to replacement by bone. The total effect is

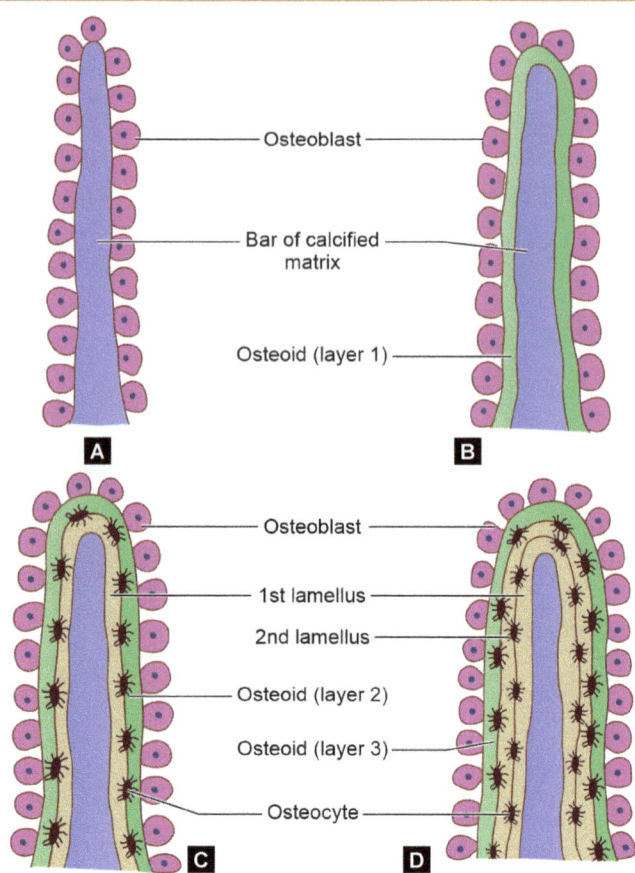

FIGS. 10.11A to D: Endochondral ossification. Stages in the formation of bony lamellae.

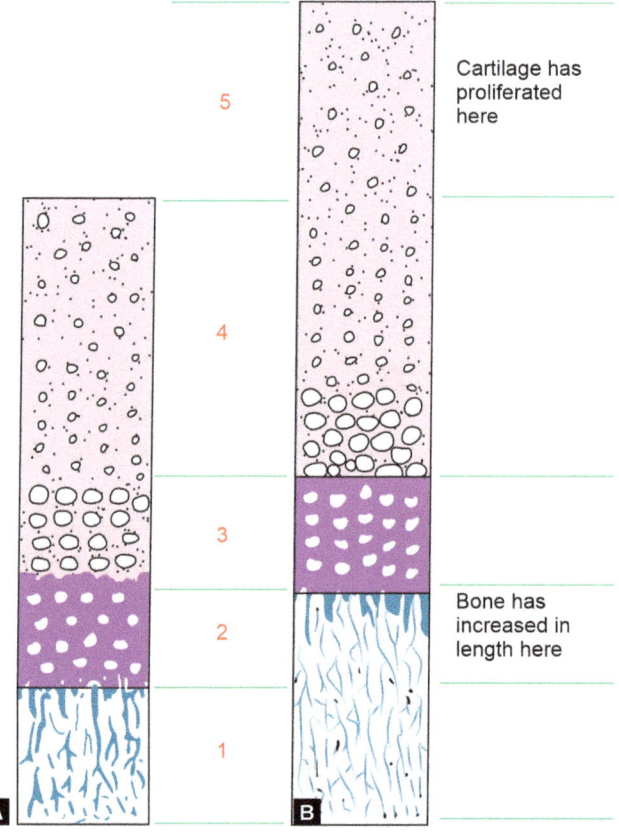

FIGS. 10.12A and B: Scheme to show the growth in length of a bone.

that the ossifying cartilage progressively increases in size.

Development of a Typical Long Bone

We may now consider how a long bone develops.

* A *mesenchymal condensation* is seen in the limb bud in the region where the bone is to be formed **(Figs. 10.13A and B)**.
* This mesenchymal condensation is converted into a *cartilaginous model*. This model closely resembles the bone to be formed. It is covered by perichondrium **(Fig. 10.13C)** that has a superficial fibrous layer and a deeper layer that has osteogenic cells.
* Endochondral ossification starts in a small area of the shaft as described above. This area is called the *primary center of ossification* **(Fig. 10.14)**.
* Gradually, bone formation extends from the primary center towards the ends of the shaft. This is accompanied by enlargement of the cartilaginous model **(Fig. 10.14)**.
* Soon after the appearance of the primary center, and onset of endochondral ossification in it, the perichondrium (which may now be called *periosteum*) becomes active. The osteogenic cells in its deeper layer lay down bone on the surface of the cartilaginous model by *intramembranous ossification*. This periosteal bone completely surrounds the cartilaginous shaft and is, therefore, called the *periosteal collar* **(Fig. 10.14)**.
* It is first formed only around the region of the primary center but rapidly extends towards the ends of the cartilaginous model. The periosteal collar acts as a splint, and gives strength to the cartilaginous model, at the site where it is weakened by the formation of secondary areolae. We shall see that most of the shaft of the bone is derived from this periosteal collar and is, therefore, intramembranous in origin.

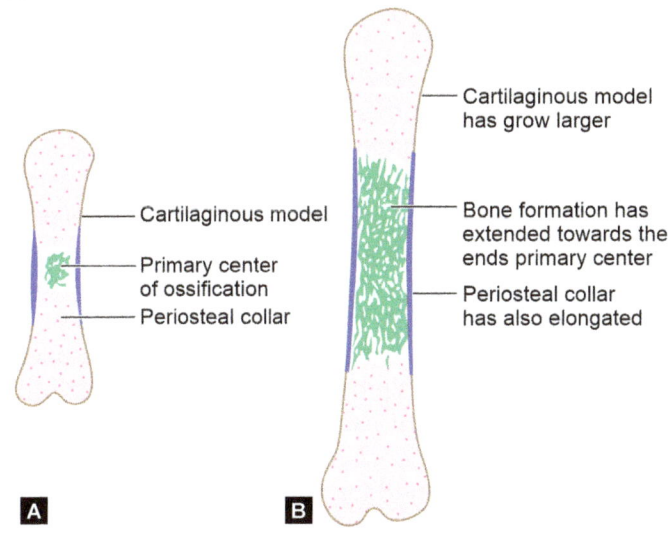

FIGS. 10.14A and B: Formation of a typical long bone: Primary center of ossification and periosteal collar.

* At about the time of birth, the developing bone consists of a part called the *diaphysis (or shaft)* (that is bony, and has been formed by extension of the primary center of ossification); and ends that are cartilaginous **(Fig. 10.15A)**. At varying times after birth, *secondary centers* of endochondral ossification appear in the cartilages forming the ends of the bone **(Fig. 10.15B)**. These centers enlarge until the ends become bony **(Fig. 10.15C)**. More than one secondary center of ossification may appear at either end. The portion of bone formed from one secondary center is called an *epiphysis*.
* For a considerable time after birth, the bone of the diaphysis and the bone of the epiphysis are separated by a plate of cartilage called the *epiphyseal cartilage*, or *epiphyseal plate*. This is formed by cartilage into which ossification has not extended either from the diaphysis or from the epiphysis. We shall see that this plate plays a vital role in growth of the bone.

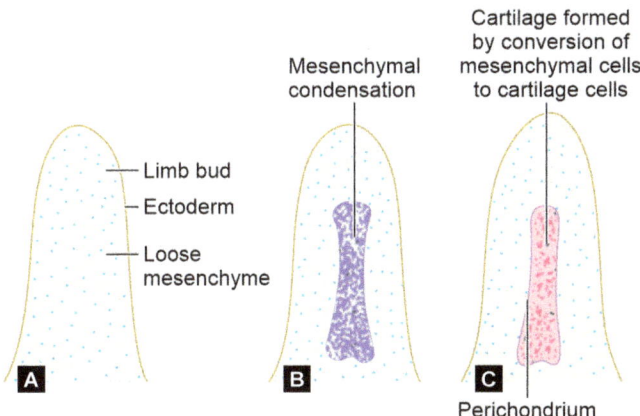

FIGS. 10.13A to C: Formation of a typical long bone: Establishment of cartilaginous model.

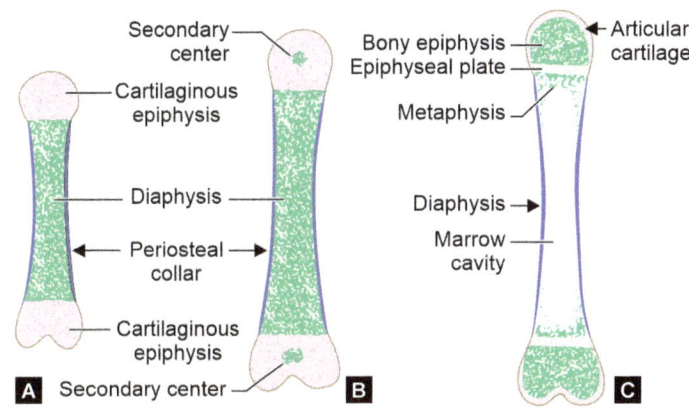

FIGS. 10.15A to C: Formation of a typical long bone: Secondary centers of ossification.

Growth of a Long Bone

A growing bone increases both in length and in thickness.

❖ The periosteum forms a layer of bone around the shaft of the cartilaginous model, known as the periosteal collar, which extends along the diaphysis. As new layers of bone are added, the periosteal bone thickens.

❖ It's important that the periosteal bone doesn't become too thick. Osteoclasts line the internal surface of the shaft, removing bone from the inside as new bone is added outside. This process allows the shaft to grow in diameter without excessively thick walls **(Figs. 10.16A to E)**. Osteoclasts also remove trabeculae in the center formed by endochondral ossification, creating a *marrow cavity*.

❖ As the shaft's diameter increases, the marrow cavity also enlarges and extends toward the ends of the diaphysis without reaching the epiphyseal plate. Most of the bone from the primary center of ossification is removed, except near the ends, leaving the shaft wall made of periosteal bone formed by intramembranous ossification.

❖ To understand how a bone grows in length, we will now have a closer look at the epiphyseal plate. Depending on the arrangement of its cells, three zones can be recognized **(Fig. 10.17)**.
  – *Zone of resting cartilage:* Here, the cells are small and irregularly arranged.
  – *Zone of proliferating cartilage:* Here, the cells are larger and are undergoing repeated mitosis. As they multiply, they come to be arranged in parallel columns, separated by bars of intercellular matrix.
  – *Zone of calcification:* Here, the cells become still larger and the matrix becomes calcified.

❖ Next to the zone of calcification, there is a zone where cartilage cells are dead and the calcified matrix is being replaced by bone. Growth in length of the bone takes place by continuous transformation of the epiphyseal cartilage to bone **(Figs. 10.17 and 10.18)** in this zone (i.e., on the diaphyseal surface of the epiphyseal cartilage). At the same time, the thickness of the epiphyseal cartilage is maintained by active multiplication of cells in the zone of proliferation.

❖ When the bone has attained its full length, cells in the epiphyseal cartilage stop proliferating. The process of ossification, however, continues to extend into it until the whole of the epiphyseal plate is converted into bone. The bone of the diaphysis and epiphysis then becomes continuous. This is called *fusion of epiphysis*.

Metaphysis

The portion of diaphysis adjoining the epiphyseal plate is called the *metaphysis*. It is a region of active bone formation and, for this reason, it is highly vascular. The metaphysis does not have a marrow cavity. Numerous

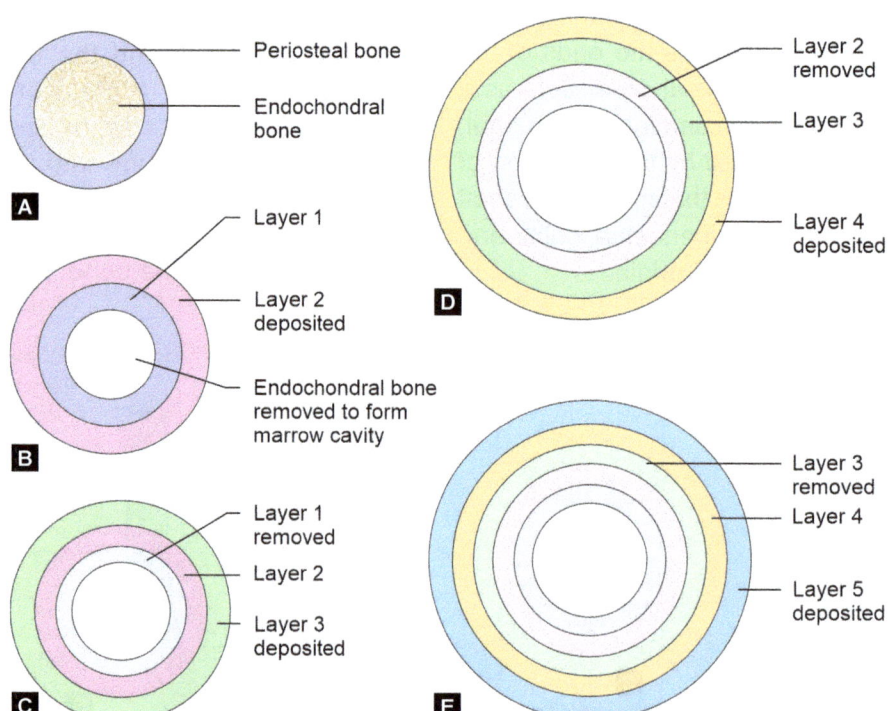

FIGS. 10.16A to E: Formation of a typical long bone: Increase in thickness. Note that the shaft is ultimately made up almost entirely of periosteal bone formed by the process of intramembranous ossification.

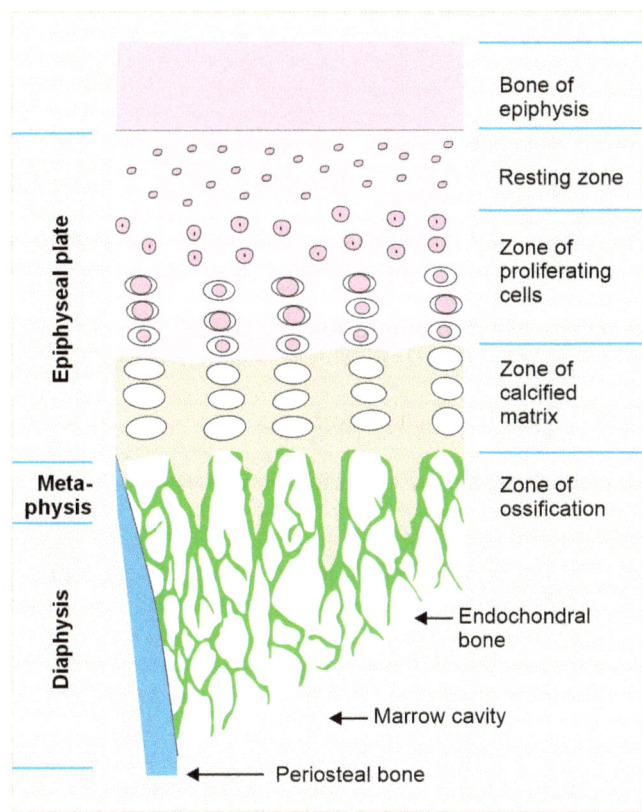

FIG. 10.17: Structure of epiphyseal cartilage.

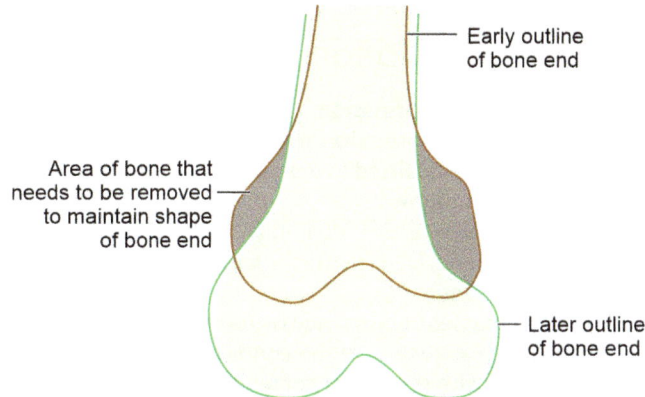

FIG. 10.19: Remodeling of bone ends during growth.

tissue. This is called *interstitial growth*. As a result, the tissue expands equally in all directions and its shape is maintained. Cartilage (and most other tissues) grow in this way.

On the other hand, bone grows only by deposition of more bone on its surface, or at its ends. This is called *appositional growth*.

Remodeling

We have seen above that when a tissue grows by interstitial growth it is easy for it to maintain its shape. However, this is not true of bone which can grow only by apposition. This will be clear from **Figure 10.19**. In this figure the brown line represents the shape of a bone end. The green line represents the same bone end after it has grown for some time. It will be clear that some areas of the original bone have to disappear if proper shape is to be maintained. This process of removal of unwanted bone is called *remodeling*.

The trabeculae of spongy bone and the Haversian systems of compact bone are so arranged that they are best fitted to bear the stresses imposed on them. This arrangement can change with change in stresses acting on the bone. This process is often called *internal remodeling*.

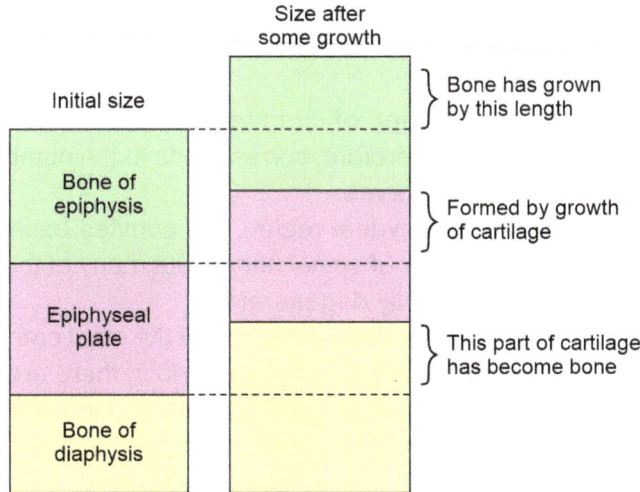

FIG. 10.18: Growth in length of bone at epiphyseal cartilage.

muscles and ligaments are usually attached to the bone in this region. Even after bone growth has ceased, the calcium-turnover function of bone is most active in the metaphysis, which acts as a storehouse of calcium. This region is frequently the site of infection.

Interstitial and Appositional Growth

Tissues grow by two methods. In some of them, growth takes place by multiplication of cells (or by increase in intercellular material) throughout the substance of the

MUSCULAR TISSUE

There are three different types of muscles. They are (1) skeletal, (2) cardiac and (3) smooth muscles.

* Skeletal muscle may be derived from somites, from somitomeres and from lateral plate mesoderm. At these sites, there are cells that are precursors of muscle. These cells divide repeatedly and finally differentiate into *myoblasts* or *premuscle cells*. Myoblasts synthesize the proteins *actin and myosin*.
* Several myoblasts fuse with each other to form multinucleated tube-like elements that are called *myotubes*.

> **Clinical correlation**
>
> **Anomalies of Bone Formation**
> Bone and cartilage formation may sometimes be abnormal as a result of various genetic and environmental factors. The anomalies may be localized to a particular part of the skeleton, or may be generalized. Some anomalies that affect the skeleton as a whole are as follows:
> - Disorderly and excessive proliferation of cartilage cells in the epiphyseal plate, or the failure of normally formed cartilage to be replaced by bone, leads to the formation of irregular masses of cartilage within the metaphysis. This is called *dyschondroplasia* or *enchondromatosis*.
> - Abnormal masses of bone may be formed in the region of the metaphysis and may protrude from the bone. Such a protrusion is called an *exostosis*, and the condition is called *multiple exostoses* or *diaphyseal aclasis*. This condition may be a result of interference with the process of remodeling of bone ends.
> - Calcification of bone may be defective *(osteogenesis imperfecta)* and may result in multiple fractures.
> - Parts of bone may be replaced by fibrous tissue *(fibrous displasia)*.
> - Bones may show increased density or *osteosclerosis*. One disease characterized by increased bone density is known as *osteopetrosis*, or *marble bone disease*.
> - In the condition called *achondroplasia*, there is insufficient, or disorderly, formation of bone in the region of the epiphyseal cartilage. This interferes with growth of long bones. The individual does not grow in height and becomes a dwarf. A similar condition in which the limbs are of normal length, but in which the vertebral column remains short, is called *chondro-osteo-dystrophy*.
> - Anomalous bone formation may be confined to membrane bones. One such condition is *cleidocranial dystosis* in which the clavicle is absent and there are deformities of the skull. On the other hand, anomalies like achondroplasia and exostoses are confined to cartilage bones.
> - Generalized underdevelopment *(dwarfism)*, or overdevelopment *(gigantism)* of bone may be present. Sometimes all bones of one half of the body are affected *(asymmetric development)*. Overdevelopment or underdevelopment may be localized, e.g., to a digit, or to a limb.

- Within these myotubes molecules of actin, myosin and other contractile proteins unite to form *myofibrils*.
- These fibrils are arranged in a definite orientation. Progressive aggregation of fibrils within the myotube pushes nuclei to the periphery. A muscle fiber is thus formed.
- Satellite cells present around muscle fibers can help in growth of fibers.

Fate of Somites

We have seen that the paraxial mesoderm becomes segmented to form a number of somites, that lie on either side of the developing neural tube.
- A cross section through a somite shows that it is a triangular structure and has a cavity **(Fig. 10.20A)**.
- The somite is divisible into three parts.
  1. The ventromedial part is called the *sclerotome*. The cells of the sclerotome migrate medially. They surround the neural tube and give rise to the vertebral column and ribs **(Figs. 10.20B and C)**.
  2. The lateral part is called the *dermatome*. The cells of this part also migrate, and come to line the deep surface of the ectoderm covering the entire body. These cells give rise to the dermis on the back of the head and trunk and to subcutaneous tissue.
  3. The intermediate part is the *myotome*. It gives rise to striated/skeletal muscle as described in the following section:

- In the cervical, thoracic, lumbar and sacral regions one spinal nerve innervates each myotome.
- The number of somites formed in these regions, therefore, corresponds to the number of spinal nerves.
- In the coccygeal region, the somites exceed the number of spinal nerves but many of them subsequently degenerate.
- The first cervical somite is *not* the most cranial somite to be formed. Cranial to it, there are:
  - The occipital somites (four to five) which give rise to muscles of the tongue and are supplied by the hypoglossal nerve.
  - The preoccipital (or preotic) somites (somitomeres), supplied by the third, fourth and sixth cranial nerves.

Development of Striated Muscle

Striated muscle is derived from somites and also from mesenchyme of the region.
- In humans, the myotomes give origin only to the musculature of the trunk, in whole or in part.
- The occipital myotomes are believed to give rise to the musculature of the tongue, while the extrinsic muscles of the eyeball are regarded as derivatives of the preoccipital myotomes.

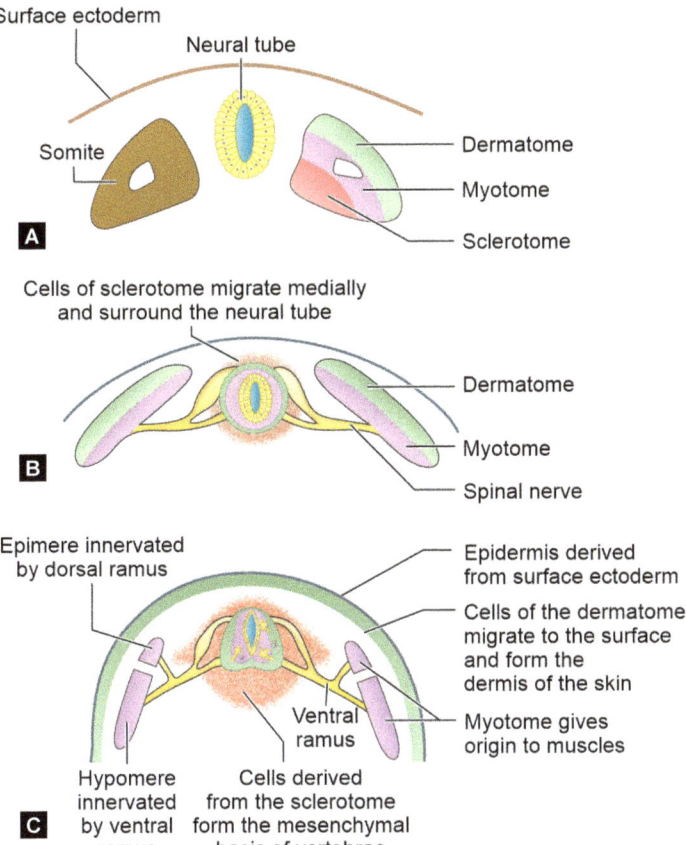

FIGS. 10.20A to C: (A) Somites lying on either side of the neural tube. Note subdivisions of somite; (B) The cells of the sclerotome have migrated medially and now surround the neural tube. The myotome is innervated by nerves growing out of the neural tube; (C) The cells of the dermatome have migrated to form the dermis of the skin.

- Soon after its formation, each myotome, in the neck and trunk, separates into a dorsal part *(epimere)* which gives rise to the muscles supplied by the dorsal primary ramus of the spinal nerve, and a ventral part *(hypomere)*, which gives origin to the muscles supplied by the ventral ramus **(Fig. 10.20C)**. The epimeres give origin to the muscles of the back (extensors of the vertebral column), while the hypomeres give origin to the muscles of the body wall and limbs.
- Some cells from the ventrolateral region of the dermomyotomes migrate into the parietal layer of lateral plate mesoderm where they form muscles of limbs, and anterolateral muscles of the neck and abdomen.

Smooth Muscle

Almost all smooth muscle is formed from mesenchyme:
- Smooth muscle in the walls of viscera (e.g., the stomach) is formed from splanchnopleuric mesoderm in relation to them.
- However, the muscles of the iris (sphincter and dilator pupillae) and myoepithelial cells of the sweat glands are derived from ectoderm.

Cardiac Muscle

This is derived from splanchnopleuric mesoderm in relation to the developing heart tubes and pericardium.

NERVOUS TISSUE

Nervous tissue consists of cells, fibers and blood vessels. Two different categories of cells are found in the nervous tissues, i.e., *neurons and neuroglial cells*.
- The neurons are cells that generate and conduct nerve impulses, while the neuroglial cells are supporting structures.
- Neurons have many processes *(axons and dendrites)*. These processes collect to form nerves.
- Blood vessels of the nervous tissue are not derived from the neural tube but enter it from surrounding *mesoderm*.
- Nervous system and specialized sense organs are derived from *neuroectoderm* which gives rise to *neural tube* and *neural crest cells*.

Formation of Neurons and Neuroglial Cells

The neurons and many neuroglial cells are formed in the neural tube:
- The neural tube is at first lined by a single layer of cells **(Fig. 10.21A)**. These proliferate to form three layers **(Fig. 10.21B)**.
- Nearest the lumen of the tube is the *matrix cell layer* (also called primitive ependymal or germinal layer). The cells of this layer give rise to nerve cells, to neuroglial cells, and also to more germinal cells.
- Next comes the *mantle layer* in which are seen the developing nerve cells, and neuroglial cells.
- The outermost layer, termed the *marginal zone*, contains no nerve cells. It consists of a reticulum

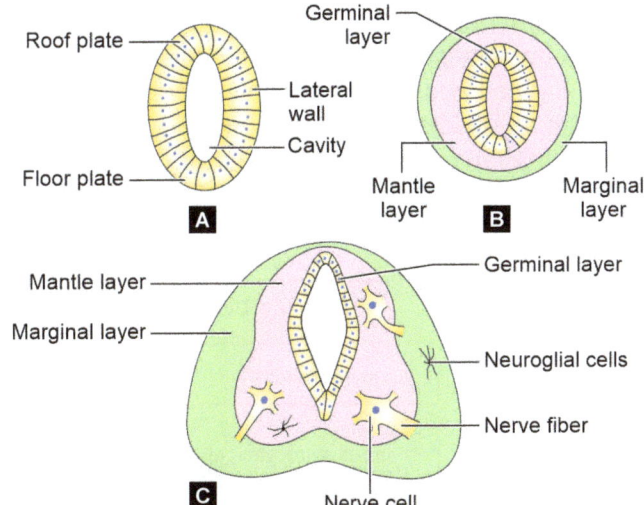

FIGS. 10.21A to C: Layers of the neural tube. Although the germinal (neuroepithelial) layer is shown as a simple epithelium, it is really pseudostratified.

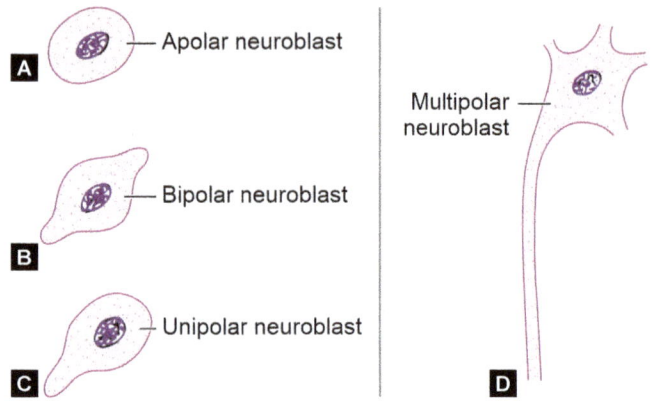

FIGS. 10.22A to D: Stages in formation of a typical neuroblast.

formed by protoplasmic processes of developing neuroglial cells *(spongioblasts)*. It provides a framework into which the processes of nerve cells developing in the mantle layer can grow.

The stages in the formation of a nerve cell are as follows:
- One of the germinal cells passes from the germinal layer to the mantle layer and becomes an *apolar neuroblast* (Fig. 10.22A).
- Two processes develop and convert the apolar neuroblast to a *bipolar neuroblast* (Fig. 10.22B).
- One of the processes of the neuroblast disappears, and it can now be called an *unipolar neuroblast* (Fig. 10.22C).
- The process of the cell (which does not disappear) now elongates, and on the side opposite to it numerous smaller processes form. At this stage, the cell is called a *multipolar neuroblast* (Fig. 10.22D).
- The main process of the multipolar neuroblast now grows into the marginal layer, and becomes the *axon* of the nerve cell (Fig. 10.21B).
- The axon can grow to a considerable length. It may either remain within the central nervous system, or may grow out of it as an efferent nerve fiber of a peripheral nerve.
- At its destination, it establishes connections, either with the cell bodies and dendrites of other neurons, or with an effector organ (e.g., muscle).
- The smaller processes of the neuroblast are the *dendrites*. These ramify and establish connections with other nerve cells.

- At first the cytoplasm of the nerve cell is homogeneous. Later *Nissl's granules* make their appearance. After their formation, neurons lose the ability to divide.

Neuroglial Cells

- Neuroglial cells are also formed from germinal cells of the ependymal layer (**Fig. 10.23**). These cells *(glioblasts)* migrate to the mantle and marginal zones as *medulloblasts* (also called *spongioblasts*), which differentiate either into *astroblasts*, and subsequently into *astrocytes*, or into *oligodendroblasts* and then into *oligodendrocytes*.
- There is a third type of neuroglial cell called *microglia*. This type does not develop from the cells of the neural tube, but migrates into it along with blood vessels. These cells are believed to be of mesodermal origin.

We have seen above that the ependymal (or neuroepithelial) cells give rise both to neuroblasts and to neuroglia. However, these two cell types are not formed simultaneously. The neuroblasts are formed first. Neuroglial cells are formed after the differentiation of neuroblasts is completed.

Formation of Myelin Sheath

- Nerve fibers, which remain within the brain and spinal cord, receive support from, and are ensheathed by, neuroglial cells.
- However, the nerve fibers, which leave the central nervous system to become constituents of peripheral nerves, acquire a special sheath called the *neurolemma*.
- This sheath is derived from some cells of the neural crest that are called *Schwann cells*.
- At a later stage of development, a large number of nerve fibers, both inside and outside the central nervous system, develop another sheath between the neurolemma and the axon. This is called the *myelin sheath*.
- The myelin sheaths of peripheral nerves are derived from the same Schwann cells that form the neurolemma.
- In the central nervous system itself, however, there are no Schwann cells and the myelin sheath is formed by neuroglial cells called *oligodendrocytes*.

Derivation of nerve cells (neurons) and neuroglial cells		
From neural tube	From neural crest	From mesenchymal cells
• Neurons • Fibrous astrocytes • Protoplasmic astrocytes • Oligodendroglia • Ependymal cells	• Schwann cells • Dorsal nerve root ganglion cells • Cells of other sensory ganglia • Neurons in sympathetic ganglia	• Microglia • Oligodendroglia

FIG. 10.23: Various types of cells are derived from neuroepithelium.

Myelinated and Unmyelinated Nerve Fibers

The relationship of an axon to a Schwann cell is illustrated in **Figures 10.24A to G**. Note the following points:

* Each axon invaginates the cytoplasm of a Schwann cell and thus comes to be completely surrounded by it **(Figs. 10.24A and B)**. Along the line of invagination, the cell membrane of the Schwann cell becomes drawn into form a double layered mesentery, like membrane called the *mesaxon* **(Fig. 10.24C)**.
* In the case of myelinated nerve fibers, the mesaxon elongates and becomes spirally wound around the axon **(Figs. 10.24D and E)**. Some fatty substances are deposited between adjacent layers of the mesaxon and, together with it, form the myelin sheath.
* In the case of unmyelinated fibers there is no elongation of the mesaxon. Several unmyelinated fibers may invaginate the same Schwann cell **(Figs. 10.24E to G)**.

Nerve fibers in different parts of the brain, and spinal cord, become myelinated at different stages of development. The process begins during the fourth month of intrauterine life, but is not completed until the child is 2–3 years old. Nerve fibers become fully functional only after they have acquired their myelin sheaths.

Formation of Blood Vessels

The blood vessels of the brain, and their surrounding connective tissue, are not derived from the neural tube. These are mesodermal in origin and invade the developing brain and spinal cord from the surrounding mesoderm.

The development of the *pia mater* and the *arachnoid mater (leptomeninges)* is not definitely understood.

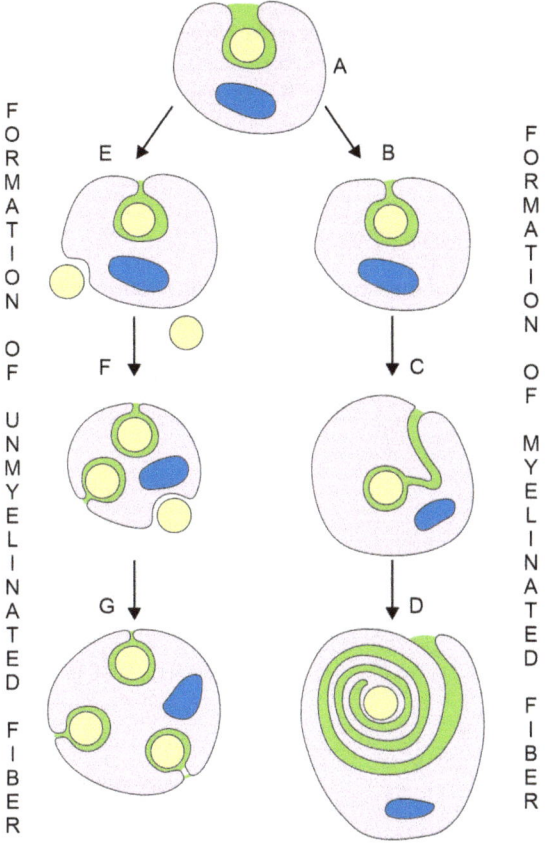

FIGS. 10.24A to G: Process of formation of (A to D) myelinated and (E to G) unmyelinated axons.

According to some researchers, these are derived from the neural crest. The dura mater develops from the mesoderm surrounding the neural tube.

HIGHLIGHTS

* **Epithelia** may originate from ectoderm, endoderm or mesoderm.
* Epithelia lining *external surfaces* of the body, and terminal parts of passages opening to the outside are derived from ectoderm.
* Epithelium lining the *gut*, and of organs that develop as diverticula of the gut, is endodermal in origin.
* Epithelium lining most of the *urogenital tract* is derived from mesoderm. In some parts, it is endodermal in origin.
* **Mesenchyme** is made up of cells that can give rise to cartilage, bone, muscle, blood and connective tissues.
* **Blood cells** are derived from mesenchyme in bone marrow, liver, and spleen. Lymphocytes are formed mainly in lymphoid tissues.
* Most **bones** are formed by **endochondral ossification**, in which a cartilaginous model is first formed and is later replaced by bone. Some bones are formed by direct ossification of membrane *(intramembranous ossification)*.
* An area where ossification starts is called a **center of ossification**. In the case of long bones the shaft (or diaphysis) is formed by extension of ossification from the *primary center of ossification*. Secondary centers (of variable number) appear for bone ends. The part of bone ossified from a secondary center is called an *epiphysis*.
* In growing bone the diaphysis and epiphysis are separated by the *epiphyseal plate* (which is made up of cartilage). Growth in length of a bone takes place mainly at the epiphyseal plate.
* The portion of diaphysis adjoining the epiphyseal plate is called the *metaphysis*.
* **Somites** undergo division into three parts. These are: (a) the *dermatome* which forms the dermis of the skin; (b) *myotome* which forms skeletal muscle; and (c) *sclerotome* which helps to form the vertebral column and ribs.
* **Skeletal muscle** is derived partly from somites and partly from mesenchyme of the region.
* Most *smooth muscle* is formed from mesenchyme related to viscera, and blood vessels.

- **Cardiac muscle** is formed from mesoderm related to the developing heart.
- **Neurons** and many *neuroglial cells* are formed in the neural tube. The myelin sheaths of peripheral nerves are derived from *Schwann cells,* while in the central nervous system they are derived from *oligodendrocytes.*

Summary

- Formation of membranous and endochondral bone **(Flowchart 10.1)**.
- Origin of muscles of human body **(Table 10.1)**.

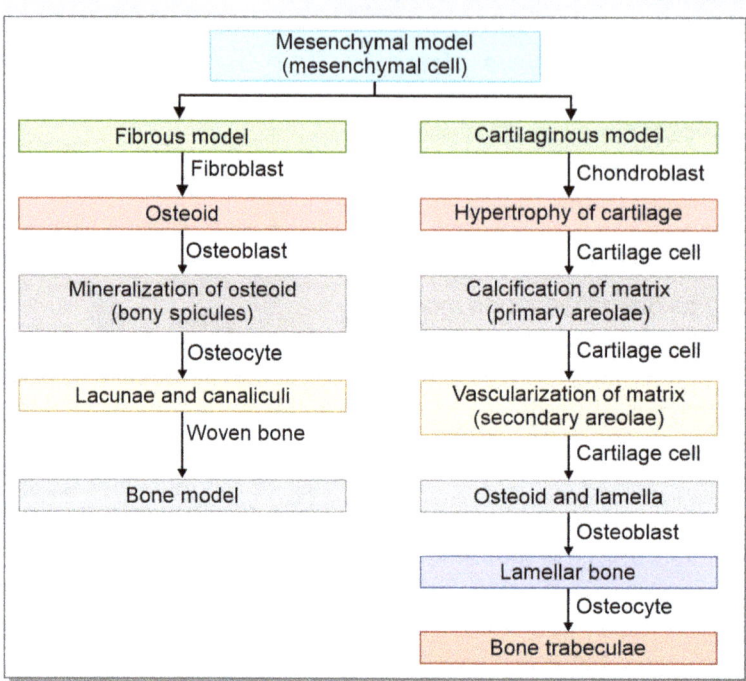

FLOWCHART 10.1: Intramembranous and endochondral ossification.

TABLE 10.1: Muscle group and structures they are derived from.

Muscle group	Derived from
Muscles of head and neck	
• Extraocular muscles	• Prechordal mesoderm, somitomeres 1–3
• Muscles of mastication	• First pharyngeal arch (mesoderm), Somitomere 4
• Facial expression muscles	• Second pharyngeal arch (mesoderm), Somitomere 6
• Sternocleidomastoid and trapezius	• Occipital somites 2–5
• Infrahyoid muscles	• C1–C3 myotomes
• Tongue muscles	• Occipital myotomes (except palatoglossus, which is from the fourth pharyngeal arch)
Muscles of the Thorax	C3–C7 myotomes (contribute to intercostal muscles)
Muscles of the abdomen	T1-L5 myotomes
Muscles of the back	Epaxial muscles derived from the dorsal portion of myotomes. All spinal myotomes (cervical, thoracic, lumbar, sacral)
Muscles of the limbs	Limb bud mesoderm (from lateral plate mesoderm)
• Upper limb muscles	Somitic mesoderm (C5-T1 myotomes)
• Lower limb muscles	Somitic mesoderm (L2-S3 myotomes)
Diaphragm	Septum transversum, pleuroperitoneal membranes, dorsal mesentery of the esophagus, and body wall mesoderm, C3fC5 myotomes (contribute to the phrenic nerve)

TEST YOUR UNDERSTANDING

REVIEW QUESTIONS

1. What are the types of glands? Discuss their formation.
2. Enumerate the derivatives of mesenchymal cells.
3. Discuss the stages in the formation of nerve cells.
4. Describe the stages in intramembranous ossification.
5. Describe the stages in endochondral ossification.

MULTIPLE CHOICE QUESTIONS

1. All the following are true about metaphysis, *except*:
   A. Highly vascular
   B. No marrow cavity
   C. Store house of calcium
   D. No active bone formation
2. The most common site of infection in a bone:
   A. Epiphysis
   B. Diaphysis
   C. Metaphysis
   D. Epiphyseal plate
3. Smooth muscle of iris is developed from:
   A. Intermediate mesoderm
   B. Somatic mesoderm
   C. Splanchnic mesoderm
   D. Neurectoderm
4. Spongioblast cells develops from:
   A. Mantle layer
   B. Matrix layer
   C. Neural crest cells
   D. Marginal layer
5. Neuron bodies present outside CNS are derived from:
   A. Ectoderm
   B. Primitive streak
   C. Notochord
   D. Neural crest cells
6. A newborn presents with craniosynostosis, where premature fusion of cranial sutures occurs. Which embryological tissue primarily contributes to the formation of cranial bones?
   A. Mesenchyme
   B. Cartilage
   C. Epithelium
   D. Nervous tissue
7. A newborn presents with congenital absence of the radius bone. Which embryological process primarily contributes to the formation of the radius?
   A. Endochondral ossification
   B. Intramembranous ossification
   C. Myogenesis
   D. Neurogenesis
8. During embryonic development, limb muscles originate from which specific embryological structures?
   A. Sclerotomes and myotomes
   B. Somites and neural crest cells
   C. Endoderm and mesoderm
   D. Ectoderm and neural tube

Answers: 1. D 2. C 3. D 4. D 5. D
6. A 7. A 8. A

Integumentary System (Skin and its Appendages, Mammary Gland)

CHAPTER 11

COMPETENCIES COVERED/LEARNING OUTCOMES

The student should be able to:

AN9.3	Describe development of breast (mammary gland).
AN72.1	Discuss skin and its appendages.

The integumentary system, primarily consisting of the skin, undergoes a complex and highly regulated process of development during organogenesis. Originating from the ectoderm and mesoderm, the skin evolves to form a protective barrier, sensory interface, and thermoregulatory organ. Skin is also the largest organ of the human body.

In this chapter we are going to study the embryonic origins, differentiation pathways, and the formation of skin and its various appendages along with development of mammary glands.

SKIN

The skin is derived from diverse components **(Fig. 11.1)**, i.e., (1) surface ectoderm, (2) underlying mesoderm, and (3) neural crest cells. The development of skin starts during the first 30 days of embryonic period.

Epidermis

- The epidermis originates from the surface ectoderm and starts as a single layer **(Fig. 11.2A)**.
- By the second month, it forms two layers: *Periderm/epitrichium* (superficial flat cells) and *basal/germinative layer* (deep cuboidal cells) **(Fig. 11.2B)**. Around the 11th week, the basal layer cells proliferate, creating a *third intermediate layer*.
- The basal layer, also known as the *stratum germinativum*, proliferates to form the various layers of the epidermis **(Fig. 11.2C)**.
- From 3rd to 5th month, cell proliferation of epidermis results in a typical stratified squamous epithelium with five layers (strata): *Stratum germinativum, stratum spinosum, stratum granulosum, stratum lucidum, stratum corneum* **(Fig. 11.2D)**. Keratinization of periderm results in formation of stratum corneum.
- The epidermis includes various other cells: *keratinocytes* and nonkeratinocytes like *melanocytes, Langerhans cells, and Merkel cells*.
- By the end of the 5th month, continuous keratinization, desquamation, and replacement of peridermal cells by those from the basal layer occur.
- **Vernix caseosa:** Whitish, sticky substance layer that covers a newborn's skin. It forms when the superficial

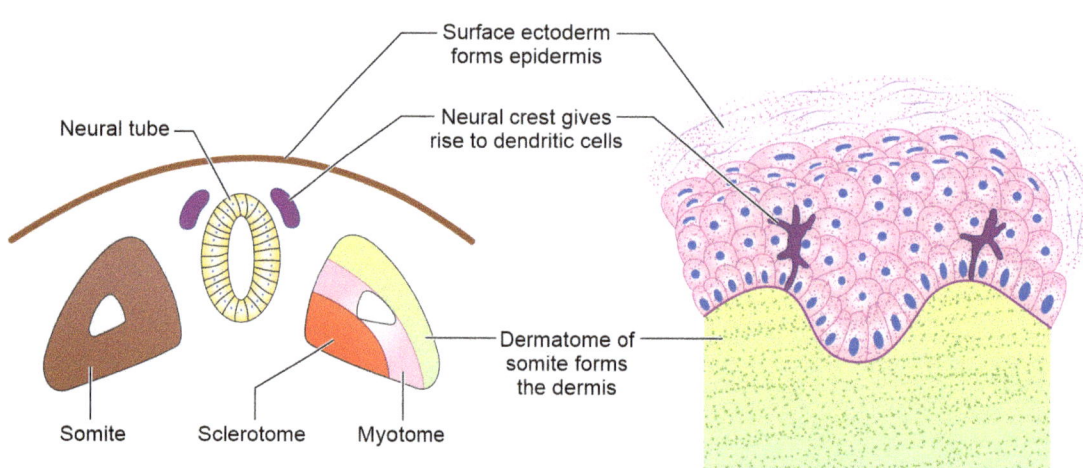

FIG. 11.1: Derivation of components of the skin.

Chapter 11: Integumentary System (Skin and its Appendages, Mammary Gland)

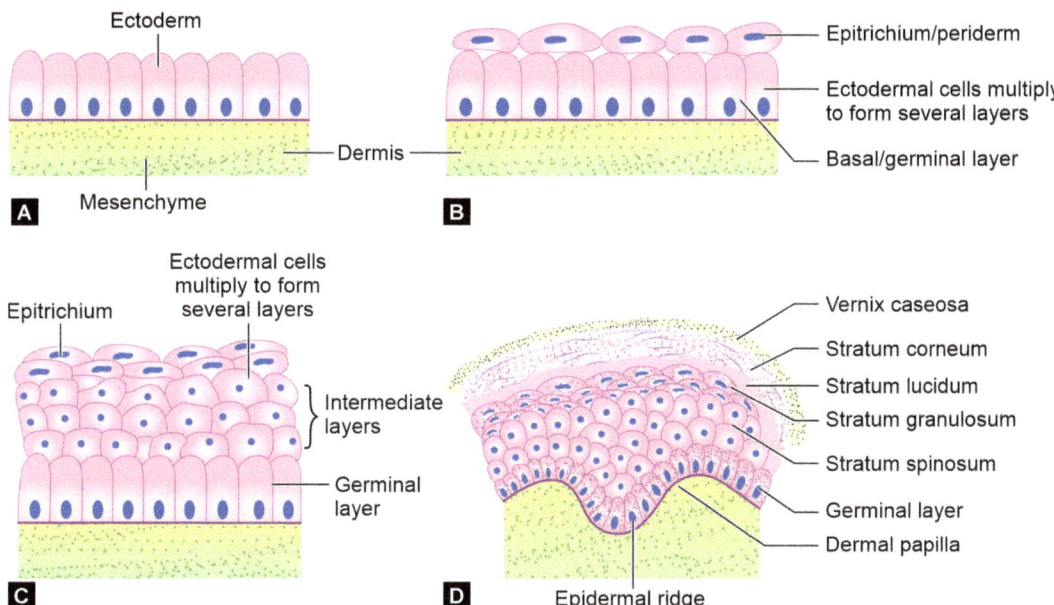

FIGS. 11.2A to D: Stages in the development of the epidermis.

layers of the epidermis shed and mix with sebaceous gland secretions. This coating protects the newborn infant's skin **(Fig. 11.2D)** from being macerated by amniotic fluid and facilitates process of parturition.
- After 5th month, the periderm disappears as cells are casts off and enter the amniotic fluid. The stratum corneum replaces the periderm.
- Stratum germinativum extends into the developing dermis, forming *epidermal ridges*. These ridges appear by the 11th week and become permanent by the 18th week.
- At birth, all layers of the adult epidermis are present.
- **Melanoblasts, or dendritic cells**, are derived from the neural crest (3rd month). These cells move to the dermoepidermal junction and become *melanocytes*, which produce melanin pigment, giving skin and hair their color.
- **Merkel and Langerhans cells:** Merkel cells, originating from the surface ectoderm, and Langerhans cells, originating from the mesoderm (bone marrow), appear in the epidermis between 8 and 12 weeks of intrauterine life.

Dermis

The dermis is formed by condensation and differentiation of mesenchyme underlying the surface ectoderm. This mesenchyme is believed to be derived from the dermatome of somites.

Recently, it has been held as follows:
- The *dermatomes* give rise only to the dermis on the dorsal aspect of the head and trunk.

- The dermis of the limbs and that on the lateral and ventral aspects of the trunk arises from *lateral plate mesoderm*.
- The dermis over most of the head and over the anterior aspect of the neck is derived from *the neural crest*.
- The line of junction between dermis and epidermis is at first straight. Subsequently, the epidermis shows regularly spaced thickenings that project into the dermis.
- The portions of dermis intervening between these projections form the *dermal papillae*.
- Grooves on the palms, soles, and digits are created by the interlocking of these epidermal ridges and dermal papillae, called *dermoepidermal junction*.

> **NOTE**
> They form unique patterns (whorls, loops, arches) on the fingertips and toes, which are genetically determined and unique to each individual. Similar patterns also form on the palms and soles. This is used in medicolegal purpose as *fingerprinting*.
> - By 11th week, mesenchymal cells differentiate to form the collagen and elastic fibers.
> - Further, dermis differentiates into two layers: superficial papillary layer and deep reticular layer.

Clinical correlation

Anomalies of Skin
- **Aplasia:** A condition where the skin fails to develop in certain regions.
- **Dysplasia:** Abnormal development or structure of the skin. It can be of various types like congenital growths of the skin or may be part of maldevelopment of various ectodermal derivatives including hair, teeth, sweat glands and sebaceous glands.

Pigment Disorders
- **Albinism:** A autosomal recessive condition where the skin, hair, and eyes lack pigment because melanocytes are unable to synthesize melanin.
- **Piebaldism:** A rare autosomal dominant disorder with patchy areas of absence of hair pigment (patches of white hair on forehead—white forelock) due to disordered development of melanocytes. Mutations in *CD117* gene results in this condition.
- **Vitiligo:** An autoimmune disorder characterized by patchy loss of pigment in the skin, hair, and oral mucosa. It is due to degeneration of already existing melanocytes.
- **Waardenburg syndrome:** A genetic disorder caused by defects in the migration and proliferation of neural crest cells, which give rise to melanocytes. It presents as white patches of skin and hair, iris of different colors and deafness (loss of pigment cells in stria vascularis of cochlea). It may be due to mutations in *PAX3* gene.
- **Congenital melanocytic nevi:** These are caused by an overgrowth of melanocytes in epidermal layer.

Keratinization Defect
- **Ichthyosis:** An autosomal recessive or X-linked disorder which present as hyperkeratinization of the skin.
- **Harlequin fetus:** Severe form of excessive keratinization results in a striking and often severe appearance in newborns.

APPENDAGES OF SKIN

The appendages of the skin are associated structures that are derived from epidermis and dermis and serve a specific function, e.g., heat loss prevention, sensation. These include nails, hairs and glands.

Nails

The nails develop from the surface ectoderm and start around 10th week. The ectoderm at the tip of each digit becomes thickened to form a *primary nail field*.
- Subsequently, this thickening migrates from the tip of the digit onto its dorsal aspect and is surrounded by U-shaped *nail folds* of ectoderm. Nail folds results in terminal structures like *nail bed* and *nail groove*.
- The cells in the most proximal part of the nail field proliferate to form the *root of the nail*. Here the cells of the germinal layer multiply to form a thick layer of cells called the *germinal matrix*. As the cells in this matrix multiply, they are transformed into the *nail substance/nail matrix* which corresponds to the stratum lucidum of the skin **(Fig. 11.3)**.
- Initially, the stratum corneum covers the entire surface of the nail but eventually disappears, except over the proximal part of the *nail plate*.
- The epidermis overlapping the proximal part of the nail plate is called the *eponychium*, while the epidermis beneath the free edge of the nail is called the *hyponychium*.

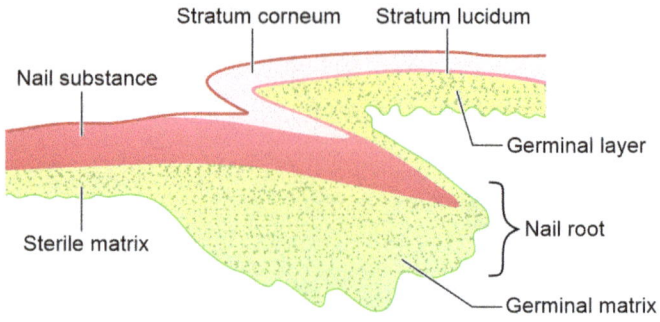

FIG. 11.3: Derivation of a nail.

Clinical correlation

- **Anonychia:** Nails may be absent. Occasionally, they may show over development.
- **Dermatoglyphics:** Researching the patterns of epidermal ridges found on the tips of fingers and toes.

Hair

- Hair is also derived from surface ectoderm. At the site where a *hair-follicle* is to form, the germinal layer of the epidermis proliferates to form a cylindrical mass, that grows down into the dermis **(Figs. 11.4A and B)**.
- The lower end of this downgrowth becomes expanded and is invaginated by a condensation of mesoderm, which forms the *papilla* **(Figs. 11.4C and D)**.
- The hair itself is formed by proliferation of germinal cells overlying the papilla. As the hair grows to the surface, the cells forming the wall of the downgrowth surround it and form the *epithelial root sheath*.
- An additional *dermal root sheath* is formed from the surrounding mesenchymal cells.
- A thin band of smooth muscle *(arrector pili)* is formed by mesodermal cells. It gets attached to the dermal root sheath. A typical hair follicle is thus formed **(Fig. 11.4E)**.
- As the hair root grows, the hair follicle is pushed outside of the skin as *shaft of hair*. The hair and shaft gets keratinized.
- **Lanugo:** They are fine, lightly pigmented hair that first appears and with which vernix caseosa is stick to skin.
- These hairs are replaced by coarser hair during prenatal period. Hairs that grow throughout life are called *angora*.

Clinical correlation

Hair Distribution Abnormalities
- **Congenital alopecia:** This condition involves the absence of hair on the scalp, and it may also affect the eyebrows and eyelashes.
- **Atrichia:** Absence of hair on any part of the body, typically associated with other ectodermal abnormalities such as defects in the teeth and nails.
- **Hypertrichosis:** Characterized by an overgrowth of hair, which can be localized (such as in the lumbar region covering spina bifida occulta) or generalized across the body.

Chapter 11: Integumentary System (Skin and its Appendages, Mammary Gland)

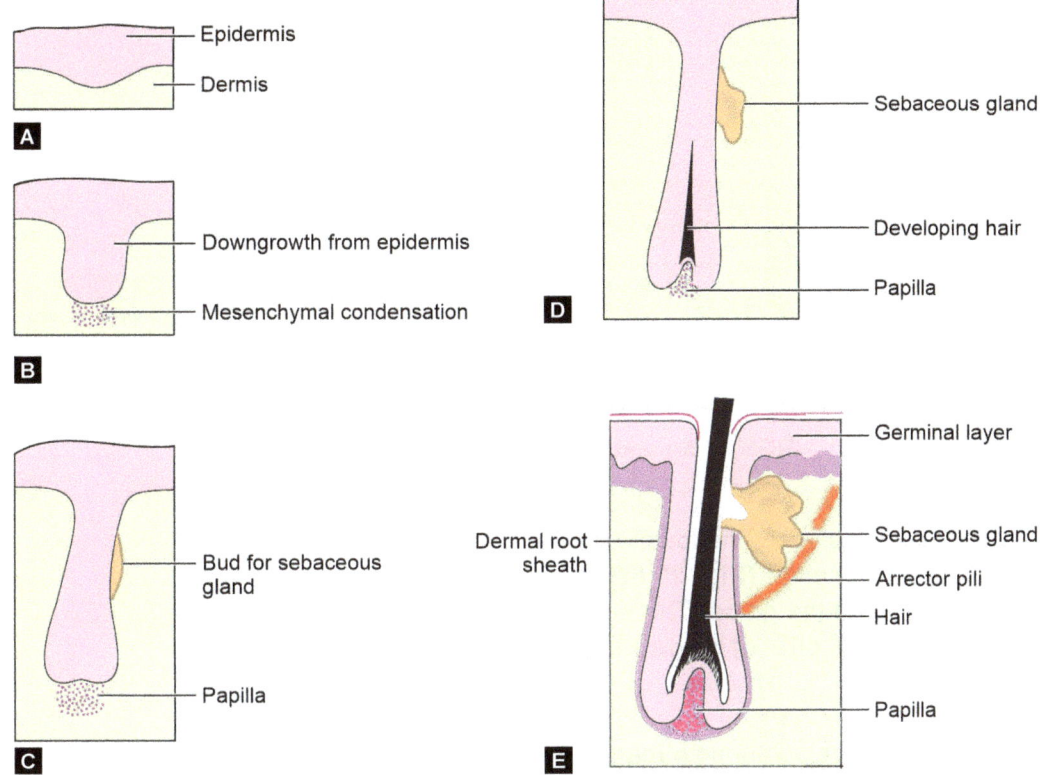

FIGS. 11.4A to E: Development of a hair follicle.

> **Molecular and Genetic Basis of Skin Development**
> - In the presence of Wnt signaling and absence of response to fibroblast growth factor (FGF) signaling, ectodermal cells express bone morphogenetic proteins (BMPs) and become committed to developing into the epidermis.
> - Cells that do not respond to Wnt signaling may receive inhibitory signals for BMP and FGF from the underlying mesenchyme, which facilitates the development of skin appendages.
> - *PAX3* genes are active in the migration of neural crest cells and their differentiation into melanoblasts and melanocytes, starting their function of producing melanin pigment.

Glands of skin

There are two types of skin glands: Sebaceous and sweat glands. Sweat glands are of further three types: Eccrine, apocrine and specialized apocrine (mammary) glands. They are summarized in **Table 11.1**.

Sebaceous Glands

- A sebaceous gland is formed as *a bud* arising from ectodermal cells forming the wall of a hair follicle.
- These buds grow into the adjacent dermis, branching into *primordia of alveoli and associated ducts*.
- The central cells of the alveoli degenerate, producing oily *sebum* which is released into hair follicle onto the skin's surface.
- Some stages in the formation of a sebaceous gland are shown in **Figures 11.4C to E**.

Sweat Glands

There are two types of sweat glands: (1) the *eccrine* and (2) *apocrine*.
- **Eccrine sweat gland** develops as a downgrowth from the epidermis into underlying dermis around 20 weeks of IUL **(Fig. 11.5A)**. The downgrowth is

TABLE 11.1: Glands of skin.

Gland	Location	Function
Sebaceous glands	Near the hair follicle	Waterproof for the surface for protection
Eccrine sweat glands	Deep dermis	Maintenance of body temperature
Apocrine sweat glands	Near hair follicles in armpit, groin, around nipple	Their secretions are odor producing and sexual attractant (emotional)
Ceruminous glands	External auditory canal	Production of earwax
Mammary glands	Pectoral region	Secretion of milk after parturition

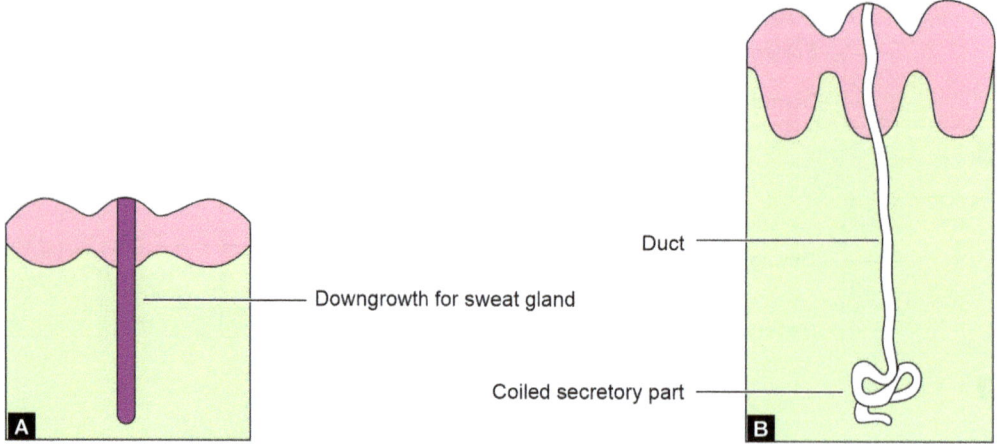

FIGS. 11.5A and B: Development of a sweat gland.

at first solid but is later canalized. The lower end of the downgrowth becomes coiled **(Fig. 11.5B)** and forms the *secretory part* of the gland. The straight part forms *the duct* and site of beginning of downgrowth forms the *pore of the duct* of sweat gland.

❖ **Apocrine sweat glands** develop during puberty and are located in the axilla, areolae of nipples, and pubic and perineal areas. They form from hair follicles as buds and open into the hair follicles. They are called apocrine because a portion of the secretory cell is shed during secretion. They secrete lipids, proteins and *pheromones* in the sweat which have peculiar odor.

MAMMARY GLANDS

❖ Mammary glands are modified/specialized apocrine sweat glands and are ectodermal in development.
❖ During 7th week, the ectoderm thickens on each side of the embryo along line that extends from the axilla to the inguinal region to form *mammary ridges or lines* **(Fig. 11.6)**. Most of these lines disappear except in thoracic/pectoral region.
❖ In the region where the mammary gland is to form, a thickened mass of epidermal cells is seen projecting into the dermis as *primary buds* **(Fig. 11.7A)**.
❖ From this thickened mass, 16–20 solid outgrowths arise, and grow into the surrounding dermis as *secondary buds* **(Figs. 11.7B and C)**.
❖ The thickened mass of epidermis (and the outgrowths), are now canalized **(Fig. 11.7D)**.
❖ The *secretory elements (alveoli)* of the gland are formed by proliferation of the terminal parts of the outgrowths. The proximal end of each outgrowth forms one *lactiferous duct*.

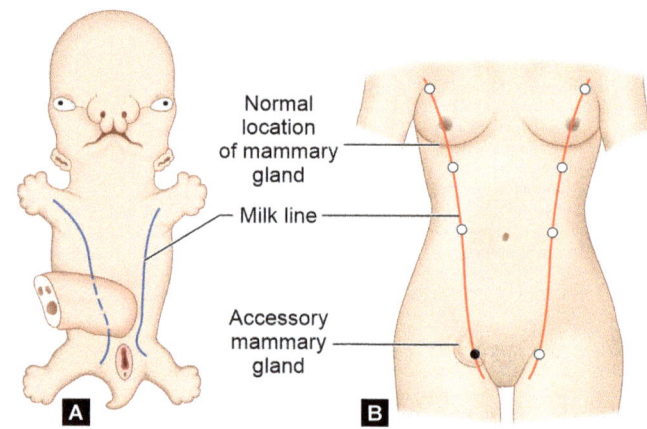

FIGS. 11.6A and B: Mammary ridge/line. (A) The mammary line passing from the axilla to the inguinal region in fetus; (B) Adult mammary gland in pectoral region and accessory mammary gland in inguinal region.

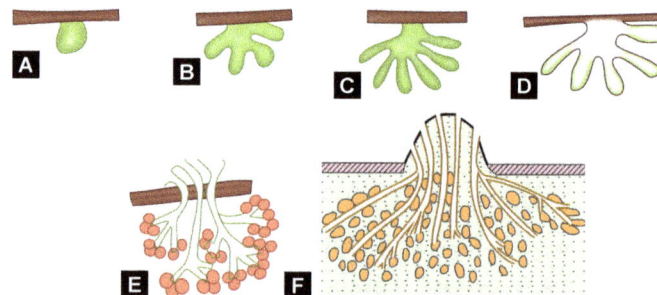

FIGS. 11.7A to F: Stages in the development of the mammary gland.

❖ The ducts at first open into a pit formed by cavitation of the original epithelial thickening. However, the growth of underlying mesoderm progressively pushes the wall of this pit outwards, until it becomes elevated above the surface and forms the *nipple* **(Figs. 11.7E and F)**.
❖ The mammary gland remains rudimentary in the male. In females, the ducts and secretory elements undergo extensive development during puberty and pregnancy.

Chapter 11: Integumentary System (Skin and its Appendages, Mammary Gland)

Clinical correlation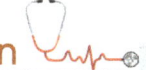

Developmental Anomalies of the Mammary Glands
- **Amastia:** Absence of mammary gland on one or both sides.
- **Athelia:** The nipple may be absent.
- **Polythelia and polymastia:** Supernumerary nipples can occur anywhere along the milk line. They may remain rudimentary (polythelia) or develop into accessory mammary glands (polymastia). Accessory breasts can also be found away from the milk line, including the neck, cheeks, femoral triangle, and vulva.
- *Accessory breasts* may be found away from the milk line. They have been observed in the neck, cheeks, femoral triangle and vulva.
- **Inverted or crater nipple:** The nipple may fail to form resulting in lactiferous ducts opening into a pit. This causes difficulty in suckling.
- **Size variations:** The mammary gland may be abnormally small (micromastia) or abnormally large (macromastia).
- **Gynecomastia:** The male breast may enlarge similarly to a normal female breast and may even produce milk.

TIMETABLE OF SOME EVENTS MENTIONED IN THIS CHAPTER

Age	Developmental events
7th week	Mammary line is established
8th week	Melanoblasts start appearing
1st to 3rd month	Cells of neural crest migrate to skin
2nd month	Surface ectoderm is single layered
2nd to 4th month	Surface ectoderm becomes multiple layered
3rd to 4th month	Dermal papillae are formed

Case Based Learning

Embryological Basis of Skin Disorders

Case Scenario 1
An adult male visited the dermatology outpatient department (OPD) with several white patches on the front of his leg (see figure below) that have been increasing in number and size over the past six months. There is no history of trauma such as cuts, burns, or ulceration. Additionally, there is no history of fever, jaundice, or use of any medications. What is the name of this condition? What explains the occurrence of white patches? What are the complications associated with it?

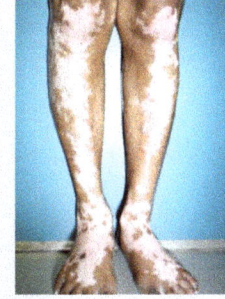

- The white patches are due to the absence of melanin pigment, a condition called vitiligo.
- Vitiligo is a pigmentary disorder of the integumentary system resulting from the destruction of melanocytes, the pigment-forming cells derived from neural crest cells. The condition is characterized by a progression in the number and area of skin patches. It must be differentiated from leukoderma, where white patches are present with a history of trauma. A thorough medical history helps rule out drug-induced or other causes. In the absence of trauma history and with other tests to rule out diabetes and hyperthyroidism, vitiligo is diagnosed.
- The exact cause of vitiligo is unknown, but it is believed to be an autoimmune disorder and may be hereditary.
- The lack of melanin increases the risk of sunburns and skin carcinoma with prolonged sun exposure. Some individuals may also experience a lack of pigmentation in the eyes and hearing loss.

Case Scenario 2
A primigravida delivered a baby, shown in Figure below. The pediatrician conducted a neurological examination, observed the eyes, and performed hearing tests. Describe your observations. What is the name of this condition? What is the basis for the tests conducted? What are the features of this condition? What is the embryological explanation?

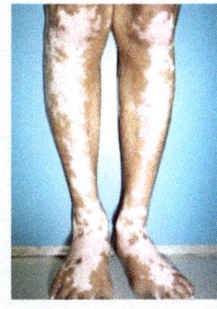

- The newborn exhibited large white patches of depigmented skin on the abdomen and both lower limbs, along with a white forelock (a patch of white hair) in the middle of otherwise black hair on the head.
- This condition is known as Waardenburg syndrome, a rare genetic disorder.
- The neurological examination is necessary to check for delays in developmental milestones and muscle tone abnormalities. The eyes were examined for the distance between the inner corners and the color of the eyes. Hearing tests were conducted to check for deafness.
- Waardenburg syndrome is characterized by pigmentation deficiencies, including white patches of skin, a white forelock, blue eyes, and sensorineural hearing loss. There are four different types of Waardenburg syndrome, each with varying features.
- The syndrome is caused by mutations in the *PAX3* gene, which affect the division and migration of neural crest cells during embryonic development. It is an autosomal dominant disorder.

Chapter 11: Integumentary System (Skin and its Appendages, Mammary Gland)

HIGHLIGHTS

- The *epidermis* is derived from surface ectoderm.
- The *dermis* is formed by mesenchyme derived from dermatomes of somites.
- **Nails** develop from ectoderm at the tip of each digit. Later, this ectoderm migrates to the dorsal aspect.
- **Hair** are derived from surface ectoderm which is modified to form hair follicles.
- **Sebaceous glands** (ectoderm) arise as diverticula from hair follicles.
- **Sweat glands** develop as downgrowths from the epidermis that are later canalized.
- **Mammary glands** arise from surface ectoderm. They are formed along a milk line extending from axilla to the inguinal region.

Summary

- Development of skin (**Flowchart 11.1**).
- Development of mammary gland (**Flowchart 11.2**).

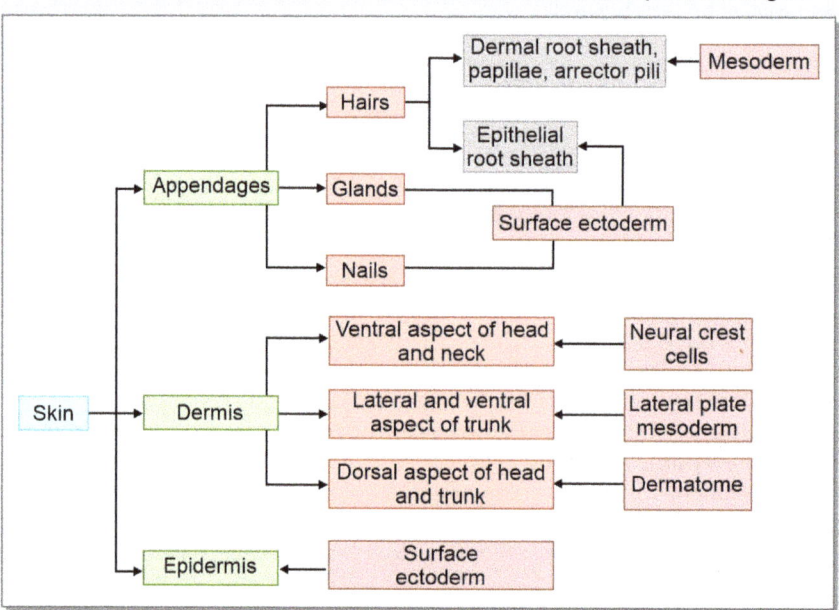

FLOWCHART 11.1: Skin—components and their developmental origin.

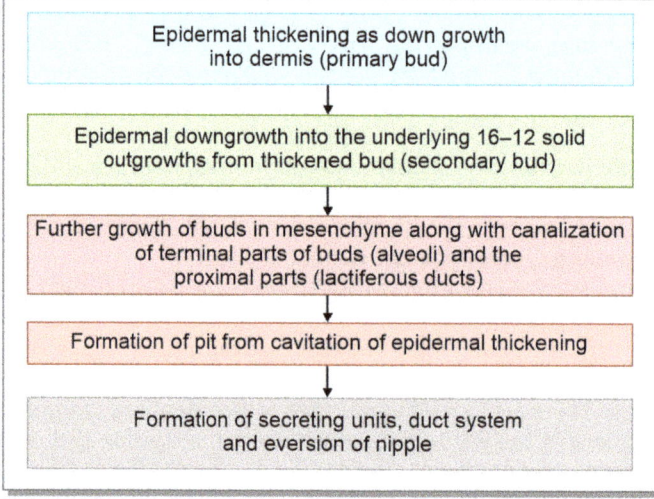

FLOWCHART 11.2: Mammary gland development.

Chapter 11: Integumentary System (Skin and its Appendages, Mammary Gland)

TEST YOUR UNDERSTANDING

REVIEW QUESTIONS

1. Discuss the development of various parts of skin.
2. Write notes on development of sweat glands.
3. Write short notes on development of nail.
4. Discuss the development of mammary glands with its applied aspect.
5. What are the types of glands that are found in skin?

EXPLAIN WHY? (REASONING QUESTIONS)

1. Child presents with areas of thick, scaly skin on the hands and feet.
2. A neonate has multiple small nodules along the groin that excrete a milky substance.
3. Amniotic fluid don't have any adverse effect on developing fetus skin.

MULTIPLE CHOICE QUESTIONS

1. All the following are derived from ectoderm, *except*:
   A. Epidermis
   B. Nails
   C. Hair follicle
   D. Arrector pili
2. Nail is a modified:
   A. Stratum corneum
   B. Stratum basale
   C. Stratum lucidum
   D. Stratum germinativum
3. Merkel cells are derived from:
   A. Neural crest cells
   B. Surface ectoderm
   C. Monocytes
   D. Mesoderm
4. When does permanent epidermal ridges of skin is formed?
   A. 11th week
   B. 18th week
   C. 28th week
   D. 20th week
5. Dermis is formed from:
   A. Somitomeres
   B. Somites
   C. Neural crest cells
   D. Epidermis
6. A newborn has a rare genetic condition causing anonychia, the complete absence of nails. This condition is linked to a mutation in a gene critical for ectodermal appendage formation. Which signaling pathway is most likely disrupted, leading to anonychia?
   A. Wnt signaling pathway
   B. Hedgehog signaling pathway
   C. Notch signaling pathway
   D. TGF-beta signaling pathway
7. An infant born with congenital ichthyosis lacks the typical vernix caseosa at birth. Considering the embryological origin and formation of vernix caseosa, which component of vernix is primarily affected in this condition?
   A. Sebaceous gland secretions
   B. Desquamated epithelial cells
   C. Amniotic fluid
   D. Placental transfer of lipids
8. A newborn with congenital ichthyosis has thick, scaly skin. What embryological process is most likely abnormal in this condition?
   A. Keratinocyte differentiation
   B. Melanocyte migration
   C. Mesenchymal condensation
   D. Neural tube closure
9. A newborn has a large area of alopecia (hair loss) on the scalp, with an underlying bony defect. Which developmental process is likely disrupted in this case?
   A. Epidermal and dermal interaction
   B. Neural crest cell migration
   C. Angiogenesis
   D. Mesodermal differentiation
10. An infant presents with a thickened, hyperkeratotic lesion on the scalp known as a sebaceous nevus. Which embryonic layer is primarily involved in the development of this lesion?
    A. Ectoderm
    B. Mesoderm
    C. Endoderm
    D. Neural crest
11. A pediatric patient is diagnosed with albinism, a condition characterized by the absence of melanin in the skin, hair, and eyes. Which cells and their embryonic origin are primarily implicated in this condition?
    A. Keratinocytes and ectoderm
    B. Melanocytes and neural crest cells
    C. Fibroblasts and mesoderm
    D. Langerhans cells and bone marrow

Answers: 1. D   2. A   3. C   4. B   5. B   6. A   7. B   8. A   9. A   10. A   11. B

CHAPTER 12

Branchial Apparatus (Pharyngeal Arches, Endodermal Pouches and Ectodermal Clefts)

COMPETENCIES COVERED/LEARNING OUTCOMES

The student should be able to:

AN43.4 Describe the development and development of congenital anomalies of branchial apparatus and thyroid gland.

We have studied about the folding of embryo in Chapter 7 along with the formation of foregut. The development of head and neck starts during that time of embryonic development.

We have now understood that after the establishment of the head fold, the foregut is bounded ventrally by the pericardium, and dorsally by the developing brain. Cranially, it is at first separated from the stomatodeum by the buccopharyngeal membrane. When this membrane breaks down, the foregut opens to the exterior through the stomatodeum.

At this stage, the head is represented as the bulging caused by the developing brain **(Fig. 12.1)**, while the pericardium may be considered as occupying the region of the future thorax. The two are separated by the stomatodeum which is the future mouth. It is, thus, apparent that a neck is not yet present.

Head and neck are formed from the complex structure known as *branchial apparatus (pharyngeal apparatus)*. It consists of pharyngeal arches, pouches, ectodermal clefts and pharyngeal membranes.

PHARYNGEAL OR BRACHIAL ARCHES

The neck is formed by the elongation of the region between the stomatodeum and the pericardium. This is achieved, partly, by a 'descent' of the developing heart. However, this elongation is due mainly to the appearance of a series of mesodermal thickenings in the wall of the cranial-most part of the foregut. These are called the *pharyngeal* or *branchial arches* **(Fig. 12.1)**.

❖ The uppermost portion of the foregut, known as the pharyngeal part, initially has a funnel-like shape **(Fig. 12.2A)**. It is dorsoventrally compressed and consists of a ventral floor, dorsal roof, and two lateral walls.

❖ A coronal section through the foregut (the part destined to form the pharynx), before the appearance of the pharyngeal arches, is shown in **Figure 12.2B**. At this stage, the endodermal wall of the foregut is separated from the surface ectoderm by a layer of mesoderm.

❖ Soon, thereafter, the mesoderm comes to be arranged in the form of six bars that run dorsoventrally in the side wall of the foregut. Each of these 'bars' grows ventrally in the floor of the developing pharynx and fuses with the corresponding 'bar' of the opposite side to form a *pharyngeal or branchial arch*.

❖ In the interval between any two adjoining arches, the endoderm extends outwards in the form of a pouch *(endodermal or pharyngeal pouch)* to meet

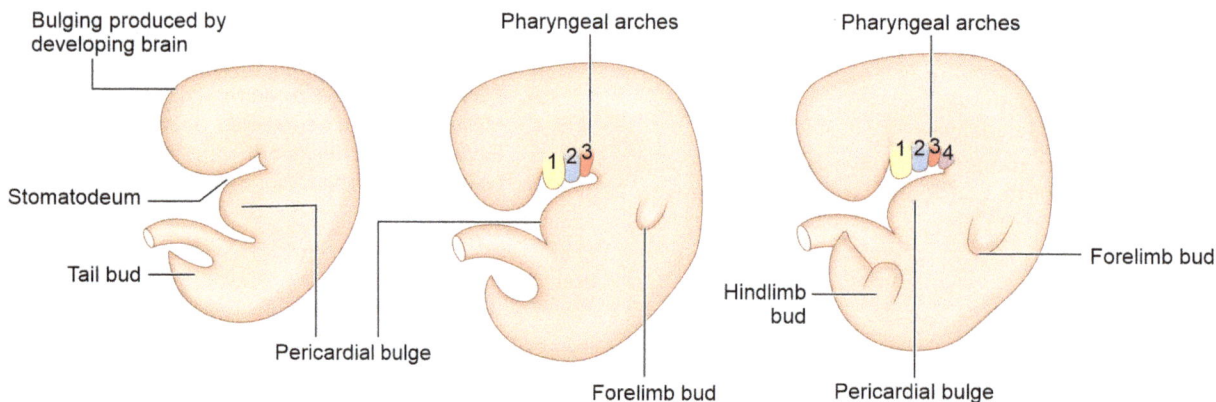

FIG. 12.1: Lateral views of embryos showing the formation of pharyngeal arches between stomatodeum and the pericardial bulge.

Chapter 12: Branchial Apparatus (Pharyngeal Arches, Endodermal Pouches and Ectodermal Clefts)

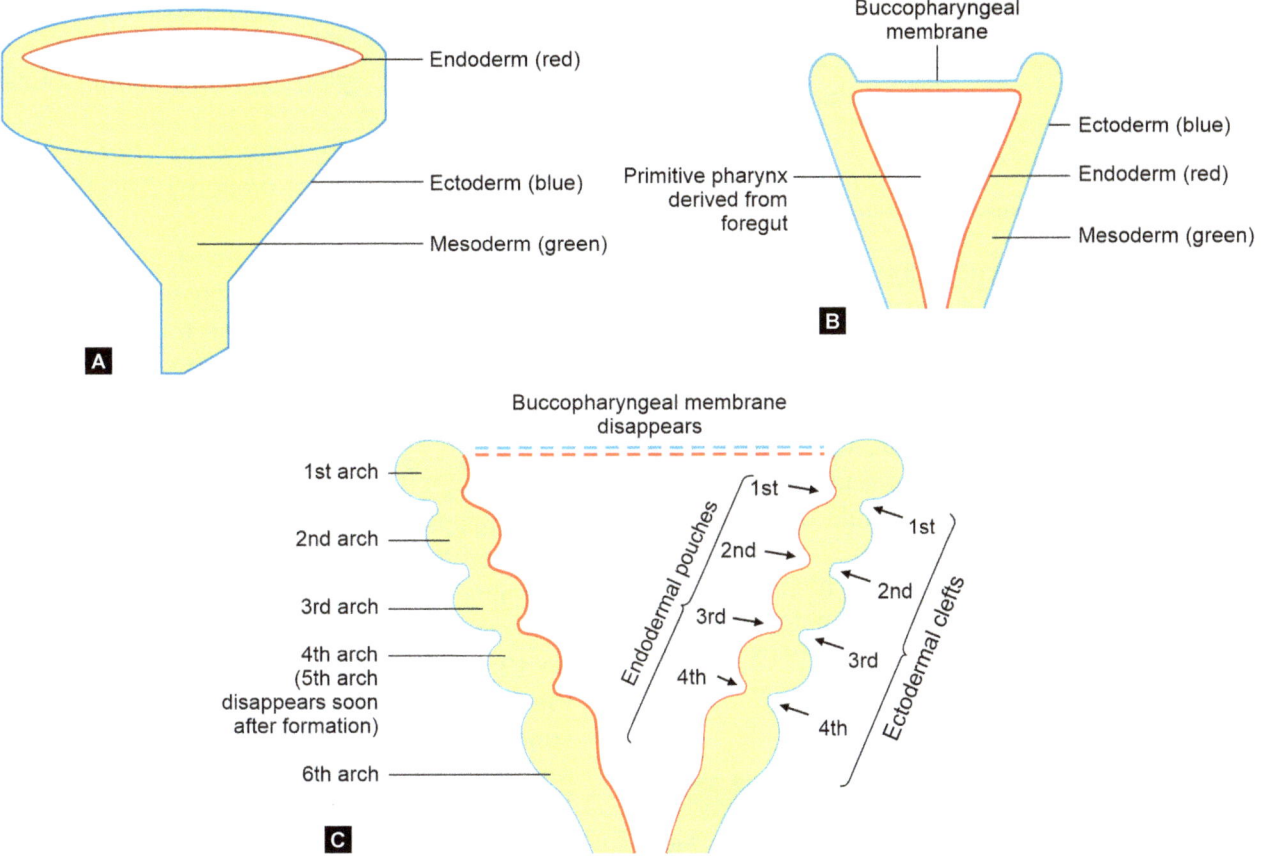

FIGS. 12.2A to C: (A) Funnel shaped cranial end of foregut; (B and C) Coronal sections through cranial part of foregut; (B) Before; (C) After formation of pharyngeal arches.

the ectoderm which dips into this interval as an *ectodermal cleft* (Fig. 12.2C).
- There are six arches which consist of mesodermal thickenings with ectodermal coverings and endodermal linings, supporting the primitive pharynx's ventral and lateral walls. By the time the anterior neuropore closes, the first and second pharyngeal arches are already formed.
- The mesoderm within the arches derives from paraxial and lateral plate mesoderm, later invaded by neural crest cells contributing to skeletal elements and connective tissue in the head and neck region.

The first arch is also called the *mandibular arch*; and the second, the *hyoid arch*. The third, fourth and sixth arches do not have special names. The fifth arch disappears soon after its formation, so that only five arches remain.

Mesoderm of each pharyngeal arches have pluripotent cells that can differentiate into following structures **(Figs. 12.3A and B)**:
- **A skeletal element**: This is cartilaginous in origin and it may remain same, may develop into bone, or may disappear. Perichondrium of disappeared cartilage can persists as ligament/raphe.

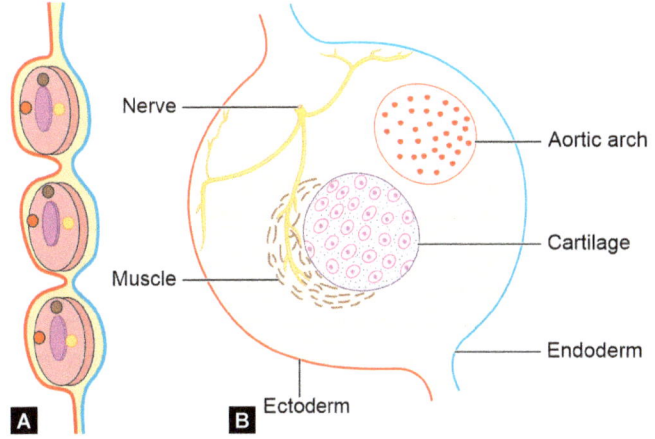

FIGS. 12.3A and B: Structures to be seen in a pharyngeal arch.

- **Striated muscle**: This muscle is supplied by the nerve of the arch (see below). In later development, this musculature may, or may not, retain its attachment to the skeletal elements derived from the arch. It may subdivide to form a number of distinct muscles, which may migrate away from the pharyngeal region. When they do so, however, they carry their nerve with them and their embryological origin can thus be determined from their nerve supply.

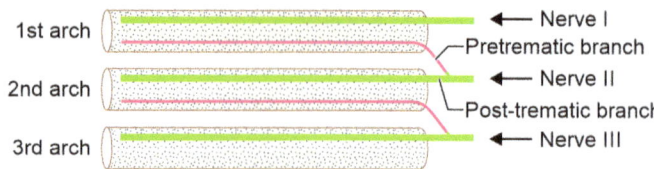

FIG. 12.4: Arrangement of nerves supplying the pharyngeal arches in some lower animals.

- **An arterial arch**: Ventral to the foregut, an artery called the *ventral aorta* develops. Dorsal to the foregut, another artery called the *dorsal aorta*, is formed. A series of arterial arches (aortic arches) connect the ventral and dorsal aortae. One such arterial arch lies in each pharyngeal arch. In a subsequent development, the arrangement of these arteries is greatly modified. The fate of the arterial arches is considered in Chapter 19.
- **Nerve of the arch**: Each pharyngeal arch is supplied by a nerve. In addition to supplying motor branches to the skeletal muscle of the arch, it supplies sensory branches to the overlying ectoderm, and endoderm **(Figs. 12.3A and B)**.

> **NOTE**
>
> In some lower animals, each arch is supplied by two nerves **(Fig. 12.4)**. The nerve of the arch itself runs along the cranial border of the arch. This is called the *post-trematic nerve* of the arch (trema = trench). Each arch also receives a branch from the nerve of the succeeding arch. This runs along the caudal border of the arch, and is called the *pretrematic nerve* of the arch. *In the human embryo, however, a double innervation is to be seen only in the first pharyngeal arch.*

DERIVATIVES OF THE SKELETAL ELEMENTS

- The cartilage of the first arch is called *Meckel's cartilage* **(Figs. 12.5A and B)**. The *incus* and *malleus* (of the middle ear) and *spine of sphenoid* are derived from its dorsal end. The ventral part of the cartilage is surrounded by mesenchyme that forms *mandible* by membranous ossification which results in cartilage entrapment and its absorption. The part of the cartilage extending from the region of the middle ear to the mandible disappears, but its sheath (perichondrium) forms the *anterior ligament of the malleus* and the *sphenomandibular ligament*. Mesenchyme of the first arch is also responsible for formation of bones of the face including the maxilla, the mandible, the zygomatic bone, the palatine bone and part of the temporal bone by membranous ossification.
- The cartilage of the second arch is called *Reichert's cartilage*, which forms the following:
  - Dorsal part forms *stapes* and *styloid process*.
  - Ventral part forms *lesser cornu* and *superior part of body of hyoid bone*.
  - *Stylohyoid ligament* (from sheath of remnant perichondrium).
  (Note that all structures listed start with 'S').
- The following structures are formed from the cartilage of the third arch:
  - Greater cornu of hyoid bone.
  - Lower part of the body of hyoid bone.
- The fourth and sixth arches together give rise to cartilages of larynx *except epiglottis* which develops from hypobranchial eminence.

NERVES AND MUSCLES OF THE ARCHES

All the muscles derived from a pharyngeal arch are supplied by the nerve of the arch and can, therefore, be identified by their nerve supply. The nerves of the arches and the muscles supplied by them are given in **Table 12.1**.

- We have already seen that these nerves not only supply muscles, but also innervate the parts of skin and mucous membrane derived from the arches. Some of the nerves (e.g., glossopharyngeal) have only a small motor component and are predominantly sensory.
- As stated above, the first arch has a *double nerve supply. The mandibular nerve is the post-trematic nerve of the first arch, while the chorda tympani (branch of facial nerve) is the pretrematic nerve.* This double innervation is reflected in the nerve supply of the anterior two-thirds of the tongue that are derived from the ventral part of the first arch.
- Sensory innervations of the nerves of arches supply as: (i) maxillary and mandibular supplies skin of face, mucous membrane of nasal cavity, oral cavity, soft palate, tongue and upper and lower teeth; (ii) sensory component of glossopharyngeal nerve supplies mucous membrane of pharynx; (iii) superior laryngeal nerve supply mucosa of larynx above vocal cord and recurrent laryngeal nerve below vocal cord.

> **NOTE**
>
> Some recent investigations suggest that mesenchyme giving rise to muscles of the pharyngeal arches is derived from paraxial mesoderm cranial to the occipital somites (i.e., from the region of the preoccipital somites); and that its organization is influenced by neural crest cells. Although paraxial mesoderm here does not form typical somites, it shows partial segmentation into seven masses of mesenchyme called somitomeres. The structures derived from the seven somitomeres and from five occipital somites that follow them, have been described as given in **Table 12.2**.

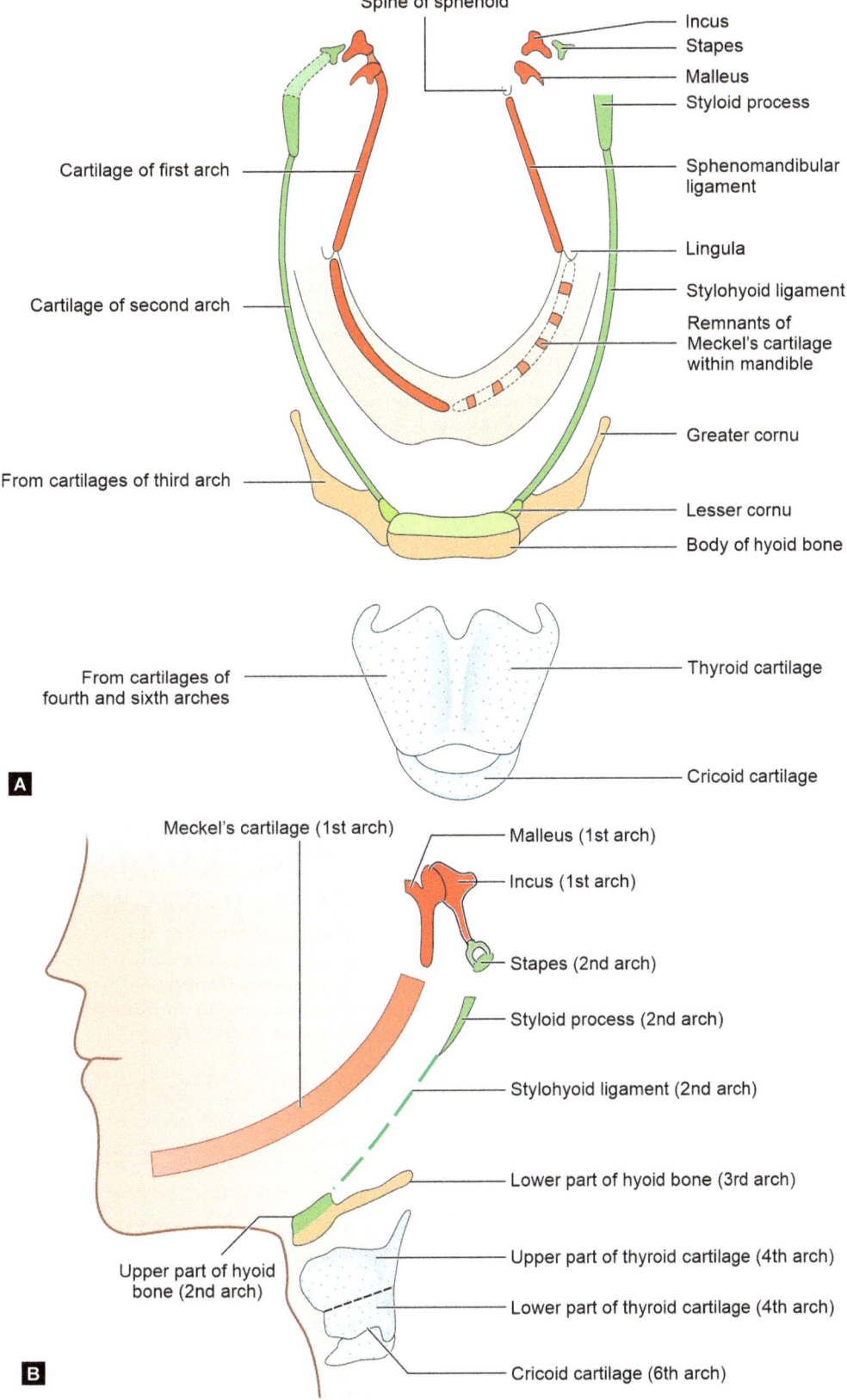

FIGS. 12.5A and B: Fate of the cartilages of the pharyngeal arches. (A) Frontal view. The left half of the figure shows an earlier stage of development. The derivatives of the first arch are shown in red, second arch in green, third arch in orange, and fourth and sixth arches in blue; (B) Side view.

TABLE 12.1: Nerves of pharyngeal arches and muscles supplied by them.

Arch	Nerve of arch	Muscles of arch
First	Maxillary (sensory) and mandibular (sensory and motor) branches of trigeminal nerve	Medial and lateral pterygoids, masseter, temporalis, mylohyoid, anterior belly of digastric, tensor tympani, tensor palati
Second	Facial nerve	Facial muscles, occipitofrontalis, platysma, stylohyoid, posterior belly of digastric, stapedius, auricular muscles, epicranius
Third	Glossopharyngeal nerve	Stylopharyngeus
Fourth	Superior laryngeal branch of vagus nerve	Muscles of larynx (cricothyroid), pharynx and intrinsic muscles of soft palate except tensor palati
Sixth	Recurrent laryngeal branch of vagus nerve	All intrinsic muscles of larynx except cricothyroid

TABLE 12.1: Muscles derived from somitomeres and somites.

Somitomere/somites	Muscles derived
Somitomere 1 and 2	Muscles supplied by oculomotor nerve
Somitomere 3	Superior oblique muscle supplied by trochlear nerve
Somitomere 4	Muscles of first pharyngeal arch supplied by mandibular nerve
Somitomere 5	Lateral rectus muscle supplied by abducent nerve
Somitomere 6	Muscles of the second pharyngeal arch supplied by the facial nerve
Somitomere 7	Stylopharyngeus (from 3rd arch) supplied by glossopharyngeal nerve
Occipital somites 1 and 2	Laryngeal muscles (from 4th to 6th arches) supplied by the vagus nerve
Occipital somites 3 to 5	Muscles of tongue supplied by hypoglossal nerve

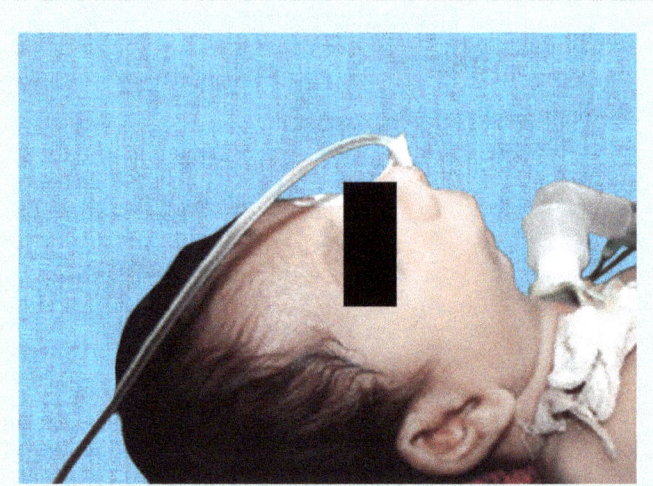

Third pharyngeal arch disorders:
- **DiGeorge syndrome:** Results from microdeletion on long arm of chromosome 22 leading to defective development of the third and fourth pharyngeal pouches which results in underdeveloped thymus and parathyroid glands. It presents as immunodeficiency, hypocalcemia, and congenital heart defects.

If we accept this view of the origin of branchial musculature, there would be no significant reason to distinguish between it and muscle derived from somites.

Clinical correlation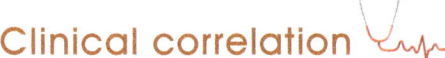

First Pharyngeal Arch Disorders
- **Treacher Collins syndrome (see figure below):** Autosomal dominant inherited disorder characterized by craniofacial deformities such as underdeveloped zygomatic bones (malar hypoplasia), mandibular hypoplasia, downward palpebral fissures and malformed external ears. Results from mutations affecting neural crest cell development.
- **Pierre Robin sequence:** Autosomal recessive inherited disorder with features of micrognathia (small jaw), glossoptosis (downward displacement of the tongue), and airway obstruction. It is often associated with cleft palate.

FATE OF ECTODERMAL CLEFTS

After the formation of the pharyngeal arches, the region of the neck is marked on the outside by a series of *grooves, or ectodermal clefts*. There are four pharyngeal clefts/grooves.
- The dorsal part of the first cleft (between the first and second arches) develops into the epithelial lining of the *external acoustic meatus* and *cuticular layer of tympanic membrane*.
- The *pinna* (or auricle) is formed from a series of swellings or hillocks, that arise on the first and second arches, where they adjoin the first cleft. The ventral part of this cleft is obliterated.
- All other clefts are obliterated.

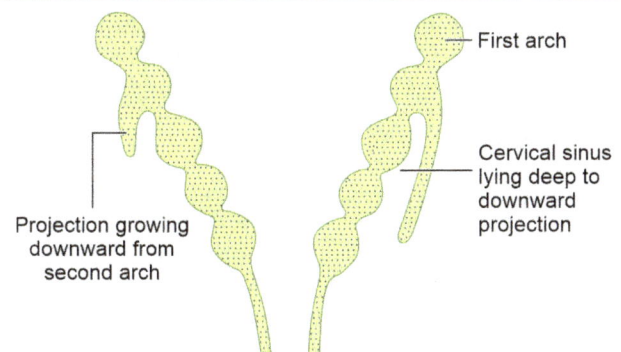

FIG. 12.6: Cervical sinus. The left half of the figure shows an earlier stage than the right half.

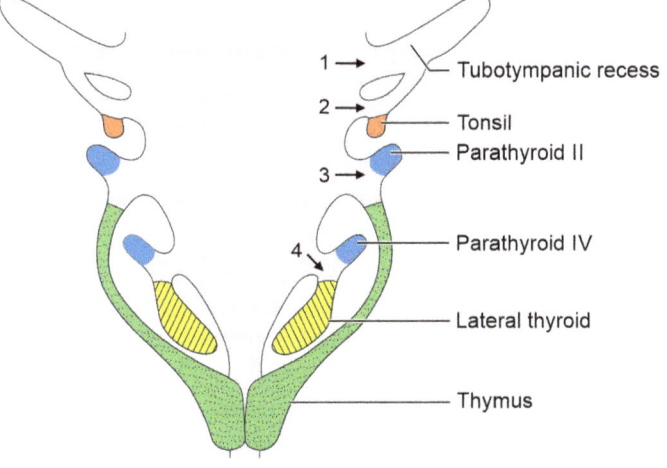

FIG. 12.7: Scheme to show the fate of the pharyngeal pouches (numbered 1 to 4).

Cervical Sinus

The second arch grows much faster than the succeeding arches and comes to overhang them **(Fig. 12.6)**. The space between the overhanging second arch and the third, fourth and sixth arches is called the *cervical sinus*.
* Subsequently, the lower overhanging border of the second arch fuses with tissues caudal to the arches *(epicardial ridge)*.
* The side of the neck (which was thus far marked by the ectodermal clefts) now becomes smooth.
* The cavity of the cervical sinus (which is lined by ectoderm) normally gets obliterated.

Clinical Importance

Congenital Anomalies of Cervical Sinus
- **Branchial cyst:** Persistence of cervical sinus as a swelling results in formation of cyst along the anterior border of sternocleidomastoid muscle. If the cyst ruptures it results in branchial sinus. The branchial cyst can be in relation to the 1st/2nd/3rd/4th branchial cleft. In relation with first cleft, there are two types of cysts, the type I and type II based on the opening of the sinus above or below the jaw line respectively.
- **Branchial sinus:** It can be external or internal. **External:** If the cyst opens outside, usually anterior to sternomastoid. **Internal:** Cyst opens into pharynx, usually in the tonsillar region.
- **Branchial/cervical fistula:** The cyst opens both externally and internally. Connects pharynx with outside.

FATE OF ENDODERMAL POUCHES

There are five pair of endodermal pouches which are evaginations between 2 arches. The derivatives of the pouches are divided into ventral and lateral. The ventral derivatives develop in the floor of pharynx and contribute for the development of tongue. Lateral derivatives except that of 1st are divided into those derived from *ventral wing* and those derived from *dorsal wing*.

The endodermal pouches take part in the formation of several important organs **(Fig. 12.7)**. These are listed below:

First Pouch

* Its ventral part is obliterated by formation of the *tongue*.
* Its dorsal part receives a contribution from the dorsal part of the second pouch, and these two together form a diverticulum that grows towards the region of the developing ear.
  This diverticulum is called the *tubotympanic recess*. The proximal part of this recess gives rise to the *auditory (pharyngotympanic) tube*, and the distal part to the *middle ear cavity*, including the *tympanic antrum* **(Fig. 12.7)**.

Second Pouch

* The epithelium of the ventral part of this pouch contributes to the formation of the *tonsil*.
* The dorsal part takes part in the formation of the tubotympanic recess.

Third Pouch

This gives rise to the *inferior parathyroid glands* (parathyroid III), and the *thymus*.

Fourth Pouch

This gives origin to the *superior parathyroid glands* (parathyroid IV), and may contribute to the *thyroid gland*.

Fifth or Ultimobranchial Pouch

A fifth pouch is seen for a brief period during development. In some species it gives rise to the *ultimobranchial body*. Its fate in man is controversial.

Caudal Pharyngeal Complex

The fifth pouch appears temporarily and incorporates into the fourth pouch, the two together forming the *caudal pharyngeal complex*. The neural crest cells migrate into this complex.

- The superior parathyroid glands develops from this complex.
- Thymic element incorporates into thymus.
- Lateral thyroid element fuses with median thyroid element of hypoglossal duct arresting thyroid migration.
- Ultimobranchial body immigrates neural crest cells that develop into *parafollicular or C cells* of thyroid gland.

Molecular regulation and genetic basis of pharyngeal arch development:
- The formation of pharyngeal arches is controlled by pharyngeal arch ectoderm. Lateral migration of pharyngeal endodermal cells forms the pharyngeal pouches.
- The migration is controlled by fibroblast growth factor (FGF-8), bone mineral protein (BMP-7), paired box gene *(PAX1)* and sonic hedgehog (Shh) gene.

PHARYNGEAL MEMBRANES

These are thin layers of tissue located between the pharyngeal pouches (endodermal origin) and the pharyngeal clefts (ectodermal origin). They are four in number.

- Each pharyngeal membrane consists of three layers: An outer ectodermal layer, an inner endodermal layer, and a thin layer of mesoderm sandwiched between them.
- Only the first pharyngeal membrane persists and differentiates to form the *tympanic membrane (eardrum)*.
- Remaining disappears during development.

DEVELOPMENT OF PALATINE TONSILS

- In the early part of the 3rd month of development, the epithelium lining the ventral part of the second pouch undergoes proliferation, forming solid cords called *tonsillar buds* **(Fig. 12.7)**. These buds extend into the surrounding mesoderm, where central cells degenerate to create hollow *tonsillar crypts*. The epithelium lining the crypts and the surrounding mesoderm together form the *palatine tonsil*.
- Between the 3rd and 5th months, lymphatic tissue infiltrates the mesoderm, originating either in situ, or from circulating blood. The tonsil's capsule develops from condensed mesoderm, contributing to its structure. As the tonsil grows, it bulges inward into the pharynx.
- The remnant of the pouch is represented by the *intratonsillar crypt*.

DEVELOPMENT OF THE THYMUS

The thymus develops from the endoderm of the third pharyngeal pouch (which also gives rise to the inferior parathyroid glands).

- Early in development, this pouch is cut off, both from the pharyngeal wall and from the surface ectoderm. After separation from the inferior parathyroid rudiment, each thymic rudiment has a **thinner cranial part** and a **broader caudal part**.
- The thinner portion forms the cervical part of the thymus. The broader parts, of the two sides, enter the thorax and become united to each other by connective tissue in front of aortic sac.
- The endodermal cells of the thymus are invaded by vascular mesoderm which contains numerous lymphoblasts. This invading mesenchyme partially breaks up the thymic tissue into isolated masses, and thus gives the organ its *lobulated appearance*.
- Bone marrow gives rise to *thymocytes* endoderm of 3rd pouch give rise to cytoreticulum and Hassall's corpuscles.
- Fragmentation of the cervical part of the thymus may give rise to *accessory thymic tissue*. Such tissue, present in relation to the superior parathyroid glands, is believed to arise from the fourth pouch.
- The thymus is relatively large at birth. It continues to increase in weight till puberty. Thereafter, it gradually undergoes atrophy.

DEVELOPMENT OF PARATHYROID GLANDS

Parathyroid glands are derived as follows:

- The inferior parathyroid glands develop from endoderm of the third pharyngeal pouch (parathyroid III).
- The superior parathyroid glands develop from endoderm of the fourth pharyngeal pouch (parathyroid IV).
- As the third pouch also gives origin to the thymus, this organ is closely related to parathyroid III. When the thymus descends towards the thorax, parathyroid III is carried caudally along with it for some distance.
- Meanwhile, parathyroid IV is prevented from descending caudally, because of the close relationship of the fourth pouch to the developing thyroid gland. As a result, parathyroid III becomes caudal to parathyroid IV. Hence, the parathyroid glands derived from the

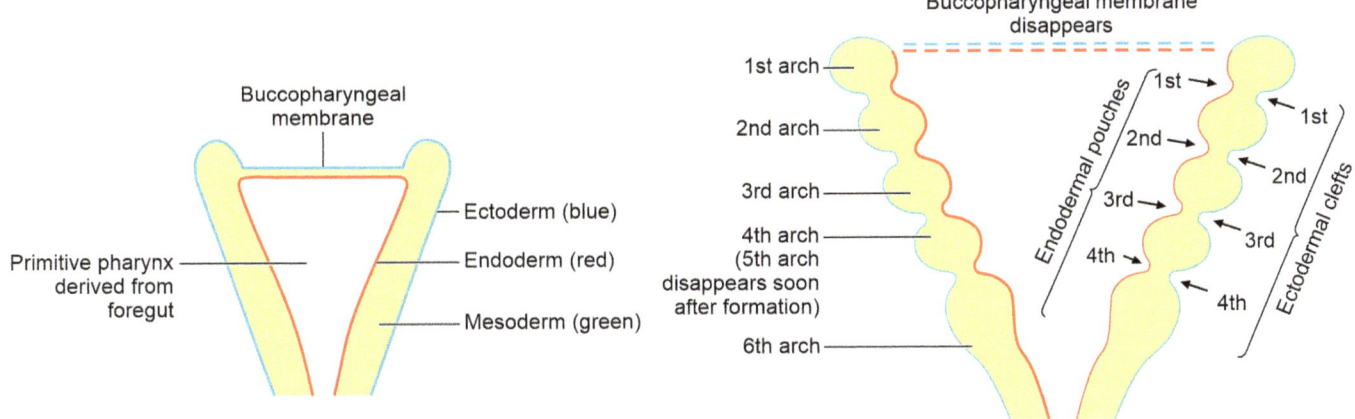

FIG. 12.8: Derivation of superior and inferior parathyroid glands. Note that the relative position of parathyroid III and IV is reversed during development.

fourth pouch become the superior parathyroid glands and those derived from the third pouch become the inferior parathyroid glands **(Fig. 12.8)**.

- In keeping with their developmental history, the superior parathyroid glands are relatively constant in position, but the inferior parathyroid glands may descend into the lower part of the neck or even into the anterior mediastinum. Alternatively, they may remain at their site of origin and are then seen near the bifurcation of the common carotid artery.

DEVELOPMENT OF THE THYROID GLAND

The thyroid gland develops mainly from the thyroglossal duct.

- *Parafollicular cells* are derived from the caudal pharyngeal complex (derived from the fourth and fifth pharyngeal pouches).
- After the formation of the pharyngeal arches, the floor of the pharynx has the appearance shown in **Figure 12.9**.
- The medial ends of the two mandibular arches are separated by a midline swelling called the *tuberculum impar*.
- Immediately behind the tuberculum, the epithelium of the floor of the pharynx shows a thickening in the middle line **(Fig. 12.10A)**. This region is soon depressed below the surface to form a diverticulum called the *thyroglossal duct* **(Fig. 12.10B)**.
- The site of origin of the diverticulum is now seen as a depression called the *foramen cecum*. The diverticulum grows down in the midline into the neck. Its tip soon bifurcates **(Fig. 12.10C)**. Proliferation of the cells of this bifid end gives rise to the *two lobes* of the thyroid gland.
- The developing thyroid comes into intimate relationship with the caudal pharyngeal complex and fuses with

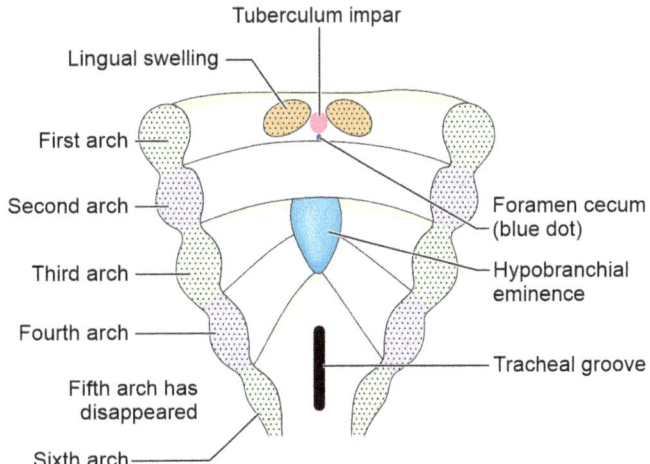

FIG. 12.9: Floor of the pharynx showing the foramen cecum from where the thyroglossal duct arises.

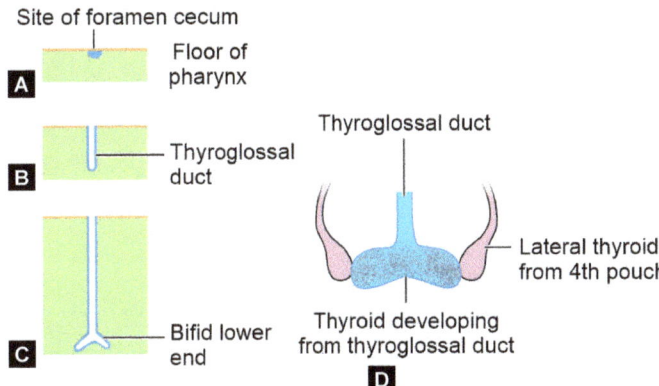

FIGS. 12.10A to D: Stages in the development of the thyroid gland.

it **(Fig. 12.10D)**. Cells arising from this complex are believed to give origin to the parafollicular cells of the thyroid which may represent the ultimobranchial body of lower animals.

Clinical correlation

Anomalies of the Thyroid Gland

A. Anomalies of Shape
- The *pyramidal lobe* is present so often that it is regarded as a normal structure. It may arise from the isthmus **(Fig. 12.11A)** or from one of the lobes **(Figs. 12.11B and C)**. It may have no connection with the rest of the thyroid, and may be divided into two or more parts **(Fig. 12.11D)**. In extent, it may vary from a short stump **(Fig. 12.11A)** to a process reaching the hyoid bone **(Fig. 12.11C)**.
- The isthmus may be, absent **(Fig. 12.12A)**.
- One of the lobes of the gland may be very small **(Fig. 12.12B)**, or absent **(Fig. 12.12C)**.

B. Anomalies of Position (Fig. 12.13)
- **Lingual thyroid:** The thyroid may lie under the mucosa of the dorsum of the tongue and may form a swelling that may cause difficulty in swallowing.
- **Intralingual:** The thyroid may be embedded in the muscular substance of the tongue.
- **Suprahyoid thyroid:** The gland may lie in the midline of the neck, above the hyoid bone.
- **Infrahyoid thyroid:** The gland may lie below the hyoid bone, but above its normal position.
- **Intrathoracic thyroid:** The entire gland, or part of it, may lie in the thorax.

Note that when thyroid tissue is present in the anomalous positions described above, an additional thyroid may or may not be present at the normal site.

C. Ectopic Thyroid Tissue
Small masses of thyroid tissue may be present at abnormal sites.
Thyroid tissue has been observed in the larynx, trachea, esophagus, pons, pleura, pericardium and ovaries. Masses of ectopic thyroid tissue have been described in relation to the deep cervical lymph nodes *(lateral aberrant thyroids)* but these are now believed to represent metastases in the lymph nodes from a carcinoma of the thyroid gland.

D. Remnants of the Thyroglossal Duct
These remnants may persist and lead to the formation of:
- **Thyroglossal cysts,** that may occur anywhere along the course of the duct. They may acquire secondary openings on the surface of the neck to form fistulae.
- **Thyroglossal fistula** opening at the foramen cecum.
- **Carcinoma** of the thyroglossal duct.

In the surgical removal of thyroglossal cysts and fistulae, it is important to remove all remnants of the thyroglossal duct. In this connection, it has to be remembered that the duct is intimately related to the hyoid bone **(Fig. 12.13)**.

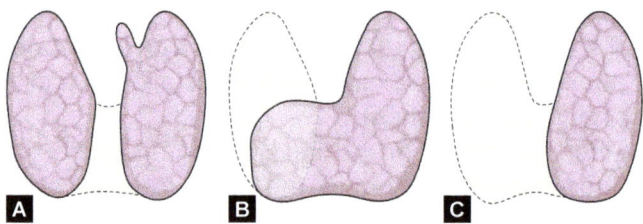

FIGS. 12.12A to C: Anomalies of the thyroid gland. The parts of the gland shown in dotted outline are missing.

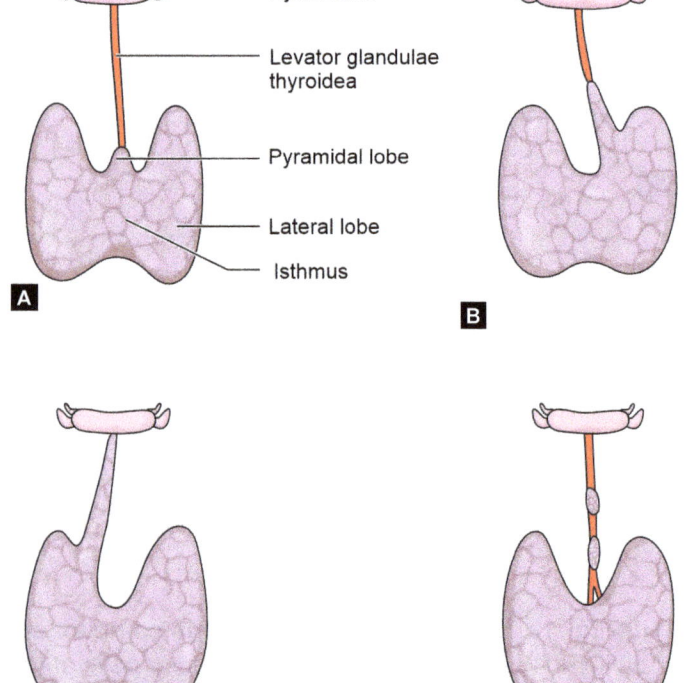

FIGS. 12.11A to D: Variations in the pyramidal process of the thyroid gland.

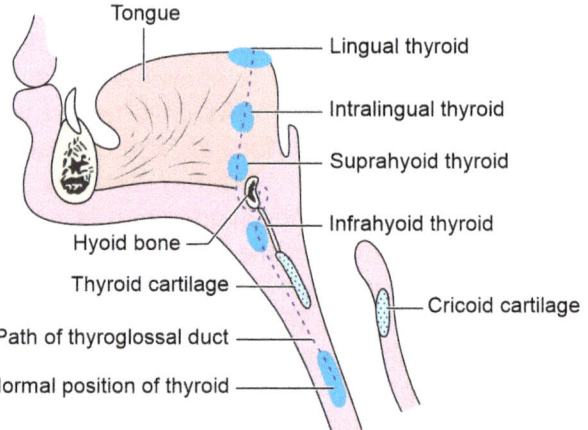

FIG. 12.13: Path of thyroglossal duct. Note that thyroid tissue may come to lie anywhere along the course of this duct.

Chapter 12: Branchial Apparatus (Pharyngeal Arches, Endodermal Pouches and Ectodermal Clefts)

TIMETABLE OF SOME EVENTS MENTIONED IN THIS CHAPTER

Age	Developmental events
4th week (22nd day)	Appearance of 1st and 2nd arches
5th week (29th day)	Four arches are seen. Thyroid, parathyroid and thymus start forming
7th week	Thyroid gland reaches its definitive position

Case Based Learning

Embryological Basis of Cervical Fistula

Case Scenario

A 7-year-old child presented to the pediatric surgeon with recurrent discharge from an opening on the right side of the neck. Examination revealed a small external opening along the anterior border of the sternomastoid muscle, from which thick discharge was spontaneously observed. Following an X-ray of the neck, the pediatric surgeon diagnosed the condition as a cervical fistula, as depicted in Figure below. What is the embryological basis for this condition? Give explanation for the position of the fistula.

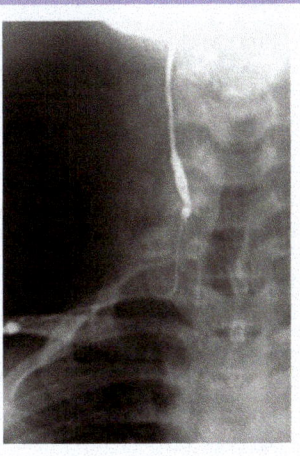

- This case involves a branchial or cervical fistula, an abnormal congenital tract connecting the skin of the neck to an internal structure due to the failure of closure of the 2nd to 4th branchial clefts.
- During embryonic development, the rapid growth of mesenchyme from the second branchial arch creates the cervical sinus between the overhanging second arch and subsequent arches. As the cervical sinus regresses, subsequent arches are covered and ectodermal clefts between the arches disappear, resulting in a smooth neck contour.
- Persistence of the cervical sinus can lead to the formation of a branchial cyst along the anterior border of the sternomastoid muscle. Rupture of the cyst can result in the formation of a branchial fistula, which may open externally or rarely internally, forming a communication between an external opening and the interior of the pharynx.
- In this particular case, the fistula is associated with the 2nd branchial cleft between the 3rd and 4th branchial arches. The 2nd branchial arch contributes to the formation of the hyoid bone, with its endodermal pouch forming the tonsil and the cleft forming the tonsillar fossa. The fistula travels between the internal and external carotid arteries, with the internal opening located at the level of the tonsillar fossa and the external opening found along the anterior border of the sternocleidomastoid muscle.

HIGHLIGHTS

- **Pharyngeal arches** are rod-like thickenings of mesoderm present in the wall of the foregut.
- At first there are six arches. The fifth arch disappears and only five remain.
- The ventral ends of the arches of the right and left sides meet in the middle line in the floor of the pharynx.
- In the interval between any two arches, the endoderm (lining the pharynx) is pushed outwards to form a series of pouches. These are called *endodermal, or pharyngeal, pouches*.
- Opposite each pouch the surface ectoderm dips inwards as an *ectodermal cleft*.
- Each pharyngeal arch contains *a skeletal element* (cartilage that may later form bone), *striated muscle* supplied by the *nerve* of the arch, and an *arterial arch*.
- The cartilage of the first arch *(Meckel's cartilage)* gives origin to the incus and malleus (of middle ear).
- The cartilage of the second arch forms the stapes, the *styloid process* and *part of the hyoid bone*.
- The cartilage of the third arch forms the *greater part of the hyoid bone*.
- The cartilages of the fourth and sixth arches give rise to the *cartilages of the larynx*.
- The *nerves of the pharyngeal arches* are as follows: First arch = mandibular; second arch = facial; third arch = glossopharyngeal; fourth arch = superior laryngeal; fifth arch = recurrent laryngeal. The muscles supplied by these nerves are derived from the mesoderm of the arch concerned.
- The *external acoustic meatus* develops from the first ectodermal cleft.
- The first endodermal pouch (and part of second) give off a diverticulum called the *tubotympanic recess*. The *middle ear* and the *auditory tube* develop from the tubotympanic recess.
- The *palatine tonsil* arises from the second pouch.
- The *inferior parathyroid gland* and the *thymus* are derived from the third pouch.
- The *superior parathyroid gland* is derived from the fourth pouch.
- The *thyroid gland* develops mainly from the thyroglossal duct. This duct is formed as a median diverticulum arising from the floor of the pharynx (at the foramen cecum).

Summary

- Derivatives of pharyngeal arches (**Table 12.3**).
- Derivatives of endodermal pouches (**Flowchart 12.1**).
- Derivatives of pharyngeal clefts and membranes (**Table 12.4**).

TABLE 12.3: Derivatives of pharyngeal arches.

Pharyngeal arch	Endodermal derivatives	Muscular components	Skeletal components	Nerve components	Artery derived
First arch	Malleus, incus, mandible	Masseter, temporalis, lateral pterygoid, mylohyoid, tensor tympani, tensor veli palatini	Maxilla, zygomatic bone, squamous part of temporal bone	Trigeminal ganglion, maxillary and mandibular nerves	Maxillary artery
Second arch	Stapes, styloid process, lesser horn and upper body of hyoid	Facial expression muscles (including orbicularis oculi, orbicularis oris), stapedius, stylohyoid	Styloid process, lesser horn of hyoid bone	Facial nerve (CN VII), vestibulocochlear nerve (CN VIII)	Stapedial artery
Third arch	Greater horn and lower body of hyoid	Stylopharyngeus	Greater horn of hyoid bone	Glossopharyngeal nerve (CN IX)	Common carotid artery
Fourth arch	Thyroid cartilage	Cricothyroid muscle, levator veli palatini	Thyroid cartilage	Superior laryngeal nerve (internal branch of CN X)	Right subclavian artery Arch of aorta (left side)
Sixth arch	Cricoid, arytenoid, corniculate, cuneiform	Intrinsic muscles of larynx (except cricothyroid)	Cricoid, arytenoid, corniculate, cuneiform cartilages	Recurrent laryngeal nerve (branch of CN X)	Ductus arteriosus (left side) Pulmonary artery (right side)

TABLE 12.4: Derivatives of pharyngeal clefts and membranes

Pharyngeal cleft/membrane	Derivatives
First pharyngeal cleft	• External auditory canal • Tympanic membrane (outer ectodermal layer)
Second pharyngeal cleft	Obliterated, may form cervical sinus leading to branchial cyst/sinus/fistula
Pharyngeal membranes	• **First:** Tympanic membrane • **Others:** Disappear

FLOWCHART 12.1: Endodermal pouches—derivatives.

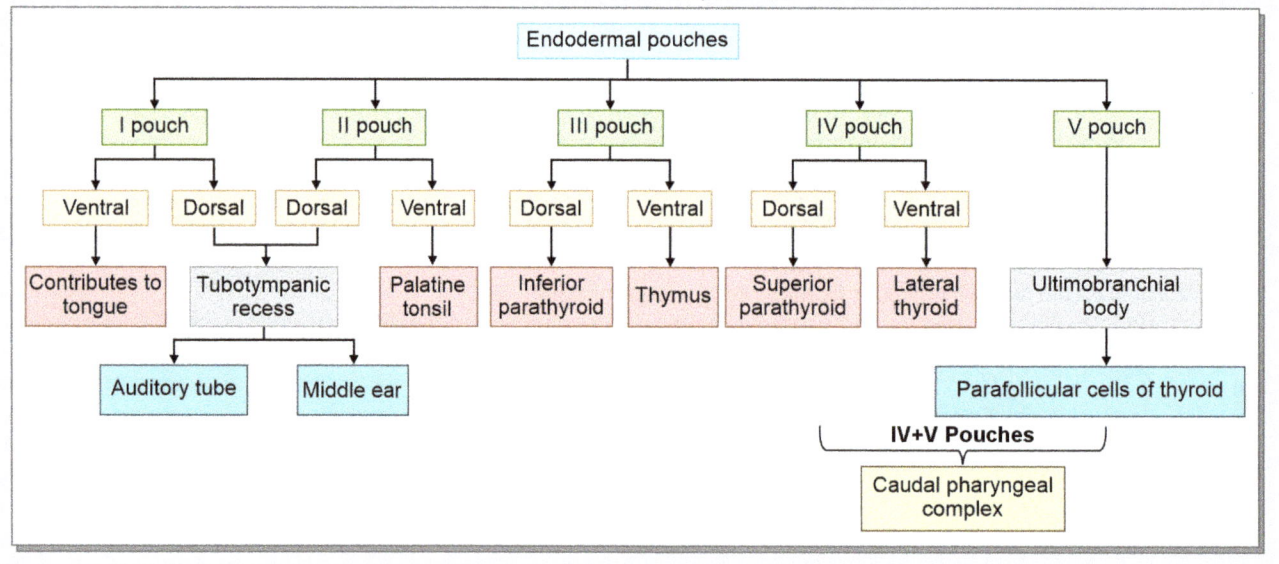

Chapter 12: Branchial Apparatus (Pharyngeal Arches, Endodermal Pouches and Ectodermal Clefts)

TEST YOUR UNDERSTANDING

REVIEW QUESTIONS

1. What are the derivatives of first pharyngeal arch?
2. Enumerate the nerves and muscles they supply of pharyngeal arches.
3. What are the skeletal elements of pharyngeal arches?
4. Describe cervical sinus and its applied aspect.
5. Discuss the derivatives of pharyngeal pouches.
6. Describe development of thymus.
7. Describe development of parathyroid glands.
8. Describe development of thyroid gland.
9. Describe development of palatine tonsil.
10. Discuss the congenital anomalies of thyroid gland.

EXPLAIN WHY? (REASONING QUESTIONS)

1. Surgeon accidentally found ectopic parathyroid gland in mediastinum during surgery.
2. Defects in the development of the first pharyngeal arch can lead to congenital anomalies.
3. Persistence of the second pharyngeal cleft can lead to the formation of lateral neck masses.
4. Ectopic thyroid tissue can be found along the path of the thyroglossal duct.

MULTIPLE CHOICE QUESTIONS

1. Palatine tonsil is derived from which endodermal pouch?
   A. 1st
   B. 2nd
   C. 3rd
   D. 4th

2. Superior parathyroid glands develop from endoderm of which pharyngeal pouch?
   A. 1st
   B. 2nd
   C. 3rd
   D. 4th

3. Parafollicular cells of thyroid gland are derived from which of the following pair of endodermal pouches?
   A. 1st and 2nd
   B. 2nd and 3rd
   C. 3rd and 4th
   D. 4th and 5th

4. All the following statements are true about derivatives of pharyngeal arches, *except*:
   A. 1st arch—malleus
   B. 2nd arch—styloid process
   C. 3rd arch—greater cornu of hyoid bone
   D. 4th arch—lesser cornu of hyoid bone

5. Identify the wrong statement about the nerves of pharyngeal arches:
   A. 1st arch—mandibular nerve
   B. 4th arch—recurrent laryngeal branch of vagus
   C. 2nd arch—facial nerve
   D. 3rd arch—glossopharyngeal nerve

6. Which pharyngeal arch of human embryo has double innervation?
   A. Fifth pharyngeal arch
   B. Fourth pharyngeal arch
   C. First pharyngeal arch
   D. Third pharyngeal arch

7. Hassall's corpuscles are derived from which pharyngeal pouch?
   A. 1st pouch
   B. 4th pouch
   C. 2nd pouch
   D. 3rd pouch

8. A newborn is found to have an accessory thyroid gland tissue located along the path of the thyroglossal duct. Which embryological structure is the source of this accessory thyroid tissue?
   A. First pharyngeal arch
   B. Second pharyngeal pouch
   C. Thyroid diverticulum
   D. Cervical sinus

9. During a routine ultrasound, a fetus is found to have a hypoplastic thymus and absent parathyroid glands. This anomaly is due to the defective development of which pharyngeal pouches?
   A. First and second
   B. Second and third
   C. Third and fourth
   D. Fourth and sixth

10. A 6-year-old child presents with a cystic mass located along the anterior border of the sternocleidomastoid muscle. This mass is most likely derived from which of the following structures?
    A. First pharyngeal arch
    B. Second pharyngeal cleft
    C. Third pharyngeal pouch
    D. Fourth pharyngeal membrane

11. A 6-year-old patient presents with recurrent infections and a midline neck mass that moves with swallowing. This mass is likely a remnant of which embryological structure?
    A. Second pharyngeal cleft
    B. Thyroglossal duct
    C. Third pharyngeal pouch
    D. Fourth pharyngeal arch

12. A neonate is diagnosed with congenital hypothyroidism and a lingual thyroid is detected. Which embryological process is most likely disrupted in this condition?
    A. Migration of the thyroid gland from the foramen cecum
    B. Formation of the thyroid diverticulum
    C. Development of the pharyngeal arches
    D. Differentiation of the thyroglossal duct

Answers: 1. B   2. D   3. D   4. D   5. B
           6. C   7. D   8. C   9. C   10. B
           11. B 12. A

Skeletal and Muscular System

CHAPTER 13

COMPETENCIES COVERED/LEARNING OUTCOMES

The student should be able to:

AN79.5	Explain embryological basis of nucleus pulposus.
AN13.8	Describe development of upper limb.
AN20.10	Describe basic concept of development of lower limb.

SKELETAL SYSTEM

The skeletal system comprises of cartilages and bones. As we have studied the formation of cartilage and bone in Chapter 10, both develop from loose tissue (mesenchyme) of the intraembryonic mesoderm. The cells of bones and cartilages are derived primarily from paraxial mesoderm, lateral plate mesoderm and neural crest cells.

Most bones of the axial skeleton are derived from *sclerotomes* of somites (paraxial mesoderm). Bones of the shoulder and hip girdle, and of the limbs, arise from *somatopleuric layer* of lateral plate mesoderm. Some bones of the face and skull are derivatives mesoderm of *pharyngeal arches* that are invaded by neural crests cells.

The skeleton is divided into the *axial skeleton* and the *appendicular skeleton*, and all bones originate from mesoderm. Based on their mode of ossification, bones can be classified as cartilaginous bones, membranous bones, or membranocartilaginous bones.

AXIAL SKELETON

The axial skeleton consists of the bones along the central axis of the body, including the skull (cranium), vertebral column, sternum and ribs. It provides structural support, protection for the brain, spinal cord, and thoracic organs, and serves as an attachment site for muscles.

Vertebral Column

The vertebral column is formed from the *sclerotomes* of the somites.
- During the 4th week of development, the cells of each sclerotome get converted into loose mesenchyme. This mesenchyme migrates medially and surrounds the notochord **(Fig. 13.1)**.

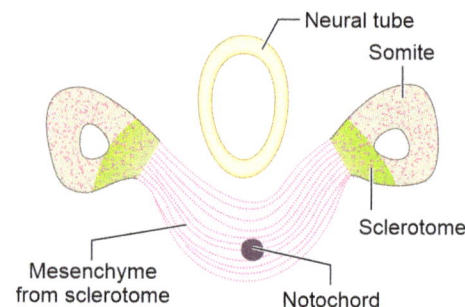

FIG. 13.1: Formation of mesenchymal basis of the body of a vertebra from a sclerotome.

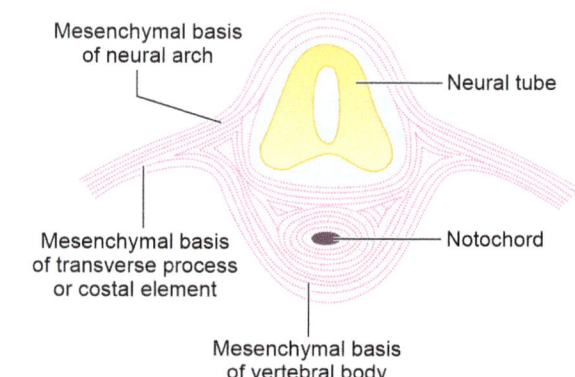

FIG. 13.2: Formation of mesenchymal basis of the neural arch and of the costal element.

- The mesenchyme then extends backwards on either side of the neural tube and surrounds it **(Fig. 13.2)**.
- Extensions of this mesenchyme also take place laterally in the position to be subsequently occupied by the transverse processes, and ventrally in the body wall, in the position to be occupied by the ribs.
- For some time the mesenchyme derived from each somite can be seen as a distinct segment **(Fig. 13.3A)**. The mesenchymal cells of each segment are at first uniformly distributed.

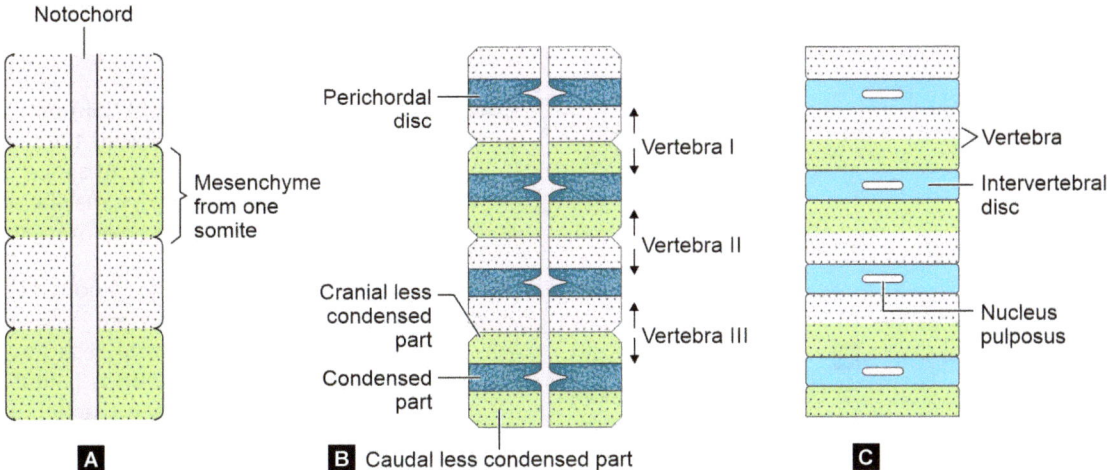

FIGS. 13.3A to C: (A) Mesenchyme derived from somites is seen in the form of segments; (B) Each segment has a central condensed part, and cranial and caudal less condensed parts; (C) A vertebra is formed by fusion of adjoining uncondensed parts of two somites. Hence it is an intersegmental structure. Each intervertebral disc is derived from the condensed part of one somite. Hence it is segmental in position.

- However, the cells soon become condensed in a region that runs transversely across the middle of the segment. This condensed region is called the *perichordal disc*. Above and below it there are less condensed parts **(Fig. 13.3B)**.
- The mesenchymal basis of the *body* (or *centrum*) of each vertebra is formed by fusion of the adjoining, less condensed parts of two segments **(Fig. 13.3C)**. The perichordal disc becomes the *intervertebral disc*.
- The neural arches and their processes are continuous with the less dense part of the sclerotomic segment. The *neural arch*, the *transverse processes* and the *costal elements* are formed in the same way as the body.
- The *interspinous and intertransverse ligaments* are formed in the same manner as the intervertebral disc.
- The notochord disappears in the region of the vertebral bodies. In the region of the intervertebral discs, the notochord becomes expanded and forms the *nucleus pulposus* **(Fig. 13.3C)**, which functions as a cushioning gel-like core providing flexibility and shock absorption to the spine.
- From the above account we may note that **(Fig. 13.4)**:
  - The vertebra is an *intersegmental* structure made up from portions of two somites. The intervertebral disc is formed at the center of the somite.
  - The transverse processes and ribs are also intersegmental. They separate the muscles derived from two adjoining myotomes.
  - Spinal nerves are segmental structures. They, therefore, emerge from between the two adjacent vertebrae and lie between two adjacent ribs.

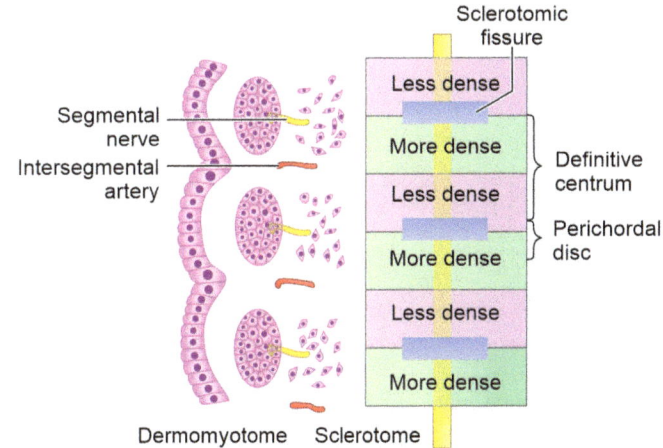

FIG. 13.4: Showing the segmental and intersegmental components of the parts of a vertebra and the nerves and arteries.

  - The blood vessels supplying structures derived from the myotome (e.g., intercostal vessels) are intersegmental like the vertebrae. Therefore, the intercostal and lumbar arteries lie opposite the vertebral bodies.

Ossification of Vertebra

- The mesenchymal basis of the vertebra is converted into cartilage by the appearance of several centers of chondrification.
- Three primary centers of ossification appear in the cartilaginous model for each vertebra; one for each neural arch and one for the greater part of the body (centrum).
- At birth the centrum and the two halves of the neural arch are joined by cartilage **(Fig. 13.5A)**. These are termed *neurocentral joints*.

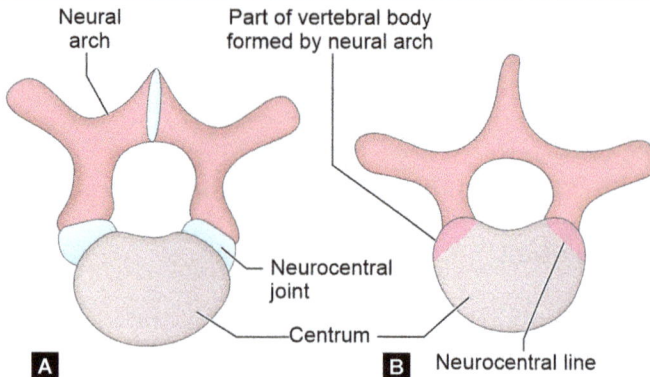

FIGS. 13.5A and B: (A) A vertebra at birth consisting of three separate pieces of bone: a centrum and two neural arches; (B) Diagram to show the neurocentral line which is the line along which body and neural arch have fused.

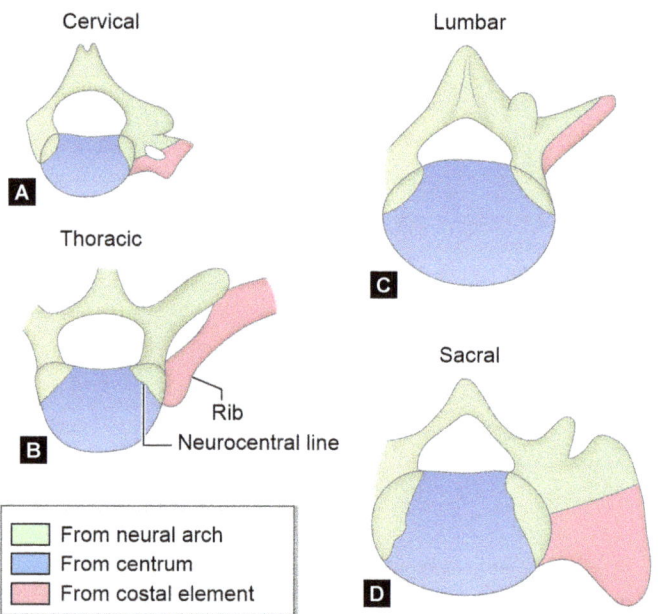

FIGS. 13.6A to D: Relative contribution to vertebrae by the centrum, the neural arch and the costal element in different regions. Note that a small part of the body of the vertebra is derived from the neural arch.

- Note that the posterolateral parts of the vertebral body are formed from the neural arch **(Fig. 13.5B)**. After the centrum and neural arch have fused, the junction between the two is indicated by the *neurocentral line*.
- In the cervical, thoracic, lumbar and sacral regions, the contributions to the various parts of the vertebrae by the centrum, neural arches and costal elements are shown in **Figures 13.6A to D**.

Molecular Regulation of Vertebra Development

Hox genes play a important role in vertebra development by specifying the identity and positional patterning of vertebrae along the anterior-posterior axis. These genes determine the unique characteristics of each vertebra segment, ensuring proper formation and alignment of the vertebral column.

Clinical correlation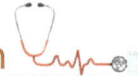

Congenital Anomalies of Vertebral Column
- One or more vertebrae may be absent, the caudal vertebrae being more commonly affected. Absence of the coccyx alone, or of the sacrum and coccyx, may be seen.
- Additional vertebrae may be present. The sacrum may show six segments.
- Part of a vertebra may be missing. Various anomalies result, depending on the part that is absent.
  - The two halves of the neural arch may fail to fuse in the midline. This condition is called *spina bifida* **(Fig. 13.7)**. The gap between the neural arches may not be obvious *(spina bifida occulta)*, or may be large enough for meninges and neural elements to bulge out of it (see meningocele and meningomyelocele). *Spina bifida aperta* is the most serious form of spina bifida, in which there open neural tube with no skin covering.
  - Spina bifida in a fetus can be recognized by ultrasound examination. Examination of amniotic fluid shows increased levels of alpha-fetoproteins (AFP) in a case with spina bifida.
  - The vertebral body may ossify from two primary centers which soon fuse. One of these parts may fail to develop, resulting in only half of the body being present. This is called *hemivertebra*. It is usually associated with absence of the corresponding rib.
  - The two halves of the vertebral body may be formed normally but may fail to fuse. The vertebral body then consists of two hemivertebrae. Sometimes the gap between the two halves is large enough for meninges and nerves to bulge forward between them *(anterior spina bifida)*.
- Two or more vertebrae that are normally separate may be fused to each other. Such fusion may occur in the cervical region *(Klippel-Feil syndrome)*. The atlas vertebra may be fused to the occipital bone *(occipitalization of atlas)*. The fifth lumbar vertebra may be partially or completely fused to the sacrum *(sacralization of 5th lumbar vertebra)*.
- Parts of the vertebral column that are normally fused to each other may be separate. The first sacral vertebra may be separate from the rest of the sacrum *(lumbarization of the first sacral vertebra)*. The odontoid process may be separate from the rest of the axis vertebra.
- The articular facets may be abnormal in orientation, or may be deficient. When there is deficiency of both the inferior articular processes of the fifth lumbar vertebra, the body of the vertebra may slip forwards over the sacrum. This is called *spondylolisthesis*.
- The vertebral canal may be divided into two lateral halves by a projecting shelf of bone, which splits the spinal cord longitudinally into two halves *(diastematomyelia)*.
- Ossification of the vertebral bodies may be defective thus reducing the total length of the spine. This can lead to the formation of dwarfs who have a short trunk but have limbs of normal length *(chondro-osteo-dystrophy)*.
- A peculiar tumor arising from cells of the primitive knot may be seen attached to the lower end of the spine. Various tissues may be seen in it. Such a growth is called a *sacrococcygeal teratoma*.

Anomalies of the vertebrae are of practical importance in that:
- They may cause deformities of the spine. The spine may be bent on itself *(congenital scoliosis)*. Deformities of cervical vertebrae may lead to tilting of the head to one side and its rotation to the opposite side *(congenital torticolis)*. This deformity may be secondary to a contracture of the sternocleidomastoid muscle.
- The spinal nerves, or even the spinal cord, may be implicated. They may be subjected to abnormal pressure leading to paralysis.
- They are frequently the cause of backache.

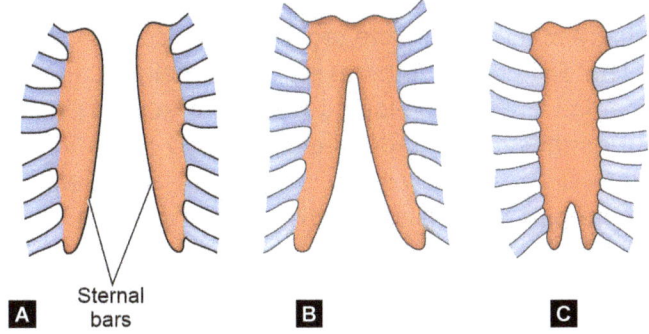

FIGS. 13.8A to C: Development of the sternum: (A) Sternal bars formed on each side of the middle line; (B) The sternal bars begin to fuse with each other at the cranial end; (C) Fusion progresses caudally.

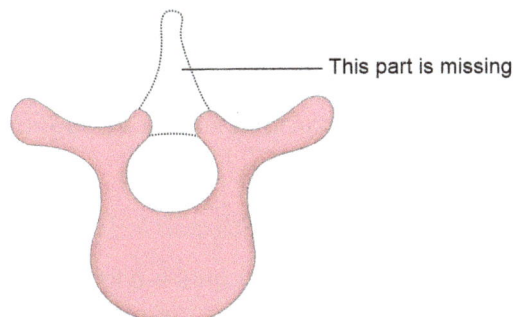

FIG. 13.7: Spina bifida produced by nonfusion of the two halves of the neural arch.

Ribs

The ribs are derived from ventral extensions of the sclerotomic mesenchyme that forms the vertebral arches. These extensions are present not only in the thoracic region but also in the cervical, lumbar and sacral regions.
- They lie ventral to the mesenchymal basis of the transverse processes with which they are continuous.
- In the thoracic region, the entire extension (called the *primitive costal arch*) undergoes chondrification, and subsequent ossification, to form the ribs.
- However, some mesenchyme between it and the developing transverse process does not undergo chondrification: it becomes loose and forms the *costotransverse joint*.
- In the cervical, lumbar and sacral regions, chondrification and ossification of the costal arch is confined to the region in immediate relationship to the transverse process.
- The bone formed from the arch is fused to the transverse process and is referred to as the *costal element* of the process. The contributions made by the costal element to the cervical, lumbar and sacral vertebrae are shown in **Figure 13.6A to D**.

Sternum

The sternum is formed by fusion of two *sternal bars* **(Fig. 13.8A)**, or *plates*, that develop on either side of the midline.

- Mesenchymal condensations forming at these sites become cartilaginous in the 7th week of intrauterine life.
- Laterally, the sternal bars are continuous with ribs. The fusion of the two sternal bars first occurs at their cranial end (manubrium) and proceeds caudally **(Figs. 13.8B and C)**.
- The manubrium and the body of the sternum are ossified, separately. The xiphoid process ossifies only late in life.

Clinical correlation

Anomalies of the Sternum and Ribs
- Some ribs that are normally present may be missing. Unilateral absence of a rib is often associated with hemivertebra.
- **Accessory ribs may** be present. Such a rib may be attached to the seventh cervical vertebra *(cervical rib)*, or to the first lumbar vertebra *(lumbar rib)*.
- When the fusion of the two sternal bars is faulty, the body of the sternum shows a partial or even a complete *midline cleft*. Minor degrees of nonfusion may result in a bifid xiphoid process or in midline foramina. Transverse clefts may also occur.
- In the condition called *funnel chest (pectus excavatum)*, the lower part of the sternum and the attached ribs are drawn inwards into the thorax. The primary defect is that the central tendon of the diaphragm is abnormally short.
- The upper part of the sternum (and related costal cartilages) may project forwards in midline as seen in birds. This condition is called *pigeon chest (pectus carinatum)*.

Skull

The skull is developed from mesenchyme surrounding the developing brain. This mesenchyme comes into close relationship with the following structures that also contribute to the development of the skull:
- Cranial to the first cervical somite there are four *occipital somites*. The mesenchyme arising from the

sclerotomes of these somites helps to form part of the base of the skull in the region of the occipital bone.
- The developing internal ear (otic vesicle), and the region of the developing nose, are surrounded by mesenchymal condensations called the *otic and nasal capsules* respectively. These capsules also take part in forming the mesenchymal basis of the skull.
- The first branchial arch is closely related to the developing skull. It soon shows two subdivisions, called the *mandibular and maxillary processes*.
- The skull is divided into two parts: (1) the *neurocranium* and (2) *viscerocranium*. The neurocranium forms the bones that encloses the brain and protects it. The viscerocranium forms facial skeleton.
- The neurocranium is divided into *chondrocranium or cartilaginous neurocranium* that forms the bones of base of skull and *membranous neurocranium* that forms the bones of vault of skull.
- The neural crest cells enter the head mesoderm and both together contribute for facial skeleton (viscero/ splanchnocranium) and membranous neurocranium.
- The chondrocranium or base of skull up to pituitary gland is formed by occipital sclerotomes and the part rostral to it is formed by neural crest cells.

Chondrocranium (Base of Skull)

- Base of the developing cranium is formed by fusion of several cartilages. The cartilaginous centers appear in cranial base during 2nd month.
- The fusion of the cartilages forms the various part of base of skull (chondrocranium) as shown in **Figure 13.9**.
- Some bones of the skull are formed in membrane, some in cartilage, and some partly in membrane and partly in cartilage, as listed below.

Membranous Neurocranium (Vault of Skull)

Intramembranous ossification occurs in the mesenchyme at the sides and top of the brain forming calvaria (cranial vault), which also receives contribution from neural crest cells.

Viscerocranium (Facial Skeleton)

The viscerocranium is divided into a *cartilaginous part* and a *membranous part*.

Bones that are Completely Formed in Membrane

- The *frontal and parietal bones* are formed in relation to mesenchyme covering the developing brain.
- The *maxilla* (excluding the premaxilla), *zygomatic* and *palatine* bones, and part of the *temporal* bones, are formed by intramembranous ossification of the mesenchyme of the maxillary process.
- The *nasal, lacrimal* and *vomer* bones are ossified in the membrane covering the nasal capsule.

Bones that are Completely Formed in Cartilage

The *ethmoid* bone and the *inferior nasal concha* are derived from the cartilage of the nasal capsule. The

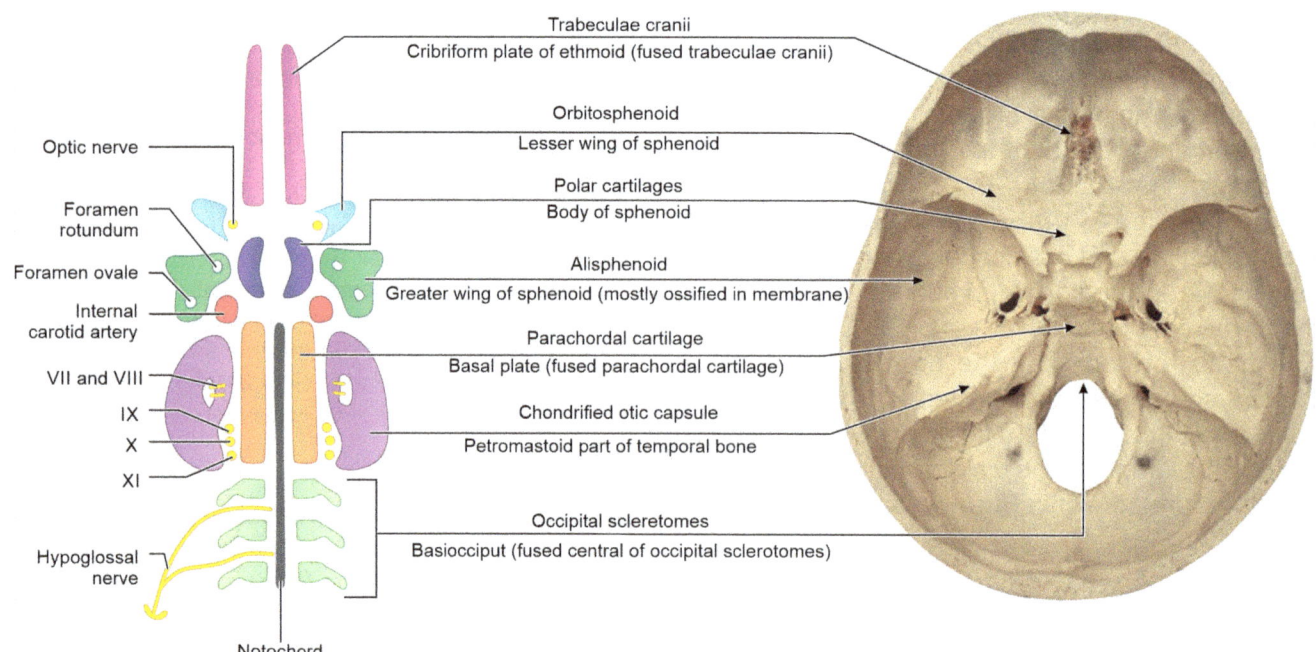

FIG. 13.9: Developmental components of chondrocranium and their derivatives.

septal and alar cartilages of the nose represent parts of the capsule that do not undergo ossification.

Bones that are Partly Formed in Cartilage and Partly in Membrane

- **Occipital:** The interparietal part (lying above the superior nuchal lines) is formed in membrane; the rest of the bone is formed by endochondral ossification.
- **Sphenoid:** The lateral part of the greater wing, and the pterygoid laminae, are formed in membrane; the rest is cartilage bone.
- **Temporal:** The squamous and tympanic parts are formed in membrane. The petrous and mastoid parts are formed by ossification of the cartilage of the otic capsule. The styloid process is derived from the cartilage of the second branchial arch.
- **Mandible:** Most of the bone is formed in membrane in the mesenchyme of the mandibular process. The ventral part of Meckel's cartilage gets embedded in the bone. The condylar and coronoid processes are ossified from secondary cartilages that appear in these situations. The development of the hyoid bone has been described in Chapter 12.

Clinical Importance

Fetal Skull
- The fetal skull develops from mesenchymal cells through intramembranous ossification.
- Initially, the skull bones are separated by areas of non-ossified membranous tissue persist between developing bones, forming *fontanelles and sutures*, which allow for flexibility during birth and accommodate rapid brain growth.
- The two important fontanelles are *Bregma* and *Lambda*.
- After birth, these bones gradually ossify and begin to fuse, forming the structure of the adult skull.
- An *open fontanelle* in an infant indicates that the cranial bones have not fully fused, leaving a soft, membranous gap. This should be monitored to assess developmental growth.

Clinical correlation

Anomalies of the Skull
- The greater part of the vault of the skull is missing in cases of *anencephaly*. This can happen be due to neural tube closure failure during the 3rd to 4th week of embryonic development. This defect leads to the absence of a major portion of the brain, skull, and scalp, and is associated with environmental and genetic factors affecting neural tube formation.
- **Encephalocele** is a neural tube defect characterized by the herniation of brain tissue and meninges through a small skull defect leading to varying degree of neurological impairment.

- The skull may show various types of deformity. In one syndrome, deformities of the skull are associated with absence of the clavicle *(cleidocranial dysostosis)*. Premature union of the sagittal suture gives rise to a boat-shaped skull *(scaphocephaly)*. Early union of the coronal suture results in a pointed skull *(acrocephaly)*. Asymmetrical union of sutures results in a twisted skull *(plagiocephaly)*. When the brain fails to grow the skull remains small *(microcephaly)*.
- The bones of the vault of the skull may be widely separated by expansion of the cranial cavity in *congenital hydrocephalus*.
- In a rare congenital condition called *Hand-Schuller-Christian* disease, large defects are seen in the skull bones. The primary defect is in the reticuloendothelial system; the changes in the bones are secondary.
- Several genetic disorders of craniofacial development have been described. One syndrome caused by under development of the first branchial arch is *mandibulofacial dysostosis*.

APPENDICULAR SKELETON

The appendicular skeleton consists of bones that form the limbs and their girdles, including the shoulder girdle (scapula and clavicle) and pelvic girdle (hip bones). These bones provide attachment points for muscles, enabling movement and supporting the body's mobility and stability during locomotion.

Development of Limbs

The bones of the limbs, including the bones of the shoulder and pelvic girdles, are formed from mesenchyme of the limb buds which appears at 4th week of IUL. With the exception of the clavicle (which is a membrane bone), they are all formed by endochondral ossification.

- The *limb buds* are, paddle-shaped, outgrowths that arise from the side-wall of the embryo at the beginning of the second month of intrauterine life **(Fig. 13.10)**. Each bud is a mass of mesenchyme covered by ectoderm.

- At the tip of each limb bud, the ectoderm is thickened to form the *apical ectodermal ridge (AER)*. This ridge has an inducing effect on underlying mesenchyme causing it to remain undifferentiated and to proliferate. Areas away from the apical ridge undergo differentiation into cartilage, muscle, etc.
- Sometimes two *AER* are formed on a limb bud. This results in formation of a supernumerary limb.

- The mesenchyme of limb buds is derived from (the parietal layer of) the lateral plate mesoderm. This mesenchyme gives rise to bones, connective tissue and some blood vessels. The muscles of the limbs are derived from myotomes of somites which migrate into the limbs.

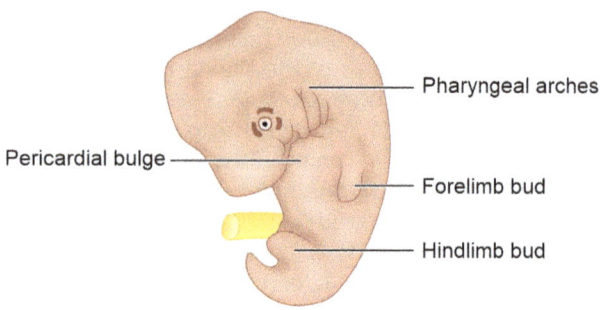

FIG. 13.10: Embryo showing limb buds.

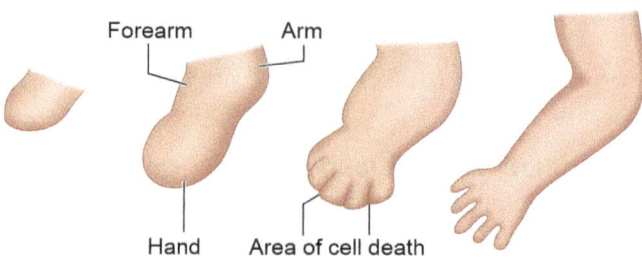

FIG. 13.11: Stages in differentiation of the forelimb bud.

- The *forelimb buds* appear a little earlier than the *hindlimb buds*. As each forelimb bud grows, it becomes subdivided by constrictions into arm, forearm and hand. The hand itself soon shows outlines of the digits. The interdigital areas show cell death because of which the digits separate from each other **(Fig. 13.11)**. Similar changes occur in the hindlimb (thigh, leg and foot).
- While the limb buds are growing, the mesenchymal cells in the buds form cartilaginous models, which subsequently ossify to form the bones of the limb.
- The limb buds are at first directed forward and laterally from the body of the embryo **(Fig. 13.12)**. Each bud has a *preaxial (or cranial) border* and a *postaxial border* **(Fig. 13.13)**. The thumb and great toe are formed on the preaxial border.
- The radius is the preaxial bone of the forearm. In a later development, the forelimb is adducted to the side of the body **(Fig. 13.11)**. The original ventral surface forms the anterior surface of the arm, forearm and hand.
- In the case of the lower limb, the tibia is the preaxial bone of the leg. Adduction of this limb is accompanied by medial rotation with the result that the great toe and tibia come to lie on the medial side. The original ventral surface of the limb is represented by the inguinal region, the medial side of the lower part of the thigh, the popliteal surface of the knee, the back of the leg and the sole of the foot.
- The forelimb bud is derived from the part of the body wall belonging to segments C4, C5, C6, C7, C8, T1 and T2. It is, therefore, innervated by the corresponding spinal nerves. The hind limb bud is formed opposite the segments L2, L3, L4, L5, S1 and S2.

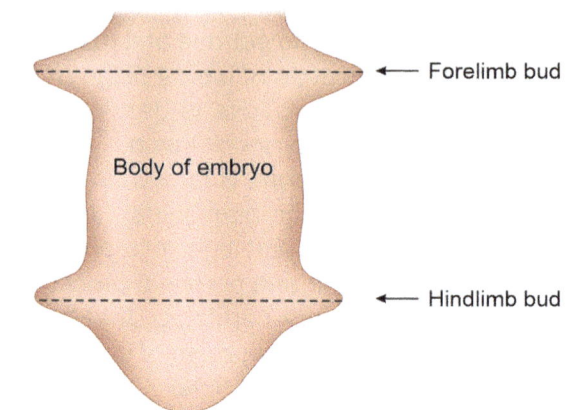

FIG. 13.12: Scheme to show that the longitudinal axis of the limb buds is transverse to the long axis of the embryonic body.

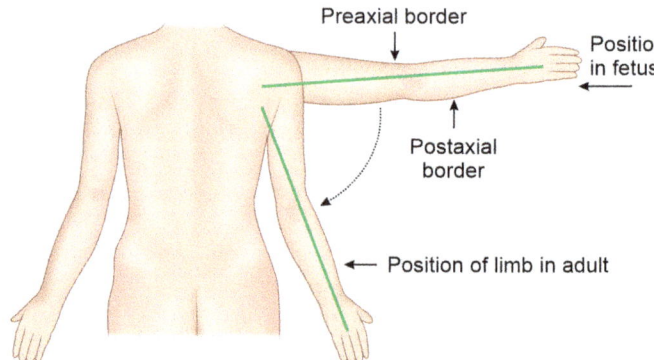

FIG. 13.13: Scheme showing that with 'adduction' of the embryonic limb, the preaxial border becomes the lateral border.

Molecular Regulation of Limb Bud Development

- **Hox** genes help in specifying the positional identity along the anterior-posterior and proximal-distal axes of limb buds.
- **Apical ectodermal ridge (AER):** It determines proximal and distal segments. It is essential for limb bud development. Removal of it leads to failure of growth and differentiation of limb called *phocomelia*.

Joint

The tissues of joints are derived from mesenchyme intervening between developing bone ends during 6th to 7th week of IUL. This mesenchyme may differentiate into fibrous tissue, forming a *fibrous joint (syndesmosis),* or into cartilage forming a *cartilaginous joint*. In the case of some cartilaginous joints *(synchondrosis or primary cartilaginous joints)* the cartilage connecting the bones is later ossified, with the result that the two bones become continuous. This is seen, typically, at the joints between the diaphyses and epiphyses of long bones.

At the site where a *synovial joint* is to be formed, the mesenchyme is usually seen in three layers. The two outer layers are continuous with the perichondrium covering the cartilaginous ends of the articulating bones. The middle layer becomes loose and a cavity is formed in it. The cavity comes to be lined by a mesothelium that forms the synovial membrane **(Figs. 13.14A to D)**. The capsule, and other ligaments, are derived from the surrounding mesenchyme.

Clinical correlation

Anomalies of Limbs
- One or more limbs of the body may be partially, or completely, absent *(phocomelia, amelia)*. These conditions may be produced by ingestion of harmful drugs. The extremities are most susceptible to teratogens during the 4th to 7th weeks; and slightly less susceptible in the 8th week.
- Part of a limb may be deformed. *Deformities* are most frequently seen in the region of the ankle and foot, and are of various types. In the most common variety of deformity, the foot shows marked plantar flexion (equinus: like the horse), and inversion (varus). Hence this condition is called *talipes equinovarus*, or *club foot*.
- **Congenital strictures, congenital amputations or congenital contractures** may be present.
- There may be abnormal fusion (bony or fibrous) between different bones of the limb. Adjoining digits may be fused *(syndactyly)*. The phalanges of a digit may be fused to one another *(synphalangia)*.
- A digit may be abnormally large *(macrodactyly)*, or abnormally short *(brachydactyly)*. In *arachnodactyly*, the fingers are long and thin *(spider fingers)*.
- Supernumerary digits may be present *(polydactyly)*. A digit (most commonly the thumb) may have an *extra phalanx*.
- The palm or sole may show a deep longitudinal *cleft (lobster claw)*.
- The limbs may remain short in *achondroplasia.*
- Sometimes the bone ends forming a joint are imperfectly formed *(congenital dysplasia)*. This can lead to *congenital dislocation*. The hip joint is most commonly affected.

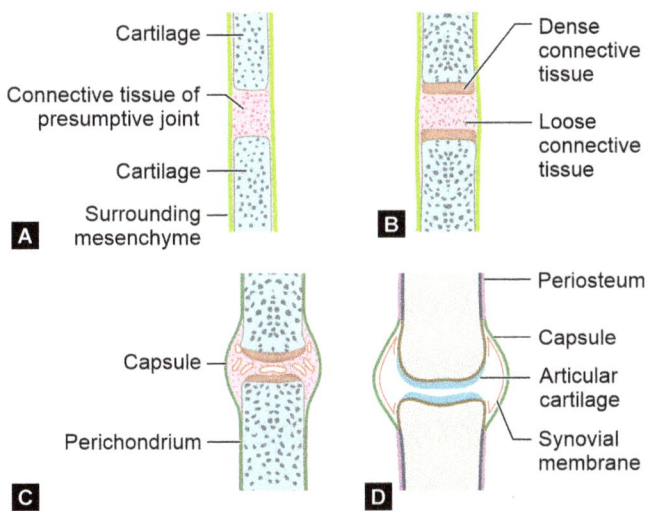

FIGS. 13.14A to D: Development of a synovial joint.

TIMETABLE OF SOME EVENTS MENTIONED IN THIS CHAPTER

Age	Developmental events
4th week (26th day)	Forelimb bud appears
4th week (28th day)	Hindlimb bud appears
5th week	Limbs become paddle shaped
6th week (36th day)	• Formation of future digits can be seen • Cartilaginous models of bone start forming
7th week	Rotation of limbs occurs
8th week (50th day)	• The elbow and knee are established • The fingers and toes are free • Primary centers of ossification are seen in many bones
12th week	Primary centers of ossification are seen in all the long bones

MUSCULAR SYSTEM

The majority of the skeletal muscles develop from somites. The cardiac and smooth muscles develop from splanchnic mesoderm. The myogenesis of skeletal, cardiac and smooth muscle are described in Chapter 10. In this chapter, the development of skeletal musculature of body will be considered.

SKELETAL MUSCLE

- Each myotome connects with a segmental nerve, meaning a muscle's nerve supply can indicate its embryological origin. On this basis, it would be presumed that all the musculature of the body walls and limbs is derived from the myotomes and has subsequently migrated to these regions.
- In humans, myotomes mainly form trunk muscles. Occipital myotomes are thought to develop into tongue muscles, while preoccipital myotomes form the extrinsic eye muscles.
- After formation, myotomes in the neck and trunk split into a small dorsal part *(epimere)* and a larger ventral part *(hypomere)*.
- The epimere forms the back muscles (extensors of the vertebral column), supplied by the dorsal primary ramus of the spinal nerve.
- The hypomere forms the body wall and limb muscles (flexors), supplied by the ventral ramus of the spinal nerve. The thoracolumbar fascia separates these muscle groups.
- Cells from the ventrolateral region of the dermomyotomes migrate to the parietal layer of the lateral plate mesoderm, forming the limb and anterolateral neck and abdominal muscles.

DEVELOPMENT OF MUSCULAR SYSTEM

The musculature of the body is derived from mesoderm as described below:
- Somatic mesoderm—limb, trunk
- Branchial mesoderm—head and neck
- Splanchnic mesoderm—cardiac, smooth
- Exceptions—ectodermal
  - Musculature of iris
  - Arrectores pilorum of skin
  - Myoepithelial cells of ducts of sweat glands

Developmentally the skeletal musculature of the body can be divided into *branchial arch derived* and *somite derived* muscles.

Branchial Arch Derived Musculature

Muscles of head and neck and face are derived from pharyngeal arches. They are already discussed in Chapter 12.

Somite Derived Skeletal Musculature

The somite derived musculature distribution is divided as follows **(Fig. 13.15)**:

Extraocular Muscles of the Eyeball

These muscles develop from three preoptic/preoccipital myotomes surrounding the developing eyeball. They are innervated by three cranial nerves:
1. The 3rd cranial nerve (oculomotor nerve) supplies the inferior oblique, levator palpebrae superioris, and the medial, superior, and inferior recti muscles.
2. The 4th cranial nerve (trochlear nerve) supplies the superior oblique muscle.
3. The 6th cranial nerve (abducens nerve) supplies the lateral rectus muscle.

Muscles of the Tongue

- All intrinsic and extrinsic tongue muscles, except the palatoglossus, originate from four occipital myotomes. These muscles are innervated by the 12th cranial nerve (hypoglossal nerve), which forms from the fusion of precervical nerves. The palatoglossus muscle is innervated by the vagus nerve.
- The occipital myotomes migrate into the developing tongue (contributed by 1st to 3rd pharyngeal arches) in the floor of mouth.

Body Wall (Trunk)

They are derived from segmental myotomes of somite origin as discussed earlier.

Limb Muscles

- During the 5th week of development, mesodermal cells from the myotomes migrate into the developing limb buds.
- Upper limb muscles originate from segments C4 to T2. Lower limb muscles originate from segments L1 to S3.

Diaphragm

- The diaphragm's musculature develops from C3 to C5 myotomes and is innervated by the phrenic nerves, which enter the septum transversum.
- The transversus layer of the thorax is displaced by the downward growth of the lung buds, contacting the septum transversum to form the thoracoabdominal diaphragm.

Other Muscles

The 2nd sacral to 1st coccygeal myotomes form the pelvic diaphragm, the external anal sphincter, and the striated muscles of the genital organs.

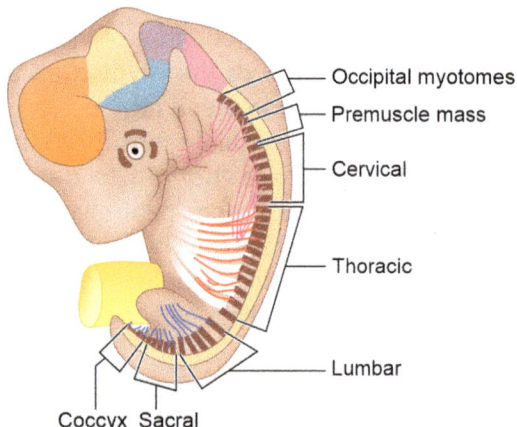

FIG. 13.15: Myotomic segment derived muscles of the body.

Case Based Learning

Embryological Basis of Anencephaly
A 30-year-old primigravida presented to obstetric OPD at 13th week and. She was advised transabdominal fetal ultrasound. The ultrasound picture (see **Figs. 13.16A and B**) presented fetus with absence of skull cap. It was diagnosed as an anencephalic fetus. The woman was advised to terminate pregnancy. The terminated fetus can be seen in the **Figures 13.16A and B**. Give the embryological explanation in this case.

Chapter 13: Skeletal and Muscular System

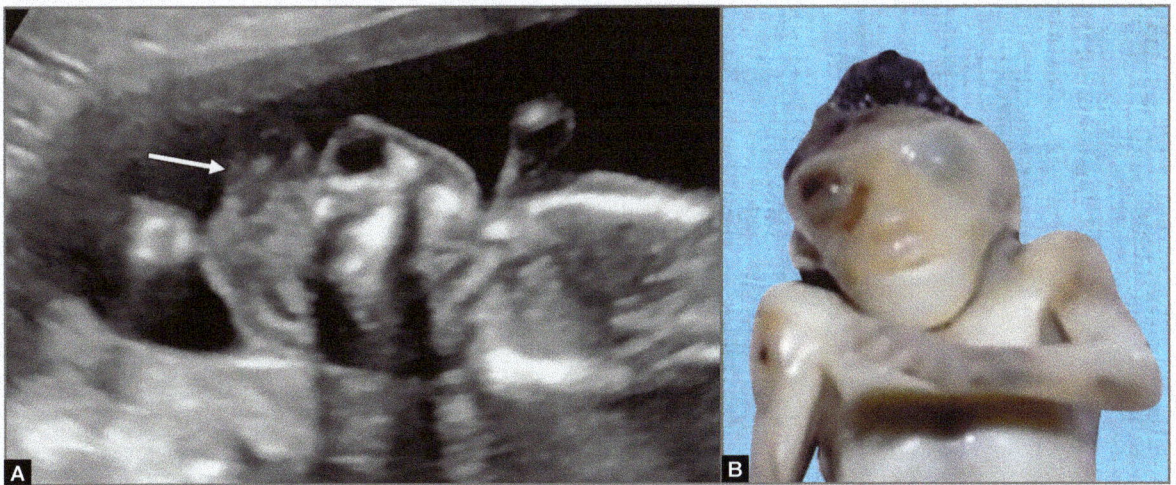

FIGS.13.16A and B: Anencephaly: USG and aborted fetus.

(Reproduced with permission from Dr Piyush Gupta. Source: A. Ranjith Kumar Manokaran and Jaya Shankar Kaushik, Chapter 24 and B. Shubha R Phadke and Ranjana Mishra, Chapter 27. In: Gupta P, UG Textbook of Pediatrics, Jaypee Brothers Medical Publishers Pvt Ltd, 2023).

- In the ultrasound, absence of the skull vault was found, i.e., an anencephalic fetus.
- The ultrasound image of the anencephalic fetus presented bulging eyes.
- Failure of closure of the cephalic part of neural tube and nonformation of vault of skull resulted in this condition.
- The neural tissue is disorganized due to exposure to amniotic fluid that caused necrosis of nervous tissue.
- Since it is a singleton, anencephalic pregnancy termination of pregnancy was be advised as the anencephalic fetus has no chance of survival.
- A 100% diagnosis of anencephaly can be made by prenatal ultrasound.
- In cases where it is a multiple gestation with dichorionic and diamniotic pregnancy with one normal fetus, the pregnancy is continued with care.

HIGHLIGHTS

- The *vertebral column* is derived from the sclerotomes of somites. Each sclerotome divides into three parts: (1) cranial; (2) middle; and (3) caudal.
- A *vertebra* is formed by fusion of the caudal part of one sclerotome and the cranial part of the next sclerotome. It is, therefore, intersegmental in position.
- The middle part of the sclerotome forms an *intervertebral disc*, which is therefore segmental in position.
- The *sternum* is formed by fusion of right and left sternal bars.
- The skull is divided into *neurocranium and viscerocranium*. Viscerocranium forms the facial skeleton. The neurocranium forms the bones around the brain.
- The neural crest cells enter the head mesoderm and both together contribute for facial skeleton (viscero/splanchnocranium) and membranous neurocranium. The *chondrocranium* or base of skull rostral to the level of pituitary gland is formed by neural crest cells. The part posterior to it is formed by occipital sclerotomes.
- The *skull* develops from mesenchyme around the developing brain. Some skull bones are formed in membrane (e.g., parietal); some partly in membrane and partly in cartilage (e.g., sphenoid); and a few entirely in cartilage (e.g., ethmoid).
- The *mandible* is formed in membrane from the mesenchyme of the mandibular process.
- Limbs are first seen as outgrowths *(limb buds)* from the side wall of the embryo. Each bud grows and gets subdivided to form parts of the limb.
- **Limb bones** develop from mesenchyme of the limb buds. Joints are formed in intervals between bone ends.
- All muscles of the body develop from mesoderm *except* muscles of iris, arrectores pilorum of skin and myoepithelial cells lining ducts of sweat glands.
- **Skeletal muscle** is derived partly from somites and partly from mesenchyme of the region.
- Most *smooth muscle* is formed from mesenchyme related to viscera and blood vessels.
- **Cardiac muscle** is formed from mesoderm related to developing heart.

Summary

- Development of vertebra (**Flowchart 13.1**).
- Somites and their derivatives (**Table 13.1**).

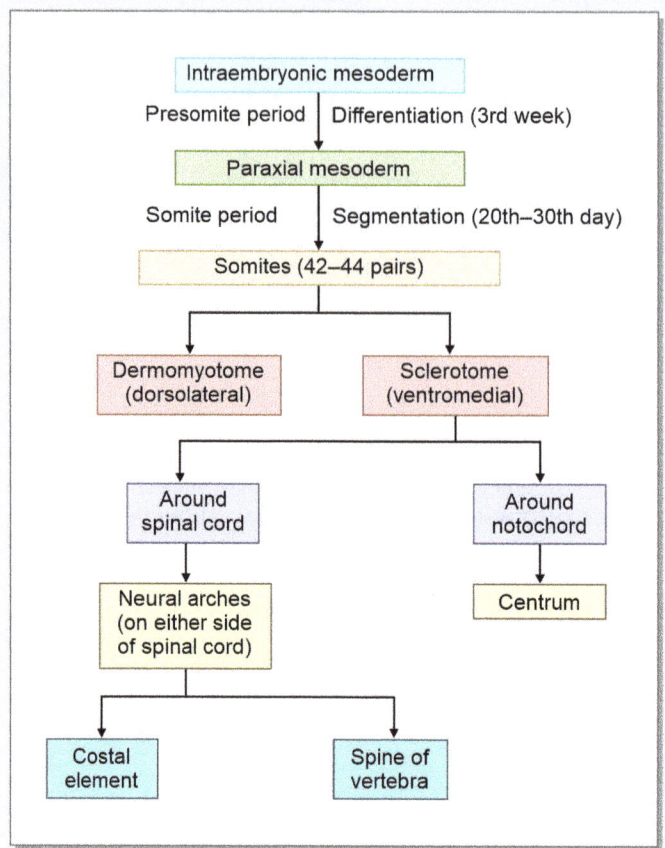

FLOWCHART 13.1: Development of vertebra.

TABLE 13.1: Somites and their skeletal and muscular derivatives.

Somites	Number of pairs	Skeletal derivatives	Muscular derivatives
Preoccipital	3	Base of skull	Extraocular muscles of eyeball
Occipital	4–5		Tongue musculature *except* palatoglossus
Cervical	8	Vertebra	Striated muscles of trunk, diaphragm, limbs
Thoracic	12	Vertebra and ribs	Intercoastal muscles and muscles of anterolateral wall of abdomen
Lumbar	5	Vertebra	Quadratus lumborum, Iliac and psoas muscles
Sacral	5	Vertebra	Pelvic diaphragm and anal muscles
Coccygeal	8–10	Vertebra	Pelvic diaphragm and anal muscles

Chapter 13: Skeletal and Muscular System

TEST YOUR UNDERSTANDING

REVIEW QUESTIONS

1. Explain development of vertebra.
2. Write short notes on development of sternum.
3. Discuss developmental components of chondrocranium and their derivatives.
4. Write short notes on development of synovial joint.
5. Discuss the development of limbs.

MULTIPLE CHOICE QUESTIONS

1. Perichordal disc is the precursor of:
   A. Nucleus pulposus   B. Annulus fibrosus
   C. Centrum   D. Neural arch
2. Following bones are formed partly in membrane and partly in cartilage, *except*:
   A. Occipital   B. Sphenoid
   C. Mandible   D. Zygomatic
3. All the following are derived from somites, *except*:
   A. Tongue muscles
   B. Erector spinae
   C. Pharyngeal muscles
   D. Muscles of perineal pouches
4. Which structure divides the paraxial mesoderm into somitomeres and somites?
   A. Otic capsules   B. Optic capsules
   C. Occiput   D. Atlas vertebra
5. All tongue muscles develops from occipital myotomes, *except*:
   A. Genioglossus   B. Palatoglossus
   C. Hyoglossus   D. Styloglossus
6. During embryonic development, which structure initially forms the template for the formation of the axial skeleton, including the vertebrae and ribs?
   A. Notochord
   B. Neural crest cells
   C. Paraxial mesoderm
   D. Lateral plate mesoderm
7. A patient exhibits a congenital anomaly where the lower limb bones are abnormally short and bowed, with associated joint deformities. Which embryological defect is most likely responsible for this condition?
   A. Defect in limb bud initiation
   B. Abnormalities in limb bud patterning
   C. Disruption in endochondral ossification
   D. Failure of limb bud outgrowth
8. A newborn presents with a defect where the frontal bones of the skull fail to fuse, resulting in a prominent midline gap (fontanelle). Which embryological process is most likely disrupted in this condition?
   A. Intramembranous ossification
   B. Endochondral ossification
   C. Mesenchymal condensation
   D. Neural crest cell migration
9. A patient presents with a congenital condition characterized by the absence of the pectoral muscles on one side of the chest. Which embryological structure is primarily responsible for the development of these muscles?
   A. Dermatome   B. Myotome
   C. Sclerotome   D. Syndetome

10. Match the following:

    Column I
    A. Occipitalization of atlas
    B. Sacralization of 5th vertebra
    C. Lumbarization of 1st sacral vertebra
    D. Spondylolisthesis
    E. Funnel chest
    F. Pigeon chest
    G. Plagiocephaly
    H. Hand-Schuller-Christian disease
    I. Lobster claw
    J. Syndactyly

    Column II
    1. Fused digits
    2. Deep cleft in palm or lumbar sole
    3. Fusion of L5 to sacrum
    4. Projection forwards of sternum and costal cartilages
    5. Twisted skull
    6. Large defects in skull bones
    7. Fusion of atlas with occipital bone
    8. Drawing inwards of ribs and sternum
    9. Body of L5 slipping over the sacrum
    10. Separation of 1st sacral vertebra from the rest

Answers: 1. B   2. D   3. D   4. A   5. B
           6. A   7. C   8. A   9. B
           10. A.7   B.3   C.10   D.9   E.8   F.4   G.5   H.6   I.2   J.1

Face, Nose and Palate

CHAPTER 14

COMPETENCIES COVERED/LEARNING OUTCOMES

The student should be able to:

AN43.4 Describe the development and developmental basis of congenital anomalies of face and palate.

In chapter 7 we have seen that during 4th week of development after the formation of head fold, there are two prominent bulgings that appeared on the ventral aspect of the developing embryo, separated by the stomatodeum **(Fig. 14.1)**. They are:
- Developing brain cranially
- Pericardium caudally

The floor of the stomatodeum is formed by the buccopharyngeal membrane, which separates it from the foregut. On each side, the stomatodeum is bounded by first (mandibular) arch.

Soon, mesoderm covering the developing forebrain proliferates and forms a downward projection that overlaps the upper part of the stomatodeum. This downward projection is called the *frontonasal process* **(Fig. 14.2)**.

The pharyngeal arches are laid down in the lateral and ventral walls of the most cranial part of the foregut (*refer* **Fig. 12.1**). These are also in very close relationship to the stomatodeum.

The development of face, nose and palate occurs through differentiation of these two, i.e., frontonasal process and mandibular arch.

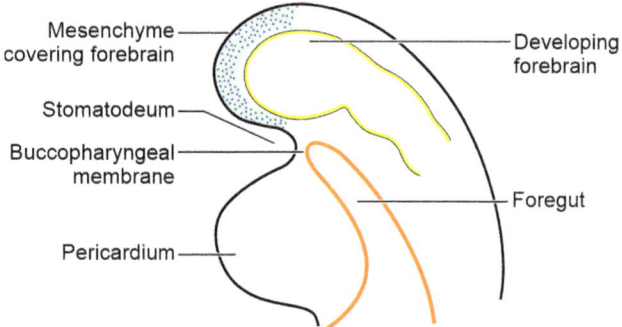

FIG. 14.1: Head end of an embryo just before formation of the frontonasal process.

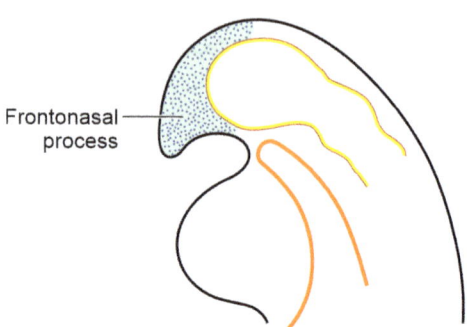

FIG. 14.2: Formation of frontonasal process.

DEVELOPMENT OF FACE

With further growth, mandibular arch forms the lateral wall of the stomatodeum **(Fig. 14.3A)**. This arch gives off a bud from its dorsal end. This bud is called the *maxillary process* **(Fig. 14.3B)**. It grows ventromedially cranial to the main part of the arch which is now called the *mandibular process*.

Now we can say that, face develops from following three structures:
1. Frontonasal process
2. Two mandibular processes
3. Two maxillary processes

Since, nose is part of developing face, we shall discuss the developing elements of nose here. The ectoderm overlying the frontonasal process soon shows bilateral localized thickenings, that are situated a little above the stomatodeum **(Fig. 14.4A)**. These are called the *nasal placodes*. The formation of these placodes is induced by the underlying forebrain. The placodes soon sink below the surface to form *olfactory/nasal pits* **(Fig. 14.4B)**. The pits are continuous with the stomatodeum below.

The mesenchyme around the edges of each pit are proliferated and raised above the surface: the medial

Chapter 14: Face, Nose and Palate

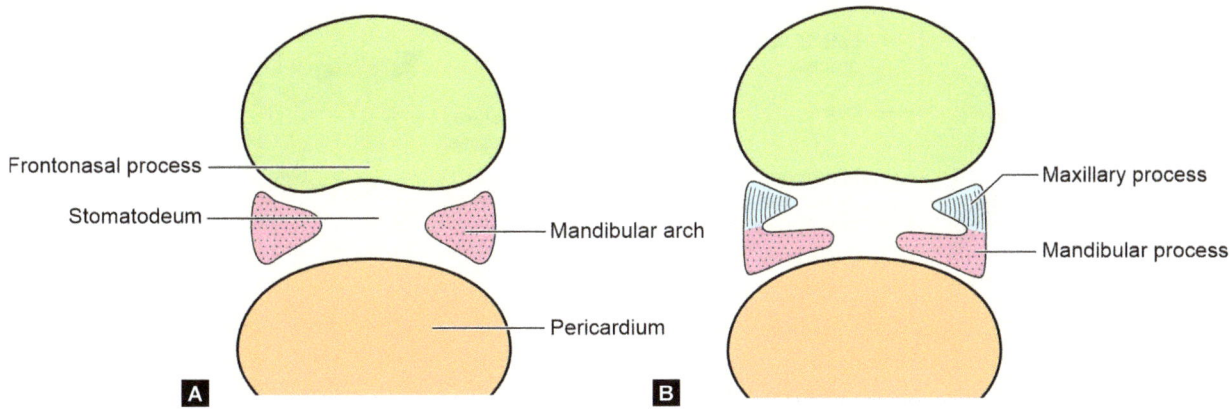

FIGS. 14.3A and B: Development of face: Formation of mandibular and maxillary processes.

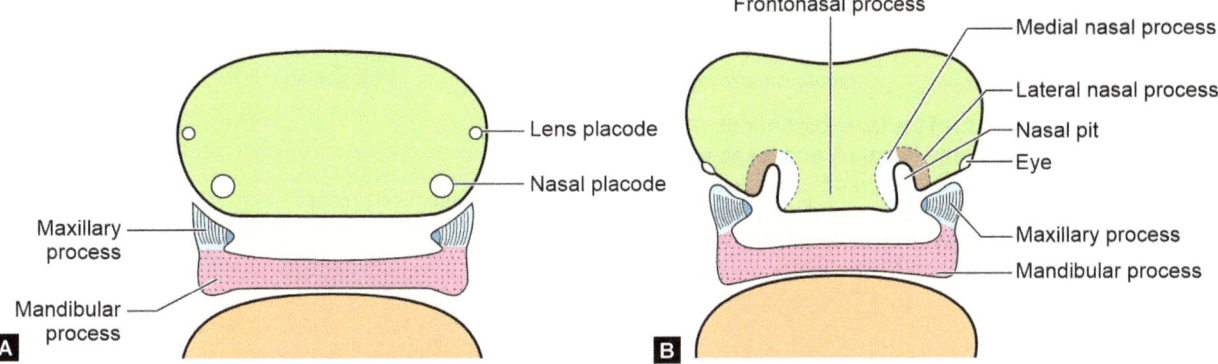

FIGS. 14.4A and B: Development of face (continued): (A) The right and left mandibular processes fuse and form the lower boundary of the future mouth. The nasal placodes appear over the frontonasal process. The lens placode appears; (B) The nasal placode is converted into the nasal pit. Elevations of the pit form the medial and lateral nasal processes.

raised edge is called the *medial nasal process* and the lateral edge is called the *lateral nasal process*.

Lets discuss the development of various parts of face.

Development of Lower Lip

- The *mandibular processes* of the two sides grow towards each other **(Fig. 14.3B)**, and fuse in the midline **(Fig. 14.4A)**.
- They now form the lower margin of the stomatodeum. If it is remembered that the mouth develops from the stomatodeum, it will be readily understood that the fused mandibular processes give rise to the *lower lip*, and to the *lower jaw* **(Fig. 14.7)**.

Development of Upper Lip

- Each *maxillary process* now grows medially and fuses, first with the *lateral nasal process* **(Figs. 14.5A and B)**, and then with the *medial nasal process* **(Figs. 14.6A and B)**. The medial and lateral nasal processes also fuse with each other. In this way the nasal pits (now called *external nares*) are cut off from the stomatodeum.
- The maxillary processes undergo considerable growth **(Figs. 14.6A and B)**. At the same time the frontonasal process becomes much narrower from

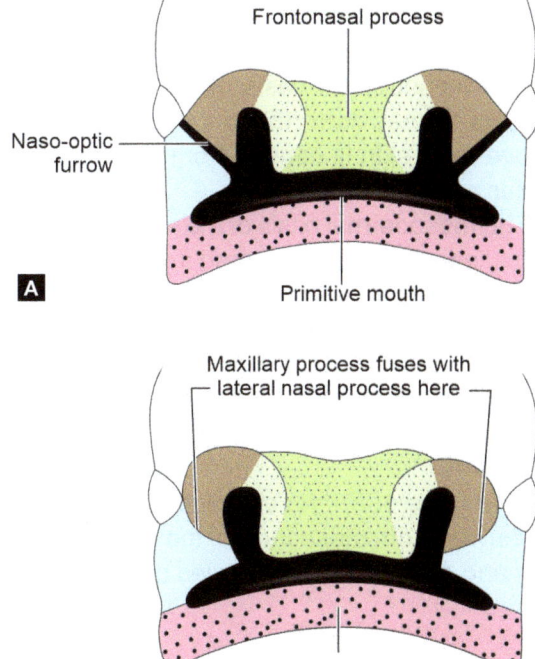

FIGS. 14.5A and B: Development of the face (continued): (A) The right and left nasal pits come close to each other. The lateral nasal process is separated from the maxillary process by the naso-optic furrow; (B) The maxillary process fuses with the lateral nasal process obliterating the naso-optic furrow.

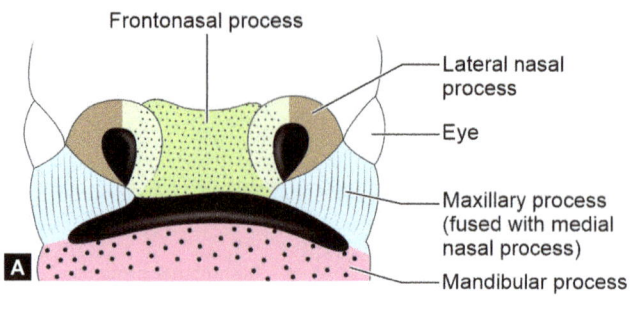

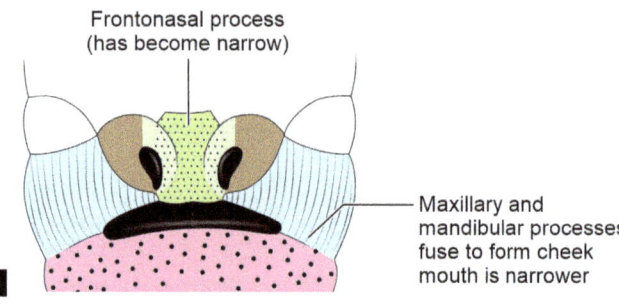

FIGS. 14.6A and B: Development of the face (continued): (A) The maxillary process extends below the nasal pit and fuses with the medial nasal process. In this way the nasal pit is separated from the stomatodeum; (B) The maxillary and mandibular processes partly fuse to form the cheek. With growth of the maxillary processes the nasal pits come closer to each other.

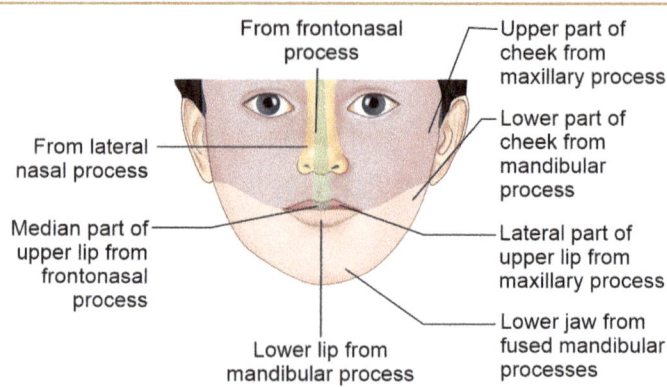

FIG. 14.7: Derivation of parts of the face.

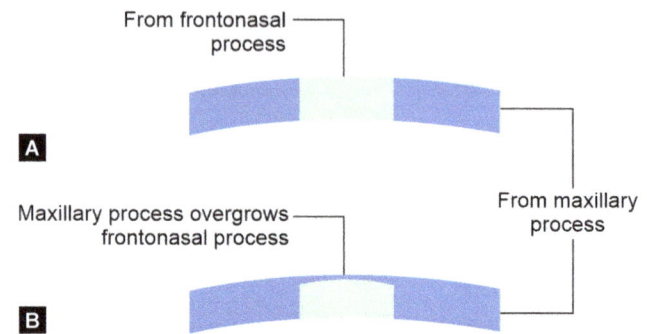

FIGS. 14.8A and B: Formation of upper lip: Scheme to show how the maxillary process 'overgrows' the frontonasal process.

side to side, with the result that the two external nares come closer together. Frontonasal process forms the *forehead* and *bridge of the nose*.

- The stomatodeum is now bounded above by the *upper lip* that is derived as follows (**Figs. 14.7 and 14.8**):
  - The mesodermal basis of the lateral part of the lip is formed from the *maxillary process*. The overlying skin is derived from ectoderm covering this process.
  - The mesodermal basis of the median part of the lip (called *philtrum*) is formed from the *frontonasal process*. The ectoderm of the maxillary process, however, overgrows this mesoderm to meet that of the opposite maxillary process in the midline (**Figs. 14.8A and B**). As a result, the skin of the entire upper lip is innervated by the *maxillary nerves*.
- The *muscles of the face* (including those of the lips) are derived from mesoderm of the *second branchial arch* and are, therefore, supplied by the *facial nerve*.

Development of Cheeks

- After formation of the upper and lower lips, the stomatodeum (which can now be called the mouth) is very broad. In its lateral part, it is bounded above by the maxillary process and below by the mandibular process.

- These processes undergo progressive fusion with each other to form the cheeks (compare **Figs. 14.6A and B**; also see **Figs. 14.9 and 14.10**).
- The maxillary process fuses with the lateral nasal process. This fusion not only occurs in the region of the lip but also extends from the stomatodeum to the medial angle of the developing eye (**Figs. 14.6 and 14.9B**).
- For some time this line of fusion is marked by a groove called the *naso-optic furrow* or *nasolacrimal sulcus* (**Fig. 14.5A**).
- A strip of ectoderm becomes buried along this furrow and gives rise to the *nasolacrimal duct*.

Development of Eye

The development of the eye itself will be dealt with later, but a brief reference to it is necessary to form a complete idea of the development of the face.

- The region of the eye is first seen as an ectodermal thickening, the *lens placode*, which appears on the ventrolateral side of the developing forebrain, lateral and cranial to the nasal placode (**Fig. 14.4A**).
- The lens placode sinks below the surface and is eventually cut off from the surface ectoderm. The developing eyeball produces a bulging in this situation (**Fig. 14.5**).

Chapter 14: Face, Nose and Palate

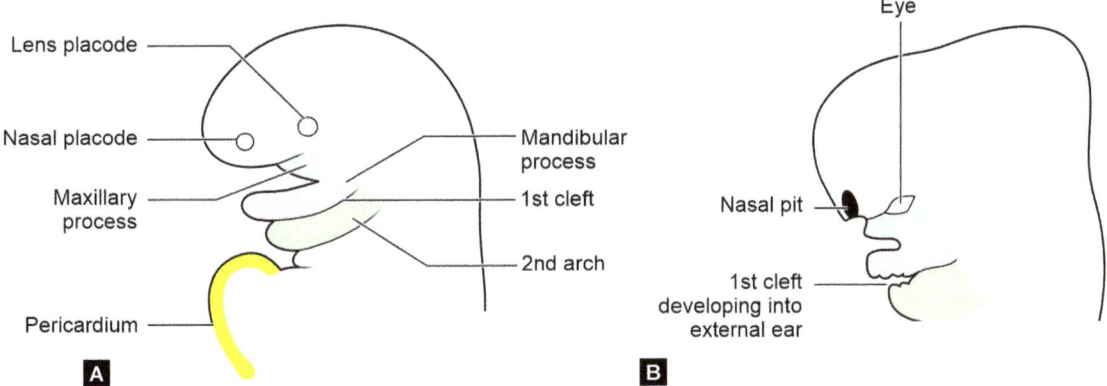

FIGS. 14.9A and B: Early stages in the development of the face as seen from the lateral aspect.

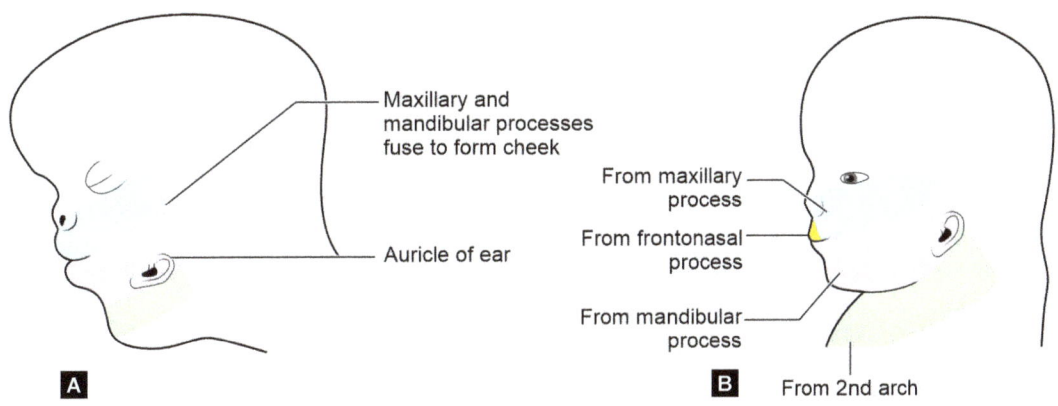

FIGS. 14.10A and B: Later stage in the development of the face as seen from the lateral aspect.

- The bulgings of the eyes are at first directed laterally (**Figs. 14.5 and 14.6**), and lie in the angles between the maxillary processes and the lateral nasal processes. With the narrowing of the frontonasal process, they come to face forwards (**Figs. 14.6 and 14.7**).
- The eyelids are derived from folds of ectoderm that are formed above and below the eyes, and by mesoderm enclosed within the folds.

External Ear

The external ear is formed around the dorsal part of the first ectodermal cleft (**Figs. 14.9A and B**).

- A series of mesodermal thickenings (often called *tubercles or hillocks*) appear on the mandibular and hyoid arches where they adjoin this cleft. The *pinna (or auricle)* is formed by fusion of these thickenings.
- From a study of **Figures 14.9 and 14.10** it will be seen that when first formed, the pinna lies caudal to the developing jaw.
- It is pushed upwards and backwards to its definitive position due to the great enlargement of the mandibular process. If the mandibular process fails to enlarge, the ears remain low down which results in *mandibulofacial dysostosis*.

Clinical correlation

Developmental Anomalies of the Face
It has been seen that the formation of various parts of the face involves fusion of diverse components. This fusion is occasionally incomplete and gives rise to various anomalies.
- **Cleft lip:** It is commonly seen in upper lip. Sometimes it is referred to *harelip* as hare upper lip has a cleft.
  - When one or both maxillary processes do not fuse with the medial nasal process, this gives rise to defects in the upper lip. These may vary in degree and may be *unilateral* (**Figs. 14.11A to C**), or *bilateral* (**Fig. 14.11D**).
  - Defective development of the lowermost part of the frontonasal process may give rise to a *midline defect* of the upper lip (**Fig. 14.11E**).
  - When the two mandibular processes do not fuse with each other the lower lip shows a defect in the midline. The defect usually extends into the jaw (**Fig. 14.11F**).

- **Oblique facial cleft:** Non-fusion of the maxillary and lateral nasal process gives rise to a cleft running from the medial angle of the eye to the mouth **(Fig. 14.12A)**. The nasolacrimal duct is not formed.
- Inadequate fusion of the mandibular and maxillary processes with each other may lead to an abnormally wide mouth *(macrostomia)* **(Fig. 14.12B)**. Lack of fusion may be unilateral: this leads to formation of a *lateral facial cleft*. Too much fusion may result in a small mouth *(microstomia)* **(Fig.14.12C)**.
- The nose may be bifid. This may be associated with median cleft lip. Both these occur due to bifurcation of the frontonasal process. Occasionally one half of it may be absent. Very rarely the nose forms a cylindrical projection, or *proboscis* **(Fig. 14.13)** jutting out from just below the forehead. This anomaly may sometimes affect only one half of the nose and is usually associated with fusion of the two eyes *(cyclops)*.
- The entire first arch may remain underdeveloped on one or both sides, affecting the lower eyelid *(coloboma type* defect), the maxilla, the mandible, and the external ear. The prominence of the cheek is absent and the ear may be displaced ventrally and caudally. There may be presence of cleft palate and of faulty dentition. This condition is called *mandibulofacial dysostosis, Treacher-Collins syndrome* or *first arch syndrome*. This is a genetic condition inherited as autosomal dominant.
- One half of the face may be underdeveloped or overdeveloped.
- The mandible may be small compared to the rest of the face resulting in a receding chin *(retrognathia)*. In extreme cases it may fail to develop *(agnathia)*.
- The eyes may be widely separated *(hypertelorism)*. The nasal bridge is broad. This condition results from the presence of excessive tissue in the frontonasal process.
- The lips may show congenital pits or fistulae. The lip may be double.

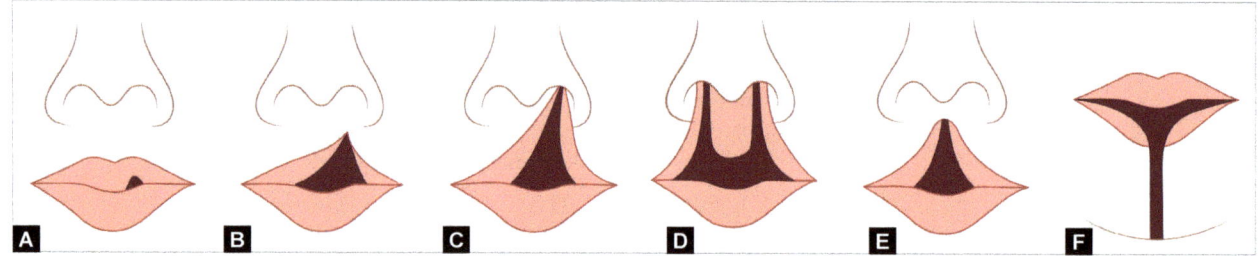

FIGS. 14.11A to F: Varieties of harelip. For explanation see text.

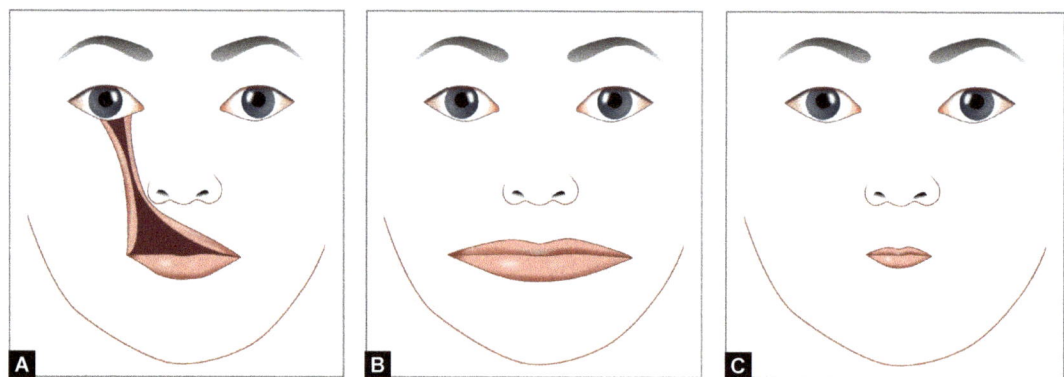

FIGS. 14.12A to C: (A) Oblique facial cleft; (B) Macrostomia; (C) Microstomia.

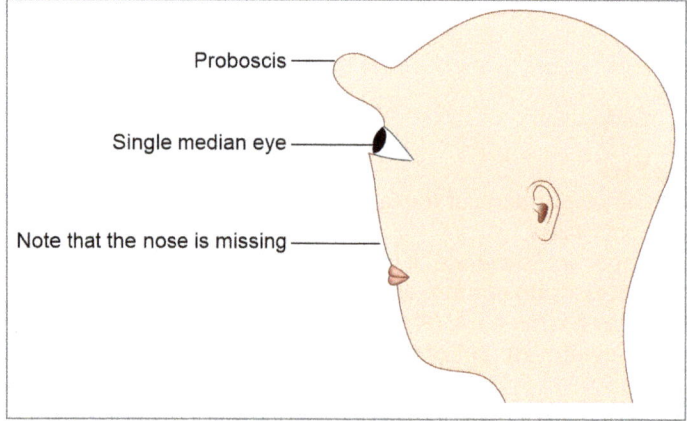

FIG. 14.13: Abnormal face showing single median eye (cyclops). A rod like projection is seen above the eye (proboscis). Also *see* **Figure 24.12B**.

DEVELOPMENT OF NOSE

The nose receives contributions from the *frontonasal process*, and from the *medial and lateral nasal processes* of the right and left sides.

* As discussed above, the external nares are formed when the nasal pits are cut off from the stomatodeum and they gradually approach each other. This is a result of the fact that the frontonasal process becomes progressively narrower and its deeper part ultimately forms the *nasal septum*.
* Mesoderm becomes heaped up in the median plane to form the *prominence of the nose*.
* Simultaneously, a groove appears between the region of the nose and the bulging forebrain (which may now be called the *forehead*) **(Figs. 14.10A and B)**.
* As the nose becomes prominent, the external nares come to open downwards instead of forwards **(Figs. 14.10A and B)**.
* The external form of the nose is thus established with the fusion of five processes as follows:
  - Frontonasal process forms the *bridge of the nose*.
  - Fused medial nasal processes form the *dorsum and tip of nose*.
  - Lateral nasal processes form the *alae of the nose*.

Development of Nasal Cavities

* The nasal cavities are formed by extension of the nasal pits. We have seen that these pits are at first in open communication with the stomatodeum **(Fig. 14.14A)**.
* Soon the medial and lateral nasal processes fuse, and form a partition between the pit and the stomatodeum. This is called the *primitive palate* **(Fig. 14.14B)**, and is derived from the frontonasal process.
* The nasal pits now deepen to form the *nasal sacs* which expand both dorsally and caudally **(Fig. 14.14C)**.
* The dorsal part of this sac is, at first, separated from the stomatodeum by a thin membrane called the *bucconasal membrane* (or *nasal fin*). This soon breaks down **(Figs. 14.14D and 14.15B)**.
* The nasal sac now has a ventral orifice that opens on the face *(anterior or external nares)*, and a dorsal orifice that opens into the stomatodeum *(primitive posterior nasal aperture)*.
* The two nasal sacs are at first widely separated from one another by the frontonasal process **(Figs. 14.15A and B)**. The narrowing of the frontonasal process, and the enlargement of the nasal cavities themselves, brings them closer together.
* The intervening tissue becomes much thinned to from the *nasal septum* **(Figs. 14.15C and D)**. The ventral part of the nasal septum is attached below to the primitive palate **(Fig. 14.15C)**. More posteriorly, the septum is at first attached to the bucconasal membrane **(Fig. 14.15D)**, but on disappearance of this membrane it has a free lower edge.
* The nasal cavities are separated from the mouth by the development of the palate, as discussed later.
* The *lateral wall* of the nose is derived, on each side, from the lateral nasal process. The *nasal conchae* appear as elevations on the lateral wall of each nasal cavity.
* The original olfactory placodes form the *olfactory epithelium* that lies in the roof, and adjoining parts of the walls, of the nasal cavity.

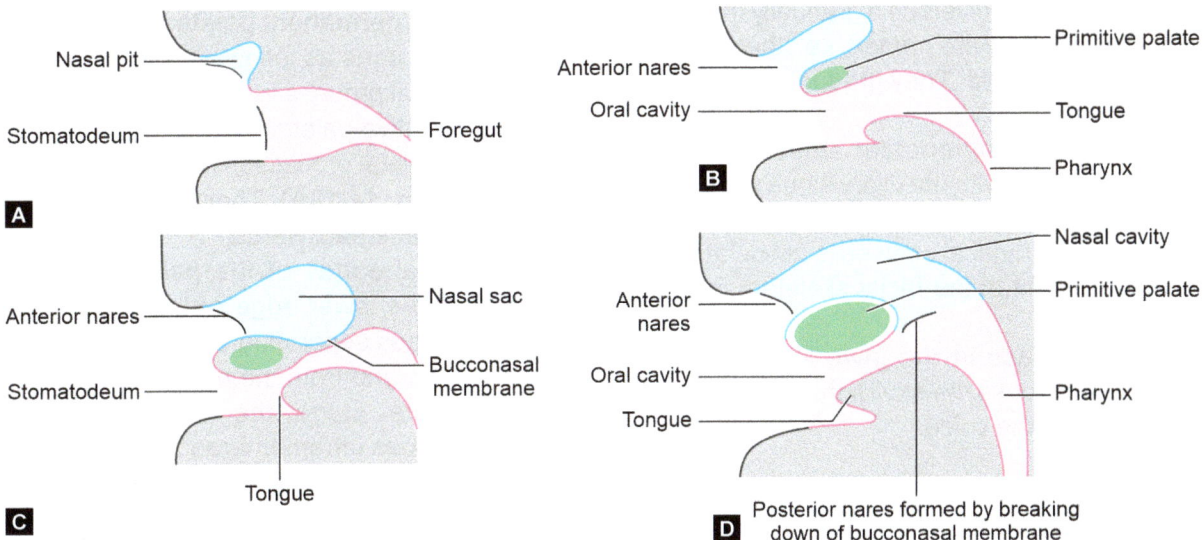

FIGS. 14.14A to D: Parasagittal sections through developing nasal cavity: (A) Nasal pit formed; (B) Nasal pit deepens. It is separated from the stomatodeum by the primitive palate; (C) The nasal pit enlarges to form the nasal sac. Posterior to the primitive palate the sac is separated from the oral cavity by the bucconasal membrane; (D) Bucconasal membrane breaks down.

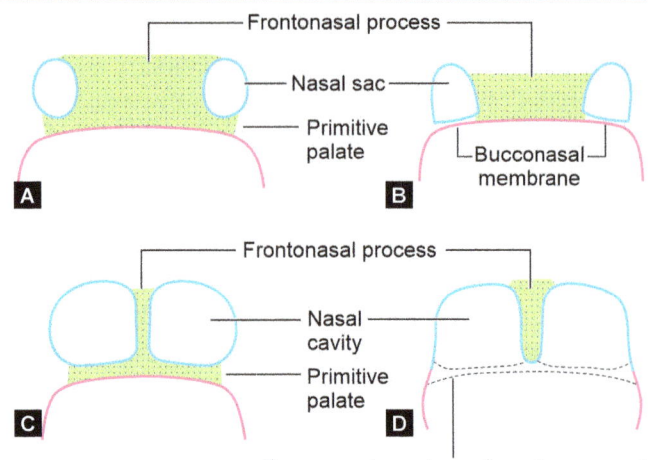

FIGS. 14.15A to D: Formation of the nasal septum. A and C are coronal sections through the anterior part of the nasal sac. B and D are sections through the posterior part: (A) Right and left nasal sacs are widely separated by the frontonasal process. Anterior part of nasal sac is separated from the stomatodeum by the primitive palate; (B) Posterior part of nasal sac is separated from the stomatodeum by the bucconasal membrane; (C) Nasal sacs enlarge and come close together. The frontonasal process is narrow and forms the nasal septum. The lower edge of the septum reaches the primitive palate; (D) Bucconasal membrane breaks down. As a result the posterior part of the nasal sac opens into the stomatodeum.

The development of various components of nasal cavity can be summarized as follows:
- Frontonasal process forms nasal septum
- Nasal pit forms the anterior nares (nostrils)
- Nasal sacs form the nasal cavity
- Bucconasal membrane forms the posterior nares (choanae) after rupture.

Development of Paranasal Sinuses

- The paranasal sinuses appear as *diverticula from the nasal cavity*. The diverticula gradually invade the bones after which they are named, i.e., the sphenoid, maxilla, frontal, ethmoid. They gradually expand and get filled with air.
- The maxillary and sphenoidal sinuses begin to develop before birth, with maxillary sinus starts at 3rd month of IUL. The other sinuses develop after birth.
- Enlargement of paranasal sinuses is associated with overall enlargement of the facial skeleton, including the jaws.
- This provides space in the jaws for growth and eruption of teeth, make the skull lighter in weight and add resonance to the voice.

Clinical correlation

Anomalies of the Nose and the Nasal Cavity
- **Cleft nose** though rare can be associated with cleft lip and palate.
- There may be *atresia of the cavity* at the external nares, at the posterior nasal aperture, or in the cavity proper. This may be unilateral or bilateral. Very rarely, there may be *total absence* of the nasal passages.
- **Congenital defects** in the cribriform plate of the ethmoid bone may lead to a communication between the cranial cavity and the nose.
- **Deviated nasal septum:** The nasal septum may not be in the middle line, i.e., it may be deflected to one side. The septum may be absent.
- Congenital midline masses like *nasal dermoid* and *nasal glioma* may be present.

DEVELOPMENT OF THE PALATE

To understand the development of the palate, let us have another look at the maxillary process.
- From **Figures 14.6 and 14.10** it will be seen that these processes not only form the upper lip but also extend backwards on either side of the stomatodeum. They can, therefore, be diagrammatically illustrated as in **Figure 14.16A**.
- If we cut a coronal section through the region (along the line XY in **Figure 14.16A**) the maxillary processes will be seen as in **Figure 14.16B**.
- Finally, if we now correlate **Figure 14.16B** with **Figure 14.15D** the relationship of the maxillary processes to the developing nasal cavity and mouth is easily understood **(Fig. 14.16C)**.
- From each maxillary process, a plate like shelf grows medially **(Fig. 14.16D)**. This is called the *palatal process*. We now have three components from which the palate will be formed. These are **(Fig. 14.17)**:
  - The two palatal processes.
  - The primitive palate formed from the frontonasal process.

The **definitive/permanent palate** is formed by the fusion of these three parts as follows:
1. Each palatal process fuses with the posterior margin of the primitive palate.
2. The two palatal processes fuse with each other in the midline **(Fig. 14.18A)**. Their fusion begins anteriorly and proceeds backwards.
3. The medial edges of the palatal processes fuse with the free lower edge of the nasal septum **(Fig. 14.18B)**, thus separating the two nasal cavities from each other, and from the mouth.
   - At a later stage, the mesoderm in the palate undergoes intramembranous ossification to form the *hard palate*. However, ossification does not extend into the most posterior portion, which remains as the *soft palate*.
   - The part of the palate derived from the frontonasal process forms the *premaxilla*, which carries the incisor teeth **(Fig. 14.19)**.

Chapter 14: Face, Nose and Palate

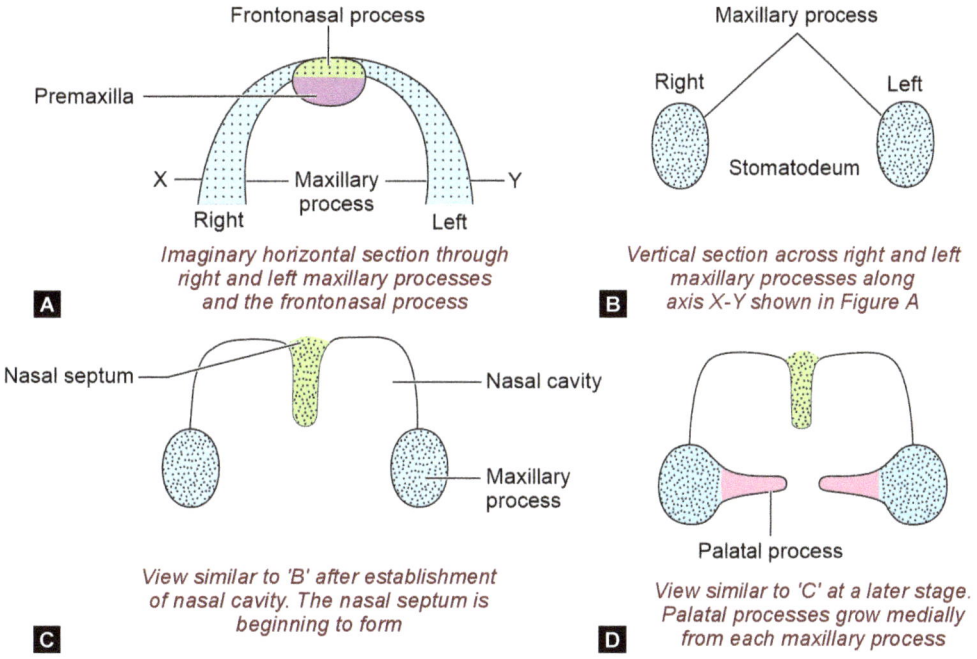

FIGS. 14.16A to D: Development of the palate.

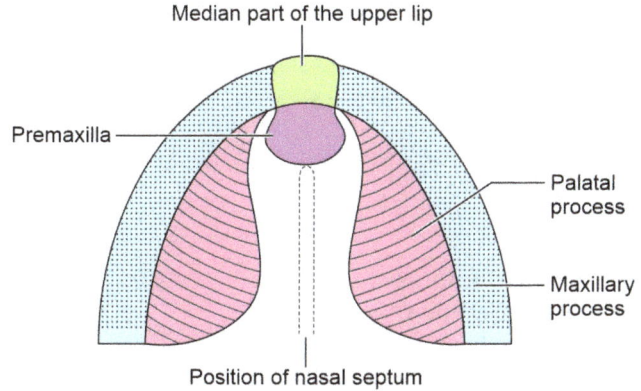

FIG. 14.17: Constituents of the developing palate as seen in a schematic horizontal section through the maxillary processes.

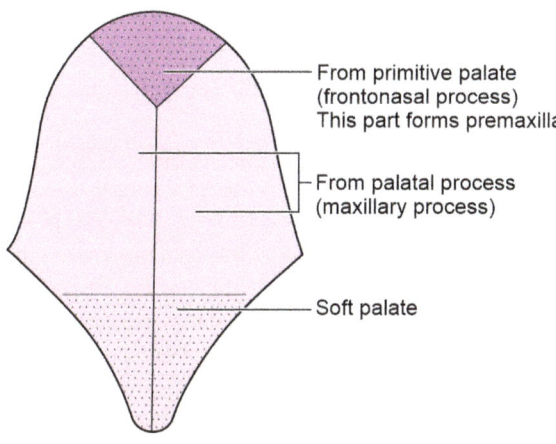

FIG. 14.19: Embryological subdivisions of the palate and the lines of fusion of these subdivisions.

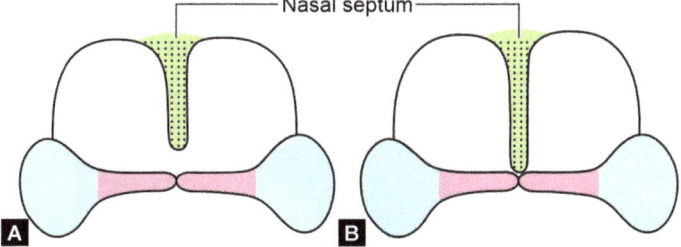

FIGS. 14.18A and B: Separation of nasal cavities from each other, and from the mouth. Compare with **Figure 14.16D**.

Clinical correlation

Cleft Palate
Defective fusion of the various components of the palate gives rise to clefts in the palate. These vary considerably in degree as illustrated in **Figures 14.20A to E**.

Complete cleft palate:
- **Bilateral complete cleft:** Failure of fusion of both palatine processes of maxilla with premaxilla. A Y-shaped cleft will be present between primary and secondary palate and between the two halves of secondary palate. It presents bilateral cleft of upper lip also (**Fig. 14.20A**).
- **Unilateral complete cleft:** Nonfusion of one side palatine process of maxilla with premaxilla. It presents unilateral cleft of upper lip (**Fig. 14.20B**).

Incomplete cleft palate:
- **Cleft of hard and soft palate:** Cleft limited to hard palate (**Fig. 14.20C**).
- **Cleft of soft palate:** Cleft limited to soft palate (**Fig. 14.20D**).
- **Bifid uvula:** Cleft limited to uvula (**Fig. 14.20E**).

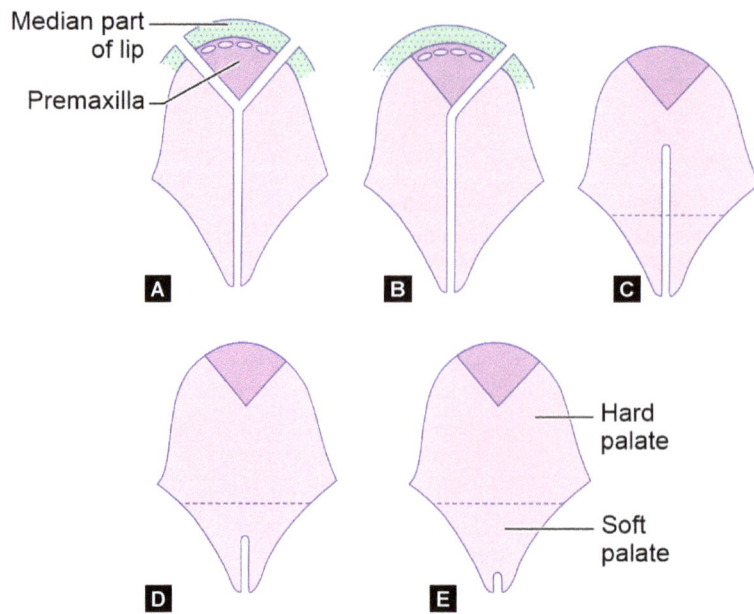

FIGS. 14.20A to E: Varieties of cleft palate: (A) Complete non-fusion, giving rise to a Y-shaped cleft, accompanied by bilateral harelip; (B) The left maxillary process has fused with the premaxilla, but not with the right maxillary process. The cleft is accompanied by unilateral harelip; (C) Midline cleft extending into the hard palate; (D) Cleft of soft palate. (E) Bifid uvula.

TIMETABLE OF SOME EVENTS DESCRIBED IN THIS CHAPTER

Age	Developmental events
4th week (28th day)	• The frontonasal, maxillary and mandibular processes can be identified. • The lens and nasal placodes are present.
5th week (31–35 days)	• The nasal pits are established.
6th week	• Tubercles for the development of pinna begins to be formed. • On each side, palatal process arise from the maxillary process.
7th week	Eyelids are established. The maxillary process fuses with the medial nasal process.
8th week	Eyes shift from a lateral to a frontal position. Bucconasal membrane ruptures.
10th week	The palatal processes and nasal septum fuse with each other.

Teratogens are likely to cause lip defects if the embryo is exposed to them during the 5th and 6th weeks. The palate is most susceptible between the 7th and 8th weeks.

Case Based Learning

Embryological Basis of Cleft lip (Fig. 14.21) and Cleft Palate
Case Scenario
A 20-day-old newborn was brought to pediatrics OPD by his mother, who appears normal, with a complaint that milk comes through the baby's nasal passages during feeding with improper grip around nipple. What could be the cause of nasal regurgitation of fluids? How can this condition be diagnosed? Describe the embryological basis and probable causes for this condition, and what advice should be given in this case? What syndromes can be associated with cleft lip and cleft palate?
- The cause of nasal regurgitation of fluids is a cleft lip and cleft palate.
- It is diagnosed through a physical examination of the mouth, nose, and palate. In this case, the baby has a cleft lip and cleft palate. There are different types of cleft palate, and it can be associated with a cleft lip.
- A prenatal ultrasound at 16–20 weeks can facilitate the diagnosis of this condition.

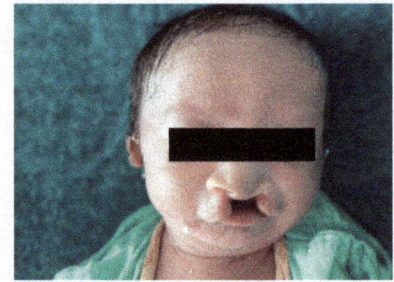

Fig. 14.21: Cleft lip
(Reproduced with permission from Dr Piyush Gupta. Source: Sriparna Basu, Poonam Singh, and Ashok Kumar, Chapter 16. In: Gupta P, UG Textbook of Pediatrics, Jaypee Brothers Medical Publishers Pvt Ltd, 2023).

- Cleft lip arises from the failure of the maxillary prominences to fuse with the medial nasal prominences during embryonic development. The four components involved in the development of the palate are the paired palatal processes of the maxillae, the nasal septum, and the premaxilla. Failure of fusion of any of these can result in cleft palate.
- Because of the cleft palate, the newborn has feeding problems, which can lead to weight loss, repeated ear infections, and speech difficulties.
- It is caused by a combination of genetic, viral, toxic, and environmental factors. Proper nutrition and prenatal vitamins during pregnancy can reduce the incidence of cleft lip and cleft palate. The use of antiepileptic drugs, especially phenytoin and valproic acid, by the mother is known to cause these defects. They can also be part of a syndrome, such as Pierre Robin, Treacher-Collins, DiGeorge, Edwards, or Patau syndrome.
- This condition is not life-threatening. Surgery is required to close the cleft within the first year of life to avoid speech difficulties and hearing problems.

HIGHLIGHTS

- The *stomatodeum* (future mouth) is a depression bounded cranially by a bulging produced by the brain, and caudally by a bulging produced by the pericardial cavity.
- Three prominences appear around the stomatodeum. These are the *frontonasal process* (above), and the right and left *mandibular arches* (first pharyngeal arches) **(Fig. 14.3A)**.
- The mandibular arch divides into a *maxillary process* and a *mandibular process* **(Fig. 14.3B)**.
- The right and left mandibular processes meet in the midline and fuse **(Fig. 14.4A)**. They form the *lower lip* and *lower jaw*.
- The *upper lip* is formed by fusion of the frontonasal process with the right and left maxillary processes. Failure to fuse completely leads to various forms of *harelip*.
- The *cheeks* are formed by fusion of (the posterior parts of) the maxillary and mandibular processes.
- The *nose* is derived from the frontonasal process.
- The *nasal cavity* is formed as follows. An ectodermal thickening, the nasal placode, appears over the frontonasal process **(Fig. 14.4A)**. The placode gets depressed below the surface to form the nasal pit **(Fig. 14.4B)**. The nasal pits enlarge to form the nasal cavity.
- **Paranasal sinuses** appear as outgrowths from the nasal cavity.
- The *palate* is formed by fusion of three components. These are the right and left palatal processes (arising from the maxillary process); and the primitive palate (derived from the frontonasal process) **(Fig. 14.19)**. Deficiency in fusion leads to various forms of *cleft palate* **(Figs. 14.20A to E)**.

Summary

- Development of face **(Flowchart 14.1)**.
- Development of palate **(Flowchart 14.2)**.

FLOWCHART 14.1: Development of different structures of face.

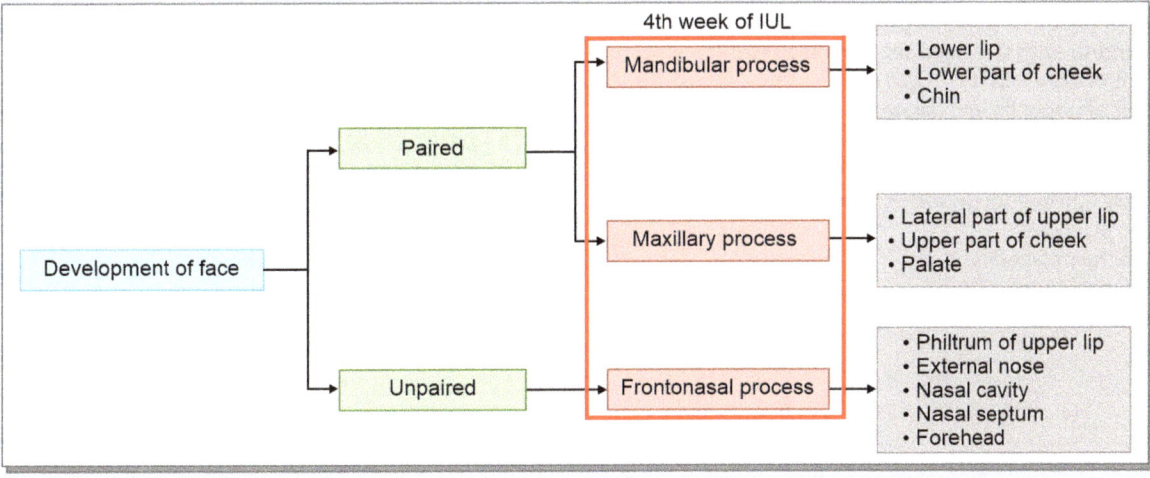

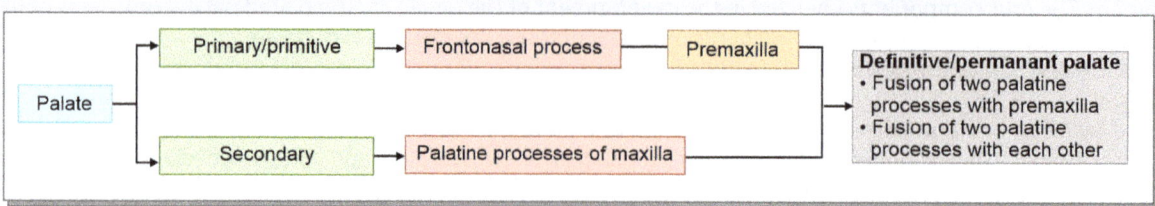

FLOWCHART 14.2: Development of palate from different processes.

 TEST YOUR UNDERSTANDING

REVIEW OR PRACTICE QUESTIONS

1. Explain the development of face.
2. Explain the development of palate.
3. Write short notes on cleft palate.
4. Describe developmental anomalies of face.
5. Write short note on cleft lip.

EXPLAIN WHY? (REASONING QUESTIONS)

1. Failure of fusion between the lateral palatine processes and the nasal septum can cause feeding and speech impairment.
2. Cleft lip is associated with cleft palate in some cases.
3. Face develops from frontonasal process and first arch but its muscles get nerve supply from facial nerve.

MULTIPLE CHOICE QUESTIONS

1. The five primordia of face development include all of the following, *except*:
   A. Paired frontonasal processes
   B. Paired maxillary processes
   C. Paired mandibular processes
   D. Unpaired frontonasal process

2. A newborn baby presented with right unilateral cleft lip. The palate is normal. Which of the following developmental defects accounts for this occurrence?
   A. Failure of fusion of right palatine process with the premaxilla
   B. Failure of fusion of right maxillary and right medial nasal processes
   C. Failure of fusion of right and left medial nasal processes
   D. Failure of fusion of both maxillary processes with the medial nasal process

3. Failure of fusion of palatine processes of maxillae with each other and/or with the nasal septum results in:
   A. Cleft of upper lip
   B. Cleft of upper lip and palate
   C. Cleft of primary palate
   D. Incomplete cleft of secondary (hard and soft) palate

4. Olfactory epithelium develops from:
   A. Otic placodes
   B. Olfactory placodes
   C. Optic placodes
   D. Nasal placodes

5. Which process of face develops from forebrain?
   A. Mandibular process
   B. Maxillary process
   C. Palatal process
   D. Frontonasal process

6. A patient with a congenital absence of the frontal sinus undergoes imaging revealing an abnormality in the development of which embryonic structure?
   A. Frontonasal prominence
   B. Lateral nasal prominence
   C. Maxillary prominence
   D. Mandibular prominence

7. During a surgical repair of a cleft palate, the surgeon uses tissue from the posterior portion of the palate to cover the defect. Which embryonic structures contribute to the formation of this tissue?
   A. Maxillary prominences
   B. Mandibular prominences
   C. Lateral palatine processes
   D. Medial nasal prominences

8. A patient presents with a unilateral cleft lip involving the philtrum and upper lip, but the palate is intact. Which embryonic structure's incomplete fusion is most likely responsible for this condition?
   A. Medial nasal prominences
   B. Lateral nasal prominences
   C. Maxillary prominences
   D. Mandibular prominences

Answers: 1. A 2. B 3. D 4. B 5. D 6. A 7. C 8. A

Alimentary System—I: Oral Cavity, Salivary Glands and Pharynx

CHAPTER 15

COMPETENCIES COVERED/LEARNING OUTCOMES

The student should be able to:

AN43.4	Describe the development and developmental basis of congenital anomalies of tongue.
AN39.1	Describe the embryological basis of nerve supply of tongue.
AN52.6	Describe the development and congenital anomalies of—foregut, midgut and hindgut.

The oral cavity, beginning at the mouth, encompasses essential structures such as teeth, tongue, salivary glands, and mucosal lining. It serves as a gateway connecting external environment with the internal body through the pharynx. This anatomical region plays a important role in functions like mastication, taste perception, speech articulation, and initial digestion processes.

In this chapter, we are going to discuss the embryological development of mouth, teeth, tongue, salivary glands, pharynx and other associated structures of oral cavity.

DEVELOPMENT OF MOUTH

The mouth is *bidermal* in development. The mouth is derived partly from the *stomatodeum (ectodermal)* and partly from the *foregut (endodermal)*. Hence its epithelial lining is partly ectodermal and partly endodermal. After disappearance of the buccopharyngeal membrane, the line of junction between the ectoderm and endoderm is difficult to define.

Primitive Oral Cavity

The *stomatodeum* is divided into two parts by the developing primitive and definitive palate.
1. **Nasal part**—forms the mucus lining of nasal cavity, nasa septum and palate.
2. **Oral part**—forms the mucus lining of cheeks, lips, gum and enamel of teeth.

The derivatives of oral part can be subdivided into those from ectoderm and those from endoderm.
- ❖ Ectodermal developmental derivatives are the major constituents. They are:
  - Epithelium lining inside of lips, cheeks and palate
  - Teeth and gums
- ❖ Endodermal derivatives are the minor constituents that contribute mainly for the floor of oral cavity. They form epithelium of:
  - Tongue, floor and soft palate
  - Palatoglossal and palatopharyngeal folds

Definitive Oral Cavity

- ❖ The following parts of definitive oral cavity are ectodermal in origin:
  1. Epithelium lining inside of lips, cheeks and palate
  2. Alveolabial sulcus
  3. Teeth and gums
- ❖ The following parts of definitive oral cavity are endodermal in origin **(Figs. 15.1A to C)**:
  1. The epithelium of the tongue
  2. Floor of oral cavity (derived from foregut)
  3. Alveolingual sulcus

Floor of Mouth

In the region of the floor of the mouth, the mandibular processes take part in the formation of three structures. These are:
1. Lower lip and lower part of cheeks
2. Lower jaw
3. Tongue
   - At first, these regions are not demarcated from each other **(Fig. 15.2A)**. Soon the tongue forms a recognizable swelling, which is separated laterally from the rest of the mandibular process by the *linguogingival sulcus* **(Fig. 15.2B)** which is endodermal.
   - Soon, thereafter, another more laterally placed sulcus makes its appearance. This is called the *labiogingival sulcus* **(Fig. 15.2C)** which is ectodermal. This sulcus deepens rapidly and the tissues of the mandibular arch lateral to it form the *lower lip* (or cheek).

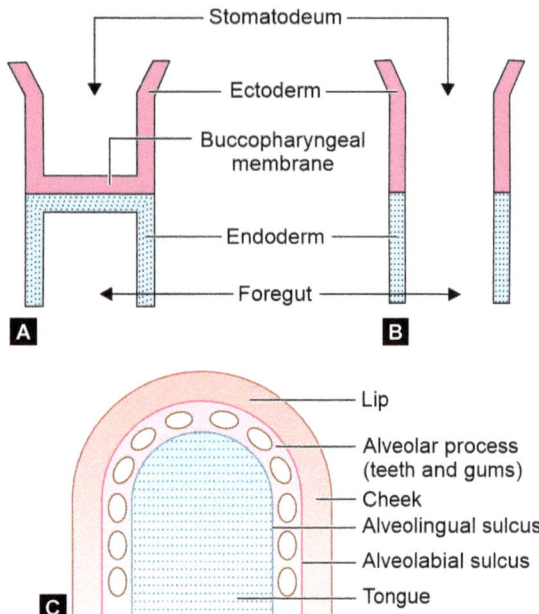

FIGS. 15.1A to C: Derivation of the ectodermal part, and endodermal part of the floor of the mouth. (A) Stomatodeum separated from foregut by buccopharyngeal membrane; (B) Buccopharyngeal membrane disappears; (C) Lips, cheeks and gums lined by ectoderm, tongue by endoderm.

- With the deepening of these two sulci, the area lying between them becomes a raised *alveolar process* (Fig. 15.2D). The alveolar process is between the labiogingival and linguogingival sulci. The alveolar process forms the jaw, and the teeth develop in relation to it. The tongue, the alveolar process (or jaw) and the lips (or cheeks) are thus separated from one another.

Roof of Mouth

- The roof of the mouth is formed by the palate. The development of the palate has already been considered.
- The alveolar process of the upper jaw is separated from the upper lip and cheek by appearance of a *labiogingival furrow*, just as in the lower jaw.
- The medial margin of the alveolus becomes defined when the palate becomes highly arched **(Figs. 15.3A to C)**.

DEVELOPMENT OF TEETH

- The teeth are formed in relation to the alveolar process. The epithelium overlying the convex border of this process becomes thickened and projects into the underlying mesoderm. This epithelial thickening is called the *dental lamina* **(Figs. 15.2C and D)**. The dental lamina is, in fact, apparent even before the alveolar process itself is defined **(Fig. 15.2C)**.
- As the alveolar process is semicircular in outline the dental lamina is similarly curved **(Fig. 15.4A)**.

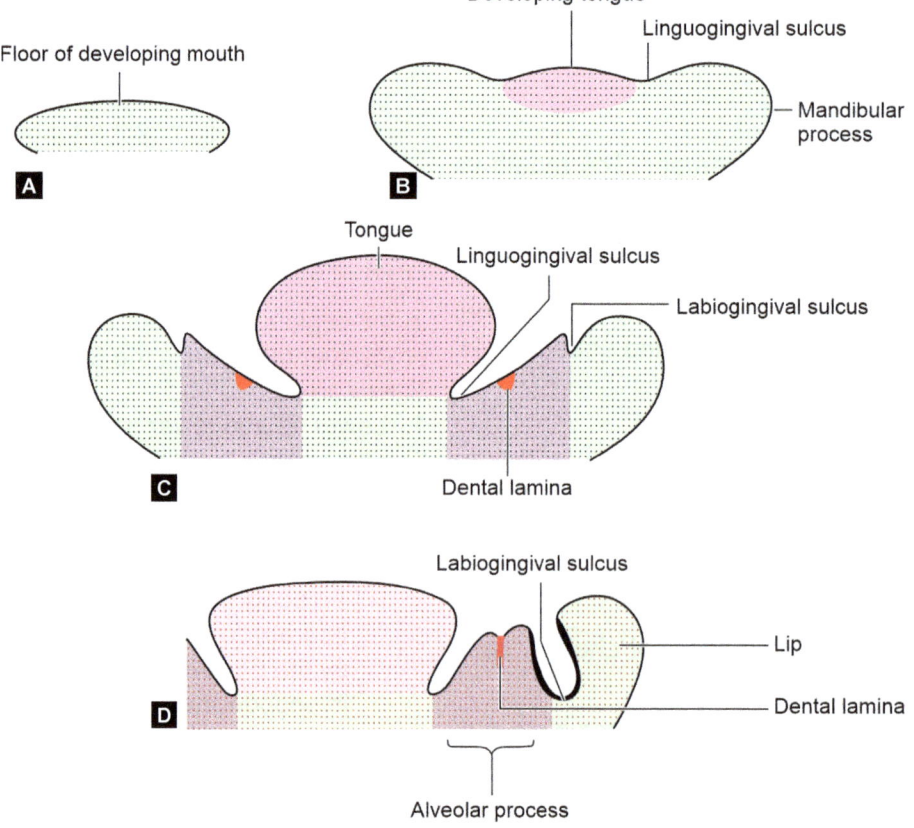

FIGS. 15.2A to D: (A) Floor of mouth formed by fused mandibular processes; (B) Linguogingival sulcus separates developing tongue from rest of mandibular processes; (C) Labiogingival sulcus separates alveolar process from lip (or cheek); (D) The dental lamina, seen in the alveolar process, gives origin to teeth.

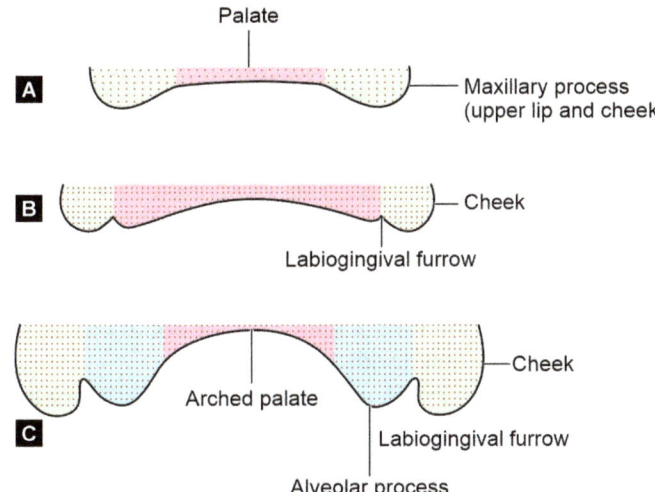

FIGS. 15.3A to C: Development of some structures seen in relation to the roof of the mouth. (A) Maxillary processes and palate; (B) Labiogingival furrow separates upper lip (or upper part of cheek) from alveolar process (of upper jaw); (C) Medial margin of alveolar process becomes distinct because of upward arching of the palate.

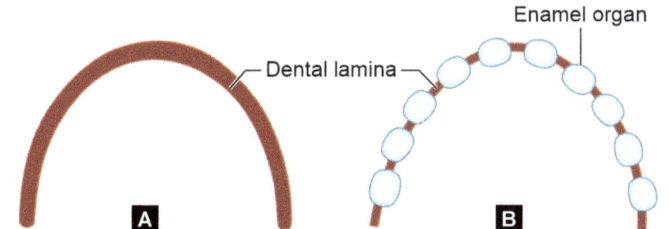

FIGS. 15.4A and B: Formation of enamel organs from dental lamina: (A) Dental lamina following the curve of the alveolar process; (B) Enamel organs formed in relation to the dental lamina.

- The dental lamina now shows a series of local thickenings, each of which is destined to form one milk tooth. These thickenings are called *enamel organs*.
- There are ten such enamel organs (five on each side) in each alveolar process (Fig. 15.4B).

The stages in the formation of an enamel organ and the development of a tooth are as follows:

- **Stage of dental lamina:** Each enamel organ is formed by localized proliferation of the cells of the dental lamina (Figs. 15.5A and B).
- **Bud stage:** During this stage, ten thickenings of dental lamina appears five on each side. These are called tooth buds/enamel organs (Fig.15.5B).
- **Cap stage:** As the enamel organ grows downwards into the mesenchyme (of the alveolar process) its lower end assumes a cup-shaped appearance (Fig. 15.5C). The cup comes to be occupied by a mass of mesenchyme called the *dental papilla* (according to some researchers, this mesenchyme is of neural crest origin).

  The enamel organ and the dental papilla together constitute the *tooth germ*. At this stage the developing tooth looks like a cap therefore, described as the *cap stage* of tooth development.

  The cells of the enamel organ that line the papilla become columnar. These are called *ameloblasts* (Fig. 15.5D).

- **Bell stage:** Mesodermal cells of the papilla that are adjacent to the ameloblasts arrange themselves as a continuous epithelium-like layer. The cells of this layer are called *odontoblasts* (Fig. 15.5E).

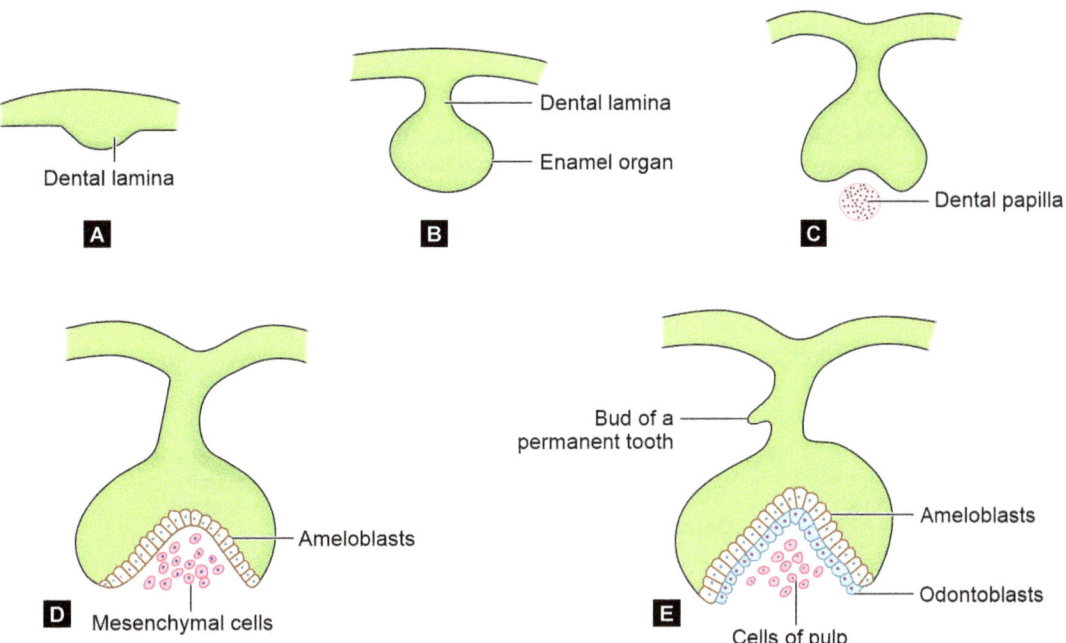

FIGS. 15.5A to E: Stages in the formation of a tooth germ: (A) Dental lamina formed by proliferation of ectoderm lining the alveolar process; (B) Deeper part of dental lamina enlarges to form enamel organ; (C) Mesodermal cells invaginate the enamel organ to form the papilla; (D) Layer of ameloblasts (ectoderm) formed from deepest cells of enamel organ; (E) Odontoblasts, derived from mesodermal cells, form a layer next to the ameloblasts.

The ameloblasts and odontoblasts are separated by a basement membrane. The remaining cells of the papilla from the pulp of the tooth. The developing tooth now looks like a bell *(bell stage)*.

- **Apposition stage:** Ameloblasts lay down enamel on the superficial (outer) surface of the basement membrane. The odontoblasts lay down dentin on its deeper surface.
  - The process of laying down of enamel and of dentin is similar to that of formation of bone by osteoblasts.
  - As layer after layer of enamel and dentin are laid down, the layer of ameloblasts and the layer of odontoblasts move away from each other **(Fig. 15.6)**.
- After the enamel is fully formed the ameloblasts disappear leaving a thin membrane, the *dental cuticle*, over the enamel. The odontoblasts, however, continue to separate the dentin from the pulp throughout the life of the tooth.
- The alveolar parts of the maxillae and mandible are formed by ossification in the corresponding alveolar process. As ossification progresses, the roots of the teeth are surrounded by bone.
- The root of the tooth is established by continued growth into underlying mesenchyme. Odontoblasts in this region lay down dentin. As layers of dentin are deposited, the pulp space becomes progressively narrower and is gradually converted into a canal through which nerves and blood vessels pass into the tooth.
- **Formation of root:** In the region of the root there are no ameloblasts. The dentin is covered by mesenchymal cells that differentiate into *cementoblasts*. These cells lay down a layer of dense bone called the *cementum*. Still further to the outside, mesenchymal cells form the *periodontal ligament* which connects the root to the socket in the jaw bone. The permanent teeth are formed as follows:
  - The dental lamina gives off a series of buds, one of which lies on the medial side of each developing milk tooth **(Figs. 15.7 and 15.8)**. These buds form enamel organs exactly as described above. They give rise to the permanent incisors, canines and premolars.
  - The permanent molars are formed from buds that arise from the dental lamina posterior to the region of the last milk tooth.

The dental lamina is established in the 6th week of intrauterine life. At birth the germs of all the temporary teeth, and of the permanent incisors, canines and first molars, show considerable development. The germs of the permanent premolars and of the second molars are rudimentary. The germ of the third molar is formed after birth. The developing tooth germs undergo calcification. All the temporary teeth and the permanent lower first molar begin to calcify before birth; the other permanent teeth begin to calcify at varying ages after birth.

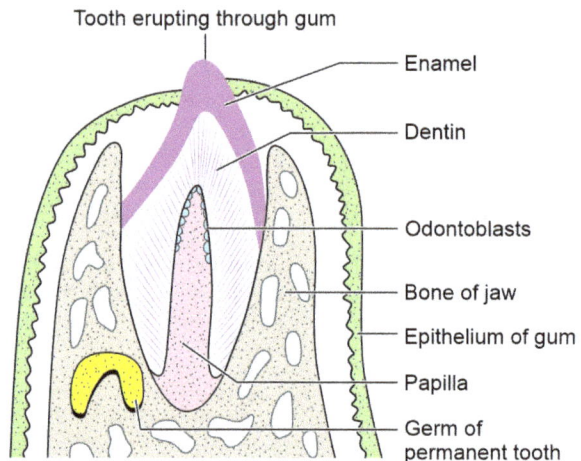

FIG. 15.7: Diagram of an erupting temporary tooth. Note its relationship to the jaw. Also observe germ of permanent tooth.

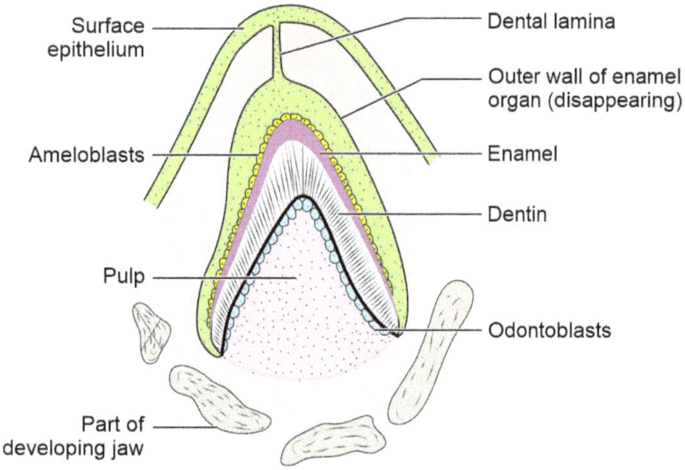

FIG. 15.6: Parts of a developing tooth. Ameloblasts lay down enamel. Odontoblasts lay down dentin. Ossification in relation to mesenchymal cells surrounding the developing tooth forms the jaw.

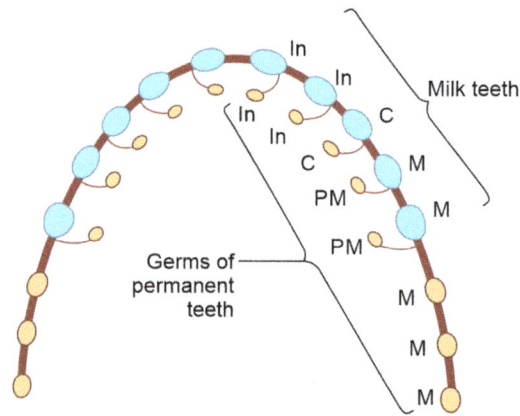

FIG. 15.8: Origin of germs of permanent teeth. Germs of permanent incisors, canines, and premolars are formed in relation to temporary teeth (as seen in **Fig. 15.7**). Permanent molars arise from the dental lamina behind the part that gives rise to temporary teeth.

The eruption of a tooth is preceded by a major development of its root. The ages at which teeth erupt vary considerably. The average age of eruption is as follows:

a. Temporary or Milk Teeth

Lower central incisor	6–9 months
Upper incisors	8–10 months
Lower lateral incisors	12–20 months
First molar	12–20 months
Canines	16–20 months
Second molars	20–39 months

b. Permanent Teeth

First molar	6–7 years
Central incisors	6–8 years
Lateral incisors	7–9 years
Premolars	10–12 years
Canines	10–12 years
Second molars	11–13 years
Third molars	17–21 years

Summary of the derivatives of dental structures are shown in **Table 15.1**.

TABLE 15.1: Summary of the derivatives of parts of a tooth.

Ectoderm	Ameloblasts → Enamel
Mesoderm (of neural crest origin)	Odontoblasts → Dentin
Mesenchyme around tooth	• Cementum • Periodontal ligament

Clinical correlation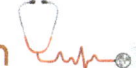

Anomalies of Teeth
- One or more teeth may be absent. Complete absence is called *anodontia*.
- *Supernumerary teeth* (extra teeth) may be present.
- Individual teeth may be abnormal. They may be too large or too small. They may have *supernumerary cusps or roots*. Alternatively, cusps or roots may be less than normal.
- *Gemination* is when a single tooth bud attempts to divide, resulting in a tooth with an enlarged or bifid crown and a single root.
- *Fusion* is when two separate tooth buds unite during development, forming a single enlarged tooth with variable crown and root structures.
- The alignment of the upper and lower teeth may be incorrect *(malocclusion)*. This may be caused by one or more of the above anomalies or by defects of the jaws.
- **Natal teeth:** Sometimes teeth can be present at birth. Most common are lower incisors which can cause injuries to nipple during breastfeeding.
- **Impaction:** Eruption of teeth may be delayed. The third molar frequently fails to erupt.
- Teeth may form in abnormal situations, e.g., in the ovary or in the hypophysis cerebri.
- There may be improper formation of the enamel or dentin of the tooth.
- **Amelogenesis imperfecta:** Defective enamel formation due to vitamin D deficiency resulting in yellow or brown color teeth.
- **Dentinogenesis imperfecta:** Chromosomal abnormality resulting in enamel degeneration.
- Certain *drugs like tetracycline* can result in yellowish discoloration teeth. Certain *infections* also affects the formation of teeth, like in case of syphilis.

DEVELOPMENT OF TONGUE

- The development of the tongue starts in the 4th month of intrauterine life.
- The tongue develops in relation to the pharyngeal arches in the floor of the developing mouth. We have seen that each pharyngeal arch arises as a mesodermal thickening in the lateral wall of the foregut and that it grows ventrally to become continuous with the corresponding arch of the opposite side **(Fig. 15.9)**.
- The medial-most parts of the mandibular arches proliferate to form two *lingual swellings* **(Fig. 15.10)**.
- The lingual swellings are partially separated from each other by another swelling that appears in the midline. This median swelling is called the *tuberculum impar*.

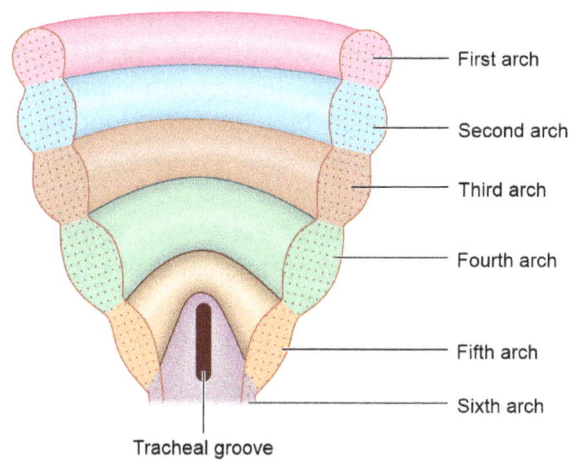

FIG. 15.9: Floor of primitive pharynx: Stage 1. Note that the right and left pharyngeal arches meet in the midline to form the floor of the pharynx.

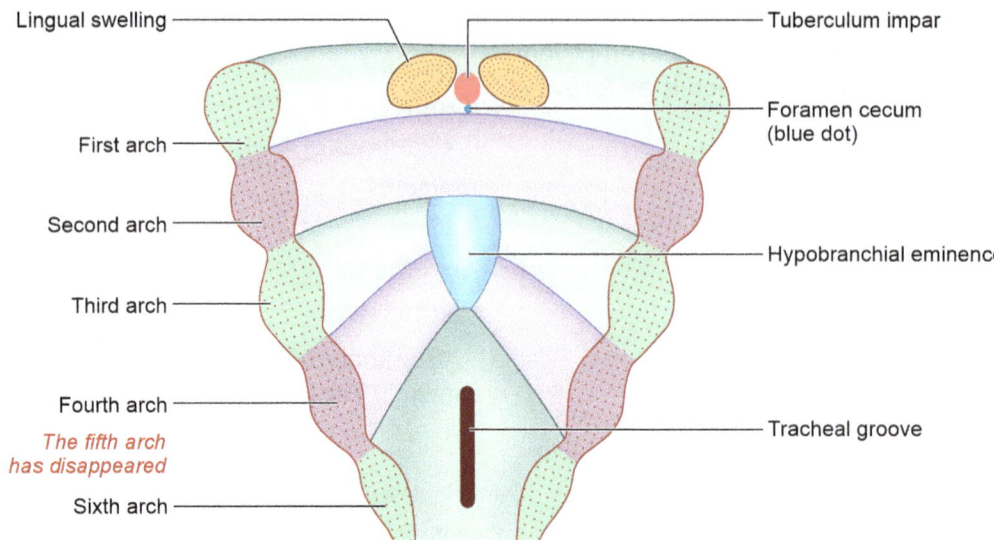

FIG. 15.10: Floor of primitive pharynx: Stage 2. The fifth pharyngeal arch has disappeared. Note the right and left lingual swellings, and the tuberculum impar formed in relation to the first arch; and the hypobranchial eminence formed in relation to the medial ends of the third and fourth arches.

- Immediately behind the tuberculum impar, the epithelium proliferates to form a downgrowth *(thyroglossal duct)* from which the thyroid gland develops. The site of this downgrowth is subsequently marked by a depression called the *foramen cecum.*
- Another, midline swelling is seen in relation to the medial ends of the second, third and fourth arches. This swelling is called the *hypobranchial eminence* **(Fig. 15.10)**. The eminence soon shows a subdivision into a cranial part related to the second and third arches (called the *copula*) and a caudal part related to the 4th arch **(Fig. 15.11A)**. The caudal part forms the *epiglottis*.

Anterior 2/3rd of Tongue

The *anterior two-third of the tongue is* formed by fusion of:
- The tuberculum impar
- The two lingual swellings
- The anterior two-third of the tongue is thus derived from the mandibular arch **(Figs. 15.11B and C)**. According to some, the tuberculum impar does not make a significant contribution to the tongue.

Posterior 1/3rd of the Tongue

The *posterior one-third of the tongue* is formed from the cranial part of the hypobranchial eminence *(copula of His)* **(Figs. 15.11A to C)**.
- In this situation, the second arch mesoderm gets buried below the surface.
- The third arch mesoderm grows over it to fuse with the mesoderm of the first arch **(Figs. 15.12A and B)**. The posterior one-third of the tongue is thus formed by third arch mesoderm.

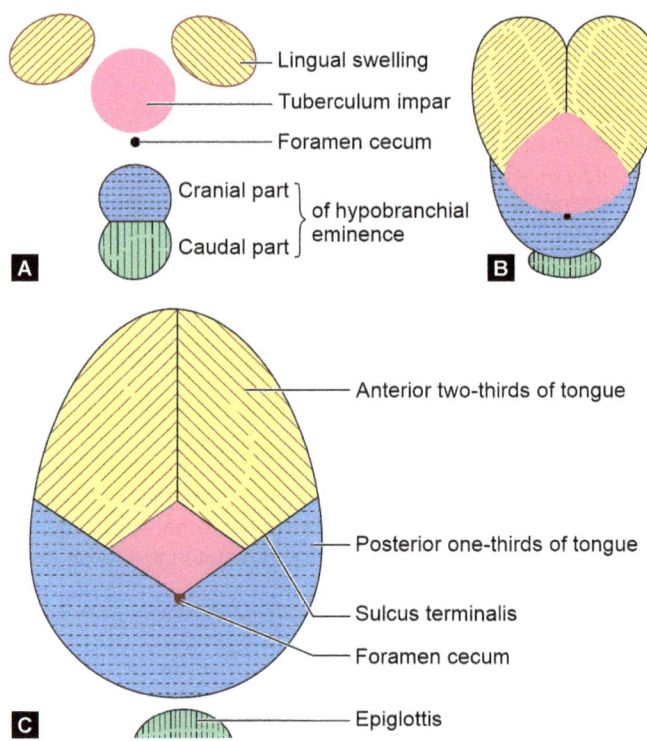

FIGS. 15.11A to C: Scheme to show the origin of different parts of the tongue.

- The *posterior-most part of the tongue* is derived from the fourth arch **(Figs. 15.12A and B)**.
- The line of junction of anterior 2/3rd and posterior 1/3rd is demarcated by inverted V-shaped *sulcus terminalis* **(Fig. 15.11C)**.

Nerve Supply of Tongue

- In keeping with its embryological origin, the anterior 2/3rd of the tongue is supplied by the *lingual branch*

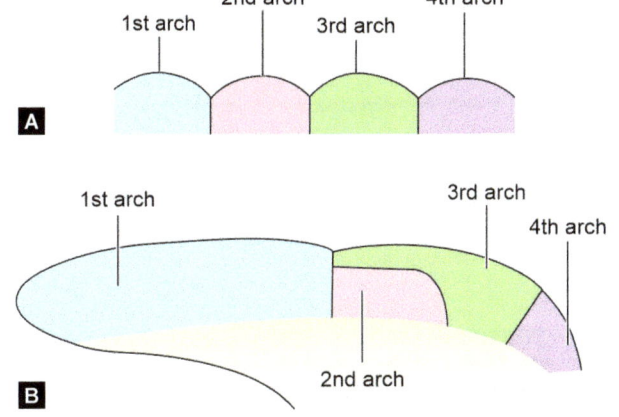

FIGS. 15.12A and B: Scheme to show how the second arch is buried by overgrowth of the third arch, during development of the tongue.

of the mandibular nerve, which is the post-trematic nerve of the first arch, and by the chorda tympani which is the pretrematic nerve of this arch.
- The posterior 1/3rd of the tongue is supplied by the glossopharyngeal (third arch).
- The posterior most part of the tongue is supplied by the superior laryngeal nerve (fourth arch).
- The musculature of the tongue is derived from the occipital myotomes except palatoglossus which is derived from 4th arch. This explains its nerve supply by the hypoglossal nerve, which is the nerve of these myotomes. Palatoglossus is supplied by vagus nerve via pharyngeal plexus.

Taste Buds

- **Taste buds** are formed in relation to the terminal branches of the innervating nerve fibers.
- The circumvallate papillae of tongue develop from the cranial part of hypobranchial eminence and migrate to the anterior aspect of sulcus terminalis, hence they are supplied by glossopharyngeal nerve.

Summary of the derivatives of the components of the tongue are shown in **Table 15.2**.

DEVELOPMENT OF SALIVARY GLANDS

The salivary glands are tubuloacinar glands comprising of secretory acini in terminal part and duct system in initial part.
- The salivary glands develop as outgrowths of the buccal epithelium into surrounding mesoderm. The outgrowths are at first solid and are later canalized.
- They branch repeatedly to form the duct system. The terminal parts of the duct system develop into secretory acini.

TABLE 15.2: Summary of the derivation of components of the tongue.

Component	Embryonic component	Sensory nerve General sensation	Sensory nerve Taste sensation	Motor nerve
Mucosa of anterior 2/3rd (oral part) Epithelium + Connective tissue	1st arch	V—mandibular lingual branch	VII—facial chorda tympani branch	
Mucosa posterior 1/3rd (pharyngeal part) Epithelium + Connective tissue	3rd arch	IX—glossopharyngeal		
Posterior most near vallecula Epithelium + Connective tissue	4th arch	X—vagus superior laryngeal nerve		
Musculature All intrinsic + All extrinsic except palatoglossus	Occipital myotomes (3–4 nos) 4th arch Palatoglossus			XII—hypoglossal X—vagus— pharyngeal branches
Papillae and taste buds	• CV and foliate: IX—glossopharyngeal • Fungiform and filiform: VII—facial			

Clinical correlation

Anomalies of the Tongue
- The tongue may be too large *(macroglossia)* or too small *(microglossia)*. Very rarely the tongue may be absent *(aglossia)*.
- **Hemiglossia** is anomaly when one of the lingual swellings fail to develop.
- The tongue may be **bifid** because of non-fusion of the two lingual swellings.
- The apical part of the tongue may be anchored to the floor of the mouth by an overdeveloped frenulum. This condition is called ankyloglossia or tongue-tie. It interferes with speech. Occasionally, the tongue may be adherent, to the palate *(ankyloglossia superior)*.
- A red, rhomboid-shaped smooth zone may be present on the tongue in front of the foramen cecum. It is considered to be the result of persistence of the tuberculum impar.

> - Thyroid tissue may be present in the tongue either under the mucosa or within the muscles. This is referred to *lingual thyroid*.
> - Remnants of the thyroglossal duct may form cysts at the base of the tongue.
> - The surface of the tongue may show *fissuring* (seen in Down syndrome).

- As the salivary glands develop near the junctional area between the ectoderm of the stomatodeum and the endoderm of the foregut, it is difficult to determine whether they are ectodermal or endodermal.

Major Salivary Glands

These consists of pairs of parotid glands, submandibular glands and sublingual glands.

Parotid Gland

- It is the first salivary gland to appear (early 6th week).
- It arises from the oral ectoderm near the angle of stomatodeum. It grows outward between maxillary process and mandibular arch in the form of ectodermal cords of cells.
- Proximal part canalizes and forms *parotid duct* that opens into the mouth. The distal part extends into the cheek mesenchyme and reaches up to the developing ear where it branches and expands to form the secreting units/alveoli of gland.
- Fusion of maxillary process and mandibular arch results in shifting of opening of parotid duct into the vestibule opposite upper second molar tooth. Capsule and connective tissue is formed from the surrounding mesoderm.

Submandibular Gland

- It appears in the later part of 6th week as an endodermal bud or outgrowth in the floor of stomatodeum at the linguogingival sulcus.
- Canalization of outgrowth occurs to form duct, acini and ductules. Duct opens on sublingual papilla.

Sublingual Gland

It appears during 8th week as multiple endodermal buds from linguogingival sulcus.

Minor Salivary Glands

- Develops around 12th week of gestation, in similar fashion as other salivary glands.
- They are small submucosal glands, distributed throughout the oral cavity mucosa except gingiva, contributing to the maintenance of oral moisture and mucosal health.

DEVELOPMENT OF TONSILS

We have studied the development of palatine tonsils in chapter 12.

Epithelial proliferations and aggregations of lymphoid tissue like palatine tonsils also give rise to the *tubal tonsils*, the *lingual tonsil* and the *pharyngeal tonsils*.

DEVELOPMENT OF PHARYNX

- Floor of pharynx is formed by fusion of ventral parts of pharyngeal arches and pouches. The floor contributes for the development of tongue, thyroid gland and lower respiratory tract.
- The pharynx is derived from the cranial most part of the foregut. The endodermal pouches are formed in relation to the lateral wall of this part of the foregut. The floor of the foregut gives rise to a midline diverticulum from which the entire respiratory system develops (*refer* Chapter 18: Body Cavities, Diaphragm and Respiratory System). Most of the endodermal pouches lose contact with the pharyngeal wall.
- The opening of the pharyngotympanic tube represents the site of origin of the tubotympanic recess. The site of the midline respiratory diverticulum is represented by the inlet of the larynx.
- With the establishment of the palate and mouth, the pharynx shows a subdivision into nasopharynx, oropharynx and laryngopharynx. The muscles forming the wall of the pharynx are derived from the third and subsequent pharyngeal arches.

TIMETABLE OF SOME EVENTS DESCRIBED IN THIS CHAPTER

Age	Developmental events
4 weeks	Tongue starts forming, i.e., two lateral lingual swelling and tuberculum impar become visible
5 weeks	Hypobranchial eminence becomes visible
6 weeks	- Dental laminae of upper and lower jaws are established. - Salivary glands starts developing
8 weeks	Enamel organs are formed
10 weeks	Enamel organ becomes cup-shaped
6 months	- Enamel and dentin have formed considerably - Formation of tongue is almost complete
Just before birth	Cementum is formed
After birth	Periodontal ligaments are formed before eruption of teeth

Chapter 15: Alimentary System—I: Oral Cavity, Salivary Glands and Pharynx

HIGHLIGHTS

- The *oral cavity* is derived partly from the stomatodeum (ectoderm), and partly from the foregut (endoderm). These two are separated by the buccopharyngeal membrane which later disappears **(Fig. 15.1)**.
- **Teeth** are formed in relation to the dental lamina **(Fig. 15.2)**. An enlargement of the lamina is formed for each tooth. It is called the *enamel organ* **(Fig. 15.5)**.
- **Ameloblasts** (derived from ectoderm) form the *enamel*. **Odontoblasts** (derived from mesoderm) form *dentin*. The *pulp* is formed by mesenchyme that invaginates into the enamel organ **(Fig. 15.5E)**.
- Three swellings appear in the floor of the pharynx, in relation to the first pharyngeal arch. These are the right and left *lingual swellings*, and a median swelling the *tuberculum impar* **(Fig. 15.10)**. Another median swelling is formed in relation to the third and fourth arches. This is the *hypobranchial eminence*.
- The *anterior two-third of the tongue* is formed from the lingual swellings and the tuberculum impar.
- The *posterior one-third of the tongue* is formed by the cranial part of the hypobranchial eminence.
- **Salivary glands** develop as outgrowths of buccal epithelium.
- The *palatine tonsil* develops in relation to the second pharyngeal pouch.
- The *pharynx* is derived from the foregut.

Summary

- Development of tooth **(Flowchart 15.1)**.
- Development of tongue **(Flowchart 15.2)**.

FLOWCHART 15.1: Development of tooth.

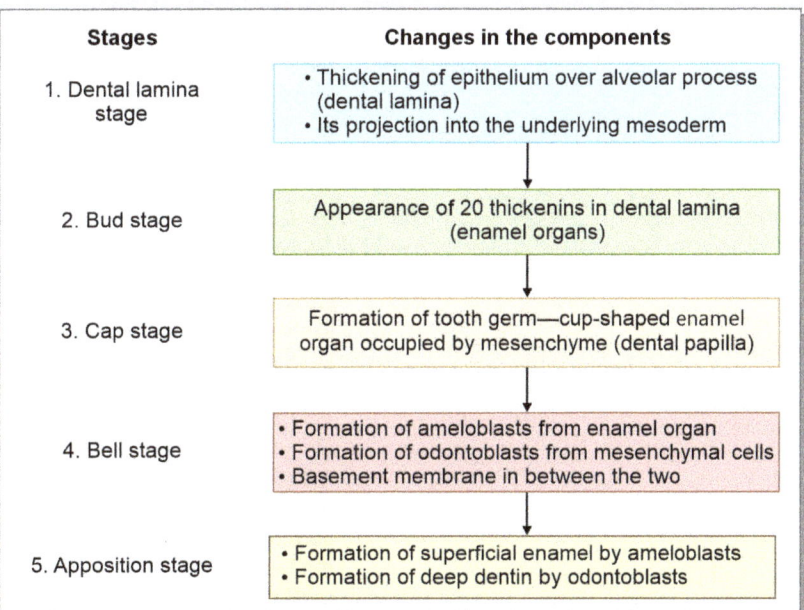

FLOWCHART 15.2: Development of tongue.

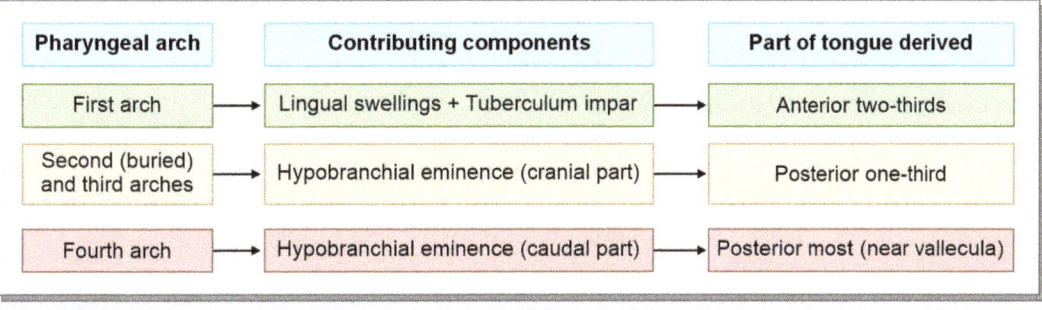

TEST YOUR UNDERSTANDING

REVIEW QUESTIONS

1. Explain the development of tongue.
2. What are the stages in the development of tooth?
3. What is the time of eruption of temporary and permanent teeth?
4. Explain the development of salivary glands.

EXPLAIN WHY? (REASONING QUESTIONS)

1. A newborn presents with multiple missing teeth (hypodontia) and a cleft tongue.
2. A patient has enamel of the teeth is improperly formed.
3. An infant is born with a congenital tooth, present at birth.

MULTIPLE CHOICE QUESTIONS

1. Tuberculum impar contributes for the development of:
   A. Thyroid
   B. Tongue
   C. Tonsil
   D. Palate
2. Foramen cecum marks the origin of:
   A. Tongue
   B. Trachea
   C. Thyroglossal duct
   D. Hypobranchial eminence
3. Copula of His refers to the development of:
   A. Tooth
   B. Diaphragms
   C. Tongue
   D. Epiglottis
4. Dentin is derived from:
   A. Ectoderm
   B. Mesoderm
   C. Endoderm
   D. Mesenchyme
5. Posterior one-third of tongue is supplied by:
   A. Nerve of third arch
   B. Nerve of first arch
   C. Nerve of fourth arch
   D. Nerve of sixth arch
6. Outgrowths of buccal epithelium forms:
   A. Enamel
   B. Dental pulp
   C. Salivary glands
   D. Tongue
7. What is the time of eruption of permanent canine and premolars?
   A. 6–7 years
   B. 10–12 years
   C. 11–13 years
   D. 17–21 years
8. A newborn is found to have a congenital absence of the submandibular salivary glands. Which pharyngeal arch contributes to the development of these glands?
   A. First pharyngeal arch
   B. Second pharyngeal arch
   C. Third pharyngeal arch
   D. Fourth pharyngeal arch
9. A pediatric patient presents with a tooth that has an enamel defect. This condition suggests an issue with which embryonic structure responsible for enamel formation?
   A. Neural crest cells
   B. Ameloblasts
   C. Odontoblasts
   D. Dental papilla
10. A 7-year-old boy is diagnosed with ankyloglossia (tongue-tie), a condition where the tongue is tethered to the floor of the mouth. Which developmental process was most likely incomplete in this case?
    A. Formation of the lingual frenulum
    B. Descent of the tongue
    C. Migration of myoblasts
    D. Fusion of lateral lingual swellings
11. A newborn presents with a small, midline oral mass that impairs feeding. Ultrasound reveals a cystic lesion at the base of the tongue. Which embryological structure is most likely involved in this condition?
    A. Second pharyngeal pouch
    B. Thyroglossal duct
    C. Rathke's pouch
    D. Fourth pharyngeal pouch
12. A 4-year-old child is brought to the clinic with complaints of difficulty in tasting bitter foods. Examination reveals an abnormality in the taste buds located on the anterior two-thirds of the tongue. Damage to which cranial nerve would most likely cause this symptom, given its role in innervating the circumvallate papillae?
    A. Facial nerve (CN VII)
    B. Glossopharyngeal nerve (CN IX)
    C. Vagus nerve (CN X)
    D. Hypoglossal nerve (CN XII)

Answers: 1. B   2. C   3. C   4. B   5. A
6. C   7. B   8. B   9. B   10. A
11. B   12. B

Alimentary System—II: Gastrointestinal Tract

CHAPTER 16

COMPETENCIES COVERED/LEARNING OUTCOMES

The student should be able to:

AN52.6 Describe the development and congenital anomalies of foregut, midgut and hindgut.

With the establishment of the head and tail folds, part of the cavity of the yolk sac is enclosed within the embryo to form the *primitive gut* (Figs. 16.1A and B). The primitive gut is in free communication with the rest of the yolk sac. The part of the gut cranial to this communication is the *foregut*, the part caudal to the communication is the *hindgut*, while the intervening part is the *midgut* (Figs. 16.1A to C).

* The communication between foregut and midgut is called *anterior intestinal portal* which later represents the termination of bile duct in the second part of duodenum. The communication between the midgut and hindgut is called *posterior intestinal portal* which later becomes the junction of right two-thirds with the left one-third of transverse colon.

* Cranially, the foregut is separated from the stomatodeum by the *buccopharyngeal membrane*. Caudally, the hindgut is separated from the proctodeum by the *cloacal membrane*. At a later stage of development, these membranes disappear, and the gut opens to the exterior at its two ends.

* The midgut during early embryonic period communicates with the extraembryonic part of yolk sac *(definitive yolk sac)* via *vitellointestinal duct*. The vitellointestinal duct disappears by 5th week of development.

* The epithelial lining of various parts of the gastrointestinal tract is of endodermal origin. In the region of the mouth and the anal canal, however, some of the epithelium is derived from the

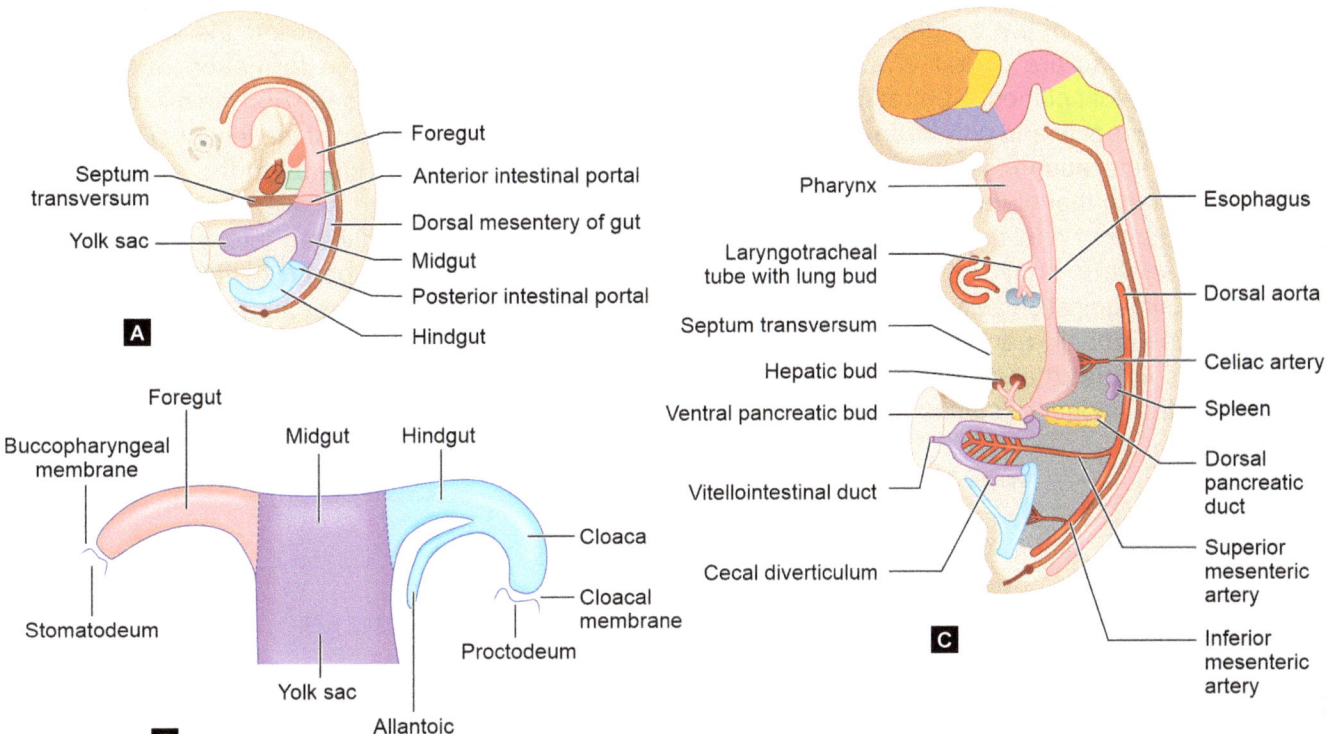

FIGS. 16.1A to C: Parts of the primitive gut.

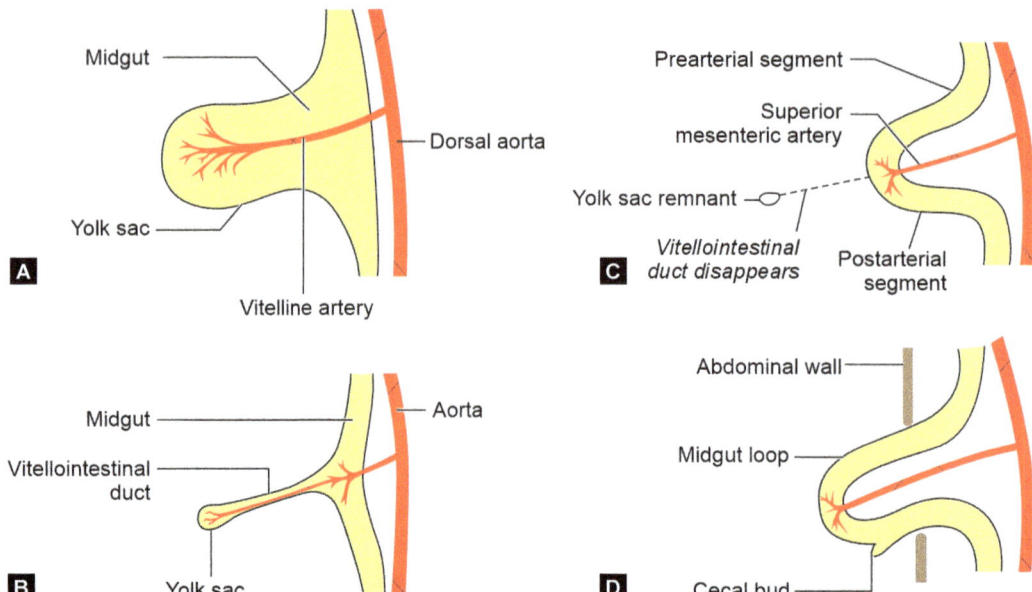

FIGS. 16.2A to D: Establishment of the midgut loop. (A) Midgut in wide communication with the yolk sac. Note vitelline artery passing from dorsal aorta to the yolk sac; (B) Yolk sac much smaller, and attached to midgut through a narrow vitellointestinal duct. The original vitelline artery gives branches to the midgut; (C) The midgut increases in length and forms a loop. The loop has a prearterial segment and a postarterial segment; (D) Midgut loop passes out of abdominal cavity. The cecal bud arises from the postarterial segment.

ectoderm of the stomodeum and of the proctodeum respectively.

- The gut is fixed to the ventral and dorsal body wall of the embryo by *ventral* and *dorsal mesenteries*.
- While the gut is being formed, the circulatory system of the embryo undergoes considerable development. A midline artery, the *dorsal aorta*, is established and comes to lie just dorsal to the gut **(Fig. 16.2)**. It gives off a series of branches to the gut.
- Those in the region of the midgut, initially, run right up to the yolk sac are called *vitelline arteries*. Subsequently, most of these ventral branches of the dorsal aorta disappear and only three of them remain. The artery of the abdominal part of the foregut is the *celiac artery*, that of the midgut is the *superior mesenteric artery* and that of the hindgut is the *inferior mesenteric artery*.
- The wide communication between the yolk sac and the midgut is gradually narrowed down **(Fig. 16.2B)** with the result that the midgut becomes tubular. Thereafter, the midgut assumes the form of a loop **(Fig. 16.2C)**. The superior mesenteric artery now runs in the mesentery of this loop to its apex. The loop has a *proximal* or *prearterial segment* and a *distal* or *postarterial segment*. A bud (called *cecal bud*) soon arises from the postarterial segment very near the apex of the loop **(Fig. 16.2D)**.
- For a few weeks, the midgut loop lie outside the abdominal cavity through the umbilical opening into a part of most proximal part of the umbilical cord. The loop is subsequently withdrawn into the abdominal cavity.
- While considering the formation of the *allantoic diverticulum*, it was seen that the diverticulum opens into the ventral aspect of the hindgut **(Fig. 16.1)**. The part of the hindgut caudal to the attachment of the allantoic diverticulum is called the *cloaca*. The cloaca soon shows a subdivision into a broad ventral part and a narrow dorsal part **(Fig. 16.3)**.
- These two parts are separated from each other by the formation of the *urorectal septum*, which is first formed in the angle between the allantois and the cloaca **(Figs. 16.4A and B)**.

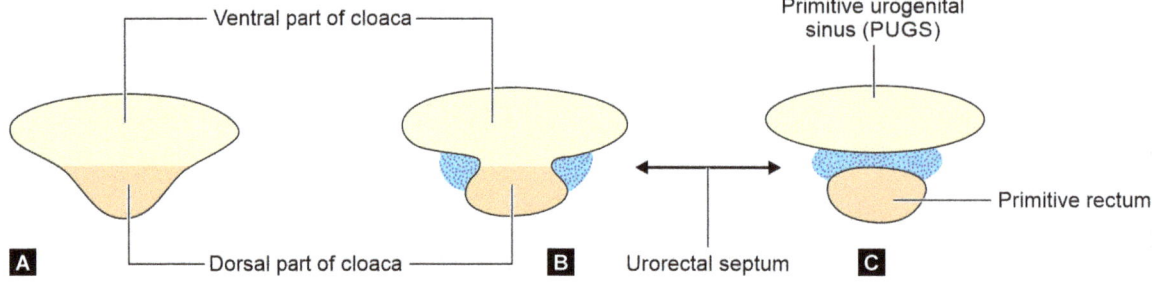

FIGS. 16.3A to C: Formation of urorectal septum as seen in transverse sections. This septum divides the cloaca into the primitive urogenital sinus and the primitive rectum.

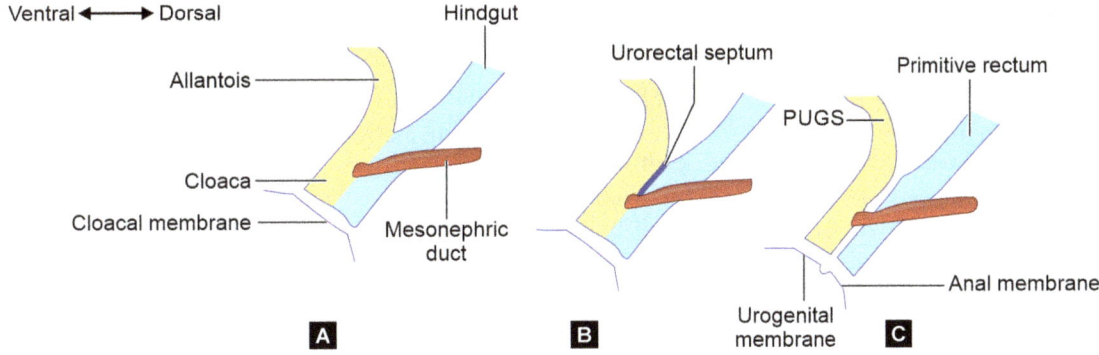

FIGS. 16.4A to C: Formation of urorectal septum as seen in longitudinal sections through the cloaca.

- The ventral subdivision of the cloaca is now called the *primitive urogenital sinus* and gives origin to some parts of the urogenital system. The dorsal part is called the *primitive rectum*. It forms the rectum, and part of the anal canal.
- The urorectal septum grows towards the cloacal membrane and eventually fuses with it **(Fig. 16.4C)**. The cloacal membrane is now divided into a ventral *urogenital membrane*, related to the urogenital sinus, and a dorsal *anal membrane* related to the rectum. Mesoderm around the anal membrane becomes heaped up with the result that the anal membrane comes to lie at the bottom of a pit called the anal pit, or proctodaeum. The anal pit contributes to the formation of the anal canal.

DERIVATIVES OF ALL THREE SEGMENTS OF THE PRIMITIVE GUT

Each one of the three segments of the primitive gut is divided into two parts. The derivatives of the gut are shown in **Figure 16.5 and Table 16.1**.
- At this stage, it might be noted that the endoderm of the foregut, midgut, and hindgut gives rise only to the epithelial lining of the intestinal tract. Smooth muscle, connective tissue, and peritoneum are derived from the splanchnic mesoderm **(Figs. 16.6 and 16.7)**.

Arteries of the Gut

Part of gut	Arterial supply	Area supplied
Foregut	Celiac artery	Lower part of the esophagus to the middle of the second part of duodenum
Midgut	Superior mesenteric artery	Middle of second part of duodenum to the junction of right two-thirds with the left one-third of transverse colon
Hindgut	Inferior mesenteric artery	The junction of right two-thirds with the left one-third of transverse colon to the upper part of anal canal

DEVELOPMENT OF INDIVIDUAL PARTS OF GUT

Foregut Development

Esophagus (Fig. 16.8)

- The esophagus is developed during 4th week of IUL from the part of the foregut between the pharynx and the stomach.
- On the ventral side, at *pharyngoesophageal junction*, laryngotracheal groove appears which bulges to form respiratory diverticulum.

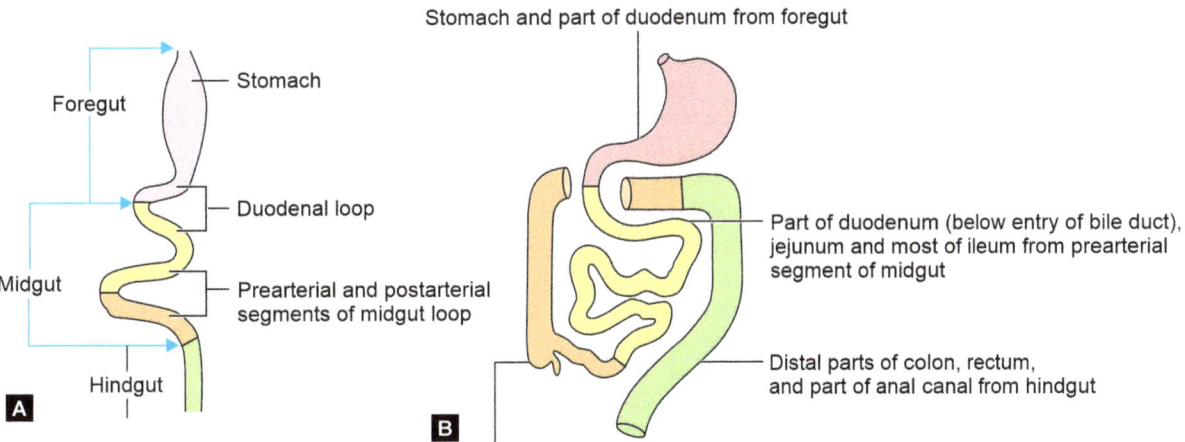

FIGS. 16.5A and B: Derivation of various parts of the gut.

TABLE 16.1: Derivatives of three segments of primitive gut.

Segment	Derivatives
Foregut: The foregut is divided into pre- and postlaryngeal parts with the development of laryngeal diverticulum from its ventral wall	• **Prelaryngeal part:** – Parts of floor of mouth including tongue – Pharynx – Salivary glands – Thyroid – Lower respiratory tract (from respiratory diverticulum) • **Postlaryngeal part:** – Esophagus – Stomach – Duodenum (proximal to ampulla of Vater) – Liver – Extrahepatic biliary system – Pancreas
Midgut: The superior mesenteric artery divides the midgut into a cranial or prearterial segment and a caudal or postarterial segment	• **Prearterial part:** – Duodenum (distal part) – Jejunum – Ileum except terminal part • **Postarterial part:** – Terminal ileum – Cecum – Appendix – Ascending colon – Right two-thirds of transverse colon
Hindgut: The appearance of allantois from the ventral wall of hindgut divides it into pre- and postallantoic parts	• **Preallantoic part:** – Left one-third of transverse colon – Descending colon • **Postallantoic part:** – Sigmoid colon – Rectum – Upper part of anal canal – Parts of urogenital system (primitive urogenital sinus derivatives)

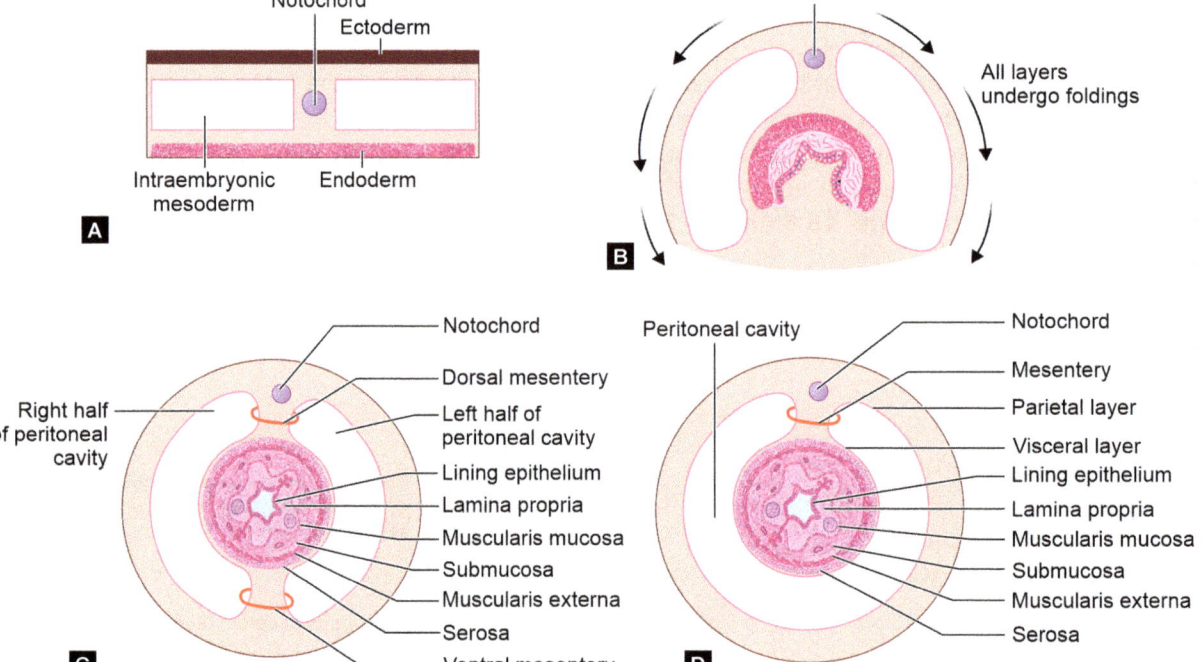

FIGS. 16.6A to D: Scheme to show how the gut is formed by lateral folding of the embryonic disc. (A) Embryonic disc before lateral folding; (B) The lateral edges of the disc grow in a ventral direction; (C and D) The edges pass medially to meet in the midline. In this way, the layer of endoderm is converted into a tube which is the future gut. The ectoderm also meets in the midline and cuts off the coelom from the exterior.

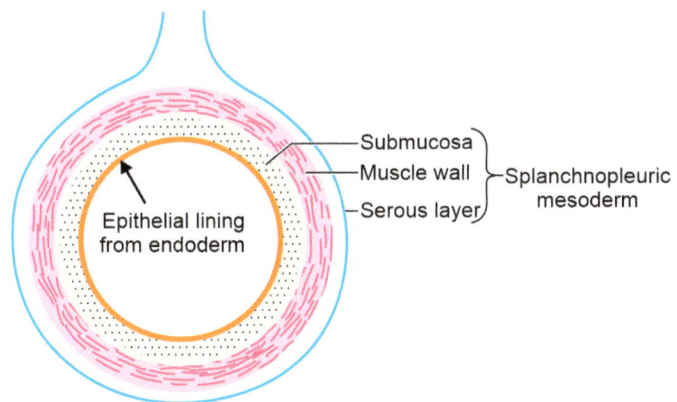

FIG. 16.7: Derivation of the coats of the gut.

- The *tracheoesophageal septum* divides the foregut into dorsal esophageal and ventral tracheal portions.
- It is at first short but elongates with the formation of the neck, with the descent of the diaphragm, and with the enlargement of the pleural cavities.
- The musculature of the esophagus is derived from splanchnic mesenchyme surrounding the foregut.
- Around the *upper two-thirds* of the esophagus, the mesenchyme forms striated muscle. Around the lower one-third, the muscle formed is smooth (as over the rest of the gut).

Clinical correlation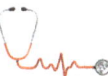

- **Esophageal atresia:** Failure of the esophagus to develop as a continuous tube, resulting in a gap (atresia) between segments. It may be associated with *tracheoesophageal fistula*. Newborns may drool saliva, choke, and have difficulty swallowing or feeding.
- **Esophageal atenosis:** Narrowing (stenosis) of the esophagus due to incomplete development or abnormal vascular tissue formation. Lower 1/3rd is most affected.
- **Tracheoesophageal fistula (TEF) (Figs. 16.9A to D):** Abnormal connection (fistula) between the esophagus and trachea which occurs due to failure of separation of tracheobronchial diverticulum and formation of tracheoesophageal septum. It is of two type proximal and distal. In most cases (86%), distal communication with trachea is there along with atresia. Clinically, the newborn vomits everything given. Diagnostic sign is presence of air in stomach.
- **Zenker's diverticulum:** Outpouching of the esophageal wall due to weakness or abnormal development in pharyngoesophageal junction.
- **Achalasia cardia:** It is a rare disorder of the esophagus characterized by difficulty in swallowing (dysphagia) due to the inability of the lower esophageal sphincter (LES) to relax properly and the loss of esophageal peristalsis. There is *bird beak sign* on barium swallow study.

Stomach

- During 4th week, the stomach is first seen as a fusiform dilatation of the foregut just distal to the esophagus. Its dorsal border is attached to the posterior abdominal wall by a fold of peritoneum called the *dorsal mesogastrium*. Its ventral border is attached to the septum transversum by another fold of peritoneum called the *ventral mesogastrium* (Figs. 16.10A, B, 16.11 and 16.12A).
- Subsequently, the liver and the diaphragm are formed in the substance of the septum transversum (Fig. 16.12C).

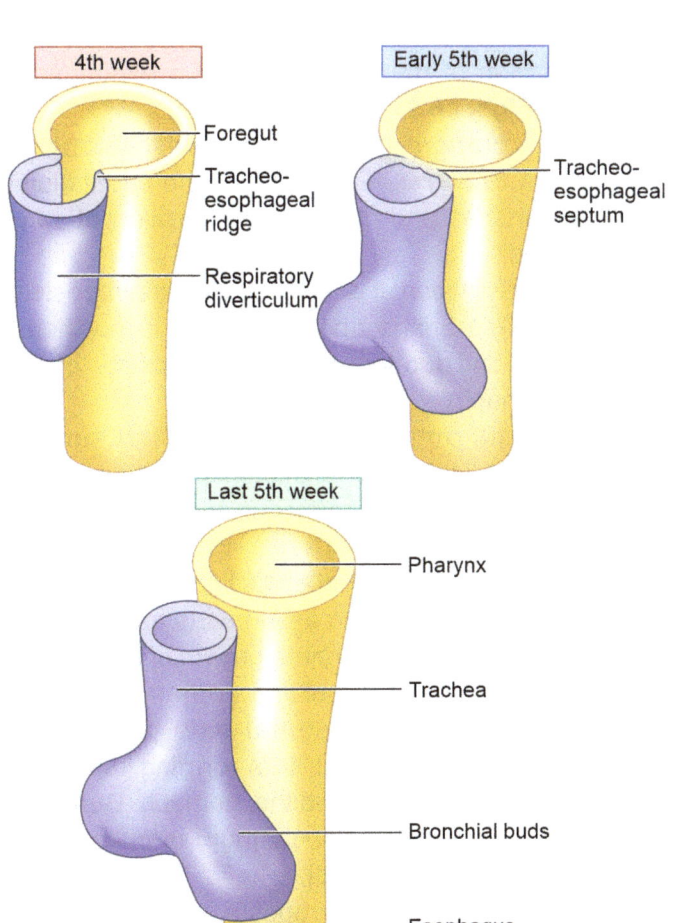

FIG. 16.8: Development of esophagus.

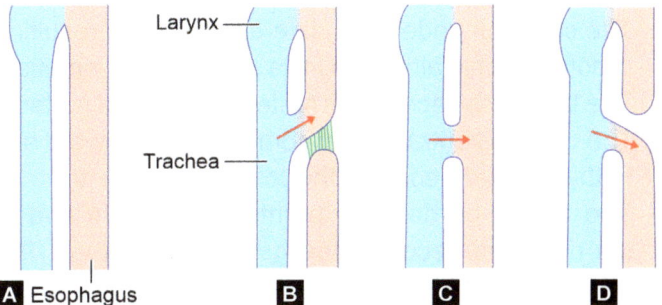

FIGS. 16.9A to D: (A) Normal arrangement of trachea and esophagus; (B to D) Various forms of tracheoesophageal fistulae.

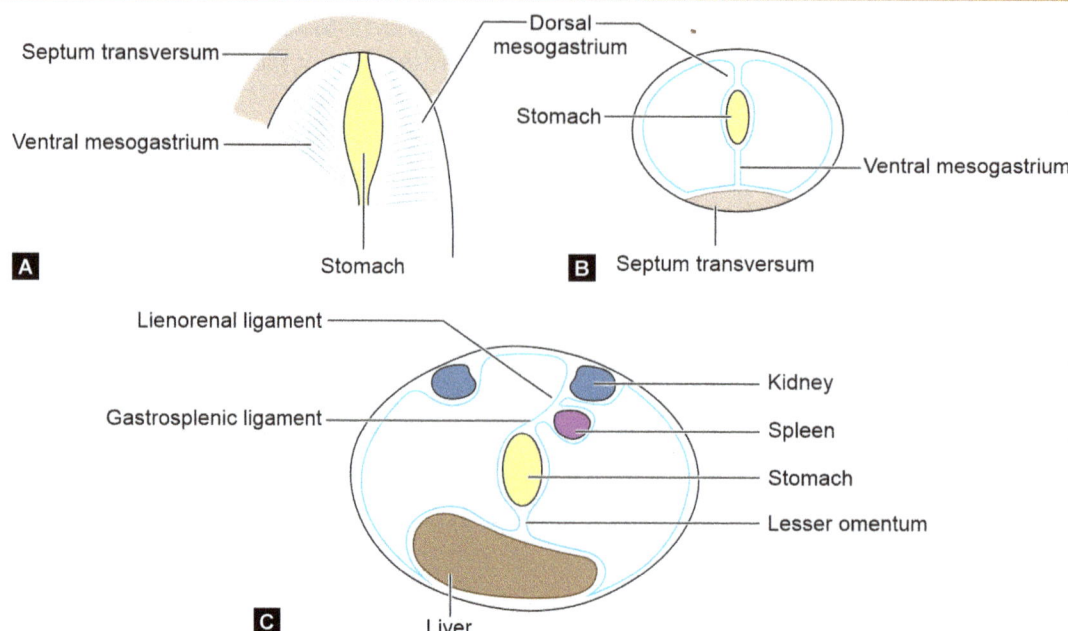

FIGS. 16.10A to C: (A) Side view of stomach showing the dorsal and ventral mesogastria; (B) Transverse section through "A" showing that the ventral mesogastrium connects the stomach to the septum transversum; (C) The most important remnant of the ventral mesogastrium is the lesser omentum. It passes from the stomach to the liver (which develops in the septum transversum). The spleen is formed in relation to the dorsal mesogastrium. Its formation divides this part of the dorsal mesogastrium into the gastrosplenic ligament and the lienorenal ligament.

- The ventral mesogastrium now passes from the stomach to the liver, and from the liver to the diaphragm and anterior abdominal wall (Fig. 16.10C). The part of the ventral mesogastrium between the liver and the stomach becomes the *lesser omentum*, while the part between the liver and the diaphragm (and anterior abdominal wall) gives rise to the *coronary*, and *falciform* ligaments.
- Similarly, the dorsal mesogastrium is divided by the development of the spleen into a part between stomach and spleen *(gastrosplenic ligament)* and a part between spleen and posterior abdominal wall called the *lienorenal ligament* (Fig. 16.10C).
- *Gastric glands* and *oxyntic glands* of stomach appear in 3rd and 4th month of IUL respectively.

Changes in Shape of Stomach

- The stomach undergoes differential growth resulting in considerable alteration in its shape and orientation. The Dorsal surface grows faster than ventral surface.
- The original ventral border comes to face upward and to the left and becomes the *lesser curvature*.
- The dorsal border now points downwards and to the right and becomes the *greater curvature*. The original left surface becomes its anterior surface and the original right surface becomes the posterior surface (Fig. 16.11).

Rotation of Stomach

- The rotation of the stomach can be explained as follows (Figs. 16.11 and 16.12):
  - *First rotation:* It is 90° clockwise along the longitudinal axis. This changes the orientation of its surfaces and changes the position of vagus nerves.
  - *Second rotation:* It is in transverse/anteroposterior axis. This brings about changes in position of fundus and duodenum and in the position of ends of stomach.
- The rotation and differential growth of surfaces explains the change in relationship of right and left vagus nerves to posteroinferior and anterosuperior surfaces respectively.
- During rotation the cranial end tilts to the left and the caudal end to the right to assume the adult position.
- Rotation and disproportionate growth of the stomach alters the position of dorsal and ventral mesogastria.
- Rotation along longitudinal axis pulls dorsal mesogastrium to the left thus forming the *lesser sac/omental bursa* behind the stomach. During this rotation, the ventral mesogastrium is pulled to the right (Figs. 16.12B and C).
- Due to rotation along anteroposterior axis, the dorsal mesogastrium bulges downward and continues to grow to form a double-layered greater omentum.

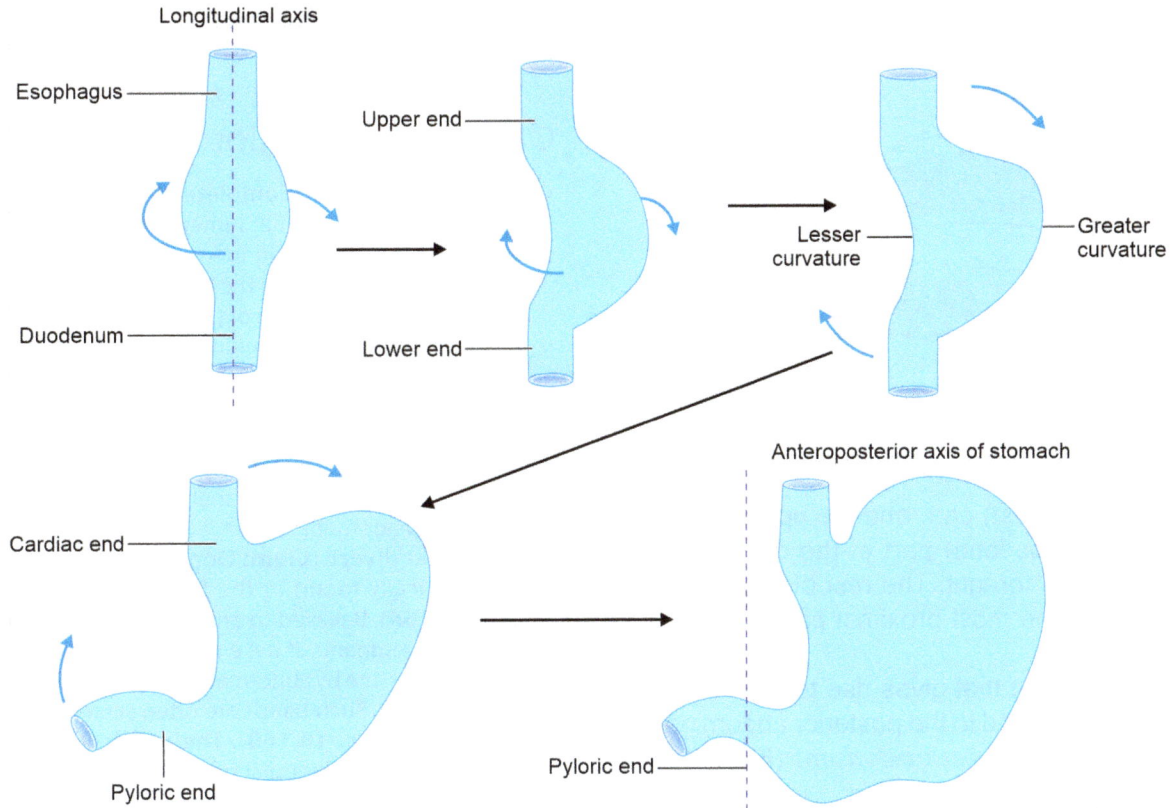

FIG. 16.11: Changes in the position and shape of stomach.

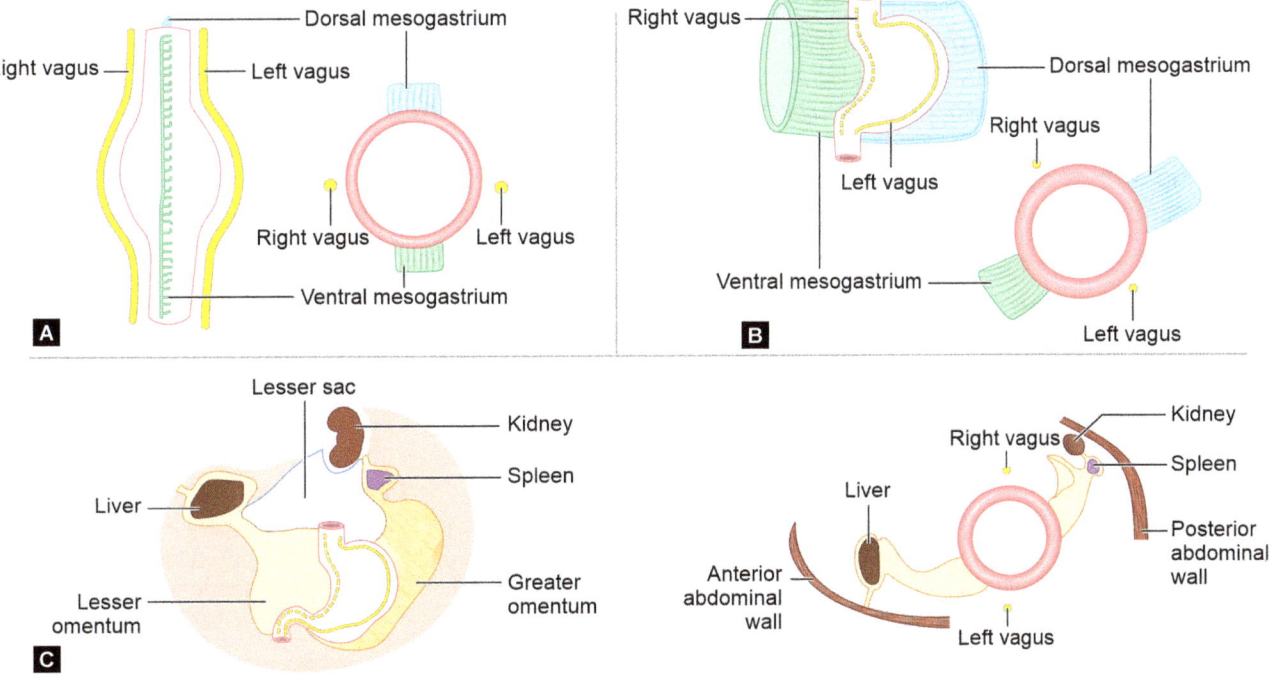

FIGS. 16.12A to C: Changes in the relation of vagus nerve and the mesogastrium to the developing stomach.

Clinical correlation

Congenital Pyloric Stenosis
- It is due to the hypertrophy of circular muscle layer in the pylorus region leading to gastric outlet obstruction **(Fig. 16.13)**. Some researchers think the primary cause of this defect is the same as in megacolon.
- Symptoms include projectile, nonbilious vomiting after feeding, persistent hunger, and weight loss.
- An *olive-shaped mass* may be palpable in the right upper abdomen.

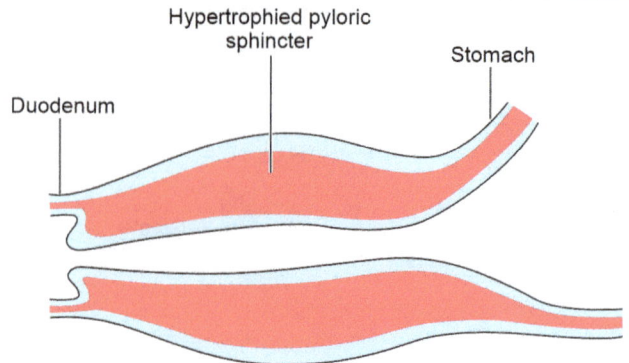

FIG. 16.13: Congenital pyloric stenosis.

Duodenum

- The superior (or first) part, and the upper half of the descending (or second) part of the duodenum are derived from the foregut. The rest of the duodenum develops from the most proximal part of the midgut (Fig. 16.14A).
- The part of the gut that gives rise to the duodenum forms a loop attached to the posterior abdominal wall by a mesentery *(mesoduodenum)* (Figs. 16.14B and C).
- Later, this loop falls to the right. The mesoduodenum then fuses with the peritoneum of the posterior abdominal wall with the result that most of the duodenum becomes retroperitoneal (Fig. 16.15).
- The mesoduodenum persists in relation to a small part of the duodenum adjacent to the pylorus. This is the part seen in radiographs as the *duodenal cap*.
- In keeping with its development, the proximal part of the duodenum is supplied by branches of the celiac artery, and the distal part by branches of the superior mesenteric artery.

Clinical correlation

- **Duodenal atresia:** Complete closure or absence of a portion of the duodenal lumen. It results from failure of recanalization of the duodenum during the 8th to 10th weeks of gestation when the lumen temporarily obliterates due to rapid proliferation of the epithelial lining. Newborns present with bilious vomiting within the first day of life, abdominal distention, and a *"double bubble" sign* on radiographic imaging.
- **Duodenal stenosis:** Narrowing of the duodenal lumen, usually in the third and fourth parts of the duodenum which is caused by incomplete recanalization or vascular accidents during development.
- **Duodenal diverticulum:** Outpouching of the duodenal wall, typically found in the 2nd part of the duodenum (Fig. 16.16A). Believed to arise from abnormal budding or persistent remnants of the embryonic foregut diverticulum.
- External pressure by abnormal peritoneal bands or abnormal blood vessels. Such bands are often seen in relation to the duodenum (Fig. 16.16B). The duodenum may also be compressed by an annular pancreas.

Midgut Development

The midgut elongates to form U-shaped intestinal loop that is suspended from the posterior abdominal wall by a short mesentery. Anteriorly, it communicates with the yolk sac by the narrow *vitellointestinal duct*. The superior mesenteric artery runs in the middle of midgut loop and divides it into a *prearterial (cranial)* and a *postarterial (caudal)* segment (Figs. 16.2A to D).

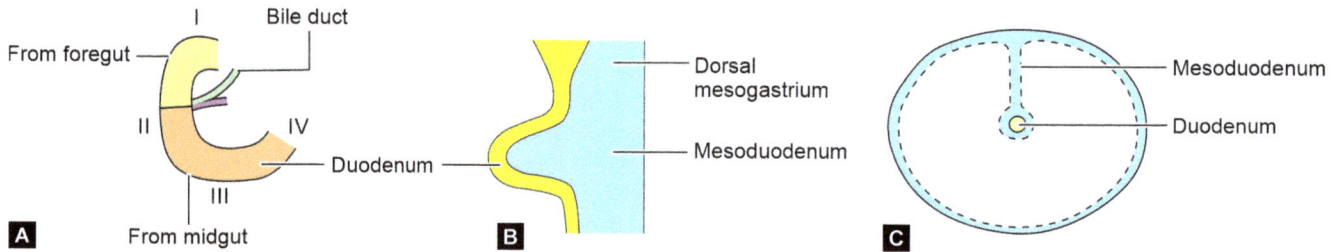

FIGS. 16.14A to C: Development of the duodenum. (A) Part of the duodenum above the entry of the bile duct is derived from the foregut, and the part below this level is derived from the midgut; (B and C) At first the duodenum has a mesentery called the mesoduodenum. As seen in "B", this is continuous, cranially, with the dorsal mesogastrium. The mesoduodenum later disappears (*see also* Fig. 16.15).

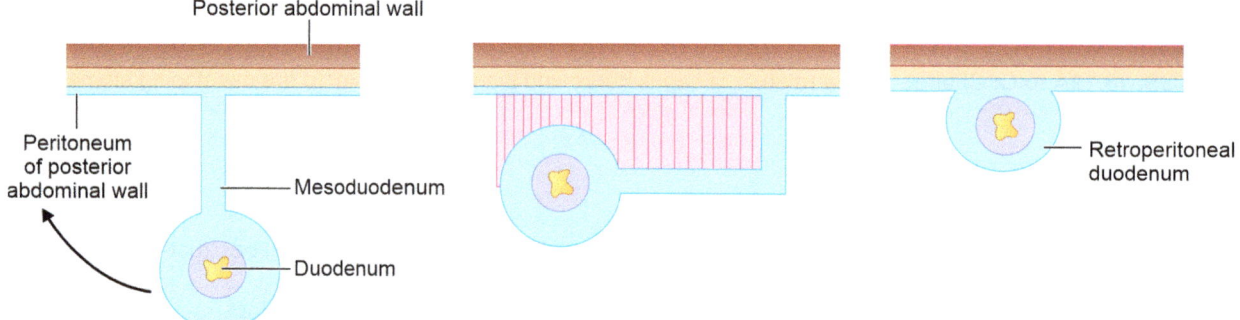

FIG. 16.15: Scheme to show how the mesoduodenum disappears. The duodenum then becomes retroperitoneal.

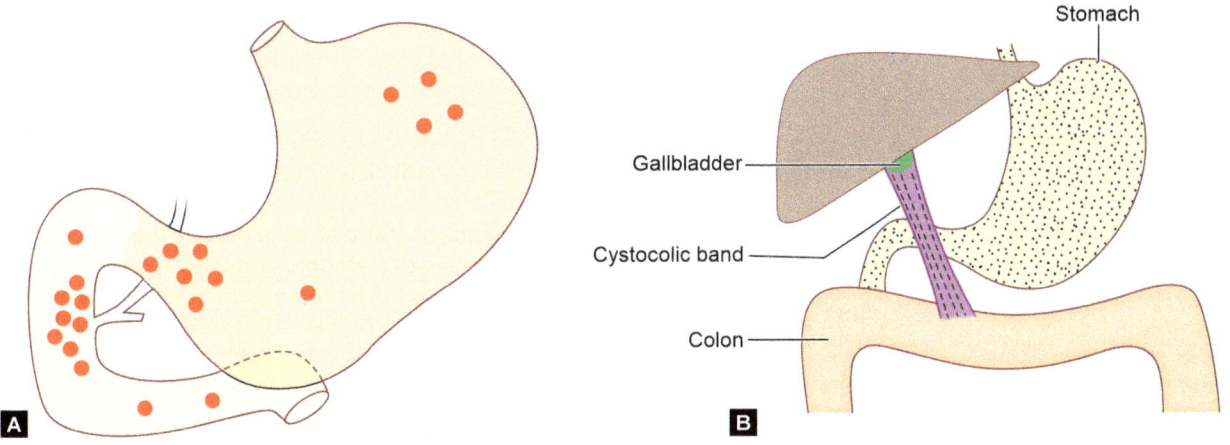

FIGS. 16.16A and B: (A) Sites at which congenital diverticula may arise from stomach and duodenum. (B) Obstruction of duodenum by a cystocolic band passing from the gallbladder to the transverse colon.

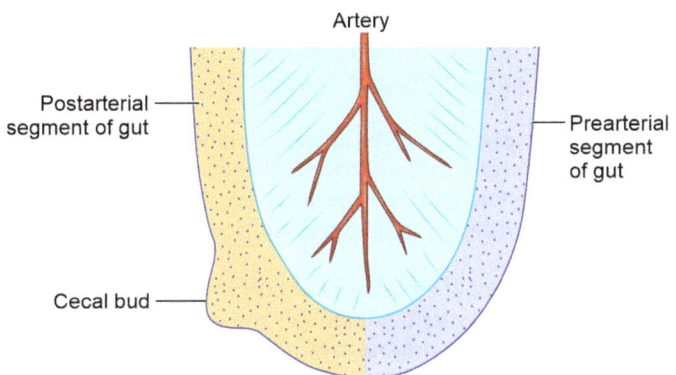

FIG. 16.17: Midgut loop. In this figure, the loop has been drawn to correspond with the orientation of the ileocecal region in postnatal life (actually, the prearterial segment is cranial to the postarterial segment).

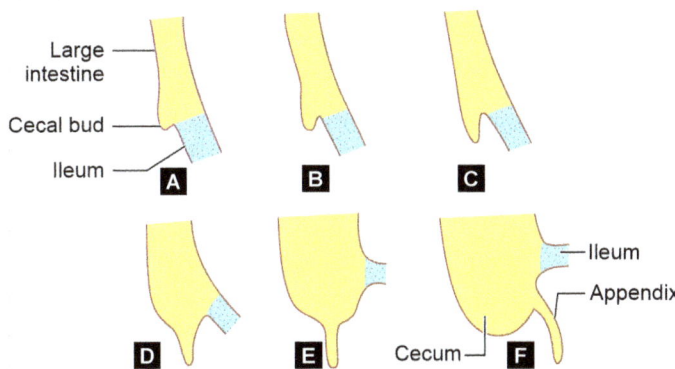

FIGS. 16.18A to F: Development of cecum and appendix. The orientation is as in **Figure 16.17**.

Jejunum and Ileum

- The jejunum and most of the ileum are derived from the prearterial segment of the midgut loop.
- The terminal portion of the ileum is derived from the postarterial segment proximal to the cecal bud **(Fig. 16.17)**.

Cecum and Appendix

- The cecal bud is a diverticulum that arises from the postarterial segment of the midgut loop **(Fig. 16.17)**. The cecum and appendix are formed by enlargement of this bud.
- The proximal part of the bud grows rapidly to form the caecum. Its distal part remains narrow and forms the appendix **(Figs. 16.18A to F)**.
- During greater part of fetal life, the appendix arises from the apex of the cecum **(Figs. 16.18A to F)**. Subsequently, the lateral (or right) wall of the cecum grows much more rapidly than the medial (or left) wall with the result the point of attachment of the appendix comes to lie on the medial side **(Figs. 16.18A to F)**.

Ascending Colon

It develops from the postarterial segment of the midgut loop **(Fig. 16.17)** distal to the cecal bud.

Clinical Importance

- **Physiological Umbilical Hernia**
  - During 3rd week of development, the prearterial segment of midgut loop elongates rapidly. Because of rapid elongation of midgut loop and rapid growth of liver and the developing mesonephric kidney, the abdominal cavity becomes too small to accommodate all the intestinal loops.
  - The midgut loop enters the extraembryonic coelomic cavity in the umbilical cord during 6th week of development. This herniation of intestinal loop is called *physiological umbilical hernia*.
- **Reduction of Physiological Umbilical Hernia**
  - During 10th week of development, the herniated midgut loop begins to return to the abdominal cavity.
  - The contributing factors for the return of midgut loop are reduction in size of developing liver, regression of the mesonephric kidney with associated expansion of abdominal cavity.

Clinical correlation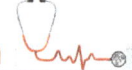

Umbilical Hernia Anomalies
- **Omphalocele/exomphalos (Fig. 16.19):** Sometimes, the coils of intestine that develop from the midgut loop remain outside the abdominal cavity. The child is born with loops of intestine hanging out of the umbilicus which may be covered with amniotic membrane. This has bad prognosis.
- **Congenital umbilical hernia:** Loops of intestine and other abdominal contents may also be seen outside the abdominal cavity for an entirely different reason. In congenital umbilical hernia, the muscle layer and skin are absent in the region of the umbilicus, creating a defect in the abdominal wall through which abdominal contents can pass. Such contents are covered with peritoneum, but in exomphalos they are covered only by amnion. This has no genetic basis when compared to exomphalos and has a good prognosis when treated timely.
- **Gastroschisis:** It is a paraumbilical, full thickness abdominal wall defect associated with protrusion of abdominal contents. This occurs when lateral folds of embryo during folding fails to fuse. On USG, one can see a defect on the right of umbilical cord and free-floating bowel loops. There is also high levels of alpha-fetoproteins during prenatal period.
- Vitellointestinal duct anomalies
    - Vitellointestinal duct normally disappears.
    - *Meckel's diverticulum* or *diverticulum ilei* is a small, persisted part of vitellointestinal duct. It is seen along the antimesenteric border of ileum which may be connected to umbilicus. It is seen in 2% of people and is 2 feet from the ileocecal junction and 2.0 inches in length. It is of surgical importance as it may undergo inflammation giving rise to symptoms like those of appendicitis. It may contain two types of ectopic tissues: pancreatic tissue, or a gastric type of mucosa in its wall (in such cases, ulceration and perforation can occur in the diverticulum).
    - Occasionally, the whole of the vitellointestinal duct, or its distal part alone, may be patent. The former conditions lead to a *fecal/vitelline fistula* communicating ileum with exterior at umbilicus. The latter condition leads to formation of an *umbilical sinus*.
    - The vitellointestinal duct may be represented by cysts *(enterocystoma* or *vitelline cyst)* or by *fibrous cords* **(Figs. 16.20A to F)**. Fibrous cords constitute a danger in later life as coils of intestine may get twisted round them leading to strangulation.
    - Remnants of the vitellointestinal duct may also give rise to growths.
- **Subhepatic cecum and appendix (Fig. 16.21):** This results due to failure of descent of cecum. This abnormal positioning occurs due to incomplete rotation and fixation of the midgut during embryonic development. Sometimes the descent of cecum is partial, or it can be excessive descent resulting in its positional variations. The cecum may remain subhepatic or may descend only to the lumbar region. Alternatively, it may descend into the pelvis **(Figs. 16.21A to C)**.

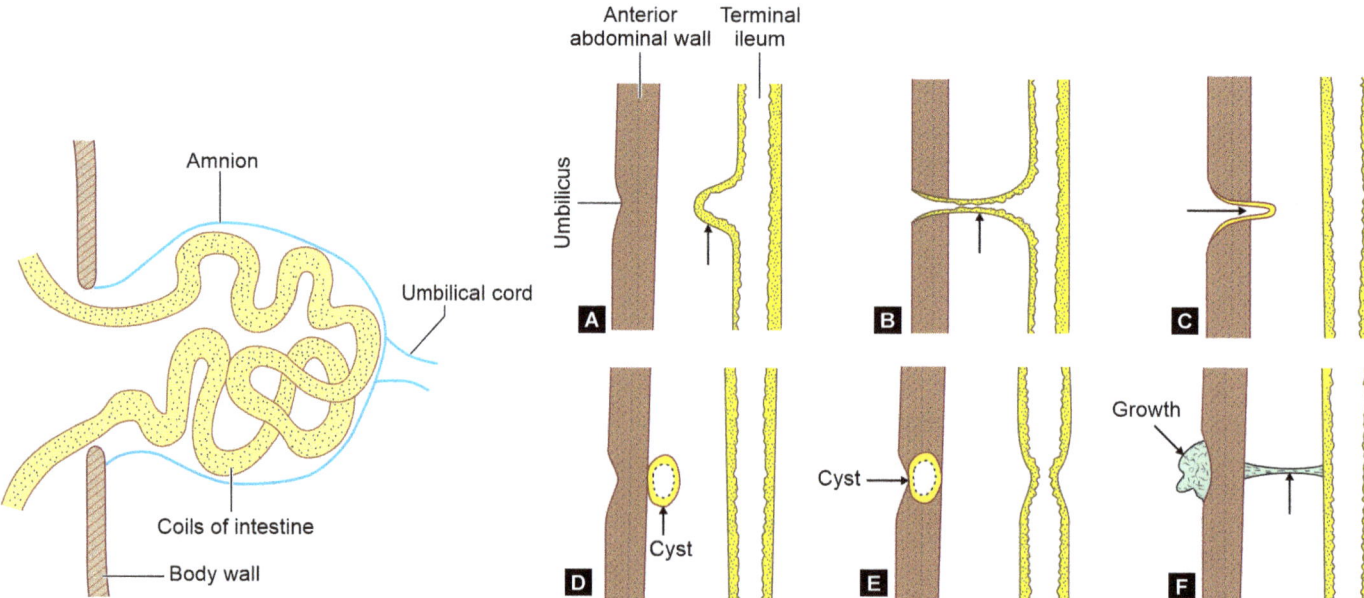

FIG. 16.19: Exomphalos. Coils of intestine derived from the midgut loop fail to return into the abdominal cavity.

FIGS. 16.20A to F: Anomalies in relation to the vitellointestinal duct (see arrows). (A) Meckel's diverticulum; (B) Patent vitellointestinal duct; (C) Umbilical sinus; (D) Cyst attached to the abdominal wall. A cyst may also be seen attached to the gut, or embedded in the abdominal wall as shown in "E"; (E) Stenosis of gut at the site of attachment of duct; (F) Vitellointestinal duct represented by a fibrous cord. An umbilical growth arising from remnants of the duct is also shown.

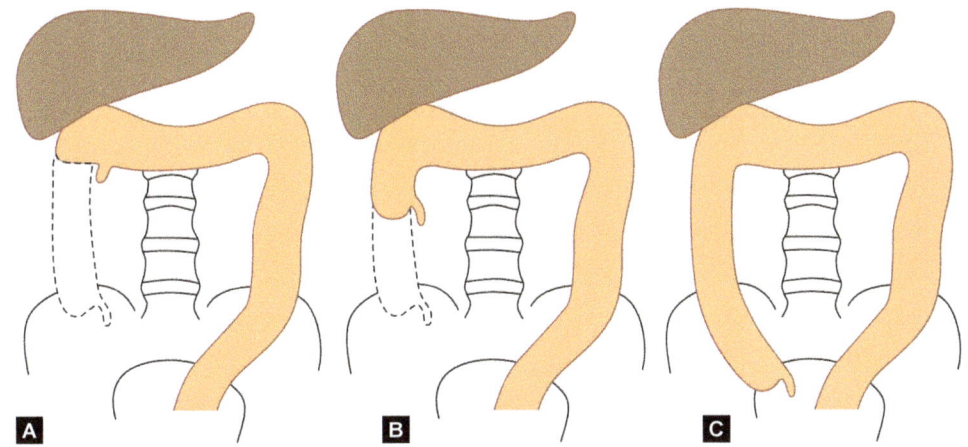

FIGS. 16.21A to C: Errors in descent of the cecum. (A) Subhepatic; (B) Lumbar; (C) Pelvic. The normal position is shown in dotted line in (A) and (B).

Hindgut Development

In the starting of chapter, we have discussed the derivatives of hindgut and its subdivisions (*refer* **Figs. 16.4A and B**). With the formation of tail fold and growth of the embryo, the urorectal septum comes into contact with the cloacal membrane dividing it into the urogenital and anal membranes.

Rupture of anal membrane creates anal opening for the hindgut dorsally. Rupture of urogenital membrane creates opening for the urogenital sinus ventrally. The point of contact of tip of urorectal septum and cloacal membrane becomes the perineal body.

Transverse Colon

- The right two-thirds of the transverse colon develop from the postarterial segment of the midgut loop. The left one-third arises from the hindgut.
- This mode of origin is reflected in its arterial supply; the right two-thirds are supplied by the superior mesenteric artery and the left one-third by the inferior mesenteric artery.

Descending Colon and Sigmoid Colon

The descending colon and sigmoid colon develop from the hindgut (postallantoic part).

Rectum

The rectum is derived from the primitive rectum, i.e., the *dorsal subdivision of the cloaca*. According to some researchers, the upper part of the rectum is derived from the hindgut proximal to the cloaca.

Anal Canal

- It develops from two components: endodermal and ectodermal. Upper two-thirds derived from the endoderm of the hindgut *(primitive rectum)* and lower one-third derived from the ectodermal proctodeum *(anal pit)* **(Figs. 16.22A to C)**.
- These two parts are initially separated by the anal membrane, which later ruptures; the junction is marked by the *pectinate line (anal valves).*
- The blood supply also differs. Superior rectal artery (branch of inferior mesenteric artery) supply the endodermal part while inferior rectal artery (branch of internal pudendal artery, from internal iliac artery) supply the ectodermal part.
- **Venous drainage:** Endodermal part drains into the portal vein (superior rectal vein) and ectodermal part drains into systemic veins (inferior rectal vein).
- The endodermal part is innervated by autonomic nerves and the ectodermal part by somatic nerves.
- Above the pectinate line, the lining epithelium is columnar epithelium and below the pectinate line is stratified squamous epithelium.

Clinical correlation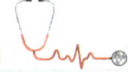

- **Congenital megacolon/Hirschsprung's disease:** It is a congenital condition characterized by the absence of ganglion cells in the myenteric and submucosal plexuses of the distal colon, leading to severe bowel obstruction. In this condition, there is a failure of these neural crest cells to migrate into the distal segments of the colon which leads to a lack of peristalsis in the affected segment, causing a functional obstruction and dilation of the proximal bowel (megacolon) **(Fig. 16.23)**.
- **Imperforate anus:** It is a congenital condition caused by stenosis or atresia of the lower part of the rectum or the anal canal. Some varieties of this condition are shown in **Figures 16.24A to D**.
- **Rectal fistula (Figs. 16.25A to H):** A rectal fistula is an abnormal connection between the rectum and another organ (such as the bladder, urethra, or vagina) or may open in perineum at abnormal site which is caused by *incomplete septation of the cloaca* and incomplete development of the urorectal septum during embryogenesis.

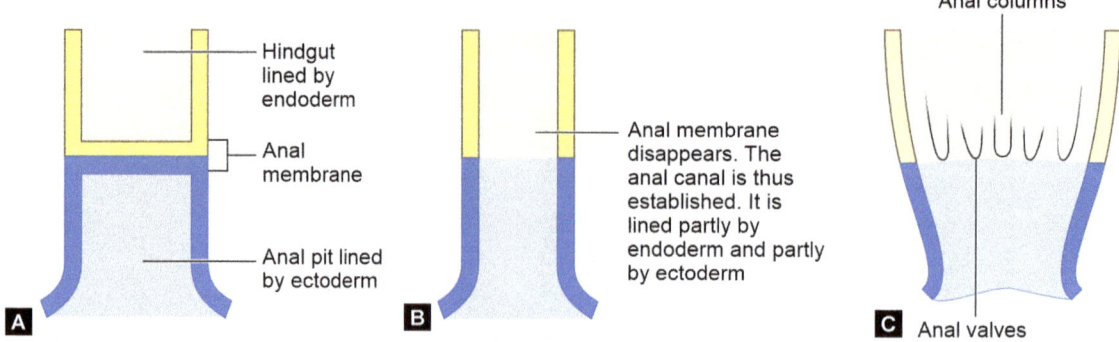

FIGS. 16.22A to C: (A) Anal membrane separates hindgut from anal pit; (B) Anal membrane disappears; (C) Scheme to show the parts of the anal canal in which the lining epithelium is derived from ectoderm or endoderm.

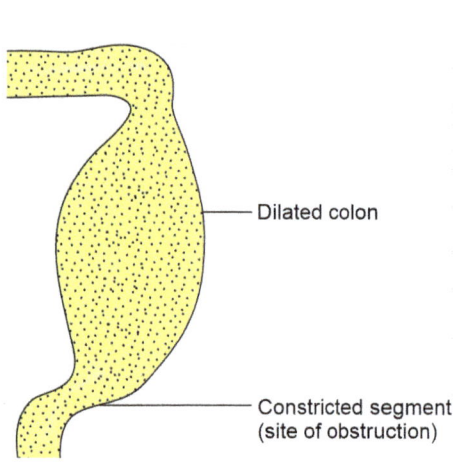

FIG. 16.23: Megacolon.

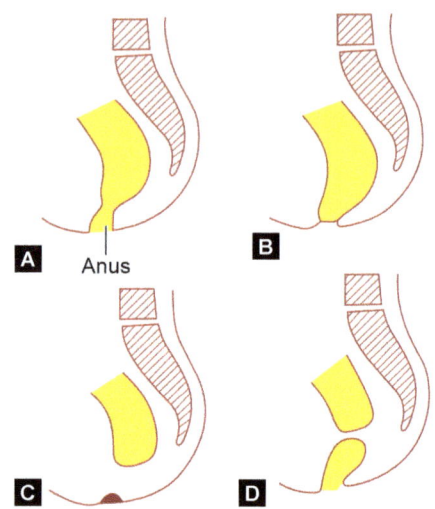

FIGS. 16.24A to D: Various types of imperforate anus. (A) Stenosis of anal canal; (B) Persistent anal membrane; (C) The proctodeum is represented by a solid mass of ectodermal cells and there is a big gap between it and the hindgut (rectum); (D) Upper and lower parts of rectum separated by a gap.

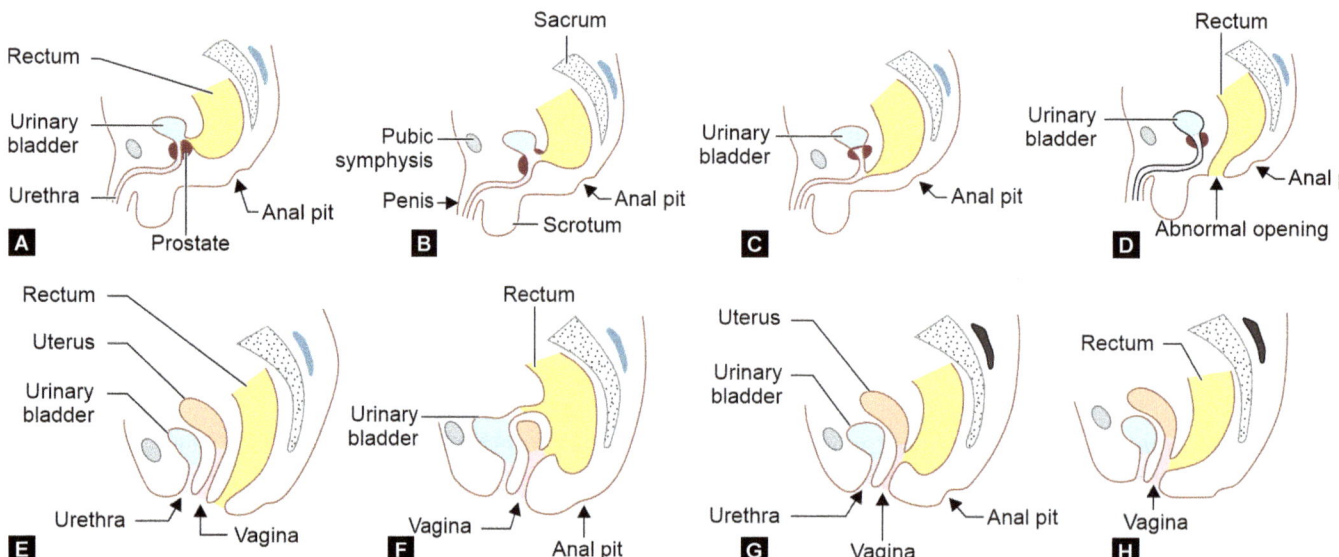

FIGS. 16.25A to H: Various types of rectal fistulae in the male [(A) Rectovesical fistula; (B) Rectourethral fistula (high); (C) Rectourethral fistula (low); (D) Ectopic anus in male] and female [(E) Ectopic anus in female; (F) Rectovesical and rectovaginal fistulae; (G) Rectovaginal fistula (high) (H) Rectovaginal fistula (low)]. The fistula may be between rectum and urinary bladder (i.e., rectovesical) as in (A) and (F), between rectum and urethra (rectourethral) as in (B) and (C), and between rectum and vagina (rectovaginal) as in (G), (H) and (F). More than one type may be present at the same time (F). The rectum may open onto the perineum at an abnormal site (D) and (E). In these cases, the anal pit is formed at the normal site.

ROTATION OF THE GUT

After its formation, the midgut loop lies outside the abdominal cavity of the embryo, in a part of the extraembryonic coelom that persists near the umbilicus. The loop has a prearterial or proximal segment and a postarterial or distal segment (**Fig. 16.26A**). Along with growth in length the midgut loop rotates around the axis of superior mesenteric artery.

When we view the midgut loop from the ventral aspect, it makes a rotation of 270° in counterclockwise direction around the axis of superior mesenteric artery. During rotation elongation of intestinal loop and coiling of jejunum and ileum also takes place. Large intestine also shows elongation but without coiling.

The total rotation of midgut can be divided into three stages of each 90°. First 90° rotation occurs during the herniation and the remaining 180° during the return of intestinal loop into the abdominal cavity.

* **First stage rotation:** Initially, the loop lies in the sagittal plane outside the umbilical ring. Its proximal segment is cranial and ventral to the distal segment (**Figs. 16.26A and 16.27A**). The midgut loop now undergoes rotation. This rotation plays a very important part in establishing the definitive relationships of the various parts of the intestine. The steps in rotation must, therefore, be clearly understood. Viewed from the ventral side the loop undergoes an anticlockwise rotation by 90°, with the result that it now lies in the horizontal plane (**Figs. 16.26B and 16.27B**). The prearterial segment comes to lie on the right side and the postarterial segment on the left of the superior mesenteric artery which forms the axis (compare **Figs. 16.26A and B**).

* **Second stage rotation:** The prearterial segment now undergoes great increase in length to form the coils of the jejunum and ileum. These loops still lie outside the abdominal cavity, to the right side of the distal limb (**Fig. 16.26C**). During the 10th week, the herniated intestinal loops return to the abdominal cavity. The reasons for return of the loop are the regression of mesonephric kidney, reduced growth of liver and expansion of abdominal cavity. The coils of jejunum and ileum (prearterial segment) now return to the abdominal cavity. As they do so, the midgut loop undergoes a further anticlockwise rotation of 90°. As a result, the coils of jejunum and ileum pass behind the superior mesenteric artery into the left half of the abdominal cavity (**Figs. 16.26D and 16.27C**). The duodenum, therefore, comes to lie behind the artery and the coils of jejunum and ileum occupy the posterior and left part of the abdominal cavity.

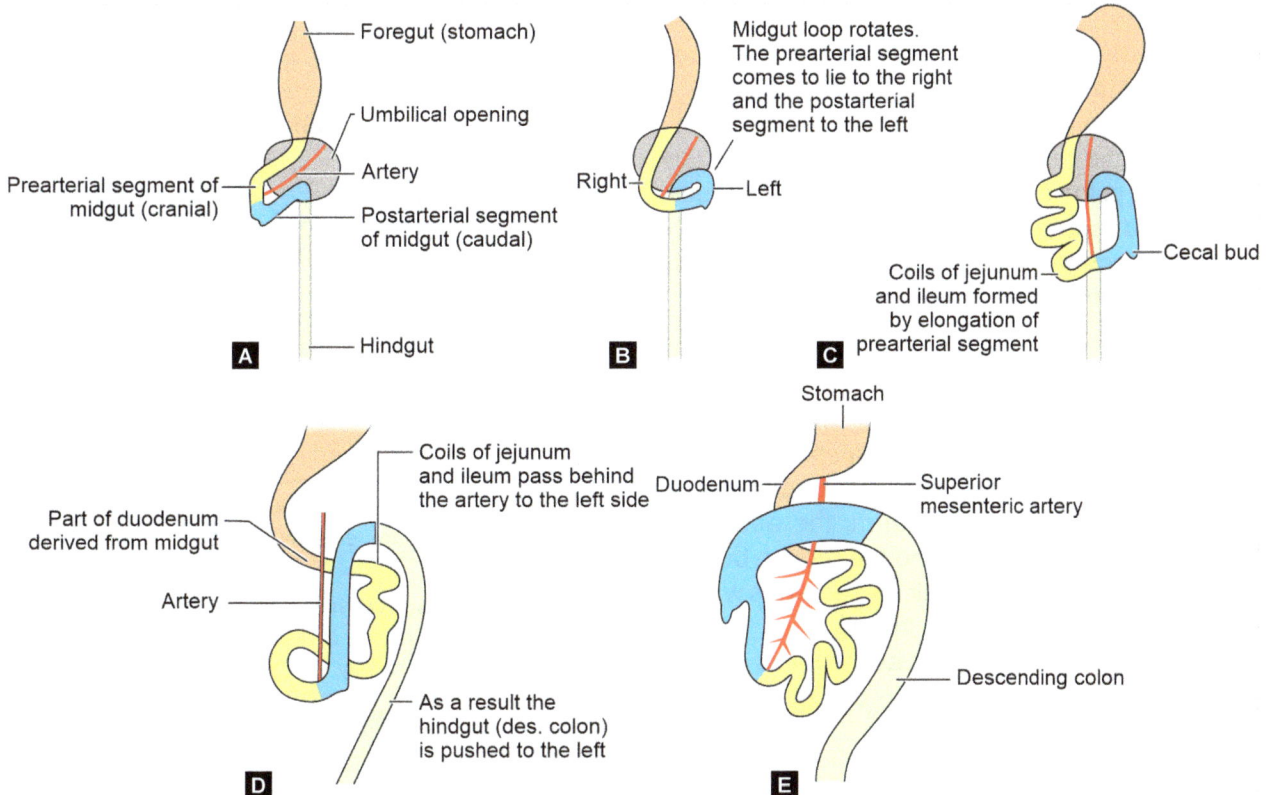

FIGS. 16.26A to E: Stages in rotation of the gut. Study these figures carefully along with the corresponding description in the text. In **Figure 16.16E**, note that the cecum moves to the right, and the transverse colon now lies in front of the superior mesenteric artery.

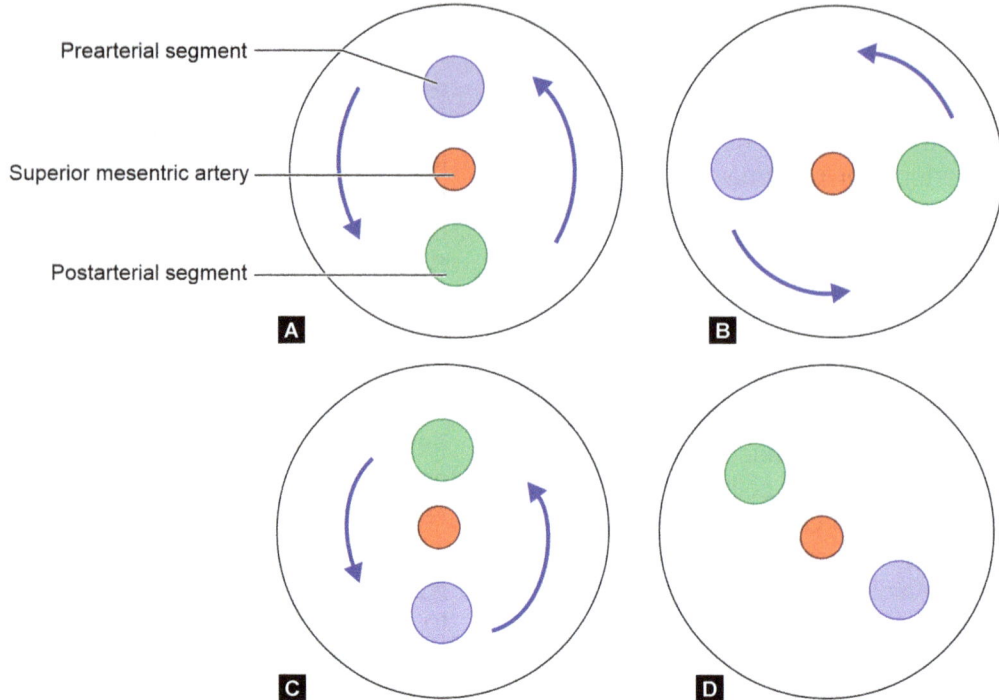

FIGS. 16.27A to D: Scheme to show the orientation of the proximal and distal ends of the midgut loop at different phases of the rotation of the gut. Arrows indicate the direction of rotation. Compare with **Figure 16.26**.

- **Third stage rotation/retraction of herniated loop:** The postarterial segment of the midgut loop returns to the abdominal cavity. As it does so, it also rotates in an anticlockwise direction of 90° **(Figs. 16.26E and 16.27D)**. With the result, the transverse colon lies anterior to the superior mesenteric artery, and the cecum comes to lie on the right side. At this stage, read the rotation of gut with **Figures 16.26 and 16.27** to understand the orientation of various parts of gut.
- At this stage, the cecum lies just below the liver, and an ascending colon cannot be demarcated. Gradually, the cecum descends to the iliac fossa, and the ascending, transverse and descending parts of the colon become distinct.

FIXATION OF THE GUT

- At first all parts of the small and large intestines have a mesentery by which they are suspended from the posterior abdominal wall. After the completion of rotation of the gut, the duodenum, the ascending colon, the descending colon and the rectum become retroperitoneal by fusion of their mesenteries with the posterior abdominal wall **(Fig. 16.15)**.
- The original mesentery persists as the *mesentery of the small intestine*, the *transverse mesocolon* and the *pelvic mesocolon*.

Clinical correlation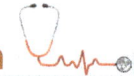

Errors of Rotation
- **Nonrotation of the midgut loop:** In this condition, the small intestine lies toward the right side of the abdominal cavity, and the large intestine toward the left **(Fig. 16.28A)**.
- **Reversed rotation:** The transverse colon crosses behind the superior mesenteric artery, and the duodenum crosses in front of it **(Fig. 16.28B)**.

Errors of Fixation
- Parts of the intestine that are normally retroperitoneal may have a mesentery. Abnormal mobility of this part of the intestine may result in its twisting. This condition is called **volvulus**. Twisting of blood vessels to the loop can lead to obstruction of its blood supply.
- Parts of the intestines, that normally have a mesentery, may be fixed by abnormal adhesions of peritoneum.

Situs Inversus
In this condition, all abdominal and thoracic viscera are laterally transposed, i.e., all parts normally on the right side are seen on the left side, and vice versa. For example, the appendix and duodenum lie on the left side, and the stomach on the right side.

Duplication of Gut Derivatives
Varying lengths of the intestinal tract may be duplicated. The duplicated part may form only a small cyst, or may be of considerable length. It may or may not communicate with the rest of the intestine **(Figs. 16.29A and B)**.

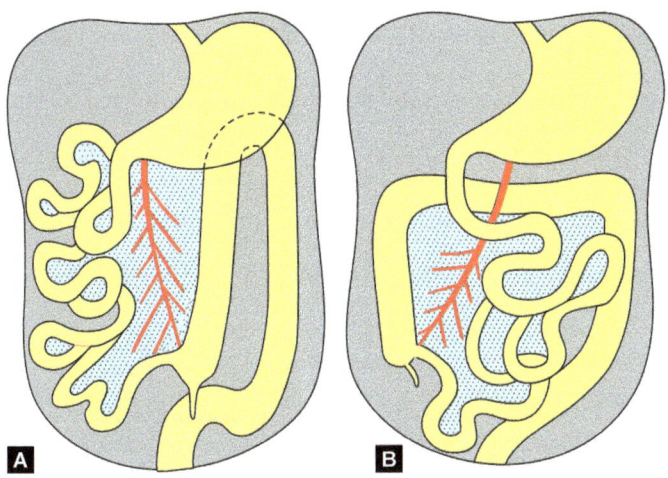

FIGS. 16.28A and B: Errors of rotation. (A) Nonrotation. Coils of small intestine lie in the right half of the abdomen, and colon in the left half; (B) Reversed rotation. The duodenum lies anterior to the superior mesenteric artery, and the colon crosses behind it.

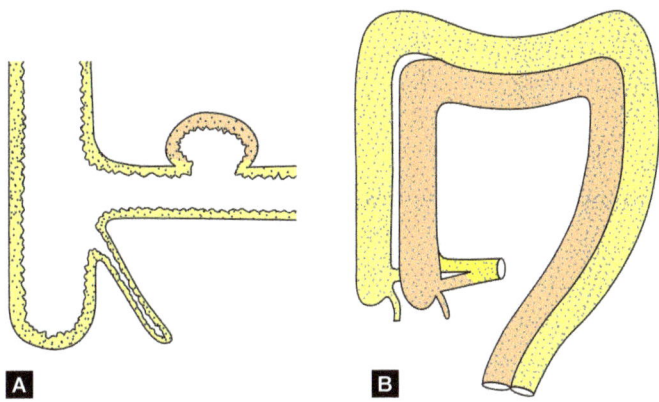

FIGS. 16.29A and B: Degrees of duplication of the gut represented by a cyst on the terminal ileum as in (A), and by duplication of the entire colon and terminal ileum as in (B).

Case Based Learning

Embryological Basis of Omphalocele

Case Scenario

A 30-year-old woman, who is pregnant for the third time with previous normal obstetric history, delivered a baby girl at 38 weeks gestation via cesarean section. Prenatal ultrasound at 20 weeks had identified an omphalocele, a congenital defect where the baby's intestines and other abdominal organs protrude outside the abdominal cavity through the base of the umbilical cord, covered by a thin membrane. The baby was immediately transferred to the neonatal intensive care unit (NICU) for further evaluation and surgical planning. Please refer to **Figure 16.30** and provide your observations and embryological explanations for this anomaly.

The observations as per the Figure 16.30 dead fetus with OEIS complex are as follows:

- **Omphalocele:** This condition is due to the failure of fusion of four ectomesodermal folds, resulting in a defect in the infraumbilical part of the anterior abdominal wall with abdominal organs lying outside. The prognosis is poor, with about 25% of affected infants dying before birth and 50–80% presenting with associated anomalies, including nearly 10% with chromosomal anomalies. In this case, associated anomalies were present. If no other defects are present and the omphalocele contains only herniated bowel, surgical correction is possible.

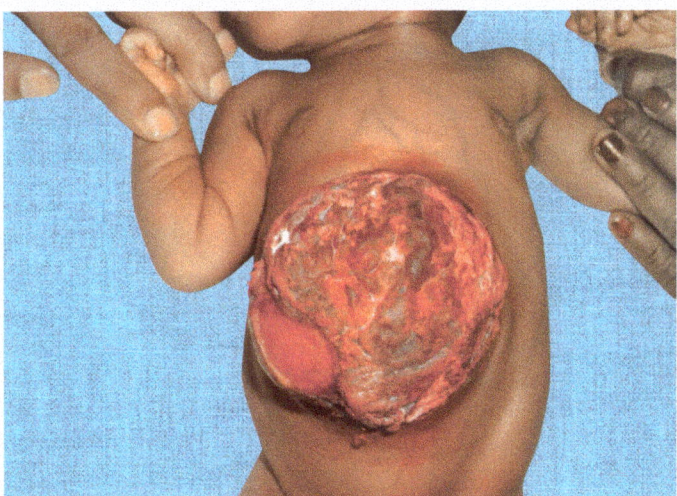

FIG. 16.30: Omphalocele.
(Reproduced with permission from Dr Piyush Gupta. Source: Ruchi Rai and DK Singh, Chapter 15. In: Gupta P, UG Textbook of Pediatrics, Jaypee Brothers Medical Publishers Pvt Ltd, 2023).

- **Omphalocele can be associated with OEIS complex** (Omphalocele, exstrophy of bladder or cloaca, imperforate anus, skeletal anomalies)
- **Biochemical:** Maternal serum AFP levels are often elevated in cases of omphalocele, as the defect allows more AFP to leak into the amniotic fluid and maternal circulation.
- **Ultrasound:**
  - Midline infraumbilical anterior abdominal wall defect, omphalocele
  - A thin, transparent membrane covering the herniated organs, distinguishing omphalocele from gastroschisis (where there is no covering membrane).

TIMETABLE OF SOME EVENTS DESCRIBED IN THIS CHAPTER

Age	Developmental events
16 days	Allantoic diverticulum starts appearing
3 weeks	Gut begins to acquire tubular form because of head and tail foldings. At the end of third week the buccopharyngeal membrane ruptures
4 weeks	The fusiform shape of the stomach becomes visible
5 weeks	Stomach rotates and dilates. Intestinal loop begins to form. Cecal bud can be identified
6 weeks	• Intestinal loop is well formed • Urorectal septum starts dividing the cloaca • Allantois and appendix become clearly visible. Stomach completes its rotation
7 weeks	• Septation of cloaca into rectum and urogenital sinus is completed • Intestinal loop herniates out of the abdominal cavity
8 week	Intestinal loop rotates counter clockwise
9 weeks	Anal membrane breaks down
3 months	• Head and tail foldings are completed • Herniated coils of intestine return to the abdominal cavity

HIGHLIGHTS

- **Endoderm,** which is at first in the form of a flat sheet, is converted into a tube by formation of head, tail and lateral folds of the embryonic disc. This tube is the gut.
- The gut consists of *foregut, midgut,* and *hindgut*. The midgut is at first in wide communication with the yolk sac. Later it becomes tubular. Part of it forms a loop that is divisible into *prearterial* and *postarterial* segments.
- The most caudal part of the hindgut is the cloaca. It is partitioned to form the *primitive rectum* (dorsal) and the *primitive urogenital sinus*.
- The *esophagus* is derived from the foregut.
- The *stomach* is derived from the foregut.
- **Duodenum:** The superior part and the upper half of the descending part are derived from the foregut. The rest of the duodenum develops from the midgut.
- The *jejunum* and *ileum* are derived from the prearterial segment of the midgut loop.
- The postarterial segment of the midgut loop gives off a cecal bud. The *cecum* and *appendix* are formed by enlargement of this bud.
- The *ascending colon* develops from the postarterial segment of the midgut loop.
- After its formation, the gut undergoes *rotation*. As a result, the cecum and ascending colon come to lie on the right side; and the jejunum and ileum lie mainly in the left half of the abdominal cavity.

Chapter 16: Alimentary System—II: Gastrointestinal Tract   187

Summary

- Derivatives of gut (**Fig. 16.31** and **Flowchart 16.1**).
- Developmental changes in the morphological parts of stomach (**Flowchart 16.2**).

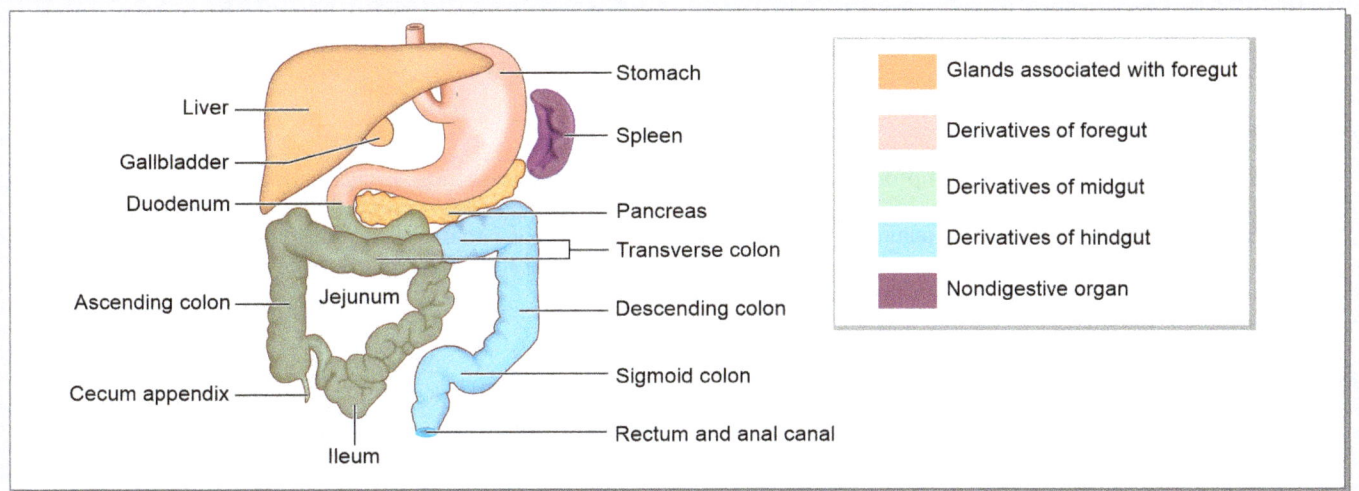

FIG. 16.31: Derivatives of gut.

FLOWCHART 16.1: Derivatives of gut.

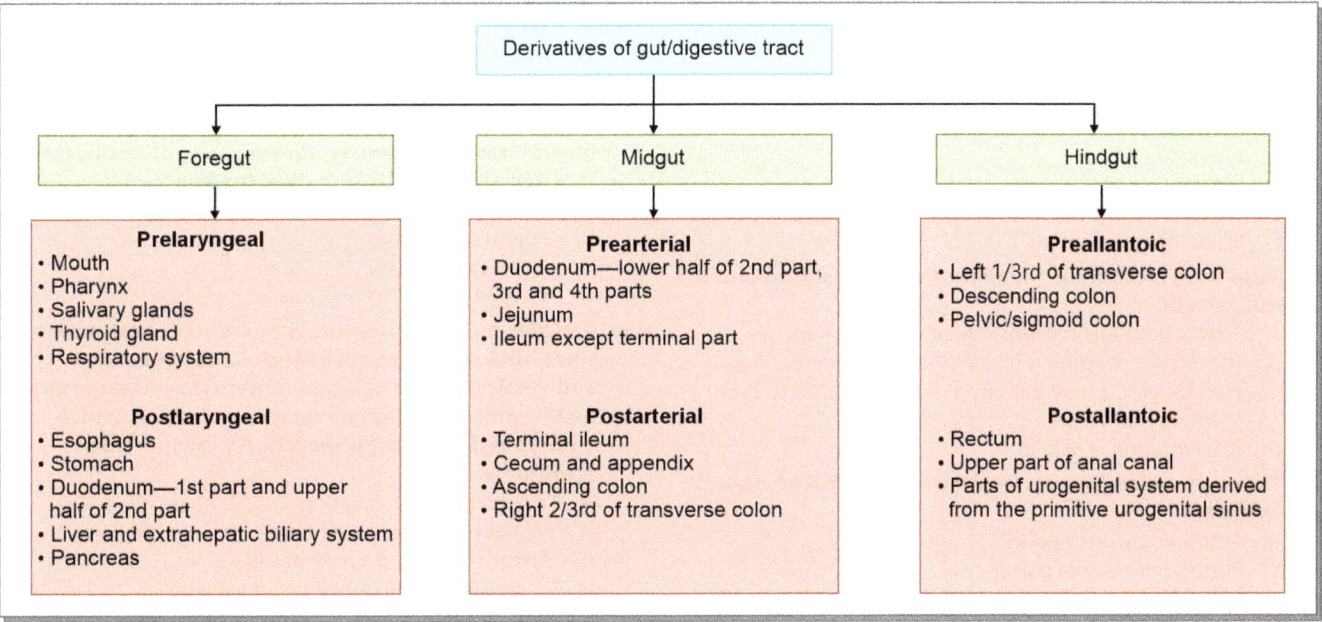

FLOWCHART 16.2: Developmental changes in morphological parts of stomach and mesogastria.

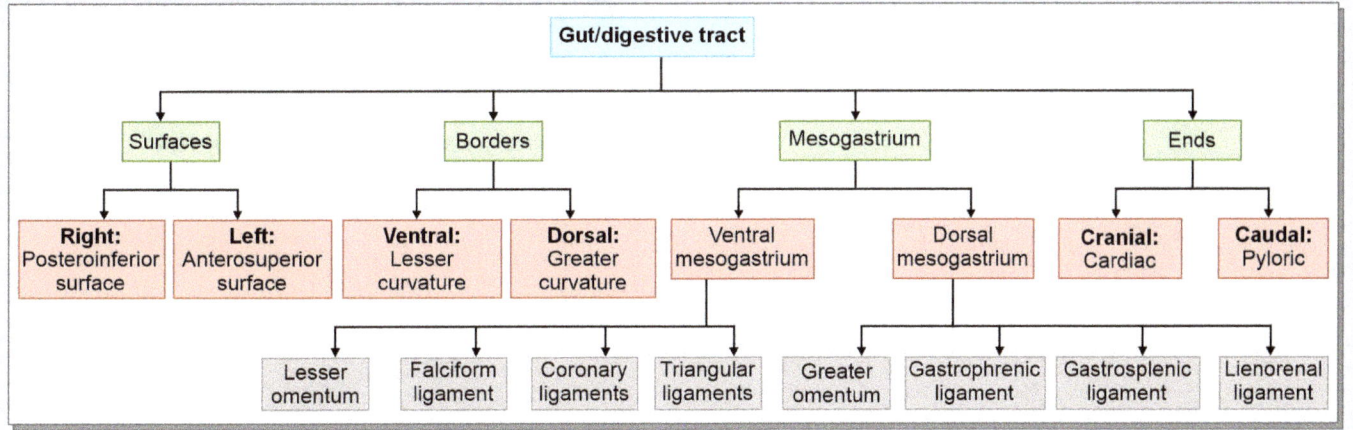

TEST YOUR UNDERSTANDING

REVIEW QUESTIONS

1. Discuss various derivatives of primitive gut.
2. Write a short note on tracheoesophageal fistula.
3. Describe development of esophagus with its clinical correlation.
4. Explain development of cecum and appendix.
5. Explain development of duodenum.
6. Discuss various congenital disorders affecting duodenum.
7. What are the stages in the rotation of gut?
8. Describe the errors in rotation of gut.

EXPLAIN WHY? (REASONING QUESTIONS)

1. Meckel's diverticulum might be symptomatic if it contains ectopic tissue.
2. Hirschsprung disease occurs due to a failure of neural crest cell migration.
3. Volvulus is more likely to occur when there is an abnormal rotation of the midgut.
4. Superior mesenteric artery is crucial for the development and functioning of the midgut.
5. The vagus nerve provides different functional control to the proximal and distal regions of the stomach.

MULTIPLE CHOICE QUESTIONS

1. **Urorectal septum develops between:**
   A. Urogenital sinus and cloaca
   B. Primitive urogenital sinus and primitive rectum
   C. Allantois and cloaca
   D. Anal canal and cloaca

2. **Physiological hernia is seen during the weeks:**
   A. 5th–12th
   B. 7th–11th
   C. 6th–10th
   D. 8th–12th

3. **Persistent part of vitellointestinal duct is called:**
   A. Allantois
   B. Cloaca
   C. Urachus
   D. Meckel's diverticulum

4. **Regarding rotation of gut all the following statements are true, *except*:**
   A. All rotations are in counterclockwise direction
   B. The axis for rotation is the superior mesenteric artery
   C. Prearterial segment of midgut loop elongates to form jejunum and ileum
   D. Total rotation is 360°

5. **The communication between the midgut and hindgut is called as:**
   A. Anterior intestinal portal
   B. Posterior intestinal portal
   C. Cloacal membrane
   D. Buccopharyngeal membrane

6. **Lower one-third of anal canal is derived from:**
   A. Primitive rectum
   B. Cloacal membrane
   C. Proctodeum
   D. Stomodeum

7. **A patient presents with symptoms of dysphagia and episodes of choking since birth. Imaging shows a blind-ending esophagus and a connection between the trachea and esophagus. Which embryological defect is responsible for this condition?**
   A. Failure of tracheoesophageal septation
   B. Anomaly in midgut rotation
   C. Defect in hindgut differentiation
   D. Abnormalities in dorsal mesentery

8. **A patient is diagnosed with Meckel's diverticulum and presents with symptoms of abdominal pain and gastrointestinal bleeding. Which embryological remnant is responsible for Meckel's diverticulum?**
   A. Vitelline duct
   B. Cloacal membrane
   C. Urorectal septum
   D. Allantois

9. **A 2-year-old child presents with chronic constipation since birth and episodes of abdominal distension and vomiting. Physical examination reveals an empty rectal vault upon digital rectal examination. Which embryological defect is most likely causing these symptoms?**
   A. Failure of foregut rotation
   B. Absence of midgut herniation
   C. Deficiency in hindgut innervation
   D. Incomplete gut vascular development

10. **A newborn is born with intestines protruding through a defect in the abdominal wall to the right of the umbilicus. Which embryological process is primarily disrupted in this condition?**
    A. Failure of midgut rotation
    B. Abnormalities in umbilical cord attachment
    C. Defect in pleuroperitoneal membrane formation
    D. Defective closure of the ventral body wall

Answers: 1. B   2. C   3. D   4. D   5. B   6. C   7. A   8. A   9. C   10. D

Liver and Biliary Apparatus; Pancreas and Spleen

CHAPTER 17

COMPETENCIES COVERED/LEARNING OUTCOMES

The student should be able to:
Note: These come under the development of the following structures developing in relations to those mentioned in competency.

| AN52.6 | Describe the development and congenital anomalies of: foregut, midgut and hindgut. |

The hepatobiliary system includes the largest gland of the body, liver along with gallbadder and bile ducts. They develops from the hepatic bud that arises from the foregut during the 4th week of development. Similarly, pancreas is also a gland that arises from endoderm of duodenum. The spleen, derived from mesoderm within the dorsal mesogastrium, begins to develop during the 5th week, playing a crucial role in hematopoiesis during fetal development.

LIVER AND BILIARY APPARATUS

THE LIVER

It has number of functions including exocrine, endocrine, hematopoietic, metabolic and phagocytic. It develops from endodermal *hepatic bud* from the ventral margin of terminal part of foregut that forms upper half of second part of duodenum.

- This bud proliferates and grows ventrally and cranially into the *ventral mesogastrium* **(Figs. 17.1A and B)** and passes through it into the *septum transversum* **(Fig. 17.1C)**.
- It further elongates and divides into a larger cranial part *pars hepatica* that forms the liver, and a smaller caudal part *pars cystica* that forms gallbladder and cystic duct **(Figs. 17.1B and C)**.
- Pars hepatica divides into right and left branches that become *right and left hepatic ducts* which contribute to form two solid *right and left lobes of the liver* **(Figs. 17.1D and E)**.
- The two lobes of the liver are of equal size during early development, but the size of left lobe reduces gradually **(Table 17.1)**. In the 3rd month of intrauterine life (IUL), the weight of liver is one-tenth of total body weight of fetus and occupies most of the upper abdomen. In the 7th month of IUL, it reduces to one-fifth of body weight. Various adult liver derivatives of different structures of developing liver are given in **Table 17.1**.

Formation of Hepatic Architecture

- The terminal parts of right and left hepatic ducts, when they reach septum transversum, clusters of cells called *hepatocytes* arise in the form of laminae. These laminae break up into interlacing columns called *hepatic trabeculae* **(Fig. 17.1E)**.
- In between hepatic trabeculae, the *hepatic sinusoids* develops from the mesenchyme of septum transversum.
- During this process, the *vitelline and umbilical veins* that are running longitudinally in the septum transversum, break up and establish communication with the hepatic sinusoids **(Fig. 17.2)**.
- Within the substance of liver, the hepatic ducts branch repeatedly and get canalized to acquire a lumen to form *intrahepatic biliary passages* **(Fig. 17.3)**.
- The hepatic trabeculae differentiate into the components of parenchyma, i.e., *liver cells* and *cells lining intrahepatic biliary system* **(Fig. 17.3)**. Septum transversum contributes to the *Kupffer cells, hematopoietic cells* and *connective tissue cells*.
- The mesoderm of the septum transversum forms the *capsule* and fibrous tissue basis of the liver.
- Reorganization of hepatic bud cells and mesenchymal cells forms the *hepatic lobule, including bile canaliculi, portal triads, and liver sinusoids* **(Fig. 17.3)**.

Formation of Peritoneal Folds of Liver

- With the rapid growth of developing liver into the septum transversum, the mesoderm of septum transversum between the liver and foregut becomes the *lesser omentum*, and the part between liver and ventral abdominal wall becomes the *falciform, triangular and coronary ligaments*.
- Lesser omentum and falciform ligament together are called *ventral mesentery/ventral mesogastrium*. Refer to Chapter 16 for more details about the ventral mesogastrium.

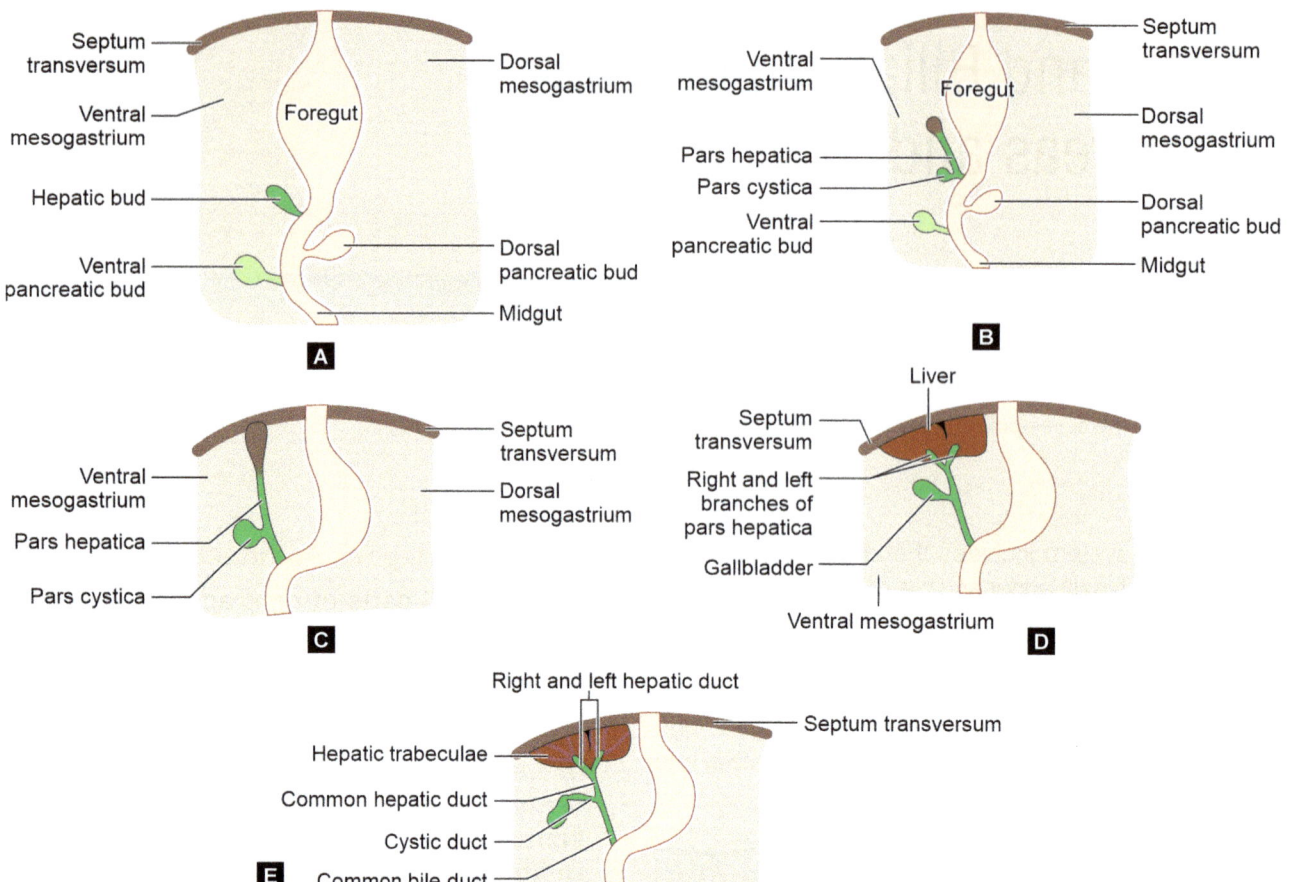

FIGS. 17.1A to E: Development of liver: (A) Origin of hepatic bud from the ventral wall of terminal part of foregut; (B) Hepatic bud growing into the ventral mesogastrium and dividing into pars hepatica and pars cystica; (C) Pars hepatica growing toward septum transversum through ventral mesogastrium; (D) Division of pars hepatic into right and left parts forming the right and left lobes of liver; (E) Formation of sheets of hepatic cells.

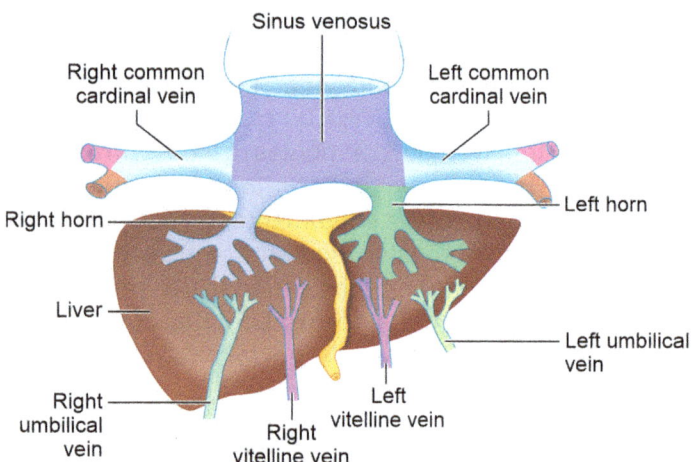

FIG. 17.2: Breaking up of umbilical and vitelline veins in septum transversum and their communication with hepatic sinusoids.

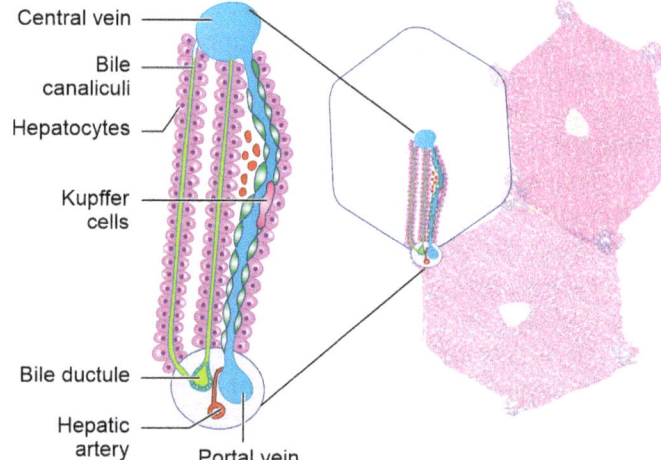

FIG. 17.3: Intrahepatic biliary apparatus. Reorganization of hepatic cells and blood vessels to form hepatic lobule, bile canaliculi, portal triad and sinusoids.

- During development, the *bare area* of the liver is triangular shaped area which forms where the liver remains in direct contact with the diaphragm and not covered by peritoneal folds which includes the falciform ligament and the lesser omentum.

Functions of Fetal Liver

- The fetal liver is an important center of blood formation *(hemopoiesis)* that begins in 6th week of IUL and continues up to birth. After birth, this function is carried out by spleen and bone marrow.

TABLE 17.1: Development of components of adult liver.

Adult component	Embryological derivative
Two lobes	Two terminal divisions of pars hepatica of hepatic bud in contact with septum transversum
Hepatic cells and intrahepatic biliary apparatus (parenchyma)	Hepatic bud (endoderm)
• Fibrous capsule of Glisson • Connective tissue cells • Kupffer's cells • Hematopoietic cells • Blood vessels	Septum transversum (intraembryonic mesoderm)
Sinusoids	Absorption and breakdown of vitelline and umbilical veins in septum transversum between hepatic trabeculae

- Bile formation begins when the fetus is about 12 weeks. The bile is responsible for the black color of the first stools *(meconium)* passed by the newborn.

Clinical correlation

Congenital Anomalies of Liver
Anomalies of liver are rare. Those that are reported in literature are **(Figs. 17.4A to E)**:
- Rudimentary left lobe **(Fig. 17.4A)**.
- Anomalous lobulation **(Fig. 17.4B)**.
- Reidel's lobe is an anatomical variant of the liver, presenting as tongue like extension of the right lobe **(Fig. 17.4C)**.
- Absence of quadrate lobe associated with absence of gallbladder **(Fig. 17.4D)**.
- Accessory liver in falciform ligament **(Fig. 17.4E)**.
- **Polycystic liver:** Failure of union of intrahepatic biliary canaliculi and ductules with extrahepatic bile ducts, results in the formation of cysts within the liver. It is usually associated with cysts in the kidney and pancreas.

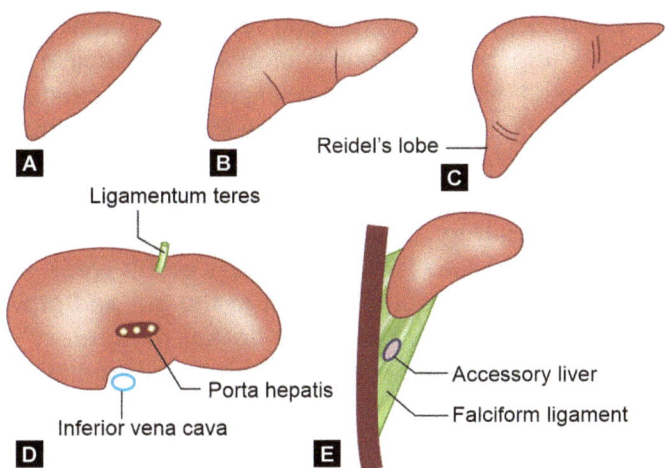

FIGS. 17.4A to E: Anomalies of the liver: (A) Rudimentary left lobe; (B) Anomalous lobation; (C) Reidel's lobe; (D) Absence of quadrate lobe associated with absence of gallbladder; (E) Accessory liver in falciform ligament.

- **Intrahepatic biliary atresia:** It is a serious anomaly and is not compatible with life unless a liver transplantation is undertaken.

GALLBLADDER AND BILIARY PASSAGES

- The pars cystica of the hepatic bud gives origin to the *gallbladder and cystic duct* **(Figs. 17.1B to E)**.
- The narrow part of hepatic bud between pars cystica and foregut forms the *common bile duct*.
- The undivided part of pars hepatica distal to the origin of pars cystica forms the *common hepatic duct* **(Fig. 17.1E)**.
- Initially, the bile duct opens on the ventral aspect of the developing duodenum. As the duodenal wall grows and rotates, the opening shifts to the dorsomedial aspect of the duodenum along with the ventral pancreatic bud (*see* **Fig. 17.16D**).

Clinical correlation

Anomalies of the Gallbladder
- **Anomalies of shape and development:**
  - *Phrygian cap:* Fundus may be folded on itself to form a cap-like structure **(Fig. 17.5A)**.
  - *Hartmann's pouch:* The wall of infundibulum may project downward as a pouch, which may be adherent to the cystic duct or even to the bile duct **(Fig. 17.5B)**.
  - *Septate gallbladder and duplication* **(Figs. 17.5C to E):** The lumen may be partially or completely divided by a septum, which may/may not extend into the cystic duct. The gallbladder may be completely or partially duplicated.
  - *Sessile gallbladder:* The gallbladder may directly open into the bile duct instead of the cystic duct **(Fig. 17.5F)**.
  - *Agenesis:* Absence of gallbladder due to failure of development of pars cystica.
  - Diverticula may arise from any part of the organ.
- **Anomalies of position:**
  - Transverse position on the under surface of right lobe, or under the left lobe.
  - *Floating gallbladder:* The gallbladder will be lined by peritoneum on all sides. It may be attached to the liver by a fold of peritoneum, or it may be completely free.
  - *Intrahepatic gallbladder:* It may be embedded in the substance of liver.

Anomalies of the Extrahepatic Duct System
- **Abnormal length:** There is considerable variation in the level at which various ducts join each other, resulting in abnormally long, or short ducts **(Figs. 17.6A to D)**.
- **Abnormal mode of termination:**
  - Cystic duct may join left side of common hepatic duct, passing either in front of it, or behind it, to reach its left side **(Figs. 17.6E to G)**.
  - Cystic duct may end in the right hepatic duct **(Fig. 17.6H)**.
  - Cystic duct may pass downward, anterior to the duodenum, before joining the common hepatic duct.
  - Bile duct may open into the pyloric, or even the cardiac end of the stomach.

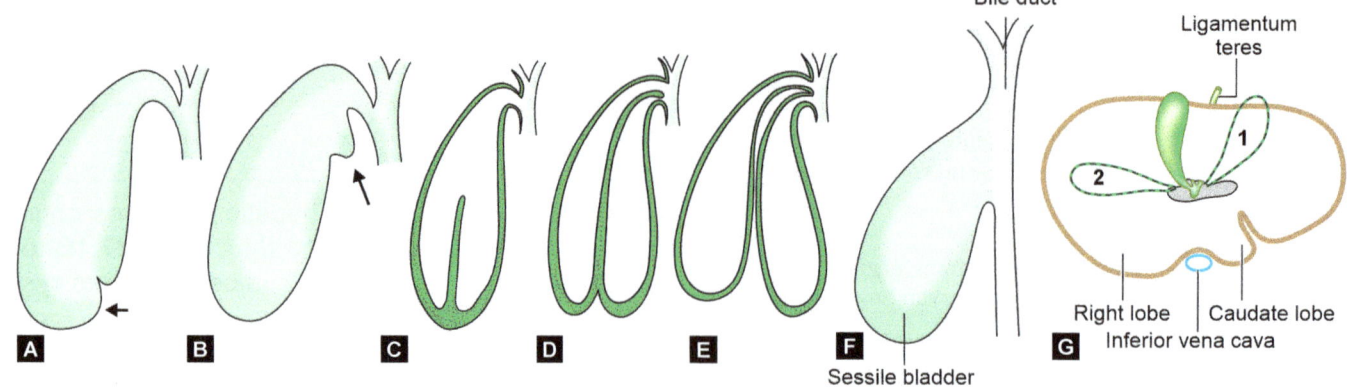

FIGS. 17.5A to E: (A) Phrygian cap; (B) Hartmann's pouch; (C to E) Duplication of gallbladder in which the lumen is partly (C and D) or completely (E) divided; (F) Sessile gallbladder in which the gallbladder may open directly into the bile duct; (G) Left-sided gallbladder (1) and transverse gallbladder (2).

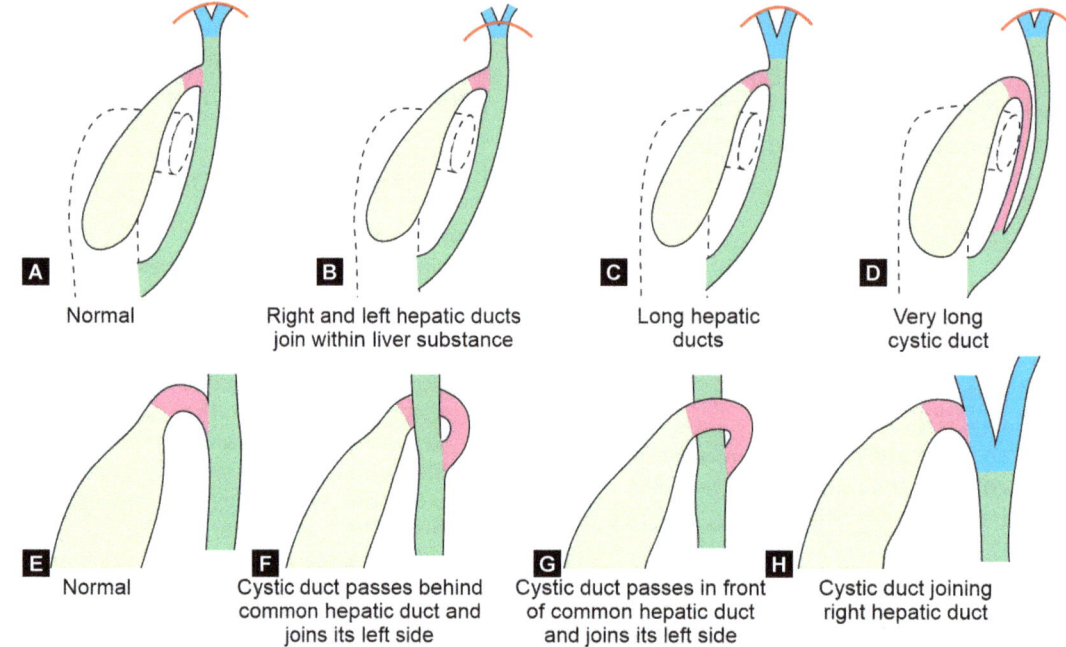

FIGS. 17.6A to H: Anomalies of extrahepatic duct system: (A) Normal; (B) Right and left hepatic ducts join within liver substance; (C) Long hepatic ducts; (D) Very long cystic duct; (E) Normal; (F) Cystic duct passes behind common hepatic duct and joins its left side; (G) Cystic duct passes in front of common hepatic duct and joins its left side; (H) Cystic duct joining right hepatic duct.

- **Atresia (Figs. 17.7A to F):** Parts of the duct system, and sometimes the whole of it, may be absent.
- **Duplication (Figs. 17.8A to C):**
  - Parts of the duct system may be duplicated.
  - Accessory ducts arising from the right lobe may terminate in the right hepatic duct, the cystic duct, the bile duct, or even directly into the gallbladder.

PANCREAS AND SPLEEN

PANCREAS

Functionally and microscopically, the pancreas is both exocrine and endocrine gland. But the developmental origin of the two structural and functional components is common. The pancreas develops from two endodermal buds the *dorsal and ventral pancreatic buds*.

- ❖ **Site of origin:** The dorsal and ventral pancreatic buds arise from the dorsal and ventral walls of terminal part of foregut (future second part of duodenum), caudal to hepatic bud **(Fig. 17.9A)** before rotation of midgut.
- ❖ The *ventral bud* arises in close relation to the hepatic bud, in the inferior angle between it and the duodenum (Fig. 17.9A).
- ❖ The *dorsal bud* is first to appear at 4th week and arises from the dorsal aspect of the gut and grows between the two layers of dorsal mesentery of duodenum. It is larger and cephalic to the ventral bud.

Development

Change in Pancreatic Buds

- ❖ Before the rotation of the duodenal loop, the ventral pancreatic bud is positioned on the ventral aspect, while the dorsal pancreatic bud is located on the

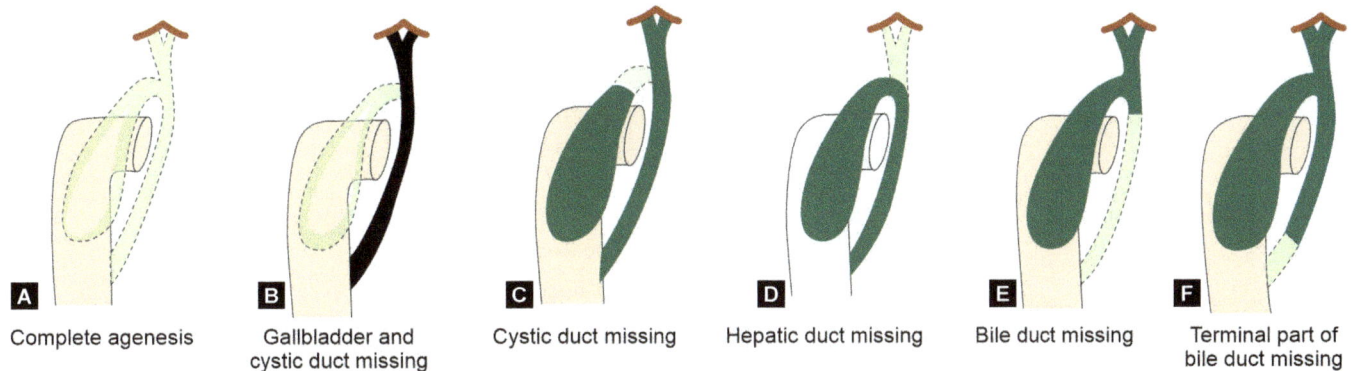

FIGS. 17.7A to F: Agenesis of parts of extrahepatic biliary tract. Missing parts indicated in light color: (A) Complete agenesis; (B) Gallbladder and cystic duct missing; (C) Cystic duct missing; (D) Hepatic duct missing; (E) Bile duct missing; (F) Terminal part of bile duct is missing.

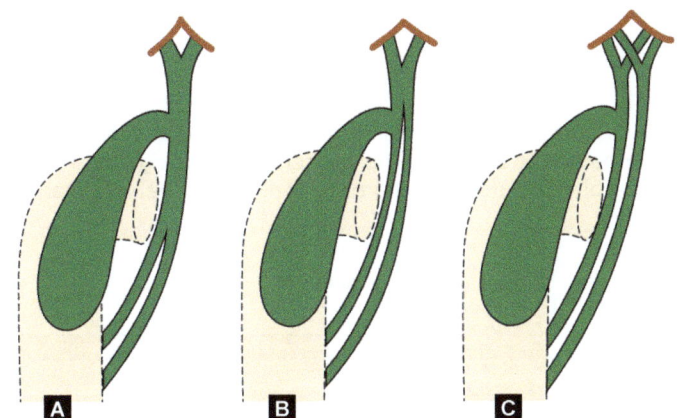

FIGS. 17.8A to C: Duplication of parts of extrahepatic biliary tract: (A) Partial duplication of bile duct; (B) Complete duplication of bile duct; (C) Complete duplication of bile duct, common hepatic duct and right and left hepatic ducts.

dorsal aspect of the duodenum (**Fig. 17.10A**). Following a 90-degree clockwise rotation of the duodenal loop to the right, the ventral pancreatic bud, along with the primitive bile duct, relocates to the right side, whereas the dorsal bud moves to the left side of the duodenum (**Figs. 17.9B and 17.10B**).

❖ Due to differential growth of wall of gut, the attachment of ventral pancreatic bud along with primitive bile duct (hepatic bud derivative) shifts to the left moving closer to the dorsal pancreatic bud (**Figs. 17.9C, 17.10C and D**).

Derivatives of Pancreatic Buds

❖ Pancreatic tissue formed from two buds fuse to form one mass in 7th week of IUL (**Figs. 17.9E and 17.10D**).

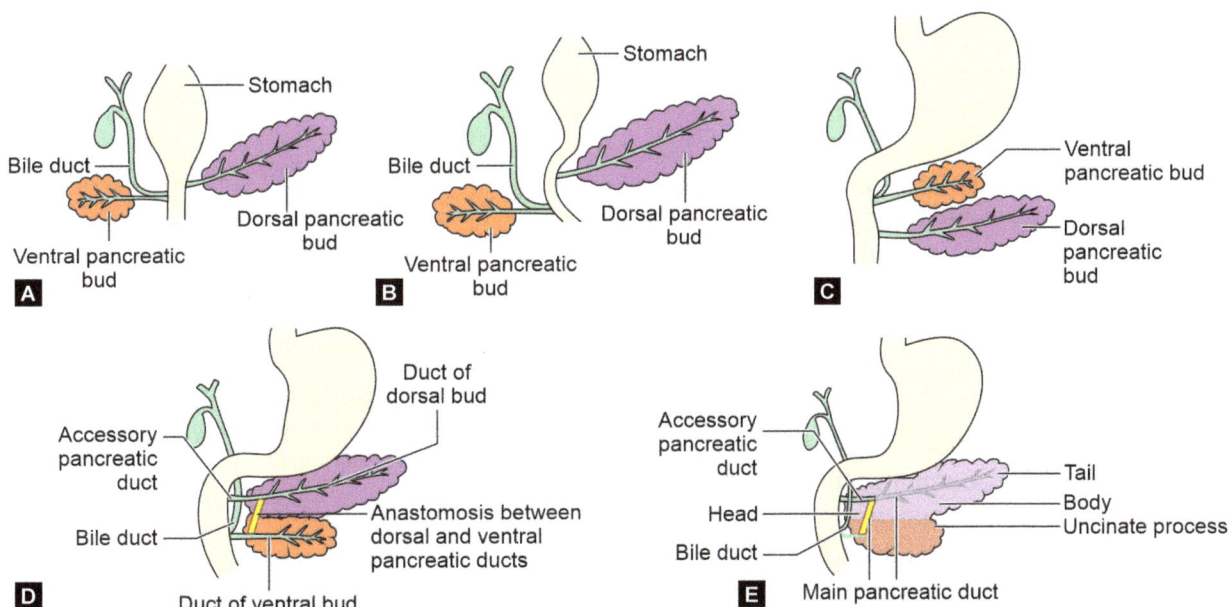

FIGS. 17.9A to E: Development of pancreas: (A) Appearance of dorsal and ventral pancreatic buds before rotation of gut; (B) Rotation of ventral and dorsal pancreatic buds with rotation of duodenal loop; (C and D) Shifting of ventral pancreatic bud to the left along with bile duct; (E) Fusion of dorsal and ventral pancreatic buds.

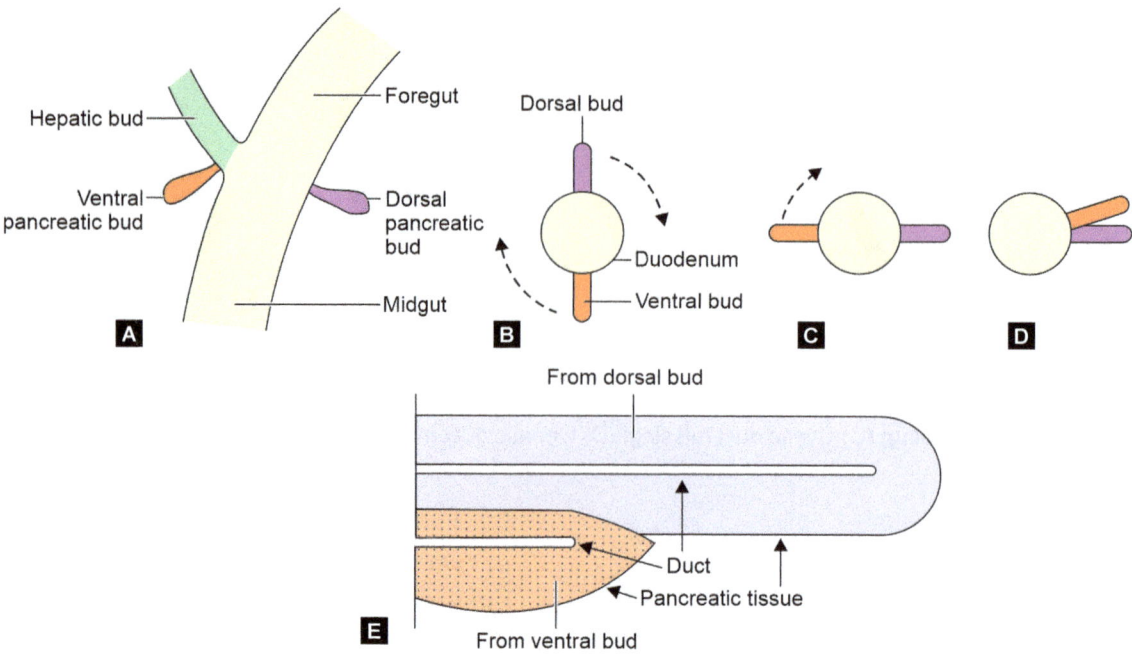

FIGS. 17.10A to E: Changes in relative position of pancreatic buds: (A and B) Initial position in which the ventral and dorsal buds lie in the direction indicated by their names; (C) Position after duodenal loop falls to the right. The ventral bud to the right and dorsal bud to the left; (D) Movement of ventral bud to the left lying close to dorsal bud with differential growth of duodenal wall. (E) Parts of pancreas derived from dorsal and ventral pancreatic buds.

- Ventral pancreatic bud forms *the lower part of head* and *uncinated process* of pancreas **(Fig. 17.9E)**.
- Dorsal pancreatic bud forms *upper part of head, neck, body and tail of pancreas* **(Fig. 17.9E)**.

Duct System of Pancreas

- Bedore anastomosis of dorsal and ventral buds, they open separately into duodenum **(Fig. 17.11A)**. The opening of dorsal pancreatic duct is 2.0 cm proximal to the opening of ventral pancreatic duct.
- With anastomoses of the two, a cross-communication between the two is established **(Fig. 17.11B)**.
- The *main pancreatic duct* is formed in its distal part, by the duct of dorsal bud, in its middle part by the oblique cross-communication between ducts of two buds and in its proximal part by the duct of ventral bud. The main pancreatic duct, therefore, opens into the duodenum at the *major duodenal papilla*, along with the bile duct **(Fig. 17.11C)**.
- The *accessory pancreatic duct* is formed by the proximal part of dorsal pancreatic duct (between the anastomosis and duodenum). It remains narrow and opens into the *minor duodenal papilla* 2.0 cm proximal to major duodenal papilla **(Fig. 17.11C)**.
- Repeated branching of the major and minor pancreatic ducts forms the interlobular and intralobular ducts and ductules **(Fig. 17.12)**.

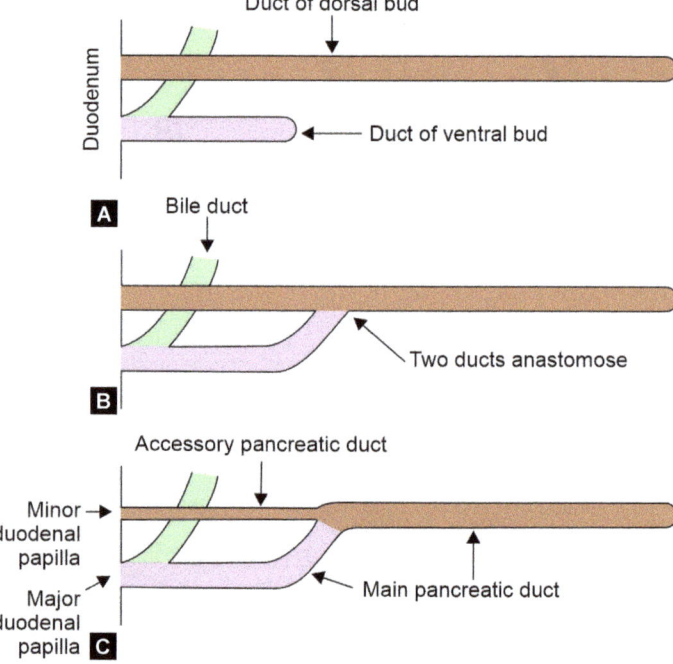

FIGS. 17.11A to C: Formation of duct system of pancreas. Distal part of main pancreatic duct is derived from the distal part of duct of dorsal bud, communication between dorsal and ventral ducts and from the duct of ventral bud. Accessory pancreatic duct is derived from the proximal part of dorsal pancreatic duct.

Secretory Elements (Fig. 17.12)

- The parenchyma develops from branching of endodermal pancreatic buds into the surrounding mesoderm which consists of exocrine and endocrine secreting units.

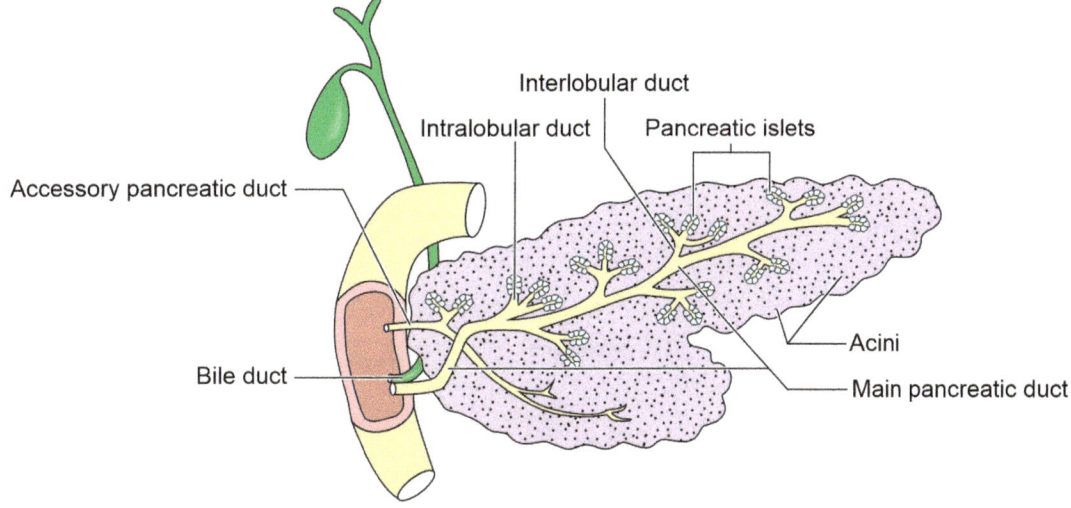

FIG. 17.12: Development of exocrine and endocrine components of pancreas. Major and minor ducts, interlobular and intralobular ducts, ductules, exocrine and endocrine units of pancreas are shown.

- The exocrine part of pancreas, consisting of acinar secreting units, develops from proliferation and reorganization of cells at the terminations (ductules) of duct system.
- The endocrine part, i.e., *islets of Langerhans*, develops from separation of groups of cells from the terminations of duct system. β-cells are more densely located in tail of pancreas.
  Though initially both buds were suspended in the respective mesogastria, due to their migration they occupy a position posterior to the peritoneum except the tail of pancreas which lies in the lienorenal ligament.

Functions of Fetal Pancreas

Endocrine function begins during embryonic period. In 7th week α-cells start secreting glucagon and by 10th week β-cells begins secreting insulin. Its exocrine function begins after birth.

Clinical correlation

Anomalies of the Pancreas
- **Annular pancreas:** It is a congenital anomaly where pancreatic tissue forms a ring around the second part of the duodenum **(Figs. 17.13A to C)**. Normally, the ventral pancreatic bud rotates and fuses with the dorsal pancreatic bud during fetal development. In this case, incomplete or abnormal rotation of the ventral pancreatic bud results in pancreatic tissue encircling the duodenum, causing varying degrees of duodenal obstruction.
  Clinical features are that of duodenal obstruction like vomiting and distention. Radiograph shows double bubble side as this condition is associated with duodenal stenosis or atresia.
  The surgical procedure for annular pancreas typically involves duodenal bypass or duodenoduodenostomy to alleviate duodenal obstruction caused by the encircling pancreatic tissue.

- **Divided pancreas (pancreas divisum):** It results from failure of fusion of parts of pancreas derived from dorsal and ventral pancreatic buds with each other **(Fig. 17.14A)**. They also have separate ductal system.
- **Accessory (ectopic) pancreatic tissue:** It may be found in stomach, duodenum, jejunum, Meckel's diverticulum, gallbladder and spleen.
- **Inversion of pancreatic ducts:** Embryonic arrangement of the ducts persists, and the greater part of the pancreas is drained by dorsal pancreatic duct through the minor duodenal papilla **(Fig. 17.14B)**.

SPLEEN

Spleen is a lymphoid organ. It develops from mesoderm in the dorsal mesogastrium, close to the developing stomach.

- It develops as a collection of mesenchymal cells in the dorsal mesogastrium to form small lobular masses of splenic tissue called *spleniculi* **(Fig. 17.15A)**.
- These lobules fuse to form a single mass of spleen. *Splenic notches* along the upper border of adult spleen indicates lobulated development of spleen.
- As the mesenchymal cells proliferate, the splenic mass projects in the left layer of dorsal mesogastrium **(Fig. 17.15B)**.
- The dorsal mesogastrium, in this region, can now be divided into a part extending from the stomach to the spleen *(gastrosplenic ligament)*, and another part extending from the spleen to the posterior abdominal wall. The latter part fuses with the posterior abdominal wall with the result that a fold of peritoneum now passes from the spleen to the left kidney *(lienorenal ligament)* **(Figs. 17.15B and C)**.

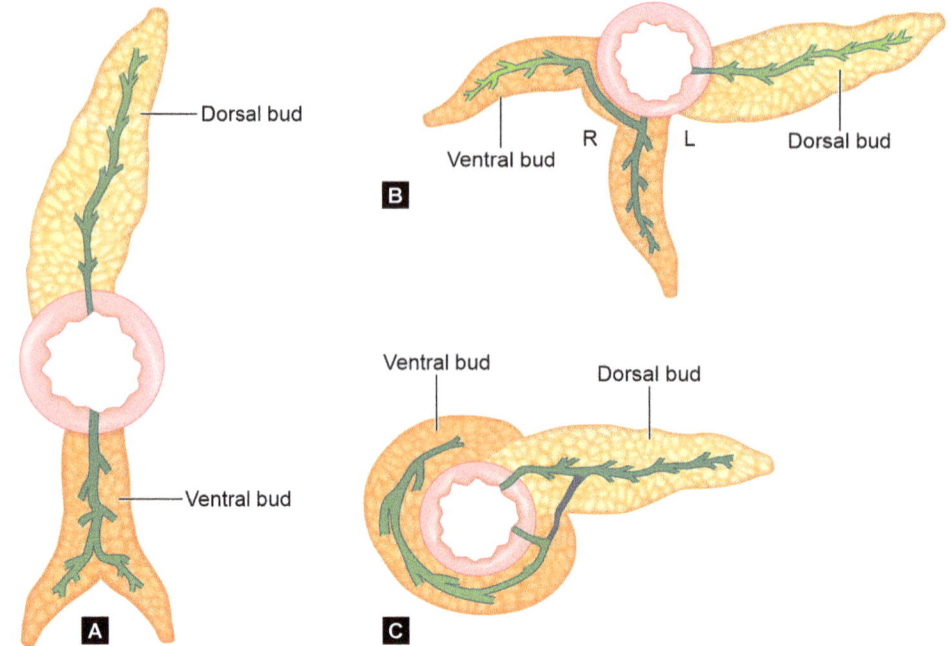

FIGS. 17.13A to C: Anomalies of pancreas—annular pancreas. Pancreatic tissue is completely surrounding the duodenum (R: right; L: left).

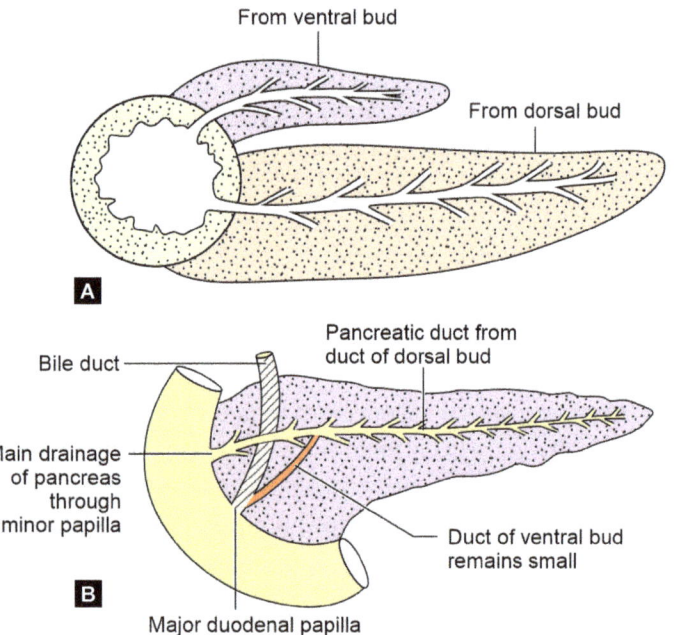

FIGS. 17.14A and B: Anomalies of pancreas: (A) Divided pancreas. The parts of pancreas arising from dorsal and ventral buds remain separate; (B) Inversion of pancreatic ducts where main pancreatic duct is formed entirely by the duct of dorsal pancreatic bud, and opens at the minor duodenal papilla. The duct of ventral bud is small.

- ❖ Because of this fusion and change in orientation of stomach, the spleen comes to lie on the left side and takes part in forming left boundary of the lesser sac of peritoneum **(Fig. 17.15D)**.
- ❖ Capsule, septa and connective tissue framework including reticular fibers develop from mesoderm. The mesenchymal cells differentiate into lymphoblasts and other blood forming cells.

Clinical correlation

Anomalies of Spleen
- The spleen may be *lobulated* due splenic lobules that are remnants of fetal splenic lobulation, persisting in adult life as variations in normal shape.
- **Agenesis** can be there.
- **Accessory spleen** may be seen:
  – At the hilum of spleen
  – In the gastrosplenic ligament
  – In the lienorenal ligament
  – Within the pancreas
  – Along the splenic artery
- **Situs inversus**—the spleen on the right side of the abdomen. The liver and pancreas are also reversed.

Chapter 17: Liver and Biliary Apparatus; Pancreas and Spleen

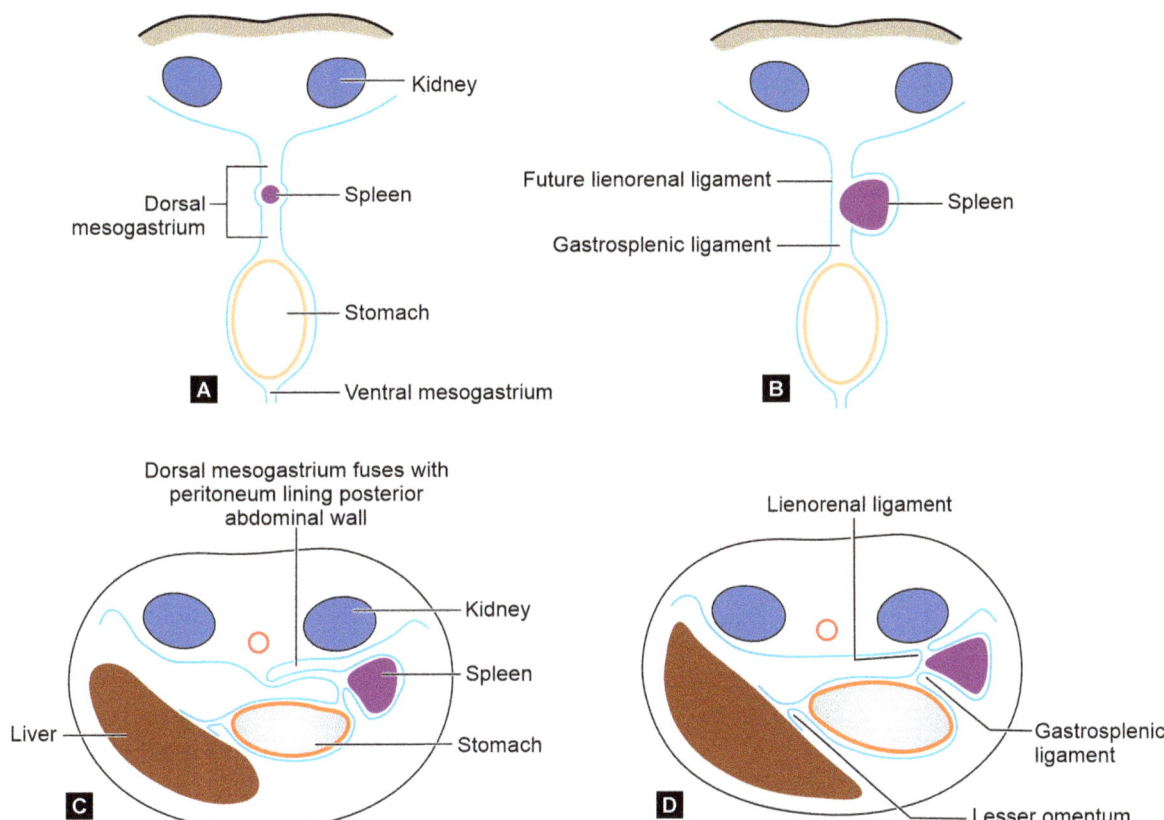

FIGS. 17.15A to D: Development of spleen: (A) Spleen appears in dorsal mesogastrium; (B) Spleen bulges into the left layer of dorsal mesogastrium. Dorsal mesogastrium division into gastrosplenic and lienorenal ligaments; (C) Fusion of dorsal mesogastrium with peritoneum of posterior abdominal wall, changing relationship of dorsal mesogastrium and lesser sac of peritoneum; (D) Change in orientation of stomach and spleen in relation to lesser sac and formation of gastrosplenic and lienorenal ligaments from dorsal mesogastrium.

TIMETABLE OF SOME EVENTS DESCRIBED IN THIS CHAPTER

Age	Developmental events
4 weeks	• Hepatic bud appears • Gallbladder bud appears • Formation of pancreatic buds (ventral and dorsal)
5–6 weeks	• Appearance of splenic lobules • Formation of hepatic cords and bile ducts • Cystic duct formation
6–7 weeks	Rotation and fusion of pancreatic buds
8–10 weeks	• Differentiation of exocrine and endocrine cells • Secretion of glucagon at 7th week • Secretion of insulin at 10th week
12 weeks	Secretion of bile

Chapter 17: Liver and Biliary Apparatus; Pancreas and Spleen

HIGHLIGHTS

- **Liver and biliary apparatus** develop from endodermal *hepatic bud*. The hepatic bud arises as an outgrowth from the ventral wall of terminal part of foregut.
- **Pancreas** develops from *two endodermal buds*, the dorsal and ventral pancreatic buds that arise at the junction of foregut and midgut. Most of the pancreas develops from dorsal bud. The ventral bud forms lower part of head and uncinated process.
- **Spleen** develops in the *mesoderm* of dorsal mesogastrium.

Summary

- Development of liver, biliary apparatus and pancreas (**Flowchart 17.1**).

FLOWCHART 17.1: Overview of development of liver, biliary apparatus and pancreas.

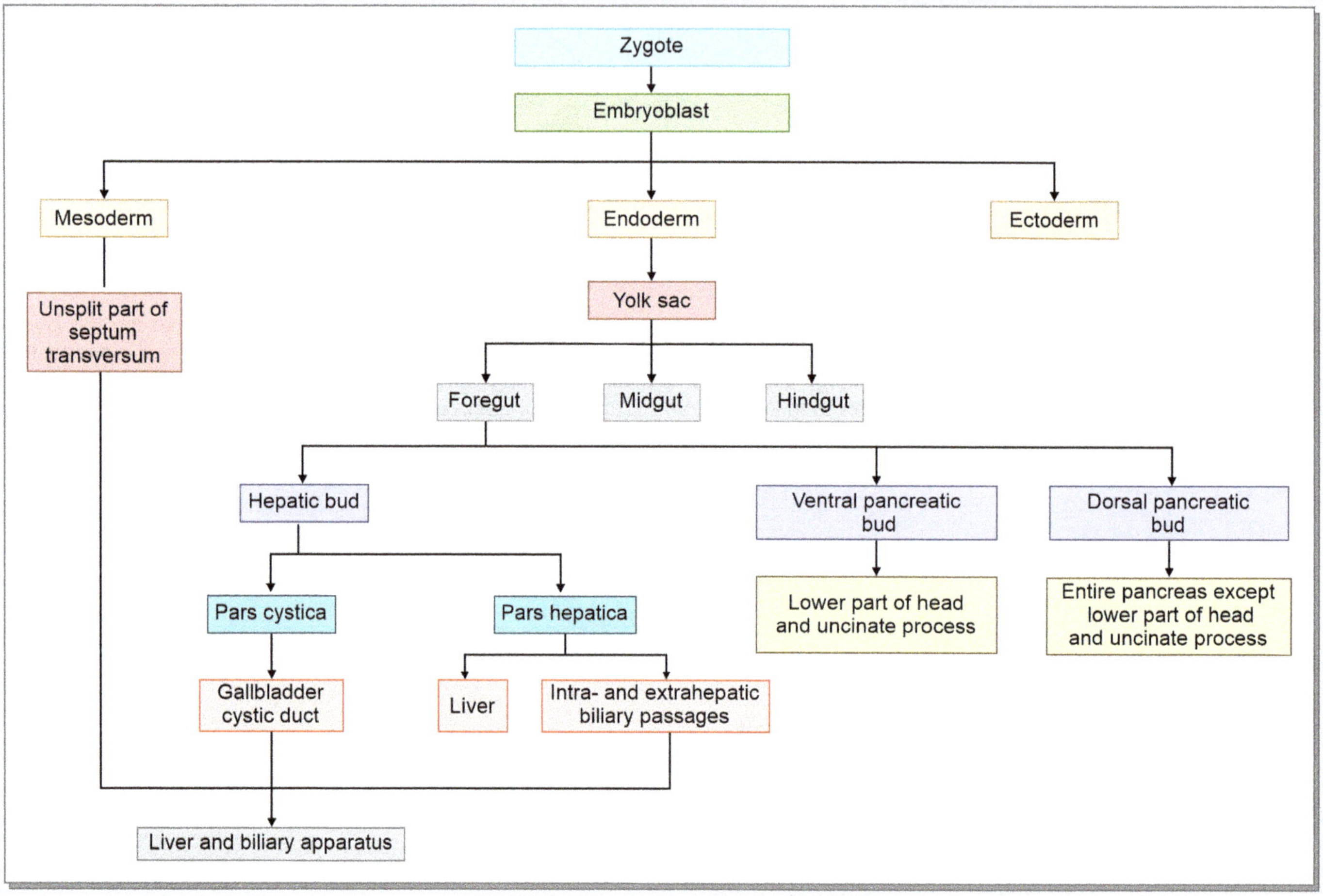

TEST YOUR UNDERSTANDING

REVIEW QUESTIONS

1. Explain the development of liver.
2. Write a short note on septum transversum.
3. Write a short note on Reidel's lobe.
4. Explain the development of extrahepatic biliary apparatus.
5. Explain the development of pancreas.
6. Explain the development of spleen.
7. Write a short note on annular pancreas.
8. Write a short note on anomalies of shape of gallbladder.

Chapter 17: Liver and Biliary Apparatus; Pancreas and Spleen

EXPLAIN WHY? (REASONING QUESTIONS)

1. There is a very large liver during embryonic development.
2. A splenic notch is considered a normal anatomical variant.
3. Abnormal development of pancreas can lead to duodenal obstruction.
4. Left lobe of liver is smaller than right lobe.

MULTIPLE CHOICE QUESTIONS

1. Accessory spleen can be found in:
   A. At the hilum of spleen
   B. In gastrosplenic ligament
   C. Along splenic artery
   D. All of the above

2. The part of pancreas that develops from the ventral pancreatic bud is:
   A. Upper part of head
   B. Body
   C. Tail
   D. Uncinate process

3. All the following are true statements about liver development, *except*:
   A. The hepatic sinusoidal endothelium is derived from vitelline and umbilical veins
   B. Kupffer cells are derived from septum transversum
   C. Hepatic duct epithelial cells are derived from splanchnic mesoderm
   D. Liver parenchyma is derived from the endoderm of hepatic bud

4. Pancreas divisum results from:
   A. Failure of fusion of dorsal and ventral pancreatic buds
   B. Duplication of pancreas
   C. Formation of single pancreatic bud
   D. Formation of more than two pancreatic buds

5. Liver weighs about one-fifth of body weight at which month of IUL?
   A. 3rd month
   B. 7th month
   C. 4th month
   D. 2nd month

6. A child is diagnosed with accessory pancreatic tissue located in the stomach. Explain the embryological basis of this anomaly.
   A. Incomplete rotation of the ventral pancreatic bud
   B. Persistence of the dorsal pancreatic duct
   C. Abnormal migration of pancreatic cells
   D. Duplication of the ventral pancreatic bud

7. A newborn presents with recurrent episodes of vomiting and failure to thrive. Imaging reveals a ring of pancreatic tissue encircling the duodenum. Which embryological event is responsible for this condition?
   A. Duplication of the dorsal pancreatic bud
   B. Incomplete fusion of the pancreatic buds
   C. Abnormal rotation of the ventral pancreatic bud
   D. Duplication of the ventral pancreatic bud

8. A 10 days child presents with jaundice and acholic stools. Imaging shows a complete absence of extrahepatic bile ducts. Which embryological process is likely disrupted in this condition?
   A. Failure of hepatic diverticulum formation
   B. Defective development of the cystic duct
   C. Abnormal migration of endodermal cells
   D. Failure of recanalization of bile ducts

Answers: 1. D 2. D 3. C 4. A 5. B
             6. C 7. C 8. A

18 CHAPTER

Body Cavities and Diaphragm

COMPETENCIES COVERED/LEARNING OUTCOMES

The student should be able to:

AN79.4	Describe the formation of intraembryonic coelom.
AN52.4	Describe the development of anterior abdominal wall.
AN52.5	Describe the development and congenital anomalies of diaphragm.

BODY CAVITIES

There are three body cavities, pericardial, pleural and peritoneal cavities, which are derivatives of the *intraembryonic coelom*. The pericardial cavity develops in relation to the heart, the pleural cavity in relation to lungs and the peritoneal cavity in relation to the abdominal viscera.

In the Chapter 6, a brief description of the formation of intraembryonic coelom (IEC) was presented. During the 3rd week of intrauterine life (IUL), with formation of this cavity the lateral plate mesoderm is split into a parietal (somatopleuric) and a visceral (splanchnopleuric) layer. The parietal and visceral layers of pericardium, pleura and peritoneum are formed from these layers of mesoderm. The mesodermal cells lining the cavities differentiate into a flattened epithelial lining called *mesothelium*. The mesothelium gives the peritoneum, pleura, and pericardium their smooth surfaces.

Formation of Serous Cavities from Intraembryonic Coelom

❖ The IEC gives rise to the serous cavities of the body. The IEC is in two halves, one on either side of the midline and joined together cranial to prochordal plate **(Figs. 18.1 to 18.3)**.

❖ Before the formation of head fold of the embryo the IEC is a horseshoe-shaped cavity which has a narrow midline portion and two lateral parts. The midline part lies caudal to septum transversum and cranial to prochordal plate near the cranial end of the embryonic disc **(Figs. 18.1 to 18.3)**. From this part of the coelom, the *pericardial cavity* is formed. The

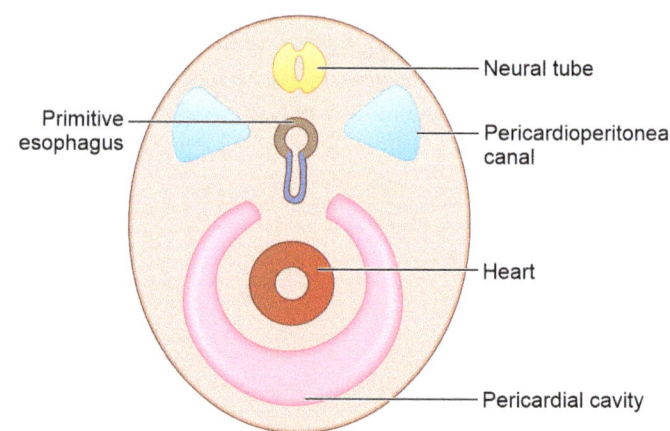

FIG. 18.2: Pericardial and pleuroperitoneal canals in relation to developing heart and foregut.

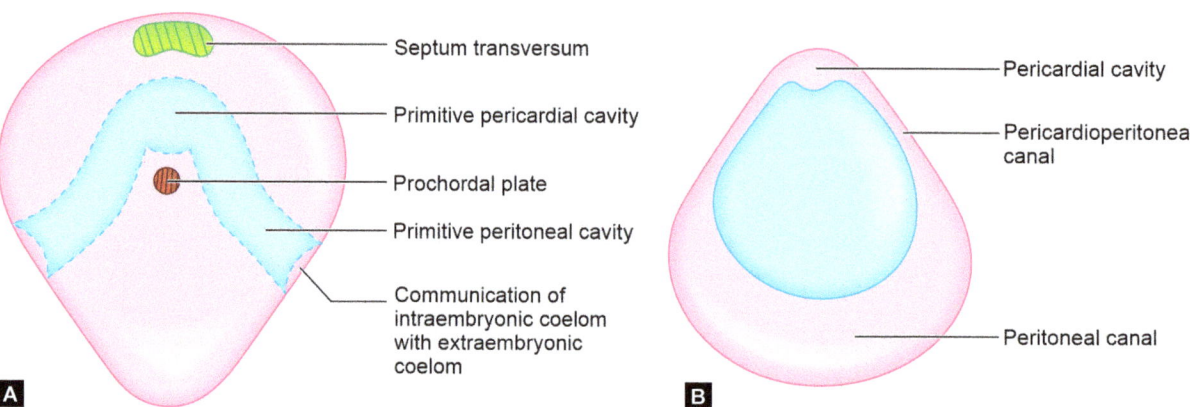

FIGS. 18.1A and B: Intraembryonic coelom and its subdivisions.

Chapter 18: Body Cavities and Diaphragm

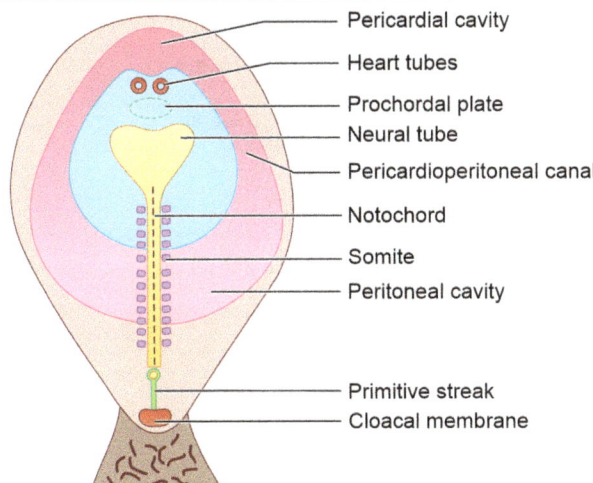

FIG. 18.3: Subdivisions of intraembryonic coelom and their location before head fold.

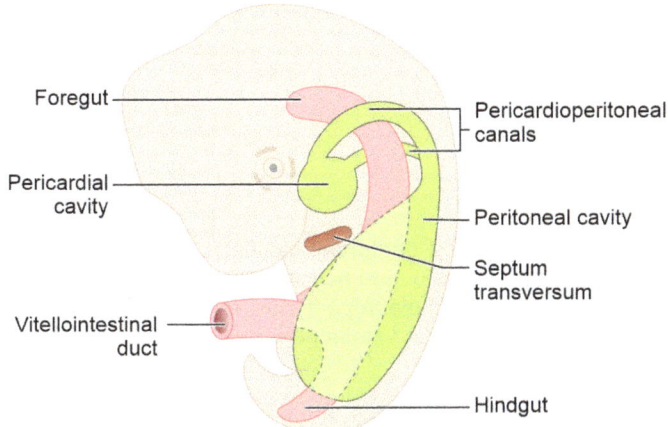

FIG. 18.4: Lateral view of embryo after head fold showing parts of intraembryonic coelom and their relationship to the gut.

two lateral limbs of the coelom form the *peritoneal cavities* (Fig. 18.3). At this stage, there is no pleural cavity as the lung buds are not developed.
- For some time, the pericardial and peritoneal cavities are connected to each other by a pair of narrow *pericardioperitoneal canals* (Fig. 18.3). The pericardioperitoneal canals undergo great enlargement to form the *pleural cavities* with elongation of lung buds. Later the two primitive peritoneal cavities fuse to form single *peritoneal cavity* (Figs. 18.4 and 18.5).

Pericardial Cavity

The midline part of intraembryonic coelom that lies near the cranial end of embryonic disc forms the pericardial cavity (Figs. 18.1 to 18.3).
- Before the formation of head fold the primitive pericardial cavity lies between the septum transversum (cranially) and prochordal plate (caudally) (Figs. 18.1 to 18.3). Between septum transversum and prochordal plate is the cardiogenic area where the primitive heart tubes

develop (Figs. 18.1 to 18.3). The heart tubes are in the floor of the developing pericardial cavity (Figs. 18.1 to 18.3).
- After the formation of head fold, the pericardial cavity and heart tube occupy a position ventral to the developing foregut, caudal to stomodeum, and cranial to the septum transversum (Fig. 18.4).

The development of pericardial cavity is closely related to the development of heart. Hence, it will be described in detail in the Chapter 20: Cardiovascular System.

Pleural Cavity

The right and left pleural cavities develop from right and left pericardioperitoneal canals (Fig. 18.4), i.e., cranial part of each limb of inverted U-shaped IEC.

Partitioning of Pleural, Pericardial, and Peritoneal Cavities

- Partitions develop in between cavities to separate definitive pericardial, pleural, and peritoneal cavities from one another.
- With the growth of lung bud into the pericardioperitoneal canal, the canal enlarges to form pleural cavity (Fig. 18.5A).
- A pair of membranous ridges appears in the cranial and caudal parts of lateral wall of pericardioperitoneal canal (Fig. 18.5B). They are:
  - A cranial *pericardiopleural fold* separates the pericardial cavity from the pleural cavities as they enlarge which later become the *pleuropericardial membranes* (Fig. 18.5C). This fold contains the common cardinal vein and phrenic nerve.
  - A caudal *pleuroperitoneal fold* enlarges and forms *pleuroperitoneal membrane* (Fig. 18.5C).

Formation of Pleural Cavity

- The pericardioperitoneal canals, connecting the pericardial and peritoneal cavities, are located dorsal to the septum transversum and on either side of the dorsal mesentery of the esophagus part of the foregut. With the formation of the head fold, the pericardial cavity moves to a position ventral to the foregut. The canals then wind backward on either side of the foregut.
- **Invagination of lung buds:** Lung buds, originating from the ventral aspect of the foregut, invaginate the pericardioperitoneal canals from the medial side.
- As lung buds enlarge to form the lungs, the pericardioperitoneal canals expand into the pleural cavities (Fig. 18.5A). Each pleural cavity communicates with the pericardial cavity through the pericardiopleural opening and with the peritoneal cavity through the pleuroperitoneal opening (Fig. 18.5B).

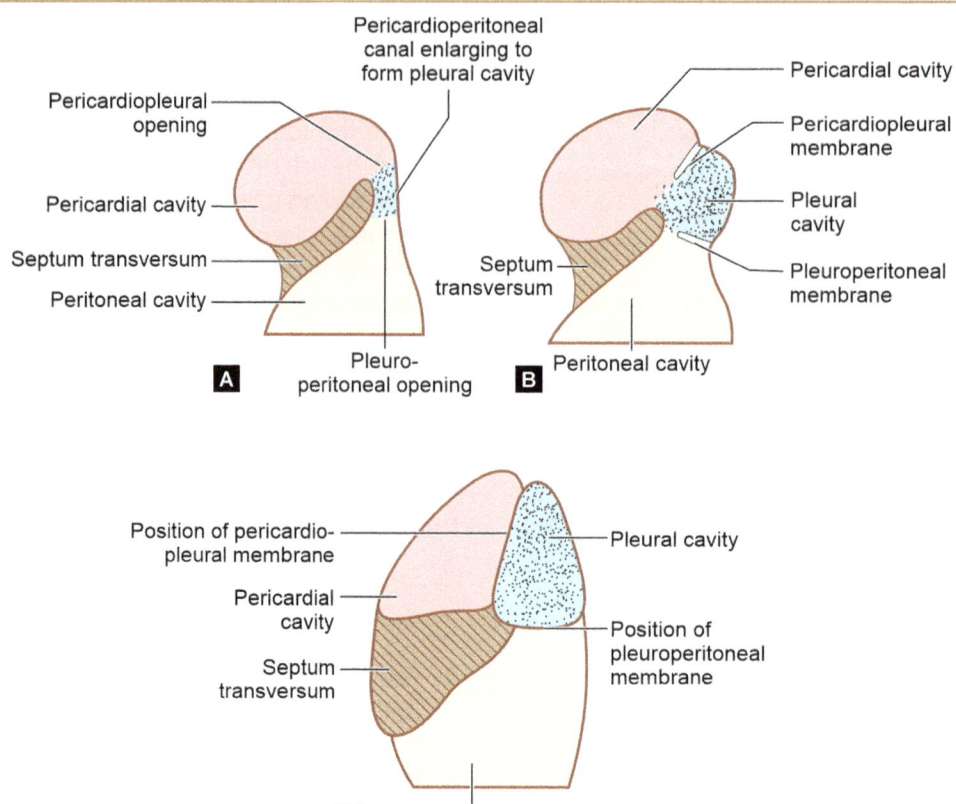

FIGS. 18.5A to C: Formation of pleural cavity and its separation from pericardial and peritoneal cavities: (A) Enlargement of pericardioperitoneal canal to form pleural cavity; (B) Communication between pleural cavity and pericardial and peritoneal cavities by pericardiopleural and pleuroperitoneal openings and formation of pleuropericardial and pleuroperitoneal folds; (C) Separation of pleural cavity from the pericardial and peritoneal cavities by formation of pericardiopleural and pleuroperitoneal membranes.

- These openings close by forming the pericardiopleural and pleuroperitoneal membranes **(Fig. 18.5C)**. These membranes are continuous with the septum transversum. The *pericardiopleural membrane* forms the lateral boundary for the *pericardiopleural opening* and contains the common cardinal vein and phrenic nerve. The *pleuroperitoneal membrane* closes the *pleuroperitoneal opening* and helps in completing the development of diaphragm.
- Initially, the pleural cavities are dorsolateral to the pericardium **(Fig. 18.6A)**. With lung expansion and heart descent, the pleural cavities extend into the body wall mesoderm, eventually lying lateral and ventral to the pericardium **(Fig. 18.6B)**. The pleural cavities also extend downward into the mesoderm forming the posterior abdominal wall and upward toward the neck **(Fig. 18.6C)**.
- With the expansion of the pleural cavity the mesoderm of the body wall splits into two parts: the outer part that forms the wall of the thorax, and an inner part over the pericardial cavity is called the *pleuropericardial membrane*. The phrenic nerve runs through this membrane and later this membrane forms the *fibrous pericardium* which explains the course of phrenic nerve over the pericardium.

Peritoneal Cavity

Peritoneal cavity is the largest cavity of the body. It is formed from the distal parts of two limbs of the horseshoe or inverted U-shaped intraembryonic coelom.
- The closure of pleuroperitoneal openings by pleuroperitoneal membranes separates the peritoneal cavity from the pleural cavities.
- With lateral folding of the embryo, the two limbs fuse to form single large peritoneal cavity but the cranial part of peritoneal cavity is still in two halves **(Figs. 18.7A and B)**.
- Up to 10th week of IUL, peritoneal cavity communicates with the extraembryonic coelom at the umbilicus **(Fig. 18.5)**. After the reduction of the physiological hernia and the return of the midgut loop into the abdomen, this communication is lost.
- The splanchnopleuric intraembryonic mesoderm forms the *visceral layer* of peritoneum while somatopleuric layer forms *parietal layer* of peritoneum.

Mesenteries of the Gut

- The line of reflection of parietal to visceral peritoneum for various gastrointestinal organs forms *mesentery*,

Chapter 18: Body Cavities and Diaphragm

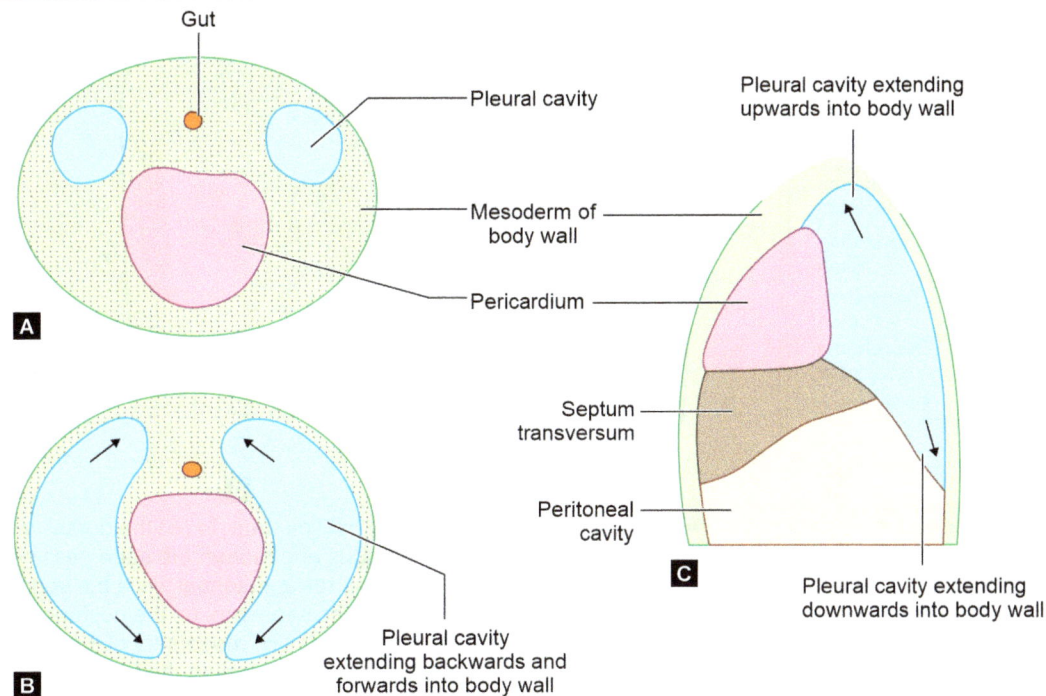

FIGS. 18.6A to C: Expansion of pleural cavities into the body wall: (A) Pleural cavities on dorsolateral aspect of pericardium; (B) Ventral and dorsal extension of pleural cavities into the body wall; (C) Upward and downward extension of pleural cavities into the body wall.

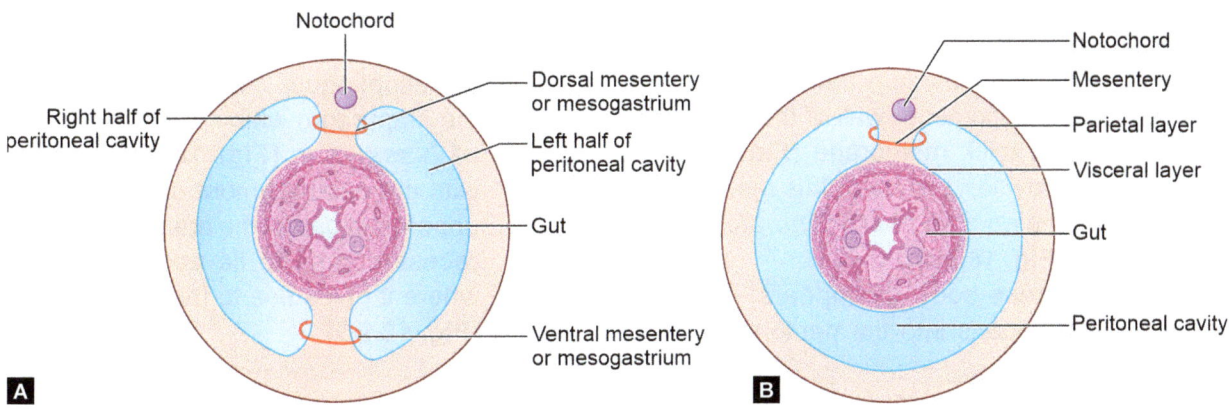

FIGS. 18.7A and B: Peritoneal cavity before (A) and after (B) lateral folding of embryo.

which is a double layer of visceral peritoneum connecting the primitive gut to the body wall, containing nerves and vessels.

- The mesentery connecting the ventral margin of primitive gut to the anterior abdominal wall is called *ventral mesentery*. It disappears except for the part connecting the distal part of foregut, i.e., caudal part of esophagus, stomach, and proximal duodenum to the anterior abdominal wall which is known as *ventral mesogastrium*. It get further splits by developing hepatic bud into a part the *lesser omentum* which connects foregut with liver, and a part connecting liver with anterior abdominal wall, the *falciform ligament*.
- Since the lower part of IEC is single, the midgut and hindgut do not have ventral mesentery.
- The mesentery that connects the dorsal margin of primitive gut to the posterior abdominal wall is called *dorsal mesentery*.
- The midline attachment of the dorsal mesentery becomes complicated due to gut rotation and parts becoming retroperitoneal, subdividing the peritoneal cavity into multiple pockets partially separated by peritoneal folds **(Figs. 18.8A to D)**.

Development of Lesser Sac or Omental Bursa

- The lesser sac, part of the peritoneal cavity behind the stomach and lesser omentum, communicates with the greater sac via the *Foramen of Winslow (epiploic foramen)* located behind the right free margin of the lesser omentum.

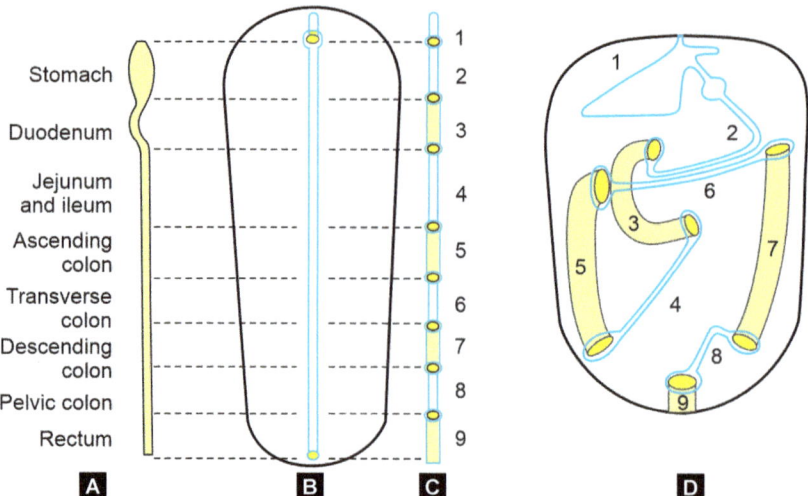

FIGS. 18.8A to D: Peritoneal relations of gut. In (A) the gut is shown as a simple midline tube. In (B) the dorsal wall of the abdomen is shown to indicate the midline attachment of the dorsal mesentery. The esophagus and rectum are seen passing through the wall. In (C) it is shown that alternate segments, i.e., 3, 5, 7 and 9 (odd numbers) become retroperitoneal while the segments 2, 4, 6 and 8 (even numbers) retain their mesentery and (D) shows the ultimate disposition of these segments on the posterior abdominal wall. (1) Represents the ventral mesogastrium, (2) The dorsal mesogastrium, (3) Duodenum, (4) The mesentery of the jejunum and ileum, (5) Ascending colon, (6) The transverse mesocolon, (7) Descending colon, (8) The pelvic mesocolon, and (9) Rectum.

- The development of lesser sac is closely related to the development of stomach.
- Three distinct processes are involved in the formation of lesser sac are:
  1. *Formation of pneumatoenteric recesses:*
     - The dorsal mesogastrium that connects the stomach to the posterior wall of the abdomen is, initially, a thick membrane **(Fig. 18.9A)**. Two small cavities appear in this membrane. These are the *right* and *left pneumatoenteric recesses* **(Fig. 18.9B)**.
     - The left recess soon disappears, and the right recess opens into the peritoneal cavity **(Fig. 18.9C)**. The cavity of the right recess now enlarges considerably and extends to the left to form the part of the *lesser sac* that lies *behind the stomach* **(Figs. 18.9D and E)**.
     - It also extends cranially on the right side of the esophagus, *behind the liver* and below the diaphragm which forms *superior recess of lesser sac* **(Fig. 18.9F)**. Subsequently, with the establishment of the diaphragm, the uppermost part of the cranial extension of right recess comes to lie above the diaphragm, where it gives rise to the *infracardiac bursa* **(Fig. 18.9G)**.

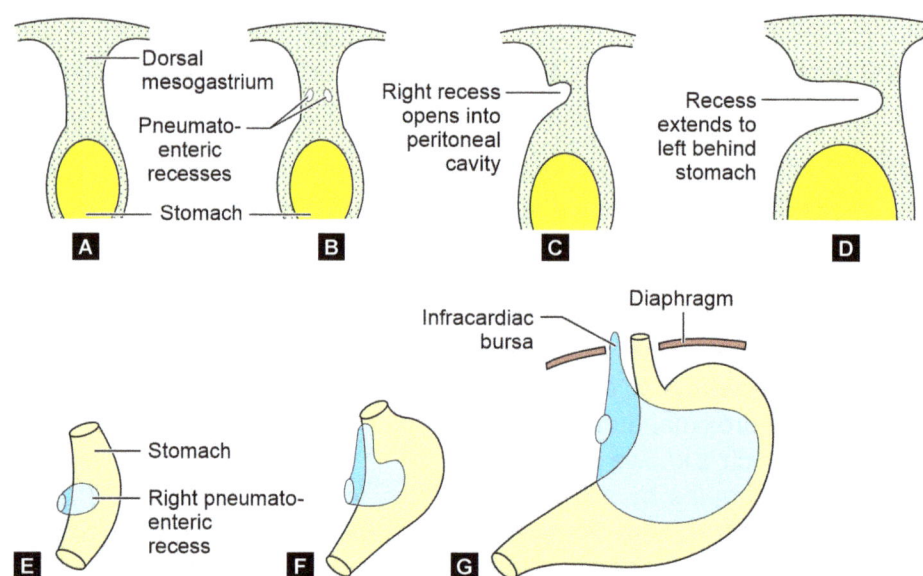

FIGS. 18.9A to G: Development of lesser sac: (A and B) Formation of right and left pneumoenteric recesses in dorsal mesogastrium; (C) Disappearance of left recess and opening of right into the peritoneal cavity; (D and E) Extension of right pneumoenteric recess to the left behind the stomach; (F) Cranial extension of pneumoenteric recess to form superior recess; (G) Extensions of the right pneumoenteric recess above the level of the diaphragm to form infracardiac bursa.

- *Formation of a part of lesser sac:*
  - While the right pneumatoenteric recess extends to the left, stomach changes its orientation, so that its posterior border (to which the dorsal mesogastrium was attached), now faces to the left. This border forms the *greater curvature*.
  - The ventral border (to which the ventral mesogastrium was attached), now faces to the right and forms the *lesser curvature* **(Figs. 18.10A and B)**. The ventral mesogastrium may now be called the *lesser omentum*.
  - As a result of this change in the orientation of the stomach, a part of the peritoneal cavity comes to lie behind the lesser omentum **(M in Fig. 18.10C)**. This part of the peritoneal cavity now forms *vestibule of the lesser sac*. It is continuous with the part of lesser sac lying behind the stomach [derived from the right pneumatoenteric recess (**N in Fig. 18.10C**)].
- *Divisions of dorsal mesogastrium and formation of lower part of lesser sac*
  - With the altered orientation of stomach **(Fig. 18.11A)** and the spleen development, the dorsal mesogastrium, which is attached to the greater curvature is subdivided into three parts **(Fig. 18.11A)**.
  - The part extending from the stomach to the diaphragm is the *gastrophrenic ligament*, from stomach to spleen is the *gastrosplenic ligament* and from the spleen to the left kidney is the *lienorenal ligament*. The latter two form the left margin of the lesser sac and the part of lesser sac extending between these ligaments is the *splenic recess of lesser sac*.
  - The part extending from the lower border of the stomach to the posterior abdominal wall **(Figs. 18.11B and 18.12A)** forms the *greater omentum*. The greater omentum undergoes enlargement which results in increasingly projection below the level of the stomach, and becomes folded on itself. The space within this fold forms the *inferior recess of the lesser sac* **(Fig. 18.12B)**.
  - The parts of lesser sac can be summarized in **Figure 18.12C**.

Development of Anterior Abdominal Wall

❖ Around the 4th week of development, lateral folding of the embryo brings the edges of the body wall toward the midline, where they fuse to form the *anterior abdominal wall*. It develops from mesoderm and ectoderm.

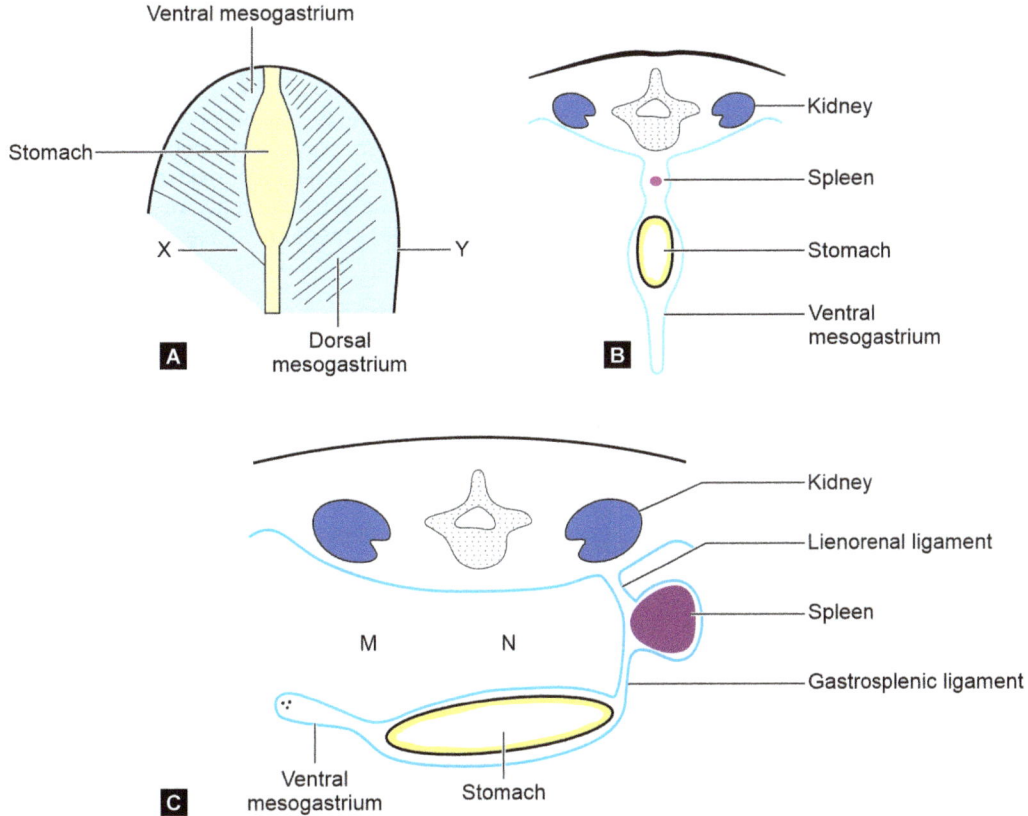

FIGS. 18.10A to C: Schemes to explain formation of the lesser sac: (A) Shows the dorsal and ventral mesogastria. Note that the ventral mesogastrium has a free border facing downward and forward; (B) The appearance if a section is cut in the plane XY in A; (C) Due to rotation of gut original ventral border of the stomach comes to lie on the right side. Two parts of the lesser sac—one derived from the right pneumoenteric recess and the part that comes to lie behind the ventral mesogastrium (lesser omentum).

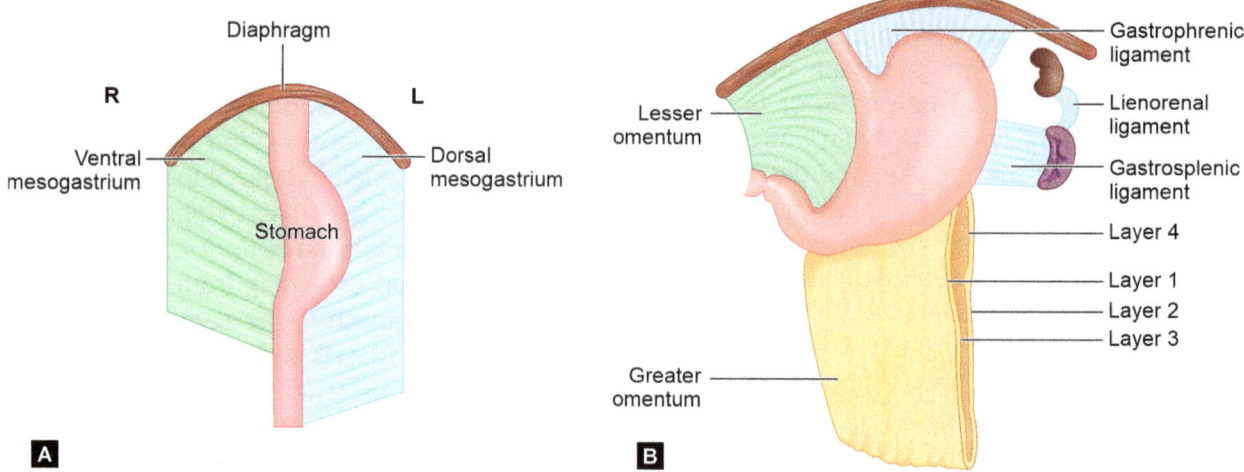

FIGS. 18.11A and B: Parts of the dorsal mesogastrium and their attachments to the stomach and to the posterior abdominal wall: (A) Attachment of dorsal and ventral mesogastria and (B) Formation of gastrophrenic, gastrosplenic, and lienorenal ligaments and greater omentum from dorsal mesogastrium. Elongation of greater omentum is shown with formation of four layers (1, 2, 3 and 4 from anterior to posterior) and cavity of lesser sac between the layers 3 and 4.

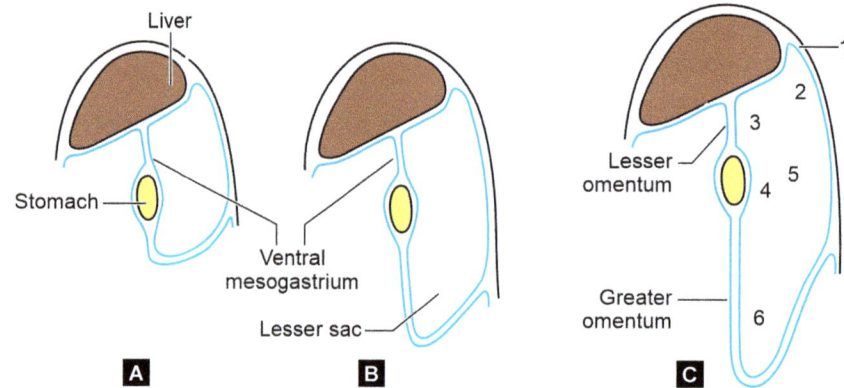

FIGS. 18.12A to C: Development of the lesser sac: Downward extension of the sac by elongation and folding of the greater omentum. The derivation of the parts numbered in (C) is (1) from cranial extension of right pneumoenteric recess above diaphragm (Infracardiac bursa), (2) cranial extension of right pneumoenteric recess on right side of esophagus (superior recess), (3) part of peritoneal cavity that comes to lie behind ventral mesogastrium, (4 and 5) right pneumoenteric recess in between gastrosplenic and lienorenal ligaments, i.e., splenic recess and (6) cavity produced by elongation and folding of greater omentum on itself (inferior recess).

- The muscles of the anterior abdominal wall originate from the myotomes of the somites which give rise to external oblique, internal oblique and transverse abdominis with vertical muscle, rectus abdominis.

DIAPHRAGM

Diaphragm is the dome-shaped musculotendinous partition that separates the thoracic and abdominal cavities. The pericardial and pleural cavities are above (or cranial to) it, whereas the peritoneal cavity is below (caudal to) it. The development of the diaphragm is, therefore, intimately related to the development of these cavities.

Development of Diaphragm

- Diaphragm is derived from **four mesodermal components** (Table 18.1). these are:
  - Septum transversum

TABLE 18.1: Embryological components of adult diaphragm.

Components of diaphragm	Embryological origin
Central tendon (tendinous part)	Septum transversum (unpaired)
Right and left crus (crura)	Dorsal mesentery of esophagus (unpaired)
Large, peripheral (posterolateral) part—costal part (muscular part)	Muscular (mesodermal) ingrowth from lateral body wall external to the part derived from pleuroperitoneal membranes
Small peripheral part—right and left (muscular part)	Pleuroperitoneal membranes (paired)
Musculature of diaphragm	Myotomic component of cervical somites C3, 4, 5

Chapter 18: Body Cavities and Diaphragm

- Pleuroperitoneal membranes
- Ventral and dorsal mesenteries of esophagus
- Mesoderm of body wall, including mesoderm around the dorsal aorta

❖ Fusion of these mesodermal components to form diaphragm. The formation of the septum transversum was considered in detail in Chapter 6.

❖ After the formation of head fold, the **septum transversum** migrates in a ventrocaudal direction and forms the thick incomplete partition between thoracic and abdominal cavities, leaving large gaps, whose components later result in diaphragm development.

❖ The partition between the thorax and the abdomen is completed when the **pleuroperitoneal canals** are closed by the formation of the pleuroperitoneal membranes **(Figs. 18.13A and 18.14A)**.

❖ During 6th week, septum transversum expands and fuses with ventral and dorsal mesenteries of esophagus and pleuroperitoneal membranes **(Figs. 18.13B and 18.14B)**. **Dorsal mesentery** of esophagus (mesoesophagus) contributes for the median portion containing the **two crura of the diaphragm**.

❖ During 9th–12th weeks of IUL the pleural cavities increase in size. Simultaneously, the diaphragm also enlarges, and this enlargement takes place at the expense of the lateral body wall **(Figs. 18.13C and 18.14C)**. Splitting of body wall tissue contributes for the peripheral parts of diaphragm outside the parts contributed by pleuroperitoneal membranes. With the result, the thorax also expands and extensions of pleural cavity into body wall forms costodiaphragmatic recess of pleura **(Fig. 18.6C)**.

❖ There is, however, considerable controversy as to how much of the diaphragm is formed from each of the constituents. According to some workers, the septum transversum forms only the central tendon, while according to others, it gives rise to almost the whole of the costal and sternal parts of the diaphragm. The crura of the diaphragm are formed from the mesoderm of the posterior abdominal wall (mesoesophagus/dorsal mesentery of esophagus), as a result of the downward extension of the pleural cavities into this region.

❖ **Innervation of diaphragm:**
  - During the 4th week of IUL, the septum transversum is at the level of C3, C4, and C5 somites. The ventral rami of these spinal nerves grow into the septum transversum and form the phrenic nerve.
  - The phrenic nerves enter the septum transversum through the pleuropericardial fold and membrane, which forms the fibrous pericardium, providing motor and sensory supply to the diaphragm's central part.
  - The diaphragm's peripheral part develops from the lateral body wall, with sensory supply from lower intercostal nerves, indicating the body wall's contribution to the diaphragm.

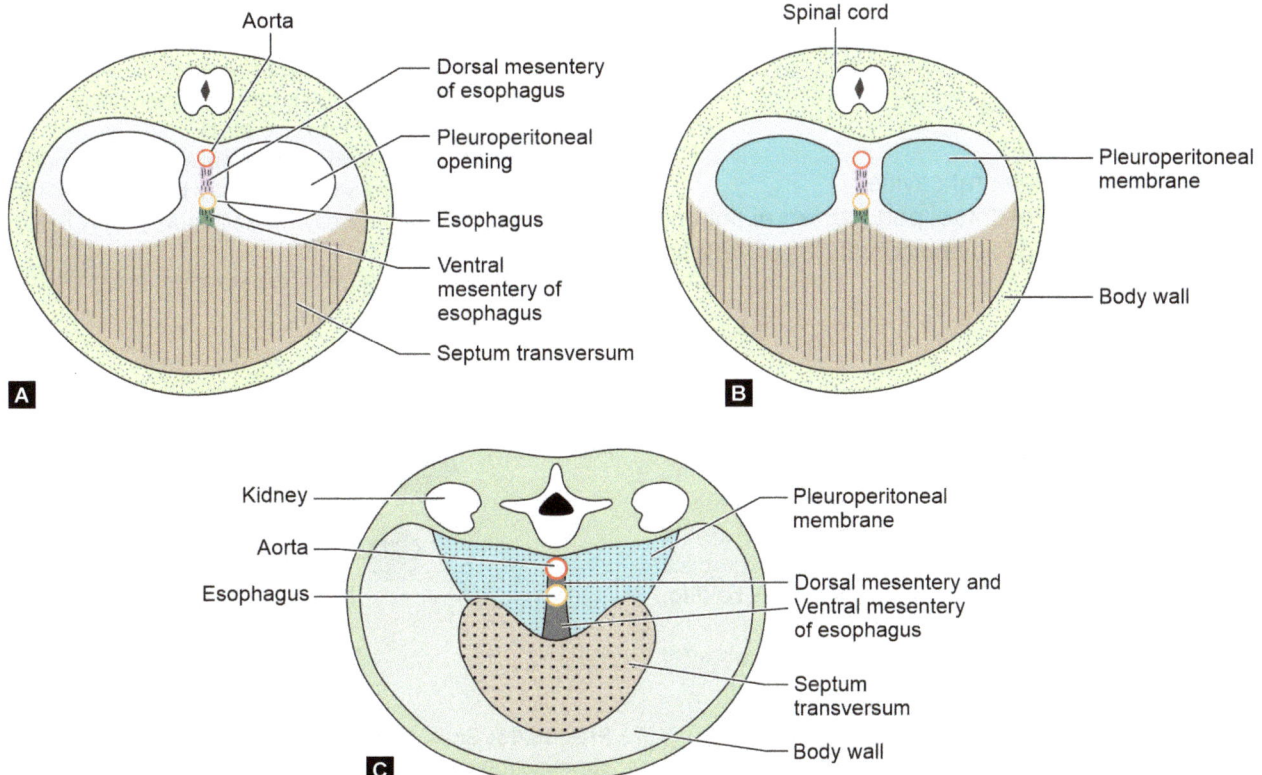

FIGS. 18.13A to C: Development of diaphragm: (A) Pleuroperitoneal canals, septum transversum and mesenteries of esophagus; (B) Closure of pleuroperitoneal canal their closure; (C) Expansion from body wall.

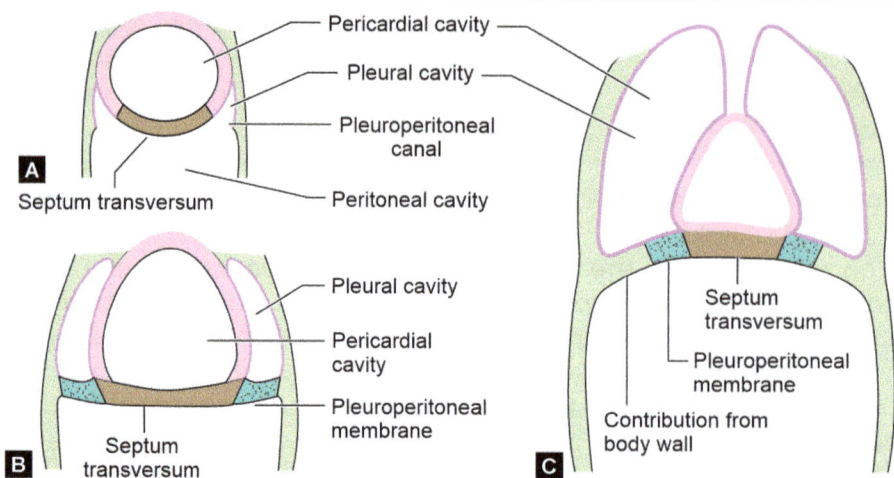

FIGS. 18.14A to C: Development of the diaphragm. Showing developmental components and how expansion of the pleural cavities into the body wall causes the wall to form part of the diaphragm.

❖ **Descent of diaphragm:**
- At first (4th week of IUL) the septum transversum is at cervical 3rd ± 5th segments.
- Later (6th weeks of IUL) the diaphragm descends to the thoracoabdominal junction opposite T7± T12 vertebra.
- At 8th week of IUL, the dorsal part of diaphragm reaches the level of T12/L1 vertebra due to rapid growth of dorsal part of body of embryo when compared to ventral part.
- When the diaphragm descends, it carries its nerve supply (phrenic nerve) with it.
- The factors responsible for descent of diaphragm are:
  - Elongation of neck
  - Descent of heart
  - Expansion of pleural cavities
  - Rapid growth of dorsal part (vertebral column) due to the head fold and curvatures of vertebral column.

Clinical correlation

Anomalies of Diaphragm
- **Diaphragmatic hernias:** Failure of development of parts of diaphragm resulting in gaps in the muscle. Abdominal contents may pass through these gaps to produce diaphragmatic hernias. Diaphragmatic hernias may be **(Fig. 18.15):**
  - *Posterolateral:* Due to failure of closure of pleuroperitoneal canal.
  - *Posterior:* Due to failure of development of crura.
  - *Retrosternal:* Due to the presence of abnormally large gap between sternal and costal parts of diaphragm. These are also known as *anterior* or *Morgagni hernia*. These account for 20% of diaphragmatic hernia.
  - *Central:* Through dome of diaphragm. These account for 2–5% of congenital diaphragmatic hernia. Occasionally one entire half (usually the left half) of the diaphragm may be absent.
  - *Posterolateral and posterior* are also known as *Bochdalek herniae*. These account for 75% of congenital diaphragmatic hernia and 75% of them are seen on left side. Abdominal contents (usually the stomach, small bowel, colon, liver or spleen) can herniate through the defect into the thoracic cavity. There will be associated hypoplasia of lung as the abnormal contents restrict the development of lung and there will be shift of mediastinum to the opposite side.
- **Accessory diaphragm:** It is rare and when present it partially subdivides the lung into two parts.
- **Congenital eventration of diaphragm:** Diaphragm may be thin and aponeurotic and may bulge upward into the thorax. The bulging may be unilateral or may be confined to a smaller area.

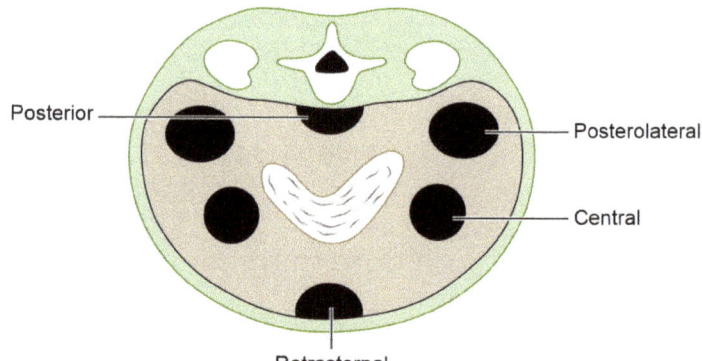

FIG. 18.15: Sites of congenital defects in diaphragm. Abdominal contents may pass through these gaps to produce diaphragmatic hernias.

Chapter 18: Body Cavities and Diaphragm

> **HIGHLIGHTS**
>
> - **Pleural, pericardial, and peritoneal cavities** develop from intraembryonic coelom. Before formation of head fold the intraembryonic coelom consists of right and left halves that are connected, across the midline, cranial to the prochordal plate.
> - **Pericardial cavity** is derived from the median midline part of intraembryonic coelom. With the formation of head fold of embryo this cavity comes to lie ventral to the foregut.
> - **Peritoneal cavity** is derived from the right and left limbs of intraembryonic coelom. After the formation of lateral folds of embryo, the two limbs unite to form single cavity.
> - **Pleural cavities** are formed from right and left pleuropericardial canals that connect pericardial and peritoneal cavities. Each pleuropericardial canal is invaginated by corresponding endodermal lung bud. Growth and expansion of lung bud leads to great enlargement of pleuropericardial canal and formation of pleural cavity.
> - **Diaphragm** develops in relation to the septum transversum. It receives contribution from pleuroperitoneal membranes, the body wall and the mesenteries of the esophagus.

Summary

- Development of diaphragm (see **Table 18.1**).
- Embryological origin of various peritoneal fold (**Table 18.2**).

TABLE 18.2: Development of various peritoneal folds.

Peritoneal fold in adult	Extent	Contents
Dorsal mesogastrium derivatives		
Gastrosplenic ligament	Stomach and spleen	Short gastric vessels and left gastroepiploic vessels
Gastrophrenic ligament	Stomach to diaphragm	Left inferior phrenic vessels
Lienorenal ligament	Left kidney to spleen	Splenic artery, tail of pancreas
Greater omentum	Between greater curvature of stomach to transverse colon	Right and left gastroepiploic vessels
Ventral mesogastrium derivatives		
Lesser omentum	Stomach and first part of duodenum to liver	• Along lesser curvature of stomach—right and left gastric vessels, gastric lymph nodes and gastric nerves • Right free margin—hepatic artery, portal vein and bile duct, hepatic plexus of nerves and lymph vessels
Falciform ligament	Liver to anterior abdominal wall	Ligamentum teres hepatis (left umbilical vein), paraumbilical veins
Coronary ligament (superior and inferior layers)	Liver to diaphragm	—
Triangular ligaments	Liver to diaphragm	—
Dorsal mesentery derivatives		
Transverse mesocolon	Transverse colon to posterior abdominal wall	Middle colic vessels
Mesentery of small intestine	Between posterior abdominal wall and small intestine (jejunum and ileum)	Superior mesenteric vessels, lymphatics, autonomic nerve plexus, lymph nodes and fat
Sigmoid mesocolon	Sigmoid colon to posterior abdominal wall	Sigmoid vessels, superior rectal vessels
Mesoappendix	Mesentery of ileum to appendix	Appendicular vessels

TEST YOUR UNDERSTANDING

REVIEW QUESTIONS

1. Discuss in brief the formation of body cavities.
2. Explain development of lesser sac.
3. Explain development of peritoneal folds.
4. Explain development of diaphragm.
5. Write a short note on congenital diaphragmatic hernia.

MULTIPLE CHOICE QUESTIONS

1. The structures passing through pleuropericardial membrane are:
   A. Common cardinal vein
   B. Phrenic nerve
   C. None of the above
   D. Both A and B

2. All the following contribute for the development of diaphragm, *except:*
   A. Pleuroperitoneal membrane
   B. Pleuropericardial membrane
   C. Septum transversum
   D. Cervical myotomes

3. All the following are derived from dorsal mesogastrium, *except:*
   A. Lienorenal ligament
   B. Gastrosplenic ligament
   C. Gastrophrenic ligament
   D. Lesser omentum

4. A newborn presents with respiratory distress. Imaging shows herniation of abdominal organs through a defect in the diaphragm into the thoracic cavity. Which embryological structure is primarily responsible for this condition?
   A. Pleuroperitoneal membrane
   B. Mesentery proper
   C. Mesocolon
   D. Falciform ligament

5. A patient presents with a rare condition where the liver is attached to the anterior abdominal wall by a visible fibrous band. This fibrous band is a remnant of which embryological structure?
   A. Ventral mesentery
   B. Dorsal mesentery
   C. Pleuropericardial membrane
   D. Mesocolon

6. A patient presents with recurrent infections of the lungs. Imaging reveals a congenital abnormality where the pleural cavity on one side is smaller than normal. Which embryological structure is likely affected in this condition?
   A. Pleuroperitoneal membranes
   B. Pericardioperitoneal canals
   C. Mesentery proper
   D. Parietal pleura

Answers: 1. D 2. B 3. C 4. A 5. A 6. D

Respiratory System

CHAPTER 19

COMPETENCIES COVERED/LEARNING OUTCOMES

The student should be able to:

AN25.2	Describe development of pleura and lung.
AN25.4	Describe embryological basis of tracheoesophageal fistula.

The respiratory system is divided into two parts *anatomically,* upper and lower respiratory tracts.
1. **Upper respiratory tract** includes nasal cavities, paranasal air sinuses, pharynx, and larynx.
2. **Lower respiratory tract** includes trachea, bronchi, terminal bronchioles, respiratory bronchioles, and alveoli.

We have discussed the development of nasal cavities, paranasal sinuses in chapter 14 and about pharynx in chapter 15. In this chapter we are going to discuss the development of larynx, and lower respiratory tract components.

OVERVIEW OF RESPIRATORY SYSTEM DEVELOPMENT

The respiratory system is *endodermal* in origin as it develops from a median *endodermal diverticulum* of the foregut *(respiratory/laryngeal diverticulum)* **(Fig. 19.1A)** and the adjacent *splanchnopleuric intraembryonic mesoderm* which forms connective tissue, cartilage and muscles.

Development of Respiratory (Laryngotracheal) Diverticulum

- During the 4th week of IUL, a groove appears on ventral pharyngeal wall, called a *laryngotracheal groove* **(Fig. 19.1B)**. The laryngotracheal groove is bordered on both sides by the 6th pharyngeal arch **(Fig. 19.2)**.
- As the laryngotracheal groove deepens, a midline evagination known as *respiratory diverticulum* or *laryngotracheal diverticulum* from the ventral wall of pharyngeal part of foregut appears **(Fig. 19.1A)**.
- This evagination is caudal to hypobranchial eminence (epiglottis) and is in the floor of developing pharynx **(Fig. 19.2)**.
- It extends in caudal direction and elongates **(Figs. 19.1B and C)**.

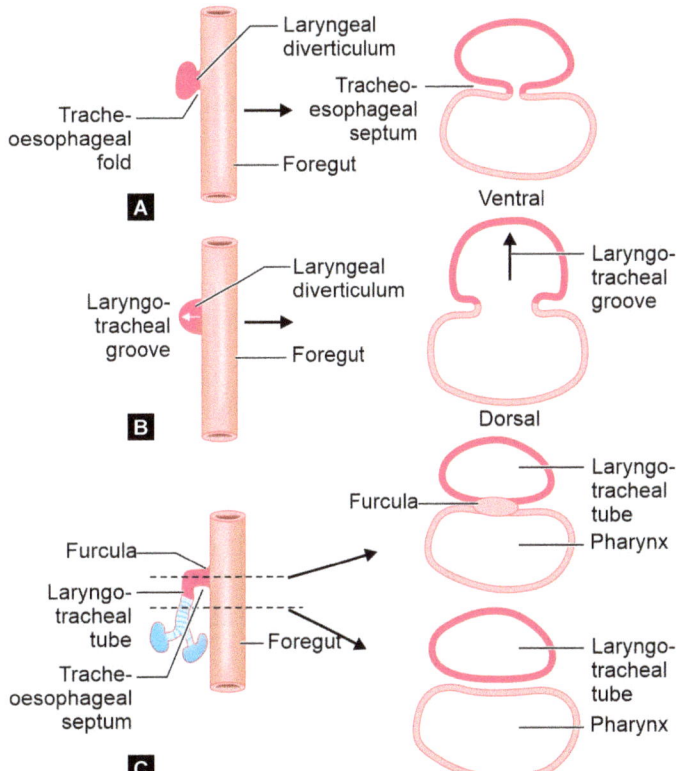

FIGS. 19.1A to C: Development of laryngotracheal or respiratory diverticulum. A median endodermal respiratory diverticulum from the ventral wall of foregut and its separation from the foregut and its subdivisions.

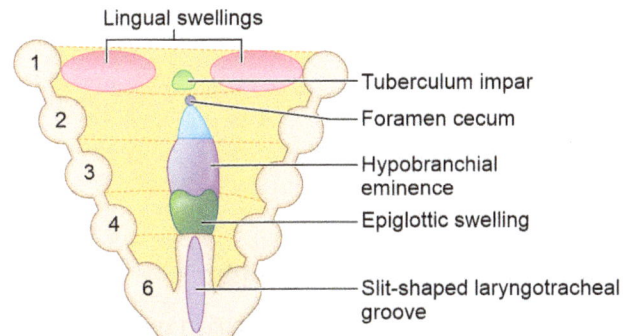

FIG. 19.2: Development of laryngotracheal groove in relation to floor of pharynx.

Derivatives of Respiratory Diverticulum

- The free caudal end grows downward to enter the thorax and becomes bifid to form the *right and left bronchial/lung buds* (Fig. 19.3A).
- Cranial to the bifurcation is *laryngotracheal tube* and it forms the *larynx* and *trachea*, while the lung buds form the *bronchi and lung parenchyma* (Fig. 19.1C and 19.3A to D).
- Each lung bud invaginates into the pericardioperitoneal canal.
- The right and left pericardioperitoneal canals form right and left *pleural cavities* (Fig. 19.3B).

Separation of Laryngotracheal Tube from the Foregut

- At the caudal part of respiratory diverticulum, two lateral folds known as *tracheoesophageal folds* grow medially and fuse to form *tracheoesophageal septum* (Fig. 19.1C). This septum separates the trachea from esophagus.
- The cranial part of the septum stops growing to form sagittal slit, the *inlet of larynx* or *furcula of His* through which the laryngotracheal tube communicates with the pharynx (Fig. 19.1C).

DEVELOPMENT OF LARYNX

The larynx develops from the cranial most part of the laryngotracheal diverticulum.

Inlet of Larynx

- The communication between the laryngotracheal tube and the pharynx persists as a slit-like orifice, the *inlet of the larynx (laryngeal inlet)* or *furcula of His* (Fig. 19.4A).

- Mesenchyme of 4th and 6th pharyngeal arches proliferates around inlet to form *thyroid, cricoid,* and *arytenoid cartilages*.
- The slit-like laryngeal inlet initially becomes U-shaped. Proliferation of mesenchyme from the 4th and 6th arches changes the U-shaped inlet into a T-shaped orifice. Reorganization of developing cartilages results in the characteristic adult shape of the laryngeal inlet (Figs. 19.4A to C).
- The caudal part of hypobranchial eminence (4th arch) forms *epiglottis* and *cuneiform cartilages*. The upper part of arytenoid swelling forms the *arytenoid* and *corniculate cartilages*, whereas the lower part of it forms the *cricoid cartilage*.

Developmental Components of Larynx

- The internal lining of larynx is derived from *endoderm*.
- The laryngeal muscles are derived from *branchial mesoderm* as indicated by their nerve supply. All intrinsic muscles by *recurrent laryngeal nerve* (6th arch) except cricothyroid which is supplied by external laryngeal branch of *superior laryngeal nerve* (4th arch).

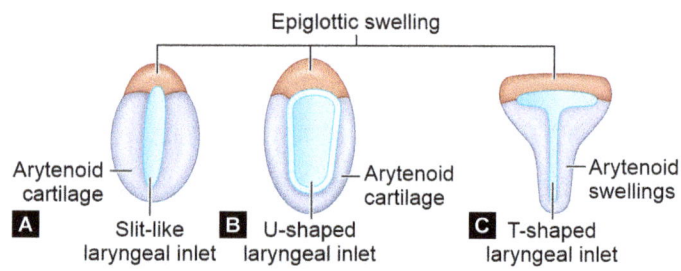

FIGS. 19.4A to C: Changes in shape of laryngeal inlet: (A) Slit-shaped (B) U-shaped; (C) T-shaped.

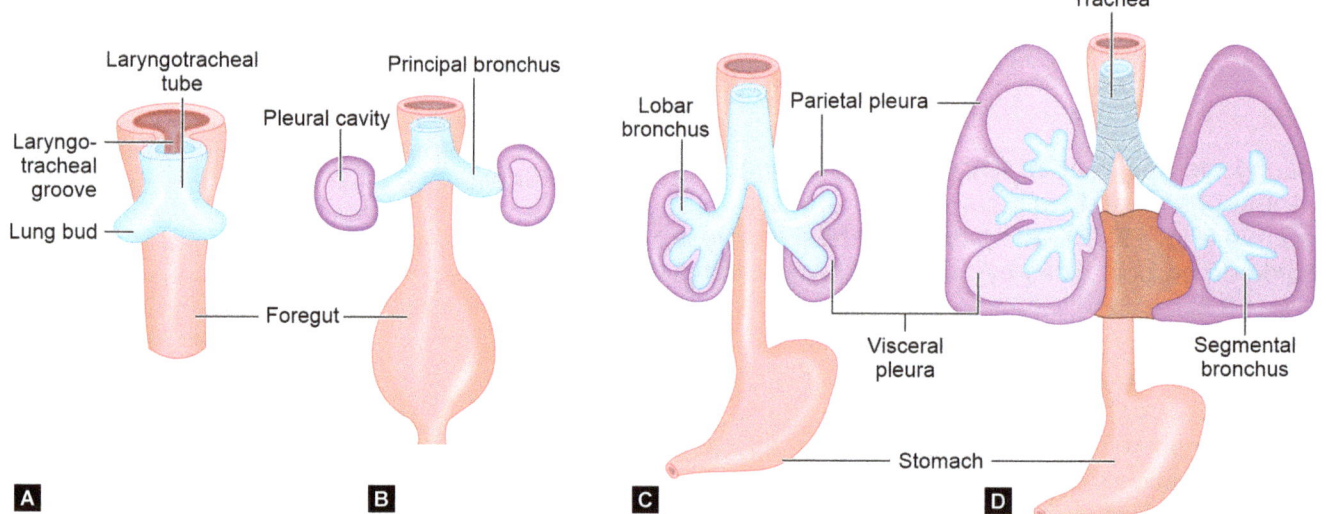

FIGS. 19.3A to D: Respiratory diverticulum growth and development: (A) Bifid respiratory diverticulum to form the right and left bronchial/lung buds; (B) Formation of principal bronchi and contact of lung buds with pleural cavity; (C) Formation of lobar bronchi and expanding lung within pleural cavity; (D) Formation of segmental bronchi.

- Initially, there will be rapid proliferation of epithelium of larynx occluding its lumen. Later vacuolation and recanalization of epithelium produces two lateral recesses known as *ventricles of larynx*.
- These recesses are bounded by endodermal folds that form an upper pair of *vestibular folds* and a lower pair of *vocal folds* which gives rise to *false* and *true vocal cords* respectively.
- The vocal folds are at the junction of 4th and 6th arches. Hence, the sensory innervation of mucosa of larynx above the vocal folds is from *internal laryngeal branch of vagus* (4th arch) whereas that part below the vocal folds is from *recurrent laryngeal branch of vagus* (6th arch).

Clinical correlation

Anomalies of Larynx
- **Laryngocele:** In this condition, the laryngeal saccule is abnormally large. It may extend beyond the larynx proper and may even form a swelling in the neck.
- **Congenital stenosis or atresia:** There may be stenosis or atresia of the larynx due to failure of recanalization of larynx. The most common site of obstruction is at vocal folds. It is also referred to *congenital high airway obstruction syndrome*.
- **Laryngeal web:** It is a thin membrane that partially obstructs the laryngeal inlet, leading to breathing and voice issues. It arises from the endodermal cells due to incomplete recanalization of the laryngotracheal tube during the 10th week of embryonic development.
- The entire larynx, or part of it (e.g., vocal cords), may be duplicated.
- **Laryngoptosis:** The larynx lies low down in the neck. Part of it may be behind the sternum. One or more of the laryngeal cartilages may be absent.

DEVELOPMENT OF TRACHEA

The trachea develops from the intermediate part of laryngotracheal tube that lies between the points of its bifurcation and the larynx. With extension of tracheoesophageal septum, the trachea elongates. At birth, the level of bifurcation of trachea lies at the lower border of 4th thoracic vertebra.

- The lining epithelium and glands of trachea forms from the endoderm of laryngotracheal diverticulum.
- The cartilage, muscle, and connective tissue of trachea develop from splanchnopleuric mesoderm surrounding laryngotracheal tube.

Clinical correlation

Anomalies of the Trachea
- **Agenesis of trachea:** Very rarely trachea may be absent. The bronchi to the lungs may arise from the blind bifurcation **(Fig. 19.5A)** or from the esophagus **(Fig. 19.5B)**.
- **Tracheoesophageal fistula (TEF):** In this condition, there is abnormal communication between esophagus and trachea. This is associated with esophageal atresia. This occurs due to defective formation of tracheoesophageal septum and failure of the tracheoesophageal ridges to fuse properly, leading to incomplete separation of the esophagus and trachea. This has also been studied in chapter 16.
  The various types of TEF are:
  – Atresia of distal esophagus with communication between proximal esophagus and trachea **(Fig. 19.5C)**.
  – Both proximal and distal parts of esophagus connected to trachea by a single passage (H type) **(Fig. 19.5D)**.
  Symptoms include coughing, choking, and cyanosis, especially during feeding.
- **Tracheal stenosis** is rare and occurs due to anterior deviation. *Tracheal atresia* may also be there due to presence of web in trachea.
- A *diverticulum* may arise from the trachea which can result in *blind bronchus*.
- **Accessory/displaced bronchi** may arise from the trachea above its bifurcation or even from the esophagus resulting in *blind bronchus*.
- May supply a mass of lung tissue *(accessory lobe)* which is not a normal part of the lungs **(Fig. 19.6A)**.
- **Tracheal bronchus:** May replace a normal bronchus (e.g., apical) in one of the lungs **(Fig. 19.6B)**.

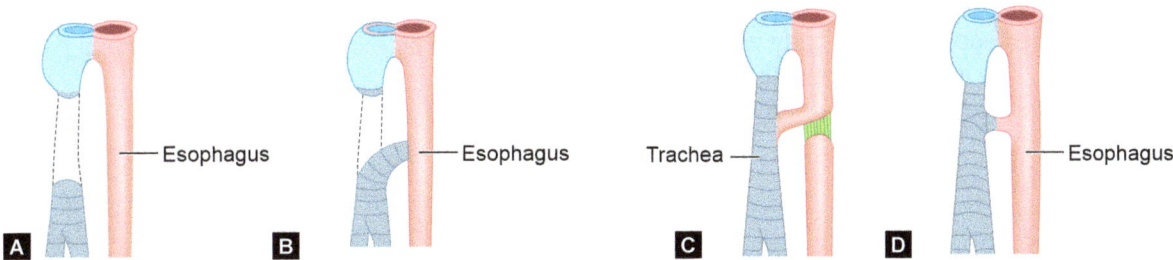

FIGS. 19.5A to D: Anomalies of trachea: (A) Agenesis of trachea—bronchi from blind bifurcation; (B) Agenesis of trachea—bronchi from esophagus; (C) Atresia of distal esophagus—communication between proximal esophagus and trachea; (D) Proximal and distal esophagus communicating with trachea by a single passage.

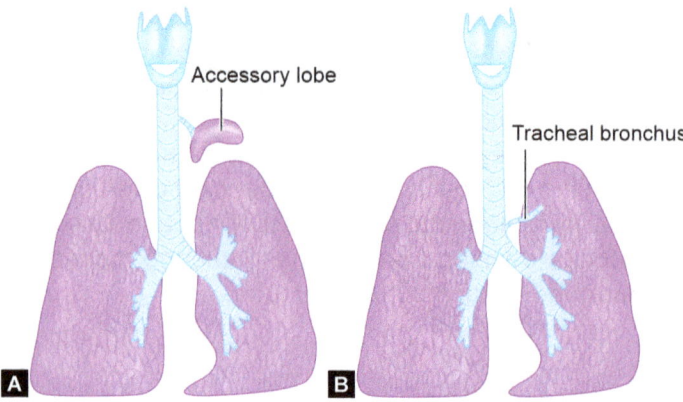

FIGS. 19.6A and B: Varieties of tracheal bronchi: (B) Supplying accessory lobe; (C) Replacing apical bronchus.

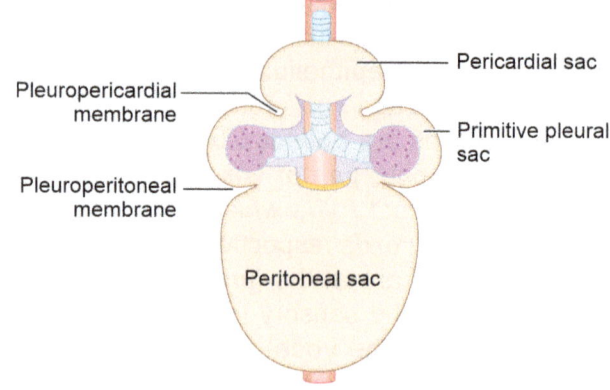

FIG. 19.7: The three coelomic cavities with pleuropericardial and pleuroperitoneal membranes separating them.

DEVELOPMENT OF LUNGS

Extrapulmonary Bronchi

During 5th week of IUL, laryngotracheal diverticulum divides to form the *right and left principal bronchi*. The right principal bronchus is larger than the left and continuous with the trachea. The left division lie more transversely **(Fig. 19.3B)**.

Intrapulmonary Bronchi and Lungs

Formation of Pleural Cavity and Pleura

- With the growth of the *respiratory diverticulum*, the lung buds come in contact with the respective *pericardioperitoneal canal* and bulge into it **(Figs. 19.3B and C)**.
- The pericardioperitoneal canals are narrow and lie on either side of the foregut. The canals are filled with gradually expanding bronchial/lung buds **(Fig. 19.7)**.
- *Pleuropericardial* and *pleuroperitoneal folds* separate the pericardioperitoneal canals from the pericardial and peritoneal cavities, respectively. This results in the formation of the *primitive pleural cavity* from that part of the pleuropericardial canal in contact with the dividing and expanding lung bud **(Fig. 19.7)**.
- The *splanchnopleuric layer* of intraembryonic mesoderm in contact with the dividing and expanding lung bud becomes the *visceral pleura*, and the *somatopleuric layer* of intraembryonic mesoderm covering the inner aspect of the body wall forms the *parietal pleura*. The space between the parietal and visceral pleura forms the *pleural cavity* **(Figs. 19.3C and D)**.

Subdivisions of Intrapulmonary Bronchi

- When both principal bronchi come in contact with the developing pericardioperitoneal canal (pleural cavity) they subdivide into secondary/*lobar bronchi* **(Fig. 19.3C)**.
- The left principal bronchus shows two subdivisions *(upper and lower)* that represent the two lobar bronchi of the left lung.
- The right principal bronchus divides into three lobar bronchi *(superior, middle, and inferior)* of the right lung.
- The parts of the lung parenchyma, developing from the lobar bronchi, are separated from one another by mesoderm which forms the connective tissue basis of the lung, cartilages, smooth muscles and also gives rise to the *pleura*.
- As the pleura lines the surface of each lobe separately, the *lobes* come to be separated by *fissures*.
- The total number of divisions of each main bronchus is about 17 by 7th month of IUL, and six more after birth to attain final shape of adult lung.
- The substance of the lung is formed by further subdivisions of the lobar bronchi.
- Each lobar bronchus further subdivides to form *segmental bronchi* in the 7th week of IUL which also forms the substance of the lungs.
- Each segmental bronchus and its surrounding mesenchyme constitute the *bronchopulmonary segment*. Each lung contains 10 bronchopulmonary segments **(Fig. 19.3D)**.
- Divisions and subdivisions of each segmental bronchus form the *bronchioles, terminal bronchioles, respiratory bronchioles, alveolar ducts and alveolar sacs, and alveoli*.
- After the establishment of the bronchial tree, alveoli are formed by expansion of the terminal parts of the tree.

Maturation of Lung

There are four stages in the maturation of lung. The ramifications of the bronchial tree pass through these stages. They are represented in **Table 19.1 and Figures 19.8A to D**. During fetal life, all subdivisions of the bronchial tree are lined by cuboidal epithelium that undergoes changes with the maturation of lung **(Table 19.1)**.

Chapter 19: Respiratory System

TABLE 19.1: Stages in the maturation of lung—morphological changes in bronchial tree and its functional importance.

Stage of lung and age of embryo/fetus/newborn	Changes in the morphology of bronchial tree and its functional importance
Pseudoglandular stage 6–16 weeks (2nd–4th month of IUL) (Fig. 19.8A)	• The lung resembles an exocrine gland, appearing like a tubuloacinar mucus gland • Bronchi divide up to the terminal bronchiole, with no development of the respiratory portion • The proximal bronchial tree is lined with columnar epithelium, while the distal part is lined with cuboidal epithelium • Surrounding mesenchymal cells differentiate into smooth muscle, cartilage, and connective tissue • Respiration is not possible; therefore, premature fetuses born at this stage cannot survive
Canalicular stage 17–26 weeks (5th–7th month of IUL) (Fig. 19.8B)	• Three generations of branching occur in the bronchial tree • Respiratory bronchioles, alveolar ducts, and a few alveolar sacs form • Vascularization of lung tissue increases with a greater capillary network in relation to future alveoli • Some cuboidal respiratory epithelial cells transform into simple squamous *type I pneumocytes* • The remaining cuboidal cells specialize into *type II pneumocytes*, functioning as stem cells and producing surfactant • A fetus born at this stage can survive if intensive care is provided
Saccular stage 27 weeks to full term (7th month of IUL to delivery) (Fig. 19.8C)	• More primitive alveoli develop • Lining epithelium of alveolar sacs changes to type I pneumocytes, while cuboidal cells lining bronchioles become thin, flat cells • Gas exchange between blood and air becomes possible in primitive alveoli • Type II cells secrete phospholipid-rich *surfactant* that reduces surface tension and prevents alveolar collapse during expiration • An intimate contact develops between the epithelium of alveolar sacs and capillaries (forming the *blood-air barrier*) to facilitate gaseous exchange • A fetus born at this stage is viable
Alveolar stage from birth to 8 years of postnatal life (Fig. 19.8D)	• Division of respiratory bronchioles forms alveolar ducts and definitive alveoli • The number of definitive alveoli increases • Surfactant production increases significantly • Rapid exchange of gases occurs between the alveolar epithelium and capillary endothelium

(IUL: intrauterine life)

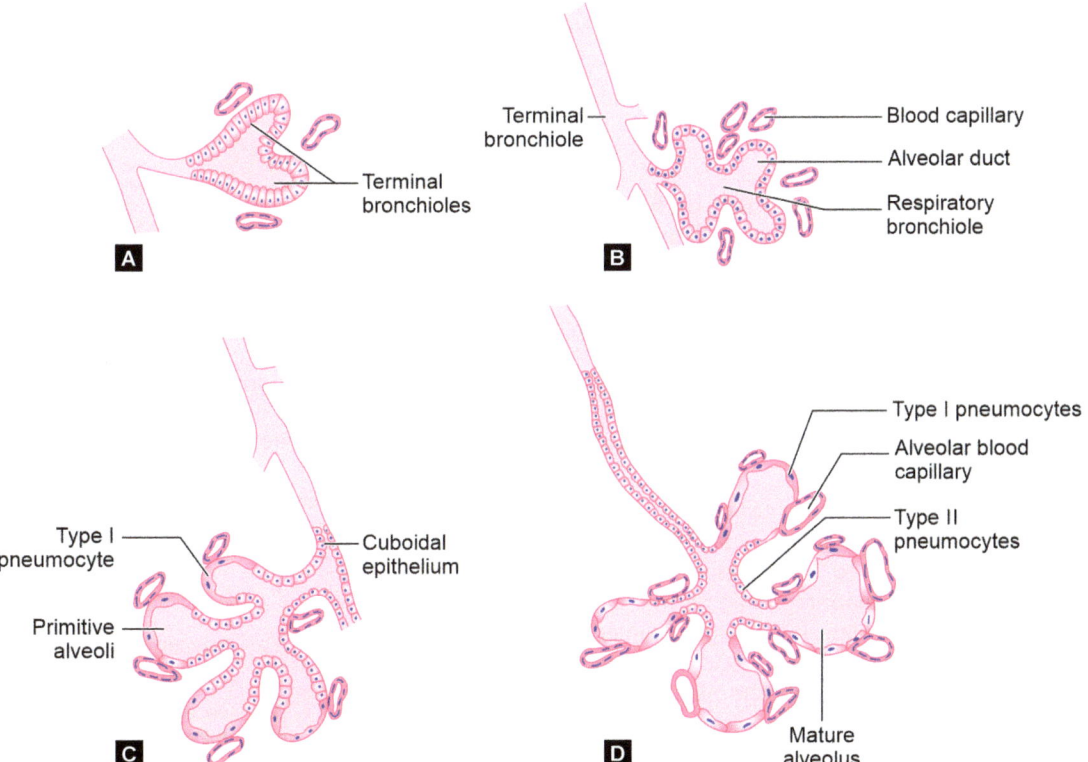

FIGS. 19.8A to D: Stages in maturation of lung: (A) Pseudoglandular stage; (B) Canalicular stage; (C) Saccular stage; (D) Alveolar stage.

Pulmonary Surfactant

- Within the respiratory passages some of the cells become specialized for production of *surfactant*. This substance is rich in phospholipids and forms a thin layer over alveoli and reduces surface tension.
- Before birth the respiratory passages are full of fluid derived from amniotic fluid which also contains surfactant. When the newborn begins to breathe, the fluid is rapidly absorbed and partly expelled. The surfactant remains as a thin layer lining the alveoli.
- This prevents collapse of alveoli during expiration. In premature babies, a deficiency of surfactant may cause difficulty in expansion of the lung and can be a cause of death of the baby.

Viable Age of Fetus

The pulmonary circulation is established early in fetal life. However, most of the blood is at first short circuited through foramen ovale and ductus arteriosus (*refer* Chapter 20 for details). The amount of blood circulating through the lungs progressively increases, and by 7th month of IUL the circulation is rich enough to provide adequate oxygen for sustaining life. Hence an infant born, thereafter, is viable (i.e., it can live).

Molecular Regulation of Development of Lungs

- The appearance of the lung bud is dependent on an increase in retinoic acid in the adjacent mesoderm.
- *TBX4* expression leads to the development of the respiratory diverticulum.
- Branching of the bronchial tree involves expression of FGFs.

Clinical correlation

Anomalies of the Lungs
- **Respiratory distress syndrome (RDS) or hyaline membrane disease (HMD):** Insufficient production of surfactant leading to collapse of lung in expiration. The newborn with this condition after birth have difficult labored breathing. The alveoli are filled with fluid high in protein content resembling glassy hyaline membrane. Due this RDS is referred to as hyaline membrane disease. This requires prenatal treatment of mothers with glucocorticoids and use of artificial surfactants and thyroxine in the premature newborn.
- **Agenesis and hypoplasia:** The whole of one lung, or one of its lobes (and associated bronchi), may fail to develop, or may remain underdeveloped. Hypoplasia of lungs is associated with congenital diaphragmatic hernia. **Lung hernia:** Part of a lung may herniate: (a) through the inlet of the thorax, (b) through a defect in the thoracic wall, (c) into the mediastinum, or (d) into the opposite pleural cavity.
- **Ectopic lung:** Either the entire lung or a lobe of it arises from trachea or esophagus. This is due to the development of respiratory buds from the foregut in addition to the main respiratory system or in place of normal lung.
- **Congenital cysts of lung:** Due to dilatation of terminal bronchi. These can be multiple and give honeycomb appearance of lung on X-ray.

Abnormalities of Lobes
- **Absence of fissures** that are normally present, leads to a reduction in the number of lobes. Absence of the transverse fissure of the right lung results in a right lung with only two lobes **(Fig. 19.9A)**.
- **Presence of abnormal fissures:**
  - A transverse fissure may be present on the left side with the result that the left lung has three lobes **(Fig. 19.9B)**.
  - The superior segment of the lower lobe may be separated **(Fig. 19.9C)**.
  - The medial basal segment *(cardiac lobe)* of the left lung may be separated by a fissure from the rest of the lower lobe **(Fig. 19.9D)**.
  - A part of the upper lobe of the right lung may come to lie medial to the azygos vein. This part is called the *azygos lobe* **(Figs. 19.10A and B)**. In this condition, the azygos vein is suspended from the wall of the thorax by a fold of parietal pleura (mesoazygos).
  - *Accessory lobes* are usually connected to bronchi that are not part of the normal bronchial tree. Such bronchi may arise from trachea (upper accessory lobe) or from esophagus (lower accessory lobe) **(Fig. 19.11)**.
- **Sequestration of lung tissue:** An area of embryonic lung tissue may separate from the tracheobronchial tree (sequestration = separation). Such tissue may form a complete lobe (lobar sequestration), which may have an independent pleural covering. In other cases, the sequestrated tissue may lie within a lobe (intralobar sequestration). The sequestered lung tissue derives its blood supply from an abnormal branch of the aorta. The condition is most frequently seen in the lower lobe of the left lung.

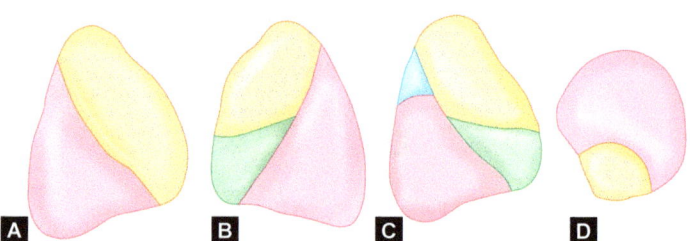

FIGS. 19.9A to D: Abnormal lobes of lungs: (A) Right lung with only two lobes; (B) Left lung with three lobes; (C) Apical segment of lower lobe is separate; (D) Separate medial basal segment.

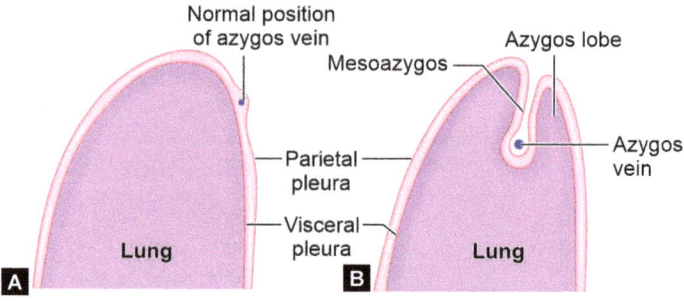

FIGS. 19.10A and B: (A) Normal relationship of azygos vein to the lung; (B) Azygos lobe of lung.

Chapter 19: Respiratory System

TIMETABLE OF SOME EVENTS DESCRIBED IN THIS CHAPTER

Age	Developmental events
4 weeks	Laryngotracheal/respiratory diverticulum formed
5 weeks	Tracheoesophageal septum forms by end
5–6 weeks	Maturation of lungs begin
36 weeks	Lung maturity/viability of fetus achieved

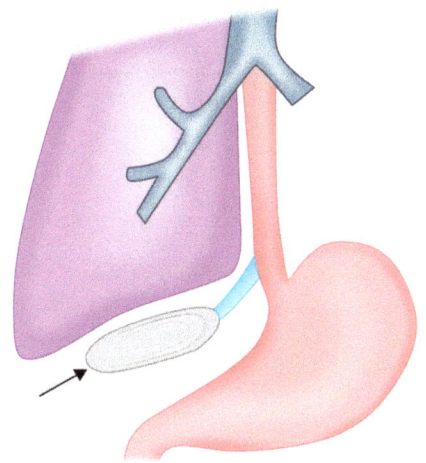

FIG. 19.11: Accessory lobe of lung (indicated by arrow) supplied by bronchus arising from esophagus.

HIGHLIGHTS

- Respiratory system develops from a median endodermal diverticulum of foregut. At its caudal end the diverticulum divides into right and left *lung buds*.
- Larynx and trachea develop from the endodermal respiratory diverticulum cranial/proximal to its division.
- Bronchial tree and alveoli of the lungs develop from repeated division of the lung buds.
- Maturity of lungs happens in four stages with which there is start of gaseous exchange process and release of surfactant.

Summary

- Development of respiratory system (**Flowchart 19.1**).

FLOWCHART 19.1: Development of respiratory system and its components.

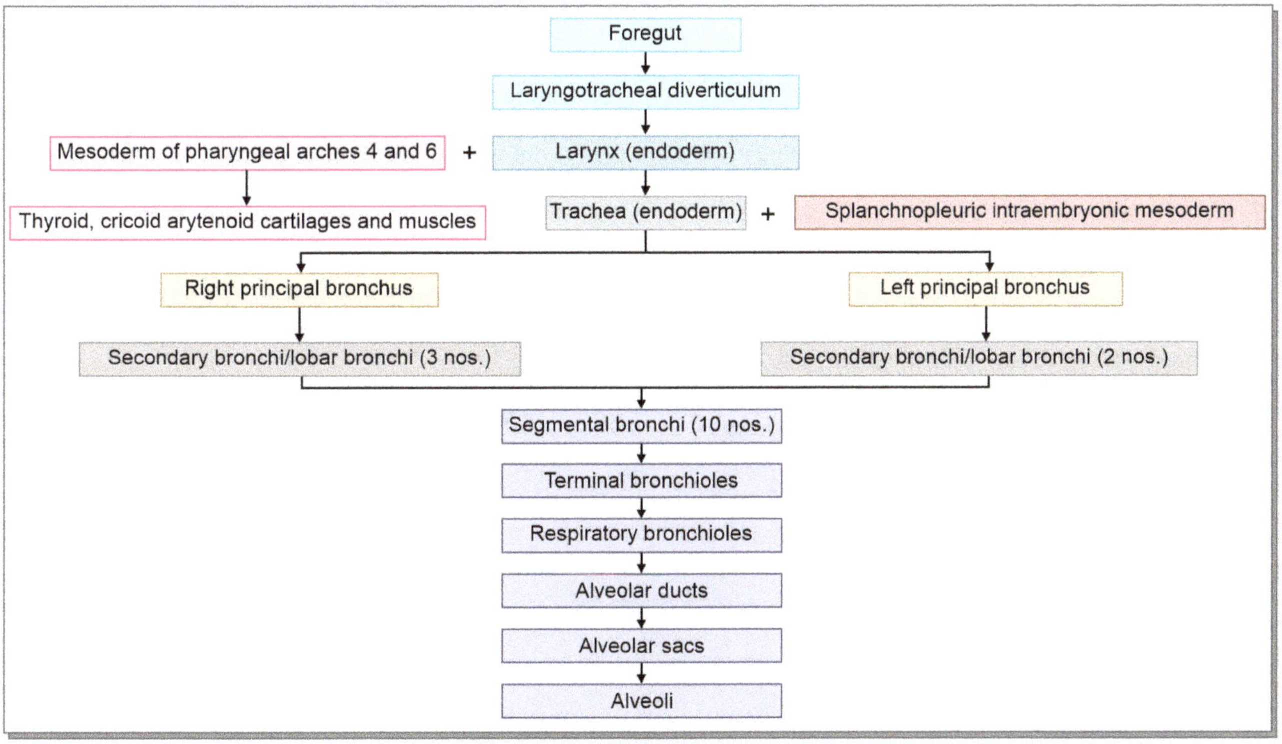

```
                          Foregut
                             ↓
                  Laryngotracheal diverticulum
                             ↓
Mesoderm of pharyngeal arches 4 and 6  +  Larynx (endoderm)
                             ↓
Thyroid, cricoid arytenoid cartilages and muscles
                     Trachea (endoderm)  +  Splanchnopleuric intraembryonic mesoderm
                     ↓                                    ↓
            Right principal bronchus           Left principal bronchus
                     ↓                                    ↓
    Secondary bronchi/lobar bronchi (3 nos.)   Secondary bronchi/lobar bronchi (2 nos.)
                             ↓
                  Segmental bronchi (10 nos.)
                             ↓
                     Terminal bronchioles
                             ↓
                    Respiratory bronchioles
                             ↓
                        Alveolar ducts
                             ↓
                        Alveolar sacs
                             ↓
                           Alveoli
```

Chapter 19: Respiratory System

TEST YOUR UNDERSTANDING

REVIEW QUESTIONS

1. Explain development of larynx.
2. Discuss subdivisions of intrapulmonary bronchi.
3. Describe the stages in the maturation of lung.
4. Write a short note on respiratory distress syndrome.
5. Write a short note on tracheoesophageal fistula.

EXPLAIN WHY? (REASONING QUESTIONS)

1. Preterm baby at 24th week of gestation was having difficulty in breathing and died.
2. There is a different nerve supply above and below vocal cords.
3. The newborn baby was choking and coughing during feeding.
4. Newborn presented with stridor during breathing.

MULTIPLE CHOICE QUESTIONS

1. Which embryonic structure gives rise to the cartilaginous framework of the larynx, including the thyroid cartilage and cricoid cartilage?
   A. Fourth pharyngeal arch
   B. Third pharyngeal pouch
   C. Laryngotracheal groove
   D. Mesenchymal condensations
   E. Thyroid diverticulum

2. Which event during lung development marks the formation of the respiratory bronchioles and initiation of gas exchange capabilities?
   A. Canalicular stage
   B. Saccular stage
   C. Alveolar stage
   D. Pseudoglandular stage
   E. Terminal sac stage

3. At approximately how many weeks of gestation does the canalicular stage of lung development begin?
   A. 4–7 weeks
   B. 8–16 weeks
   C. 17–26 weeks
   D. 27–36 weeks
   E. 37–40 weeks

4. Which structure primarily secretes surfactant, crucial for reducing surface tension in the alveoli and aiding in lung maturation?
   A. Type I pneumocytes
   B. Type II pneumocytes
   C. Alveolar macrophages
   D. Fibroblasts
   E. Endothelial cells

5. A newborn is found to have bronchogenic cysts. These cysts are remnants of which developmental structure?
   A. Foregut
   B. Hindgut
   C. Mesonephric duct
   D. Pronephros

6. During a prenatal ultrasound, a fetus is found to have a congenital diaphragmatic hernia. Which of the following complications is most likely to occur due to this condition?
   A. Pulmonary hypoplasia
   B. Tracheoesophageal fistula
   C. Laryngeal web
   D. Bronchogenic cysts

7. A preterm infant at 28 weeks' gestation is diagnosed with respiratory distress syndrome (RDS). Explain why surfactant therapy is administered in this case.
   A. Surfactant decreases the elasticity of the alveolar walls
   B. Surfactant increases the viscosity of the lung secretions
   C. Surfactant reduces surface tension in the alveoli, preventing collapse
   D. Surfactant inhibits the function of type I alveolar cells

8. A neonate with severe respiratory distress is found to have pulmonary hypoplasia secondary to oligohydramnios. What is the embryological reason for this condition?
   A. Inadequate production of amniotic fluid
   B. Excessive growth of the pulmonary arteries
   C. Premature closure of the tracheoesophageal septum
   D. Overdevelopment of bronchial cartilage

9. During an autopsy of a deceased aborted fetus, it was found that the right lung was located in the abdominal cavity, with its bronchus originating from the esophagus. What is the most likely embryological basis for this condition?
   A. Defective development of the pleuropericardial membranes
   B. Abnormal migration of neural crest cells
   C. Anomaly in the formation of the laryngotracheal diverticulum
   D. Reduced production of retinoic acid in the mesoderm adjacent to the right principal bronchus

Answers: 1. A   2. C   3. B   4. B   5. A
          6. A   7. C   8. A   9. D

Cardiovascular System

CHAPTER 20

COMPETENCIES COVERED/LEARNING OUTCOMES

The student should be able to:

AN25.2	Describe development of pleura, lung and heart.
AN25.3	Describe fetal circulation and changes occurring at birth.
AN25.4	Describe embryological basis of: (1) atrial septal defect, (2) ventricular septal defect, (3) Fallot's tetralogy.
AN25.5	Describe developmental basis of congenital anomalies, transposition of great vessels, dextrocardia, patent ductus arteriosus and coarctation of aorta.
AN25.6	Mention development of aortic arch arteries, SVC, IVC and coronary sinus.

HEART

The heart is the first organ of the body to start functioning. The development of the heart is complex and it starts as a separate vascular system at the beginning of the 3rd week to supply the nutritional needs to the embryo.

The heart (like all blood vessels) is mesodermal in origin. It is formed from splanchnopleuric mesoderm lying immediately cranial to the prochordal plate. This mesoderm constitutes the *cardiogenic area* forming the floor of the pericardial cavity. The *primitive heart tubes* develop in the cardiogenic area.

The internal surfaces of the heart and all blood vessels are lined by a layer of flattened cells called *endothelium*. *All the abovementioned components of the heart and blood vessels are of mesodermal origin.*

DEVELOPMENT OF HEART TUBE

Cardiac Progenitor Cells and Heart Fields

Cardiac progenitor cells originate in the caudal epiblast and migrate through the primitive streak into the splanchnopleuric mesoderm, forming a horseshoe-shaped *primary heart field* by days 16–18.

These cells differentiate and fuse to create the *primitive heart tube*, which later develops into the atria and ventricles. By day 21, a *secondary heart field* forms in the splanchnopleuric mesoderm ventral to the posterior pharynx, contributing to the right ventricle and outflow tracts. Proper development of these fields is crucial for the formation of a functional, four-chambered heart and the alignment of the great vessels.

Cardiogenic Area

Pharyngeal endoderm underlying primary heart field induces formation of *cardiogenic area* (Fig. 20.1) where horseshoe-shaped blood islands are formed by angiogenic clusters, which later get canalized to form endothelial lined heart tubes that are surrounded by myoblasts. Bilateral blood islands close to midline or paranotochordal region form the *dorsal aortae*.

The heart develops from angioblastic tissue that arises from splanchnopleuric mesoderm, which is, therefore, called the *cardiogenic area*. This area is between the dorsal wall of yolk sac and the floor (splanchnopleuric layer) of pericardial cavity. With the establishment of the head fold, the splanchnopleuric mesoderm and the developing heart come to lie dorsal to the pericardial cavity, and ventral to the foregut.

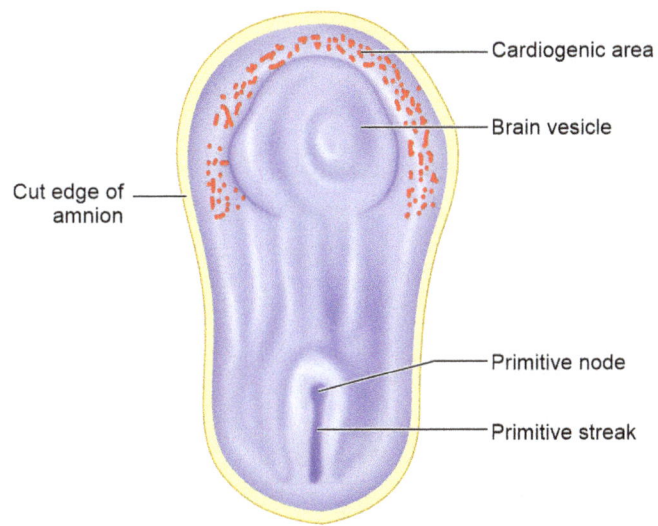

FIG. 20.1: Embryonic disc showing horseshoe-shaped cardiogenic area.

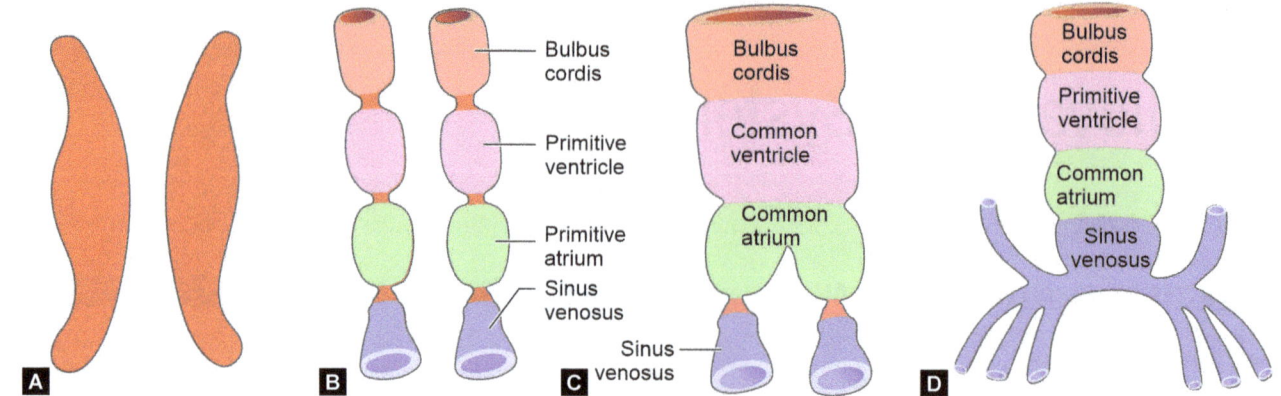

FIGS. 20.2A to D: (A) Right and left heart tubes; (B to D) Progressive fusion of tubes from cranial to caudal end. Fusion of sinus venosus is partial.

The heart is at first seen in the form of right and left endothelial heart tubes **(Figs. 20.2A to D)** that soon fuse with each other. The single tube thus formed shows a series of dilatations **(Fig. 20.3)**. These are:
- Bulbus cordis
- Ventricle (primitive ventricle)
- Atrium (primitive atrium or atrial chamber)
- Sinus venosus

Sinuatrial orifice connects the sinus venosus and atrium. The atrium and ventricle are in communication through **atrioventricular canal (AV canal)**.

The bulbus cordis lies at the **arterial end of the heart**. It is divisible into three parts, i.e., **proximal, middle and distal**. The proximal one-third is dilated and does not have any special name; the middle one-third is called the *conus*, and the distal one-third is called the *truncus arteriosus* **(Figs. 20.3 and 20.4)**. The truncus arteriosus is continuous distally with the **aortic sac**. The aortic sac is continuous with right and left pharyngeal arch arteries. These arteries arch backwards to become continuous with the right and left dorsal aortae.

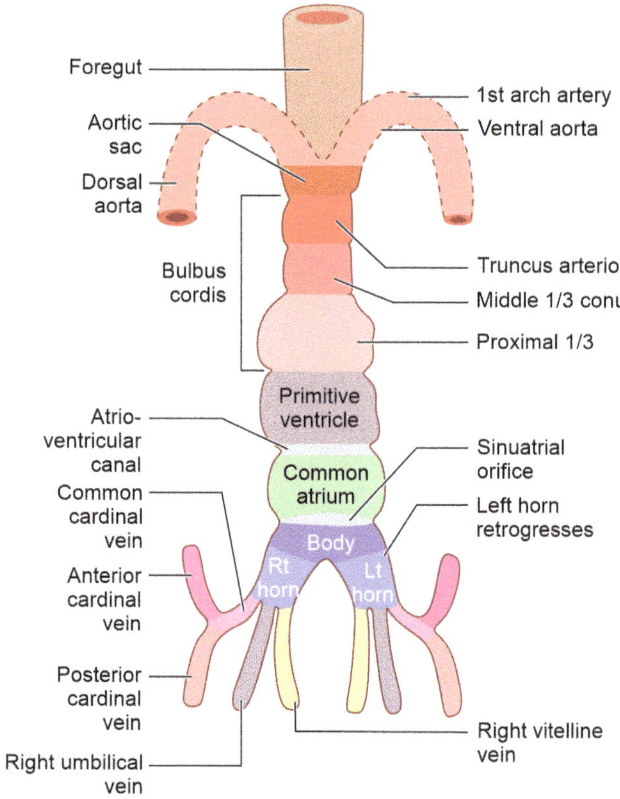

The sinus venosus lies at the **venous end of the heart**. It has right and left horns. One vitelline vein (from the yolk sac), one umbilical vein (from the placenta) and one common cardinal vein (from the body wall) join each horn of the sinus venosus.

Between 5th and 8th weeks, cardiac septations to form definitive heart occur. Simultaneous development of all the chambers takes place though they are considered separately for easy understanding. The fate of the various parts of the heart tube is summarized in **Figure 20.4**.

DEVELOPMENT OF VARIOUS CHAMBERS OF HEART

Formation of Atria

Sinus Venosus and its Absorption into the Right Atrium

- The sinus venosus is the caudal most part of the primitive heart tube, with a body and two horns (right and left). Each horn receives one vitelline vein (from the yolk sac), one umbilical vein (from the placenta), and one common cardinal vein (duct of Cuvier) from the body wall **(Fig. 20.3)**. Initially, both horns are of equal size, but due to left-to-right shunts, most blood drains into the right horn.
- The sinus venosus initially connects to the primitive atrium via a wide opening called the **sinuatrial orifice**. Grooves develop on the heart tube's lateral walls, partially separating the sinus venosus from the atrium **(Figs. 20.5A to E)**.
- The right groove remains shallow while the left groove deepens significantly **(Figs. 20.6A to C)**. This separation causes the left part of the sinus venosus

FIG. 20.3: Subdivisions of fused heart tube.

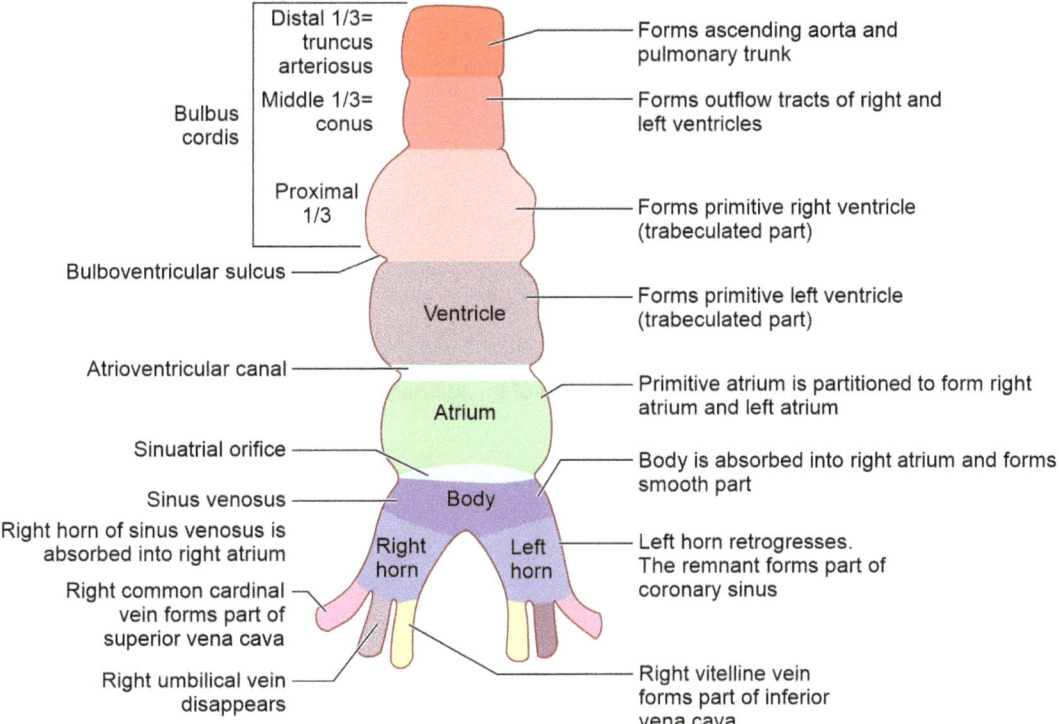

FIG. 20.4: Main subdivisions of the heart tube and their fate.

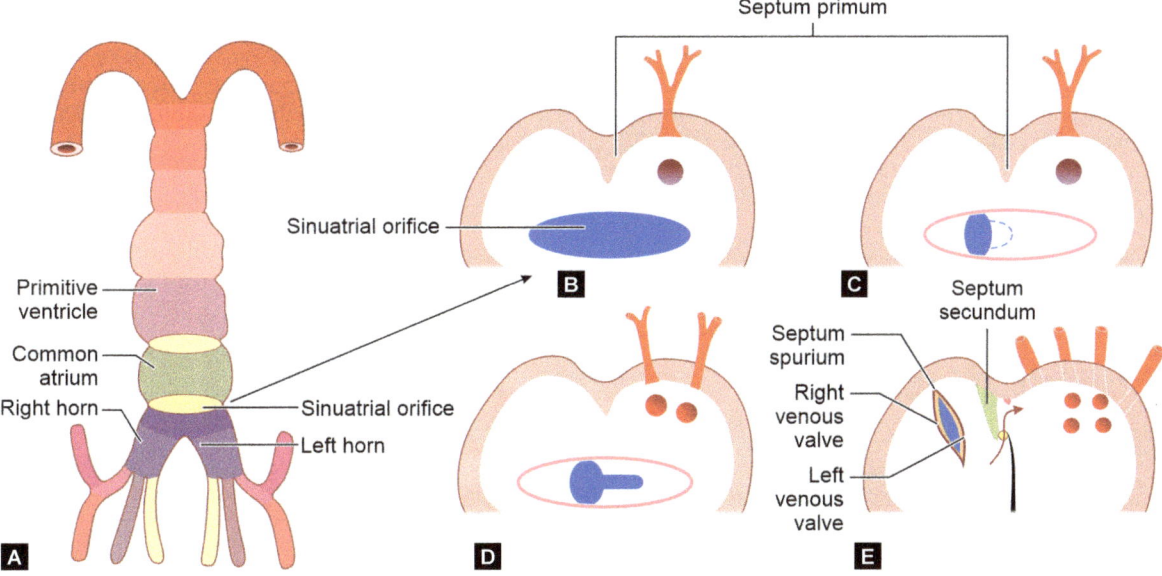

FIGS. 20.5A to E: (A) Sinuatrial orifice in heart tube. (B to E) Changes in the sinuatrial orifice. Note that firstly, the centrally placed orifice (B) shifts to the right (C). Secondly, the orifice that is at first transversely orientated becomes vertical (D). Dotted lines in (D) indicate the outline of the opening in the previous figure to show how the change occurs. (E) The right and left venous valves guarding sinuatrial orifice.

to become isolated from the atrium, with its blood now entering through the right sinus venosus. The left horn and its tributaries reduce in size, becoming part of the *coronary sinus* (Fig. 20.7).

- Initially the sinuatrial orifice is larger in size. Gradually the opening becomes narrow and changes its orientation from transverse to oval and finally to vertical with a narrow slit. The slit has right and left margins called the *right* and *left venous valves*. Cranially these two valves fuse to form a structure called the *septum spurium* (Figs. 20.5 and 20.8). Caudally it forms the *sinus septum*.
- The right common cardinal vein becomes part of the *superior vena cava* and right vitelline vein forms the terminal part of the *inferior vena cava* (Figs. 20.7 and 20.9).
- The right venous valve expands large and divides into three parts by two muscular bands, the (1) *superior*

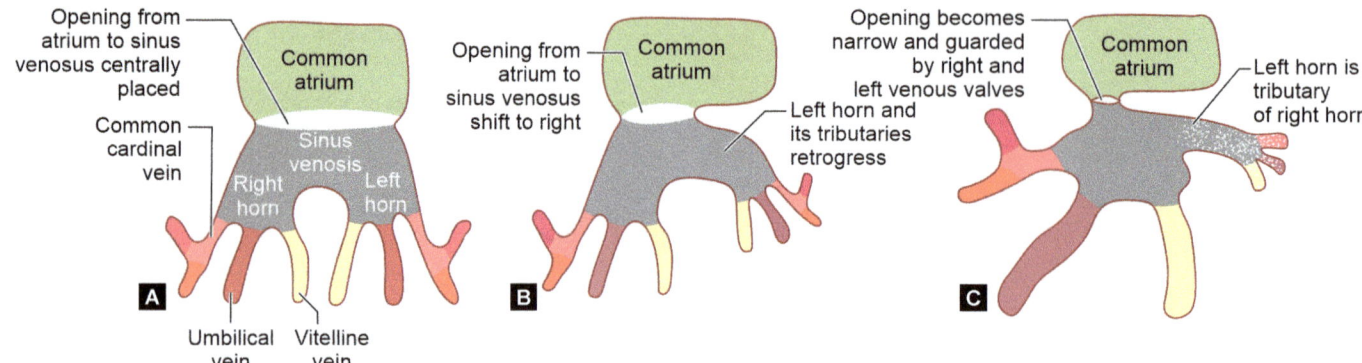

FIGS. 20.6A to C: Regression of the left horn of sinus venosus.

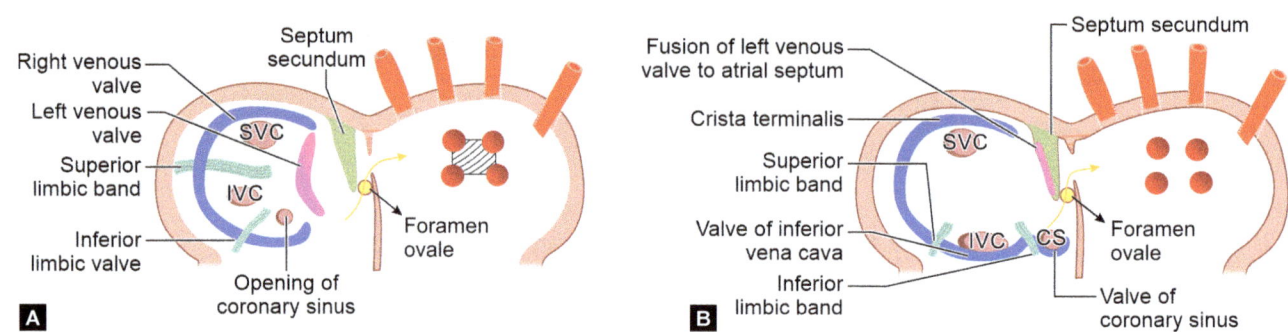

FIGS. 20.7A and B: Sinus venosus—fate of right and left venous valves. The right venous valve expands greatly and forms the crista terminalis, the valve of the inferior vena cava and the valve of the coronary sinus. The left venous valve remains small and fuses with the interatrial septum. Formation of interatrial septum. Incorporation of pulmonary veins into the left atrium are also shown in these figures. (SVC: superior vena cava; IVC: inferior vena cava; CS: coronary sinus)

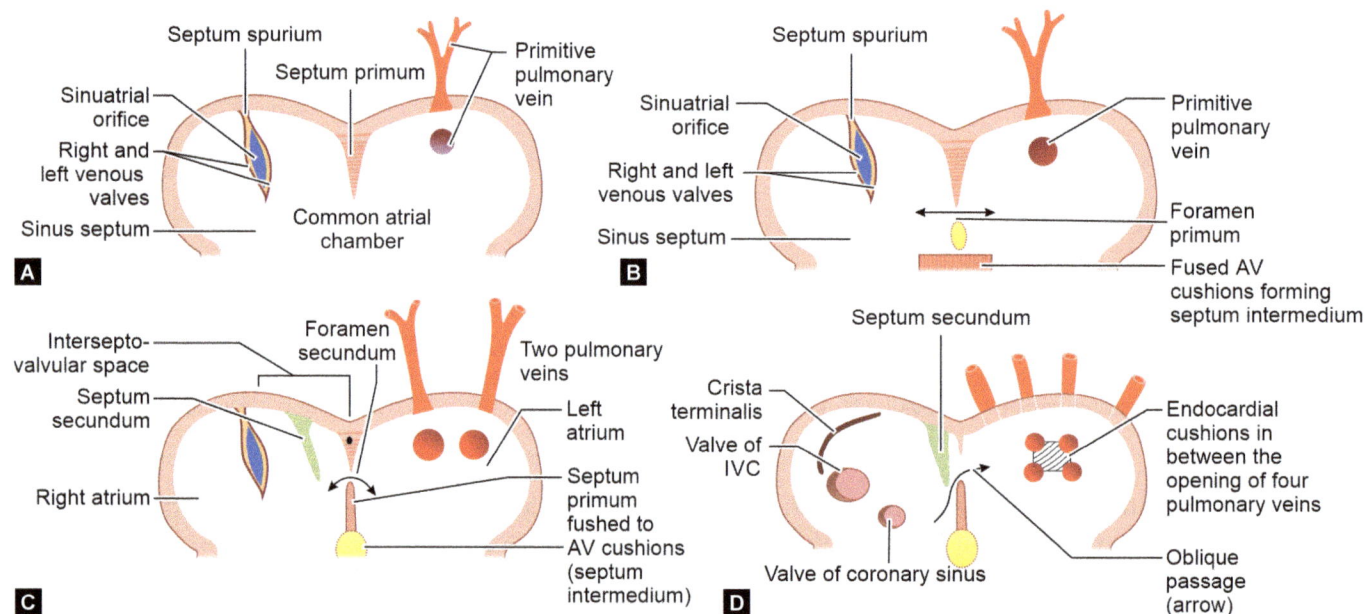

FIGS. 20.8A to D: Sinuatrial orifice and venous valves in right atrium. Formation of interatrial septum. (A) Septum primum appears; (B) Septum primum grows toward fused AV cushions (septum intermedium). The gap between them is the foramen primum; (C) Septum primum fuses with atrioventricular (AV) cushions. At the same time, the upper part of the septum primum degenerates to form the foramen secundum. The septum secundum is formed to the right of the septum primum; (D) Septum secundum overlaps the free edge of septum primum. Blood now flows from left to right through the oblique cleft between the two septa. Incorporation of pulmonary veins into the left atrium is shown. (IVC: inferior vena cava)

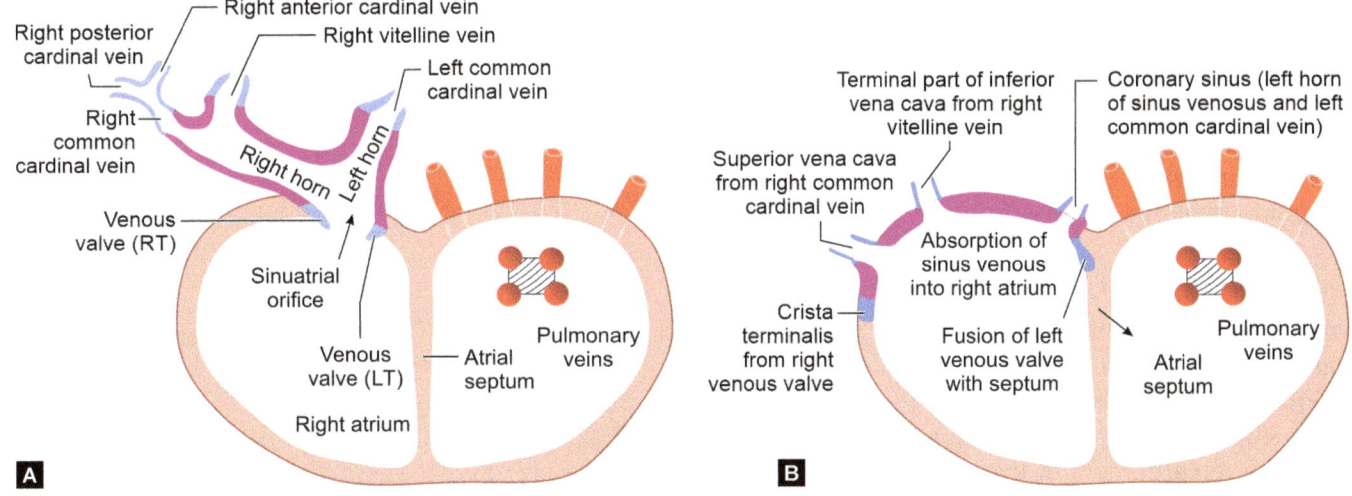

FIGS. 20.9A and B: Partitioned atrial chambers and sinoatrial orifice and pulmonary veins in partitioned atria.

and (2) *inferior limbic bands*. The three parts of the right venous valve are the (1) *crista terminalis* (Figs. 20.7A and B), (2) *valve of the inferior vena cava* and (3) *valve of the coronary sinus*. The left venous valve gets incorporated into the development of *septum secundum*.

Atrioventricular Canal

This is the communication between the common atrial chamber and ventricle. The AV canal divides into right and left halves as follows:
* Two thickenings, the *AV/endocardial cushions* appear on the dorsal and ventral walls of AV canal.
* They grow toward each other and fuse to form the *septum intermedium* (Fig. 20.10).
* The AV endocardial cushions take part in the formation of interatrial and interventricular septa, defects of which are involved in many congenital heart diseases.

Formation of Interatrial Septum

The atrial chamber undergoes division into right and left halves by formation of two septa (that later fuse) **(Figs. 20.8A to D)**.
* Pressure of bulbus cordis results in the formation of a sickle shaped fold from the roof primitive atrium. This fold is called *septum primum*. It is located exactly in the midline and is to the left of septum spurium. It grows downward toward AV canal and fuses with the septum intermedium **(Fig. 20.8A)**.
 However, note the following carefully. Throughout fetal life oxygenated blood reaches the right atrium from the placenta. This blood has to reach the left atrium, and for this purpose a communication between right and left atria is essential.
* Before the septum primum reaches and fuses with the septum intermedium, blood flows through the

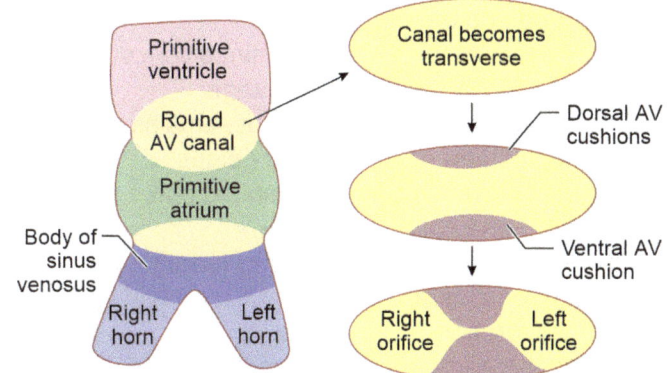

FIG. 20.10: Division of atrioventricular (AV) canal into right and left orifices.

gap between them. This gap is the *foramen primum* **(Fig. 20.8B)**.
* Before the foramen primum can be closed, it is essential that another path for flow of blood be created. This is achieved by breaking down of the upper part of the septum primum. The new gap is the *foramen secundum*. The septum primum now has a free upper edge **(Fig. 20.8C)**.
* The *septum secundum* grows down from the roof of the atrial chamber to the right of the septum primum. As it grows, it comes to overlap the free upper edge of the septum primum. The left venous valve and the cephalic attachment of septum primum get incorporated into the septum secundum **(Figs. 20.8C and D)**.
* Once the two septa overlap blood has to flow through the interval between the septa. This gap is the *foramen ovale*. It is an oblique valvular passage that allows blood to flow from right to left, but not from left to right **(Fig. 20.8D)**. This is patent throughout fetal life.
* After birth of the baby, the left atrium starts receiving oxygenated blood from the lungs. The pressure in this chamber becomes greater than that of right atrium and there is no need for flow of blood from right

atrium to left atrium. The foramen ovale is, therefore, obliterated by fusion of the septum primum and septum secundum.

- In terms of adult anatomy, the *annulus ovalis* represents the lower free edge of the septum secundum while the *fossa ovalis* represents the septum primum.

Development of Right Atrium

As described above, the main part of the right atrium is derived from the three sources:
- Right half of the primitive atrium.
- The sinus venosus is absorbed into the right atrium by great enlargement of the sinuatrial orifice **(Figs. 20.7 and 20.9)**.
- The right half of the atrioventricular canal is also absorbed into the right atrium.

Some relevant facts about the sinus venosus (and its tributaries) may be noted at this stage.
- The left horn of the sinus venosus remains very small. It becomes part of the coronary sinus.
- The right common cardinal vein becomes part of the superior vena cava.
- The right vitelline vein forms the terminal part of the inferior vena cava.
- After absorption of the sinus venosus into the right atrium, the coronary sinus and the venae cavae are seen opening into the right atrium.
- The expanded right venous valve that is partitioned by the two limbic bands that form the *crista terminalis*, *valve of inferior vena cava* and *valve of coronary sinus*. The left venous valve fuses with atrial septum.
- Note that the crista terminalis lies at the junction of the part of the right atrium derived from the sinus venosus *(sinus venarum)* and the atrium proper.

Development of Left Atrium

The left atrium is derived from the following three components **(Figs. 20.8 to 20.11)**:
1. Left half of the primitive atrial chamber.
2. Left half of the AV canal.
3. Absorbed proximal parts of the pulmonary veins.

Absorption of Pulmonary Veins into the Left Atrium

- At the time when the septum primum is just beginning to form, a single pulmonary vein opens into the left half of the primitive atrium **(Figs. 20.5A to E)**. When traced away from the heart **(Figs. 20.8 and 20.11)**, the vein divides into a right and a left branch each of which again bifurcates, to drain the corresponding lung bud.
- Gradually, the parts of the pulmonary veins nearest to the left atrium are absorbed into the atrium, with

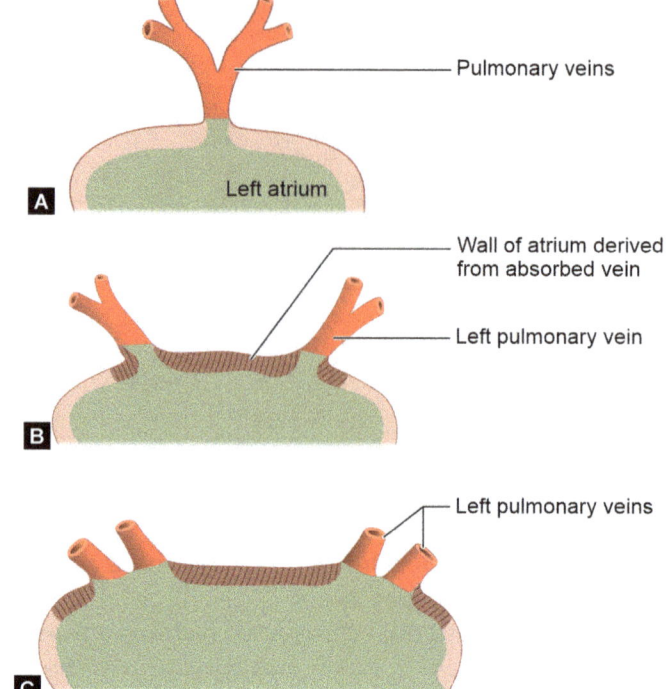

FIGS. 20.11A to C: Absorption of pulmonary veins into the left atrium. At first only one vein from the lungs enters the left atrium. The proximal part of the vein is gradually absorbed and is incorporated into the wall of the atrium. As a result of continued absorption of tributaries, four veins (two right and two left) finally open into the atrium.

result the four separate veins, two from each side, come to open into it **(Figs. 20.8 to 20.11)**.

Clinical correlation

Defective Formation of Septa
This results in the formation of abnormal passages.

Atrial septal defects (ASD)/Interatrial septal defects are the congenital condition in which there is defect in interatrial septum which causes communication between two atria. The symptoms include cyanosis and breathlessness due to mixing of oxygenated blood and deoxygenated blood. It is the most common condition affecting atria.

This condition may be of three types:
- The *septum primum* may fail to reach the AV endocardial cushions, as a result of which the foramen primum persists **(Fig. 20.12A)**. This ostium primum defect can also be caused by defective formation of AV endocardial cushions.
- The *septum secundum* may fail to develop as a result of which the foramen secundum remains wide open resulting in ostium secundum defect **(Fig. 20.12B)**.
- The septum primum and secundum may develop normally but the oblique valvular passage between them may remain patent resulting in *patent foramen ovale* **(Fig. 20.12C)**. The patency is significant only if there is shunt of blood through it. In many cases, a probe can be passed through the oblique slit *(probe patency)* but without shunt.

- Occasionally, there is *premature closure of the foramen ovale* (i.e., before birth). As a result, the right atrium and ventricle undergo great hypertrophy, while the left side of the heart is underdeveloped.
- Defective formation of septa, if marked, can lead to a two-chambered heart (cor biloculare) in which there is one common ventricle and one common atrium. Alternatively, a three-chambered heart (cor triloculare) may be seen; it may consist of a single ventricle with two atria or of a single atrium with two ventricles *(cor triloculare biventriculare)*.

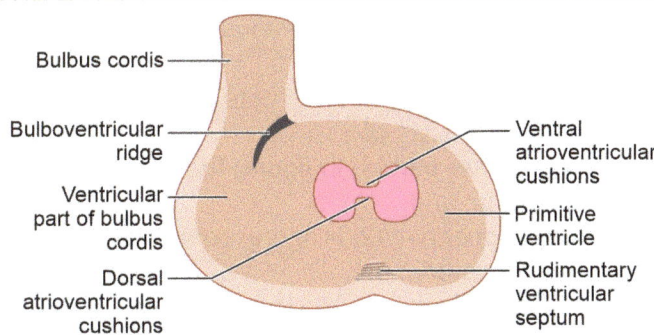

FIG. 20.13: Formation of bulboventricular cavity.

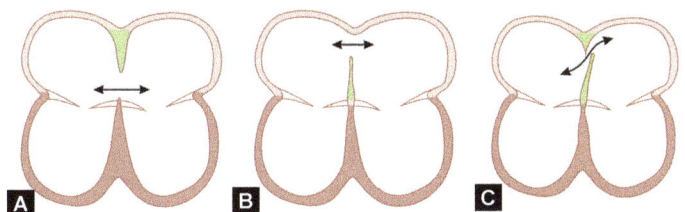

FIGS. 20.12A to C: Atrial septal defects. (A) Septum primum defect; (B) Septum secundum defect; (C) Patent foramen ovale.

Development of Ventricles

The right and left ventricles are formed by partitioning of primitive ventricle and incorporation of bulbus cordis.

Bulbus Cordis

The *bulbus cordis* is the cranial most part (arterial end) of the heart tube. It is divisible into three parts, i.e., proximal, middle and distal. The proximal is dilated and does not have any special name; the middle is called the *conus*, and the distal is called the *truncus arteriosus* (Fig. 20.3).

- The proximal part merges with the cavity of the primitive ventricle and forms the *bulboventricular chamber* (Figs. 20.4 and 20.13).
- The *conus cordis* forms the outflow part of both the ventricles. Two septa are formed which are the *proximal* and *distal bulbar septa*. The proximal bulbar septum contributes to the formation of *interventricular septum*. The distal bulbar septum separates the conus into *aortic vestibule* and *conus arteriosus/infundibulum* (Figs. 20.14A to C).
- A *spiral septum* appears within the truncus arteriosus and subdivides it into *ascending aorta* and *plumonary trunk*. The spiral septum is formed by union of right superior and left inferior *truncus swellings* or *cushions*. Orientation and fusion of these cushions takes place in such a manner that at its lower end, the pulmonary trunk lies ventral to the aorta, but as it is traced upward it comes to lie on its left side. This is because of the difference in the orientation of the spiral septum (Figs. 20.14A to C) at different levels.
    - *Proximal part*—coronal orientation and continuous with distal bulbar septum. With the result, the

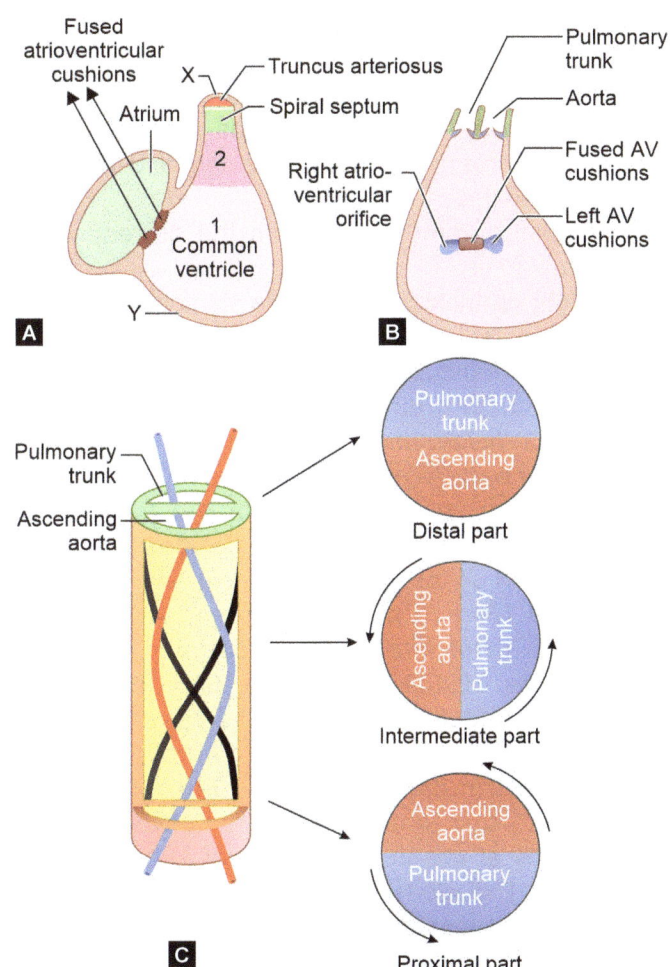

FIGS. 20.14A to C: (A) Two parts of the ventricular chamber. Part 1 lies anterior to the atrioventricular orifice. Part 2 is conical and lies higher up; (B) This is a section across the ventricle in the plane XY, shown in (A). Sections in the plane indicated by the arrow in (A) are shown in **Figure 20.15**; (C) Aorticopulmonary/spiral septum.

pulmonary trunk is anterior and the aorta is posterior.
- *Intermediate part*—anteroposterior orientation with pulmonary trunk on left and aorta on right.
- *Distal part*—again coronal orientation with aorta anterior and pulmonary trunk posterior.
- The truncus arteriosus is continuous distally with the aortic sac. The aortic sac is continuous with right and left pharyngeal arch arteries. These arteries arch

backward to become continuous with the right and left dorsal aortae.

From **Figures 20.14A to C**, note that the bulboventricular cavity consists of:
- A dilated lower part (1, in figure) that communicates with the atria; and
- A conical upper part (2, in figure) communicating with the truncus arteriosus.
- Part "1" is derived from the proximal one-third of the bulbus cordis and the primitive ventricle, while part "2" is from the conus.

Formation of Interventricular Septum

The ventricular cavity formed after the conus and proximal 1/3rd of bulbus cordis has merged into the primitive ventricle is subdivided into right and left halves in such a way that:
- Each half communicates with the corresponding atrium.
- The right ventricle opens into the pulmonary trunk and the left ventricle into the aorta.

The interventricular septum consists of three parts that develop from different sources. They are: (1) *muscular*, (2) *bulbar* and (3) *membranous* parts.
- **Muscular part:** A septum, called the *interventricular septum*, grows upward *from the floor of the bulboventricular cavity* and divides the lower dilated part of this cavity into right and left halves **(Fig. 20.15A)**. It meets the fused AV cushions *(septum intermedium)* and partially fuses with them **(Figs. 20.15A to D and 20.16A and B)**. On the external surface of the heart, the site of formation of the interventricular septum corresponds to the *bulboventricular sulcus* (see **Fig. 20.22A**). An interventricular foramen appears between the two ventricles at the upper margin of interventricular septum. The closure interventricular foramen is facilitated by septum intermedium and proximal bulbar septum **(Figs. 20.16A and B)**.
- **Bulbar part:** Two ridges, termed the *right* and *left bulbar ridges*, arise in the wall of the bulboventricular cavity (in the part derived from the conus). These ridges grow toward each other and fuse to form a *bulbar septum* **(Figs. 20.15 and 20.16)**. The bulbar septum grows downward toward the muscular part of interventricular septum but does not quite reach it, with the result that a gap is still left between the two.
- **Membranous part:** The gap between the upper edge of the interventricular septum, and the lower edge of the bulbar septum, is filled by proliferation of tissue from the right side of the AV cushions **(Figs. 20.15 and 20.16)** and the right and left bulbar ridges. The

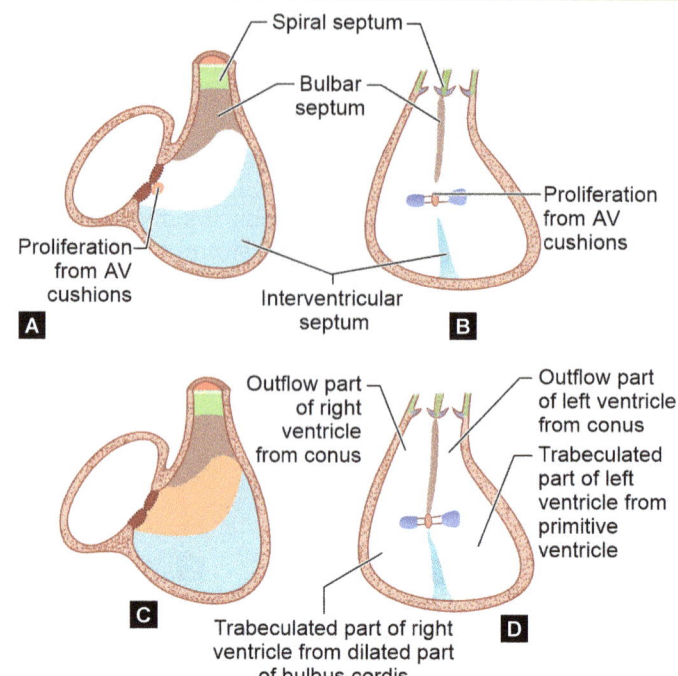

FIGS. 20.15A to D: Two stages in the formation of the ventricular septum. (B) and (D) correspond to (A) and (C) respectively. (A) Bulbar septum grows down from above, and interventricular septum grows upward from below; (C and D) The gap between the bulbar septum and the interventricular septum is filled in by proliferation from atrioventricular (AV) cushions. For explanation of orientation of these figures, see legend to **Figures 20.14A and B**.

membranous part of the interventricular septum is divisible into an anterior part, which separates the right and left ventricles, and a posterior part which separates the left ventricle from the right atrium (also called *AV septum*).
- The anterior part is derived from the proliferation of tissue from the endocardial cushions as described above. The derivation of the posterior part is shown in **Figures 20.17A and B**. It will be seen that the interatrial and interventricular septa do not meet the AV cushions in the same line. As a result, a part of these cushions separates the left ventricle from the right atrium. This part of the AV cushions forms the posterior part of the membranous septum.
- The interventricular septum is probably formed more by downward enlargement of the right and left ventricular cavities on either side of the septum, rather than by active growth of the septum itself.

Clinical correlation

Defective Formation of Septa
- **Ventricular septal defect (VSD)/ Interventricular septal defects** may be seen either in the membranous or in the muscular part of the septum **(Fig. 20.18)**. They are the most common congenital anomalies of the heart caused due to

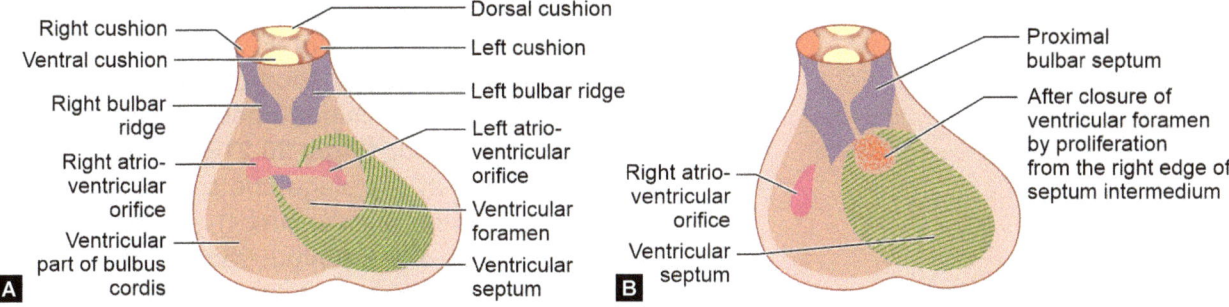

FIGS. 20.16A and B: Interior of bulboventricular cavity showing the cephalic margin of interventricular septum and its two horns and the proximal bulbar septum.

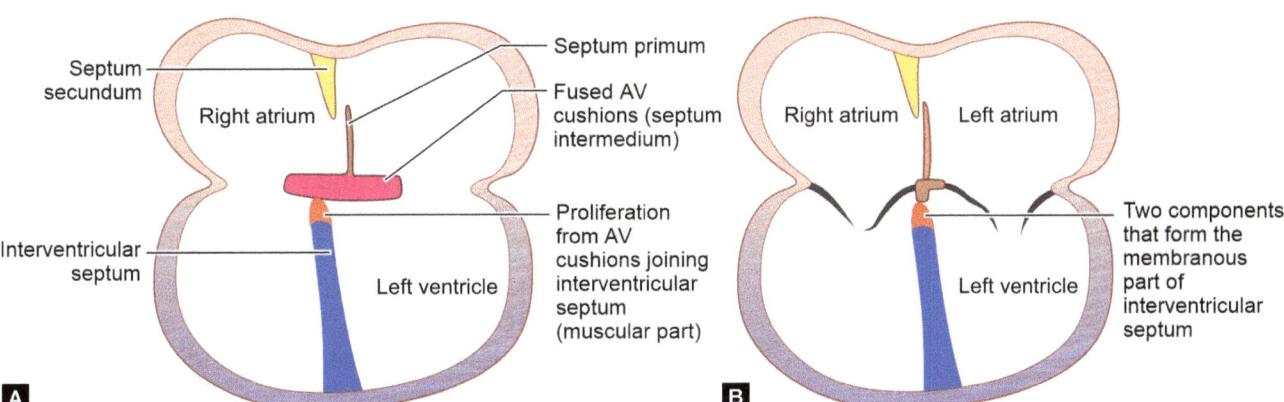

FIGS. 20.17A and B: In Figure (A) note that the interatrial and interventricular septa do not meet the atrioventricular (AV) cushions in the same plane. In Figure (B) note that the membranous part of the interventricular septum is made up of the original AV cushion between the attachment of the interatrial and interventricular septa, and of the endocardial proliferation from these cushions. The first part separates the left ventricle from the right atrium while the second part separates the two ventricles. The tricuspid valve is attached to the membranous septum at the junction of these parts. These figures are sections in the plane indicated by an arrow in **Figure 20.14A**.

failure of fusion of right and left bulbar ridges with AV cushions which forms membranous part. This results in right to left shunting. The cardiac output decreases resulting in exertion and fatigue. Rarely this condition affects muscular part.
- **Atrioventricular canal defect or persistent AV canal:** Defective formation of the AV cushions may lead to a condition in which *all four chambers of the heart may intercommunicate*. The interatrial and interventricular septa are incomplete (as the normal contributions to these septa from the endocardial cushions are lacking).
  - *Tetralogy of Fallot:* Two or more congenital heart defects may coexist. The embryological basis of the role of neural crest cells in tetralogy of Fallot lies in their contribution to the development of the conotruncal region, including the formation of the aorticopulmonary septum and proper alignment of the aorta and pulmonary trunk, defects in which lead to the characteristic features of this congenital heart defects. One classically recognized condition of this type is known as *Fallot's tetralogy*. It consists of (Fig. 20.19):
    ♦ Interventricular septal defect
    ♦ Overriding aorta
    ♦ Pulmonary stenosis
    ♦ Hypertrophy of the right ventricle
    This results in right to left shunt causing cyanosis. It's a common congenital cyanotic heart disease with symptoms including cyanosis, easy fatigability, breathlessness and paroxysmal hypercyanotic attacks.

Defects of the Spiral Septum

The spiral septum may not be formed at all. This condition is called *patent truncus arteriosus* (Fig. 20.20). Partial absence of the septum leads to communications (shunts) between the aorta and the pulmonary trunk.

Anomalies of Relationship of Chambers to Great Vessels
- **Transposition of great vessels:** The aorta arises from the right ventricle and the pulmonary trunk from the left ventricle.
- **Taussig–Bing syndrome:** The aorta arises from the right ventricle; the pulmonary trunk overrides both the right and left ventricles, there being an interventricular septal defect.
- The superior or inferior vena cava may end in the left atrium.
- The pulmonary veins may end in the right atrium or in one of its tributaries.

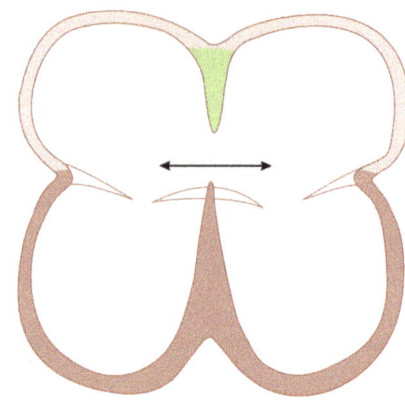

FIG. 20.18: Ventricular septal defects.

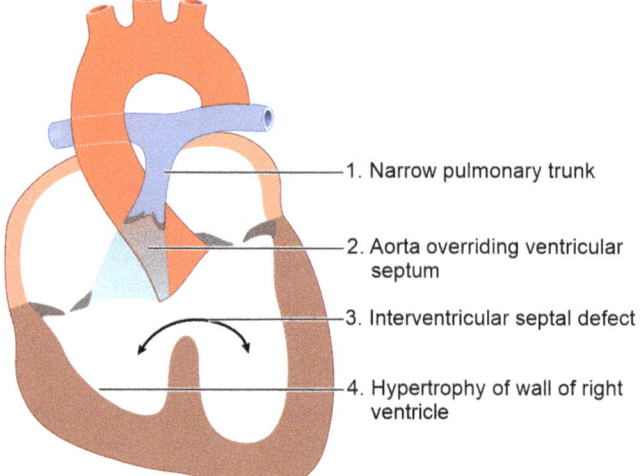

1. Narrow pulmonary trunk
2. Aorta overriding ventricular septum
3. Interventricular septal defect
4. Hypertrophy of wall of right ventricle

FIG. 20.19: Four features that constitute Fallot's tetralogy.

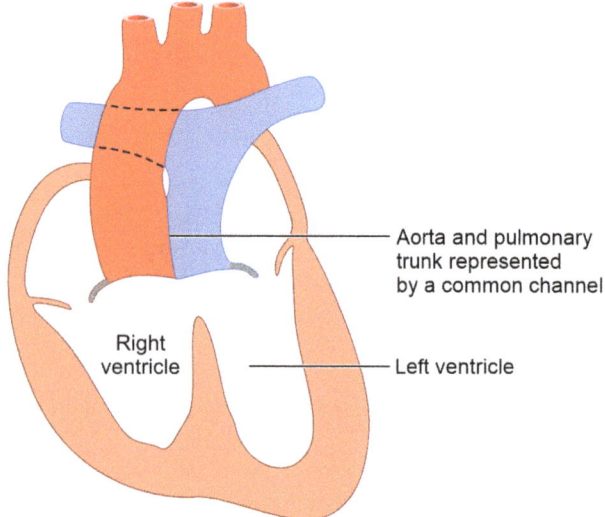

Aorta and pulmonary trunk represented by a common channel

Right ventricle

Left ventricle

FIG. 20.20: Patent truncus arteriosus. The ascending aorta and pulmonary trunk are represented by a single channel that opens into both ventricles.

EXTERIOR SHAPE OF HEART

❖ The heart tube is, for some time, is placed longitudinally and suspended from the dorsal wall of the pericardial cavity by two layers of pericardium that constitute the *dorsal mesocardium* (Fig. 20.21A).
❖ This mesocardium soon disappears and the heart tube lies free within the pericardial sac, suspended by its two ends (Figs. 20.21B and C).
❖ However, at this stage, the caudal part of the heart tube (atrium, sinus venosus) is embedded within the substance of the septum transversum.
❖ The part of the heart tube lying within the pericardial cavity is thus made up of bulbus cordis and ventricle. This part of the tube grows rapidly and, therefore, becomes folded on itself to form a "U"-shaped *bulboventricular loop* (Fig. 20.21C). Now, the primitive atrium is to the left and dorsal to primitive ventricle.
❖ Subsequently, as the atrium and sinus venosus are freed from the septum transversum, they come to lie behind and above the ventricle, and the heart tube is now "S"-shaped (Fig. 20.21D).
❖ At this stage, the bulbus cordis, and ventricle, are separated by a deep *bulboventricular sulcus* (Figs. 20.21D and 20.22). This sulcus gradually becomes shallower so that the conus, the proximal part of the bulbus cordis, and the ventricle, come to form one chamber (Figs. 20.22A to C) which communicates with the truncus arteriosus.
❖ The atrial chamber which lies behind the upper part of the ventricle, and of the truncus arteriosus, expands; and as it does so parts of it come to project forward on either side of the truncus. The sinus venosus moves away from the septum transversum and occupies a position dorsal to primitive atrium.
❖ As a result of these changes, the exterior of the heart assumes its definitive shape (Figs. 20.23A to D).

Clinical correlation

Congenital Anomalies of the Heart
Anomalies of position
- **Dextrocardia:** The chambers and blood vessels of the heart are reversed from side to side, i.e., all structures that normally lie on the right side are on the left, and vice versa (Fig. 20.24). This may be a part of the condition called situs inversus, in which all organs are transposed. When dextrocardia is not a part of situs inversus, it is usually accompanied by anomalies of the chambers of the heart, and of the great vessels. The PITX2 is the master gene for left sidedness.
- **Ectopia cordis (Fig. 20.25):** It is a rare congenital condition in which heart lies exposed, on the front of the chest, and can be seen from the outside, due to defective development of the chest wall. Death occurs in almost all cases during first day of life.

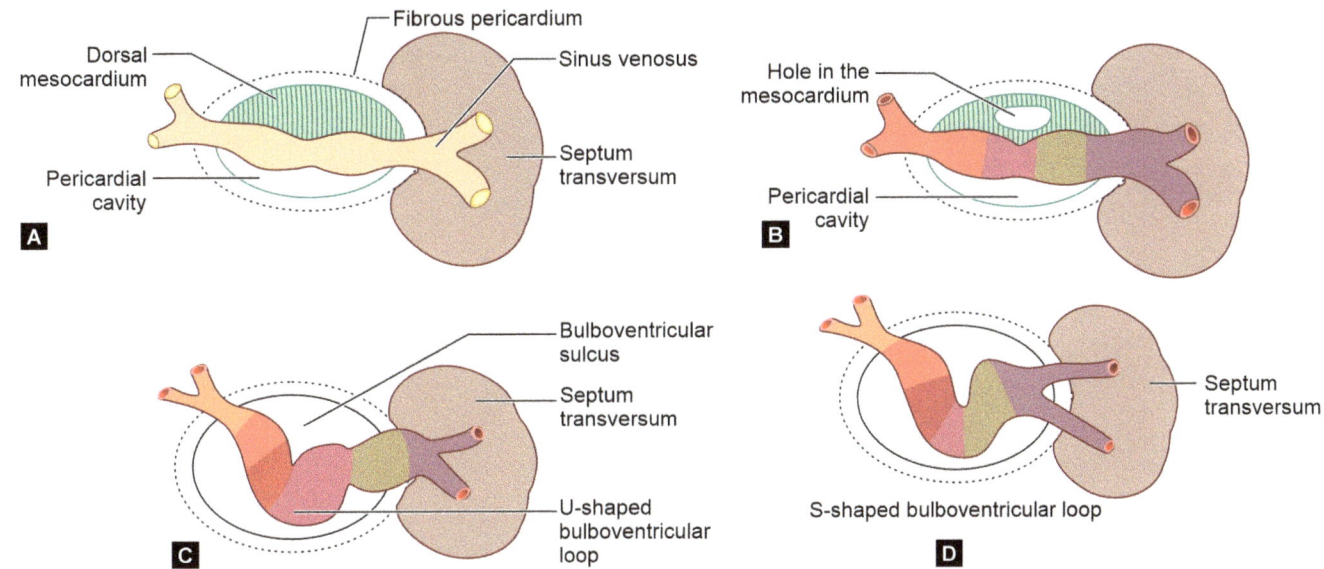

FIGS. 20.21A to D: Schemes to show the following: (A) Heart tube suspended by mesocardium; (B) Appearance of a hole in mesocardium; (C) Disappearance of mesocardium resulting in formation of transverse sinus of pericardium; In Figures (B) to (D) note gradual freeing of heart tube from septum transversum, and folding of heart tube.

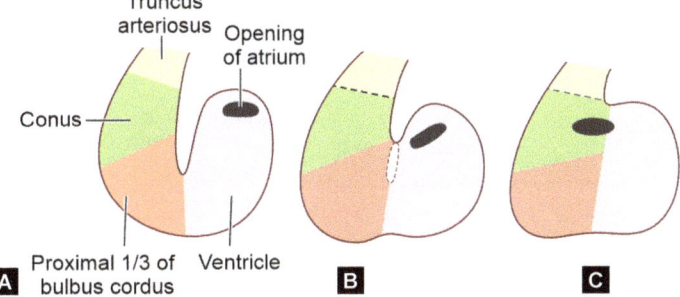

FIGS. 20.22A to C: Scheme to show incorporation of conus (and proximal dilated part of bulbus cordis) into the ventricle by disappearance of the bulboventricular sulcus. Note that the opening of atrium into ventricle gradually shifts to the center of the posterior wall of the common bulboventricular chamber. The part labeled "conus" includes the dilated part of the bulbus cordis.

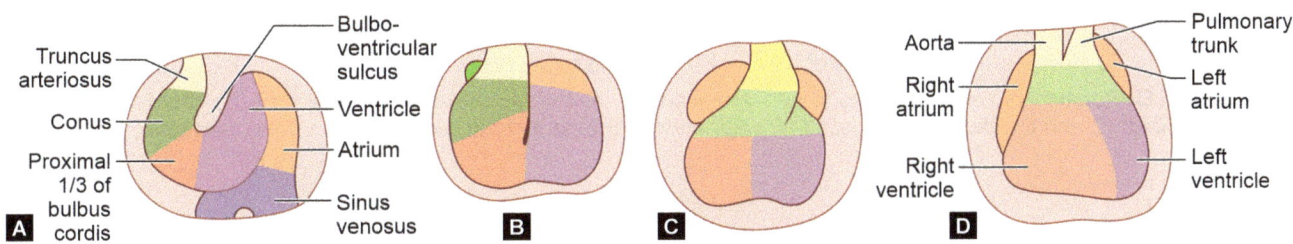

FIGS. 20.23A to D: Stages in establishment of external form of the heart.

LAYERS OF CARDIAC WALL

The cardiac wall is made up of three layers: *endocardium, myocardium, and epicardium*.
1. Endocardium forms from the wall of endothelial of heart tube.
2. Myocardium forms from splanchnopleuric mesoderm.
3. Epicardium forms from the outer cell layer of primitive heart tube.

The heart tube invaginates into the pericardial sac on its dorsal side. As it does so, the splanchnopleuric mesoderm lining the dorsal side of the pericardial cavity proliferates to form a thick layer called the *myoepicardial mantle* (or *epimyocardial mantle*) **(Figs. 20.26C and D)**. When the invagination is complete, the myoepicardial mantle completely surrounds the heart tube. It gives rise to the *cardiac muscle (myocardium)* and also to the *visceral layer of pericardium (epicardium)*. The parietal layer of pericardium is derived from somatopleuric mesoderm.

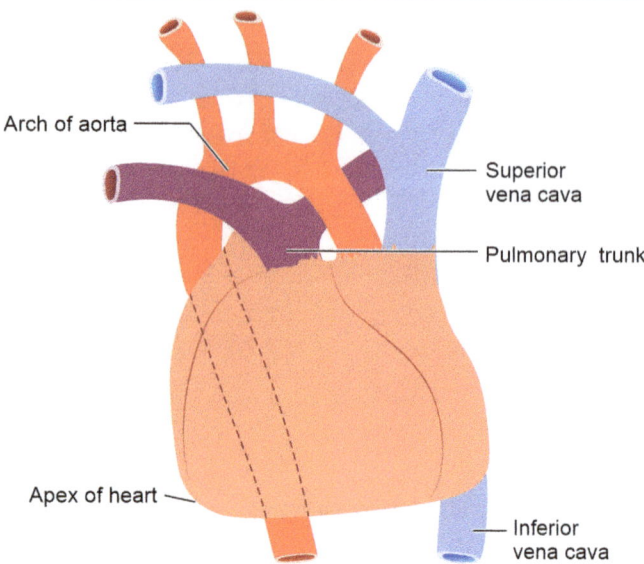

FIG. 20.24: Dextrocardia. The chambers and large blood vessels show right left reversal.

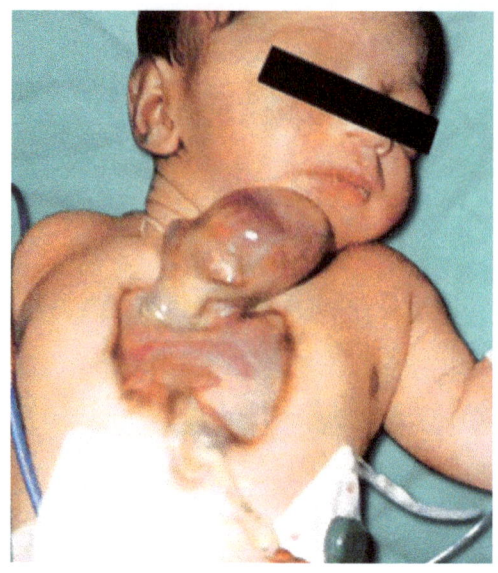

FIG. 20.25: Ectopia cordia.

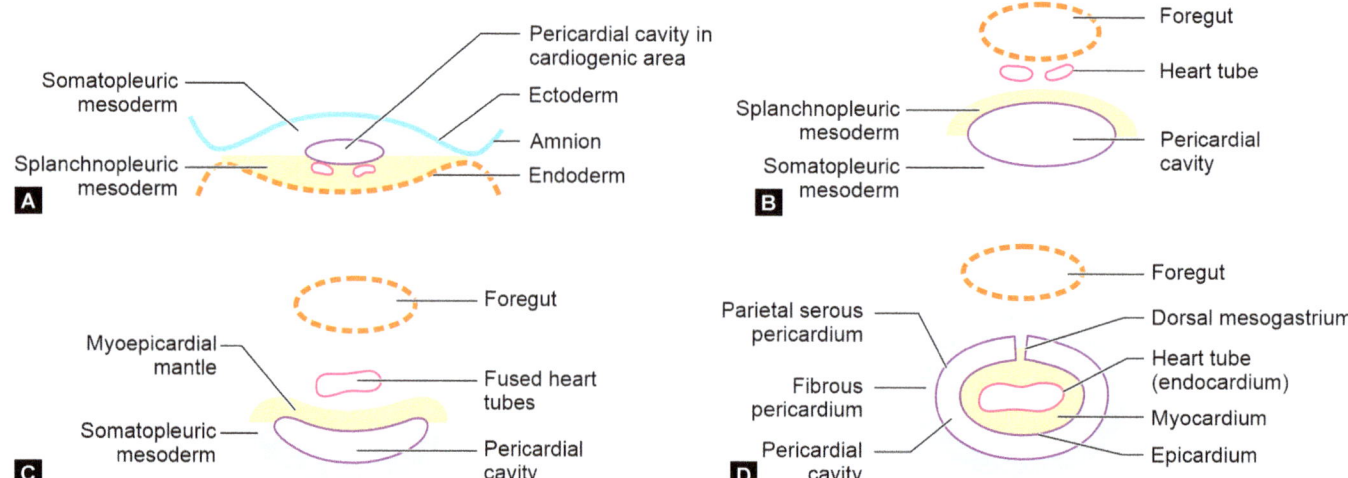

FIGS. 20.26A to D: Relationship of heart tubes to pericardial cavity. (A) Before formation of head fold; (B) After formation of head fold; (C and D) Show the process of invagination of the pericardial cavity by the single heart tube.

VALVES OF THE HEART

The *mitral* and *tricuspid* valves are formed by proliferation of connective tissue under the endocardium of the left and right AV canals. Mitral valve is *bicuspid valve*.

- The *pulmonary* and *aortic valves* are derived from *endocardial cushions* that are formed at the junction of truncus arteriosus and the conus. Two cushions, right and left, appear in the wall of the conus. They grow and fuse with each other (Figs. 20.27A to D).
- With the separation of the aortic and pulmonary openings, the right and left cushions are each subdivided into two parts, one part going to each orifice (Figs. 20.27A to D).
- Simultaneously, two more cushions, anterior and posterior appear.
- As a result, the aortic and pulmonary openings each have three cushions, from which three cusps of the corresponding valve develop.
- The pulmonary valve is at first ventral to the aortic valve (Figs. 20.27A to D). Subsequently, there is a rotation so that the pulmonary valve comes to lie ventral and to the left of the aortic valve (Figs. 20.27A to D).
- It is only after this rotation that the cusps acquire their definitive relationships (pulmonary trunk: 1 posterior, 2 anterior; aorta: 1 anterior, 2 posterior).

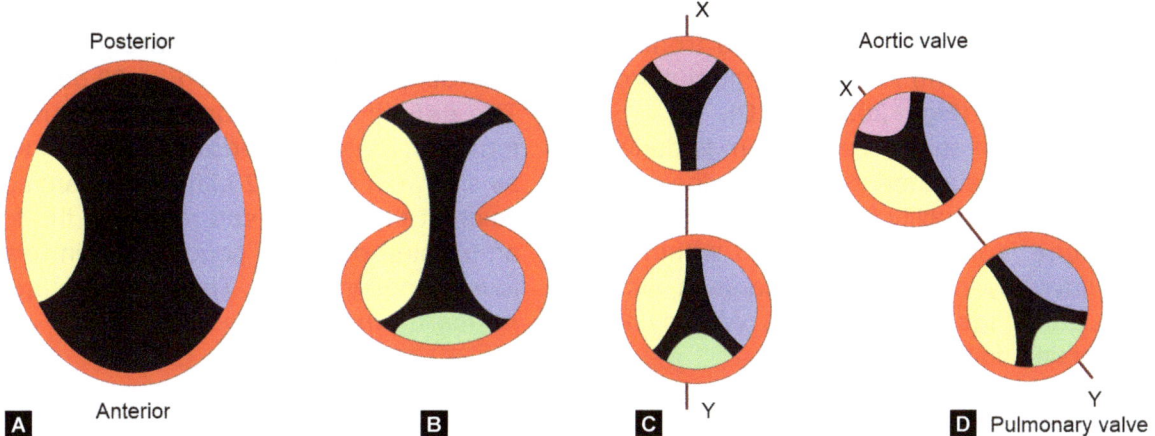

FIGS. 20.27A to D: Formation of aortic and pulmonary valves. Note that the vessels undergo an anticlockwise rotation [compare axis XY in (C and D)]. It is only after this rotation that the cusps of the aortic and pulmonary valves acquire their definitive position.

Clinical correlation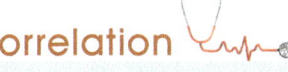

Congenital Anomalies of the Heart Valves
Atresia or stenosis
Any of the orifices of the heart may have too narrow an opening (*stenosis*), or none at all (*atresia*). The aortic and pulmonary passages may also show *supravalvular, or subvalvular, stenosis* **(Figs. 20.28A to C)**. Alternatively, the openings may be too large as a result of which the valves become incompetent.
- In *pulmonary stenosis*, the foramen ovale and the ductus arteriosus remain patent.
- In *aortic stenosis* also, the ductus arteriosus is patent and blood flows into the aorta through it.
- *Tricuspid atresia:* It is a congenital heart defect where the tricuspid valve is absent an underdeveloped right ventricle and insufficient tissue in AV cushion for formation of the valve. This is always associated with patent foramen ovale, VSD, underdeveloped right ventricle and hypertrophy of left ventricle.

Sometimes, there may be accessory cusps in the valves.

- After fusion of the two tubes, the SA node lies in the sinus venosus.
- When the sinus venosus is incorporated into the right atrium, it comes to lie near the opening of the superior vena cava.
- The *atrioventricular/SA node* and the *AV bundle of His* form in the left wall of the sinus venosus, and in the AV canal respectively.
- Fibers of AV bundle passes into ventricle and split into two sides, left and right bundle branches which are distributed through out pericardium and termed as *Purkinje fibers*.
- After the sinus venosus is absorbed into the right atrium, the *AV node* comes to lie near the interatrial septum.

> **NOTE**
>
> These nodes and Purkinje fibers are supplied by autonomic nervous system but conducting system of heart functions well before the innervation. This is due the conducting system is made up of cardiomyocytes which initiates impulses in heart through only one pathway. That's why the contraction of cardiac muscles is myogenic rather than neurogenic.

PERICARDIAL CAVITY

We have already noted several important facts about the development of the pericardial cavity, and these may be briefly recapitulated as follows:
- The pericardial cavity is a derivative of the part of intraembryonic coelom that lies in the midline, cranial to the prechordal plate.
- After the formation of the head fold, the pericardial cavity comes to lie on the ventral side of the body of the embryo.
- The heart tube invaginates the pericardial sac from the dorsal aspect **(Figs. 20.26A to D)**.

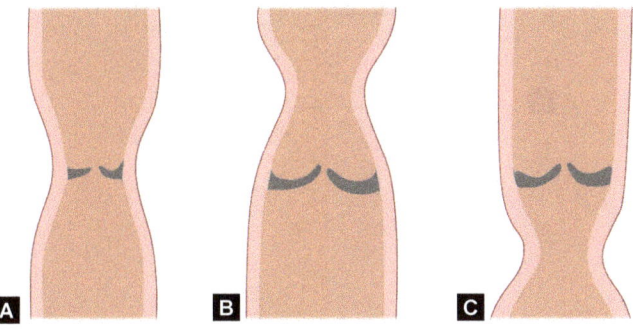

FIGS. 20.28A to C: Types of aortic stenosis. (A) Valvular; (B) Supravalvular; (C) Infravalvular.

CONDUCTING SYSTEM OF HEART

- At the stage when there are two heart tubes, a pacemaker (which later forms the *sinuatrial node or SA node*) lies in the caudal part of the left tube.

- The parietal layer of the *serous pericardium*, and the *fibrous pericardium*, are derived from the somatopleuric mesoderm lining the ventral side of the pericardial cavity **(Figs. 20.26A to D)**.
- The visceral layer of serous pericardium is derived from the splanchnopleuric mesoderm lining the dorsal side of the pericardial cavity **(Fig. 20.26D)**.
- The heart tube is initially suspended within the pericardial cavity by the dorsal mesocardium, which soon disappears **(Figs. 20.21A and B)**. We may now consider certain additional facts.
- After disappearance of the dorsal mesocardium, the visceral and parietal layers of pericardium are in continuity only at the arterial and venous ends of the heart tube **(Figs. 20.29A, B, D and E)**.
- With the folding of the heart tube, the arterial and venous ends come closer to each other. The space between them becomes the *transverse sinus of pericardium* **(Figs. 20.29C and F)**.
- A number of blood vessels are formed at the two ends of the heart tube. At the arterial end, these are the aorta and the pulmonary trunk. At the venous end, they are the superior vena cava, inferior vena cava, and four pulmonary veins **(Fig. 20.30A)**.
- The definitive reflections of the pericardium are formed merely by rearrangement of these vessels as shown in **Figure 20.30B**. Rearrangement of the veins at the venous end results in the formation of an isolated pouch of pericardium, in relation to the four pulmonary veins. This is the *oblique sinus of pericardium*.

Clinical correlation

Congenital Anomalies of the Pericardium
- **Abnormal growth:** Congenital tumors may be formed. The left atrium may be partially subdivided by a transverse septum. The myocardium may be poorly developed *(hypoplasia)*.
- The pericardium may be partially or completely absent.
- It's congenital defects in the conducting system of the heart.

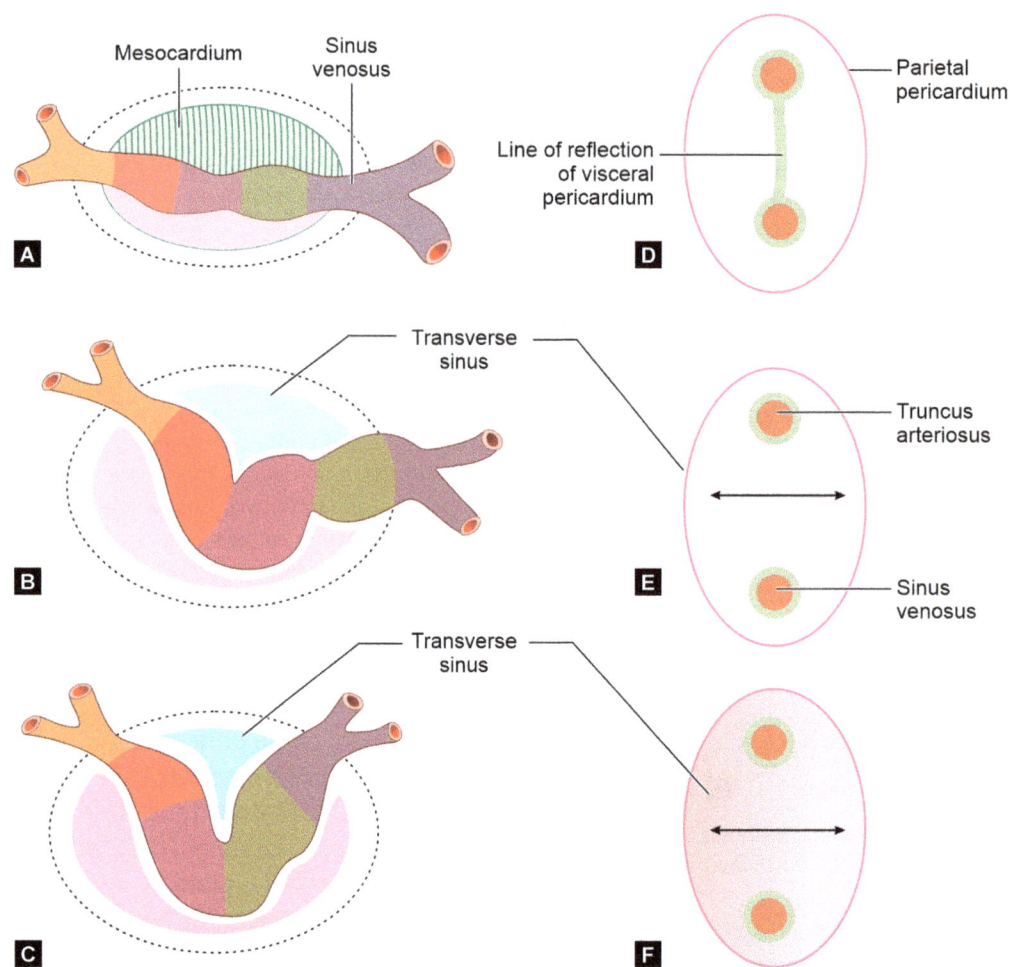

FIGS. 20.29A to F: Schemes showing the relationship of the heart tube to the pericardial sac. (A), (B) and (C) are lateral views while (D), (E) and (F) show the dorsal aspect of the interior of the pericardial sac at corresponding stages. Disappearance of the mesocardium leads to formation of transverse sinus of pericardium. Note that with the folding of the heart tube, the arterial and venous ends of the heart tube are brought closer together, and the transverse sinus comes to lie between them.

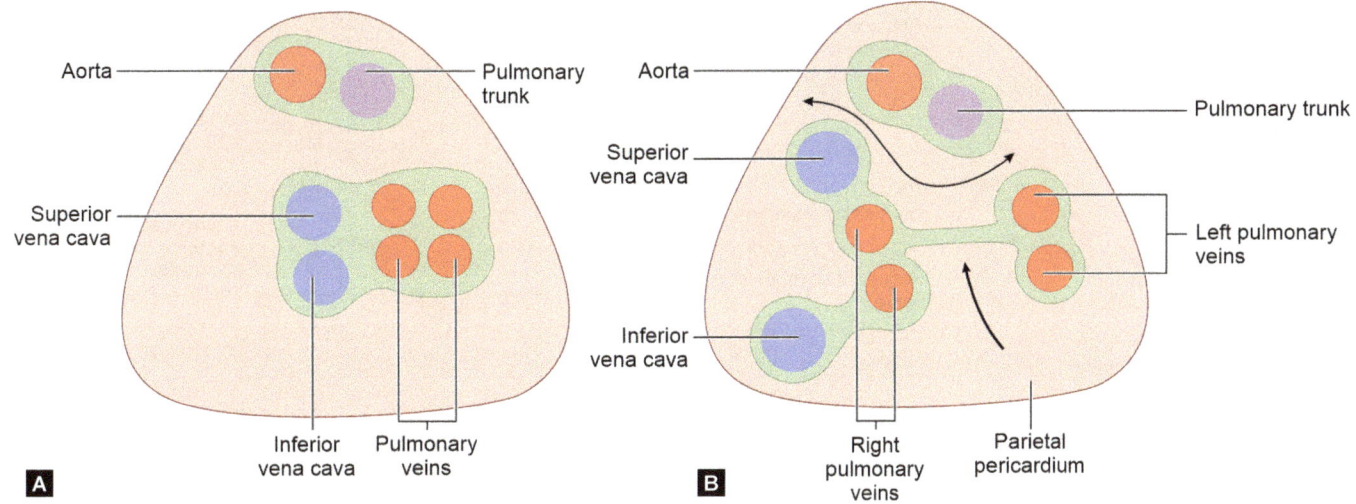

FIGS. 20.30A and B: (A) Scheme to show that the oblique sinus of pericardium is established by rearrangement of veins entering the heart. The sinus is indicated by the lower arrow in (B), the upper arrow indicates the transverse sinus.

DEVELOPMENT OF BLOOD VESSELS

In chapter 10, we have already discussed the formation of blood vessels. They develop from mesenchymal cells that are derived from mesoderm by two processes: *vasculogenesis* and *angiogenesis*.

Vasculogenesis results in the formation of major vessels of the body, i.e., dorsal aorta and cardinal vessels. All other vessels are formed by angiogenesis.

DEVELOPMENT OF ARTERIES

The first arteries to appear in the embryo are the right and left *primitive aortae*. They are continuous with the two endocardial heart tubes. Pharyngeal arch arteries formed the arteries supplying head and neck while dorsal aorta forms the remaining arteries.

Each primitive aorta consists of three parts **(Fig. 20.31A)**:
1. A portion lying ventral to the foregut *(ventral aorta)*.
2. An arched portion lying in the first pharyngeal arch forms the *first aortic arch artery*.
3. A dorsal portion lying dorsal to the gut *(dorsal aorta)*.

Pharyngeal/Aortic Arch Arteries and their Fate

* After the fusion of the two endocardial tubes, the two ventral aortae partially fuse to form the *aortic sac*, the unfused parts remaining as the *right and left horns* of the sac **(Fig. 20.31B)**.
* Successive arterial arches now appear in the second to sixth pharyngeal arches, each being connected ventrally to the right or left horn of the aortic sac and dorsally to the dorsal aorta **(Fig. 20.31C)**.
* The major arteries of the head and neck, and of the thorax, are derived from these arches as follows:
  - The greater part of the first and second arch arteries disappear **(Fig. 20.32A)**. In adult life, the

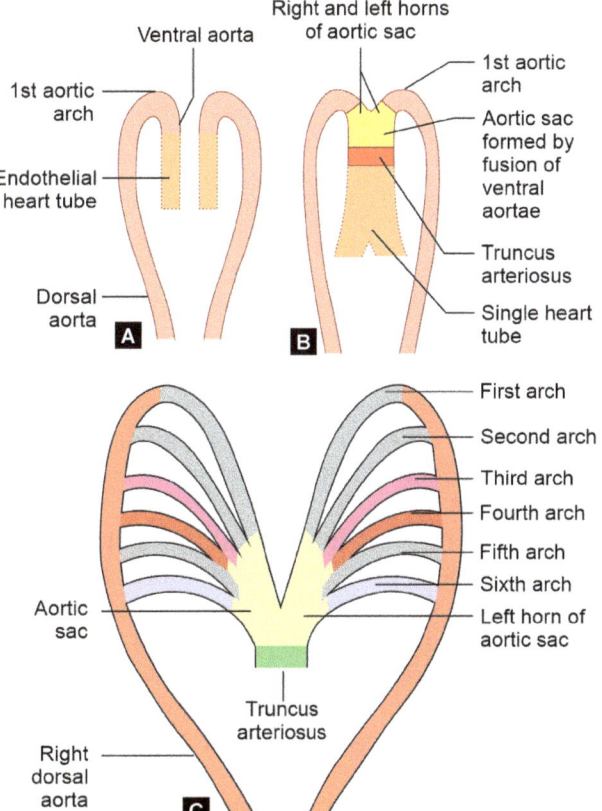

FIGS. 20.31A to C: Relation of first aortic arch to heart tubes. (A) Before fusion of heart tubes; (B) After fusion; (C) Aortic arches. Each arch connects the aortic sac to the dorsal aorta. Note that actually all arches are never present at the same time. The first and second arches have retrogressed by the time the sixth appears.

first arch artery is represented by the *maxillary artery*. The second arch artery persists for some part of fetal life as the *hyoid artery* and *stapedial artery*: it may contribute to the formation of the *external carotid artery*.
  - The fifth arch artery also disappears **(Fig. 20.32A)**.

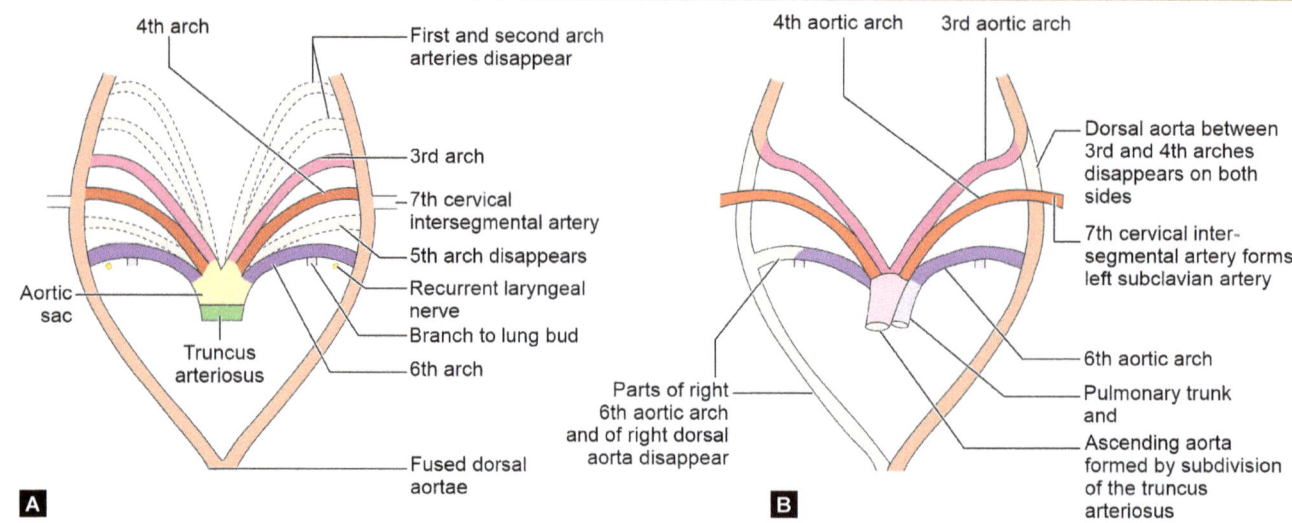

FIGS. 20.32A and B: Fate of aortic arches: (A) Disappearance of first, second and fifth arches; (B) Disappearance of ductus caroticus (on both sides), and of part of right dorsal aorta. Part of the right sixth arch also disappears.

- Now, the aortic sac is connected only with the arteries of the third, fourth and sixth arches.
- The third and fourth arch arteries open into the ventral part, and the sixth arch artery into the dorsal part of the aortic sac **(Fig. 20.32B)**.
- The spiral septum that is formed in the truncus arteriosus extends into the aortic sac; and fuses with its posterior wall in such a way that blood from the pulmonary trunk passes only into the sixth arch artery, while that from the ascending aorta passes into the third and fourth arch arteries **(Fig. 20.32B)**.
❖ Several changes now take place in the arterial arches to produce the adult pattern as follows:
  - The two dorsal aortae grow cranially beyond the point of attachment of the first arch artery **(Fig. 20.32B)**.
  - The portion of the dorsal aorta, between the attachment of the third and fourth arch arteries called *carotid duct (ductus caroticus)* disappears on both sides **(Fig. 20.32B)**.
  - Portion of right dorsal aorta, between the point of attachment of the fourth arch artery and the point of fusion of the two dorsal aortae, disappears **(Fig. 20.32B)**.
  - Each sixth arch artery gives off an artery to the developing lung bud. On the right side, the portion of the sixth arch artery between this bud and the dorsal aorta disappears. On the left side, this part remains patent and forms the *ductus arteriosus*. The ductus arteriosus carries most of the blood from the right ventricle to the dorsal aorta. It is obliterated after birth and is then seen as the *ligamentum arteriosum*.
  - Each third arch artery gives off a bud that grows cranially to form the *external carotid artery* **(see Fig. 20.33G)**.
  - The dorsal aortae give off a series of lateral intersegmental branches to the body wall. One of these, the seventh cervical intersegmental artery supplies the upper limb bud. It comes to be attached to the dorsal aorta near the attachment of the fourth arch artery **(Fig. 20.32B)**.
❖ Development of main arteries can now be summarized as follows:
  - *Ascending aorta* and the *pulmonary trunk* are formed from the truncus arteriosus **(Fig. 20.32B)**.
  - *Arch of the aorta* is derived from the ventral part of the aortic sac, its left horn, and the left fourth arch artery **(Fig. 20.33A)**.
  - *Descending aorta* is derived from the left dorsal aorta, below the attachment of fourth arch artery, along with the fused median vessel **(Fig. 20.33B)**.
  - *Brachiocephalic artery* is formed by the right horn of the aortic sac **(Fig. 20.33C)**.
  - Proximal part of the *right subclavian artery* **(Fig. 20.33D)** is derived from the right fourth arch artery, and the remaining part of the artery being derived from the seventh cervical intersegmental artery and the part of right dorsal aorta connecting the right 4th arch and right 7th cervical intersegmental arteries.
  - *Left subclavian artery* is derived entirely from the seventh cervical intersegmental artery, which arises from the dorsal aorta opposite the attachment of the fourth arch artery **(Fig. 20.33D)**.
  - *Common carotid artery* is derived, on either side, from part of the third arch artery, proximal to the external carotid bud **(Fig. 20.33E)**.
  - *Internal carotid artery* is formed by the portion of the third arch artery distal to the bud, along with the original dorsal aorta cranial to the attachment of the third arch artery **(Fig. 20.33F)**.
  - As the right third and fourth arch arteries arise from the right horn of the aortic sac, the common carotid and subclavian arteries become branches of the *brachiocephalic artery*.

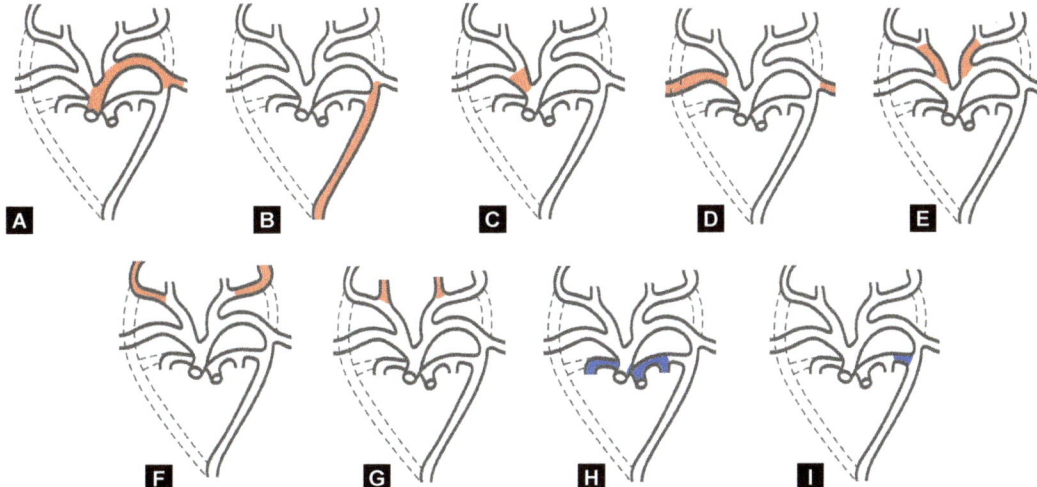

FIGS. 20.33A to I: (A) The arch of the aorta is derived from the aortic sac, its left horn, and the left 4th arch artery; (B) The descending aorta is derived from the left dorsal aorta, and fused dorsal aortae; (C) The brachiocephalic artery is derived from the right horn of the aortic sac; (D) The right subclavian artery is derived from the right 4th arch artery, right 7th cervical intersegmental artery and small part of right dorsal aorta connecting the two. The left subclavian artery is formed only from the left 7th cervical intersegmental artery; (E) The common carotid artery is derived from the proximal part of the 3rd arch artery; (F) The internal carotid artery is derived from distal part of the 3rd arch artery and dorsal aorta (cranial—most part); (G) The external carotid artery arises as a bud from the 3rd arch artery; (H) The pulmonary arteries arise from the 6th arch arteries; (I) The ductus arteriosus is derived from part of the left 6th arch artery.

- As already mentioned, the *external carotid artery* arises as a bud from the third arch artery **(Fig. 20.33G)**.
- *Pulmonary arteries* are derived from the part of the sixth arch arteries lying between the pulmonary trunk and the branches to the lung buds **(Fig. 20.33H)**.
- As already stated, the part of the left sixth arch artery, between the branch to the lung bud and the aorta, forms the *ductus arteriosus* **(Fig. 20.33I)**.
- ❖ Relationship of the main nerves of the head and neck to the arteries:
  This can be explained on the basis of the development of the arteries.
  - The nerves of the pharyngeal arches are, at first, lateral to the corresponding arteries.
- The nerves of the first, second and third arches (V, VII and IX) retain their lateral positions.
- The disappearance of the ductus caroticus enables the nerve of the fourth arch *(superior laryngeal)* to move medially, and it comes to lie deep to the main arteries of the neck.
- The nerve of the sixth arch *(recurrent laryngeal)* is at first caudal to the artery of this arch **(Fig. 20.34A)**. With the disappearance of part of the sixth arch artery, on the right side, the nerve moves cranially and comes into relationship with the right fourth arch artery (subclavian) **(Fig. 20.34B)**. On the left side, it retains its relationship to that part of the sixth arch which forms the *ductus arteriosus*. With the elongation of the neck, and the descent of the heart, these nerves are dragged downward and, therefore, have to follow a recurrent course back to the larynx.

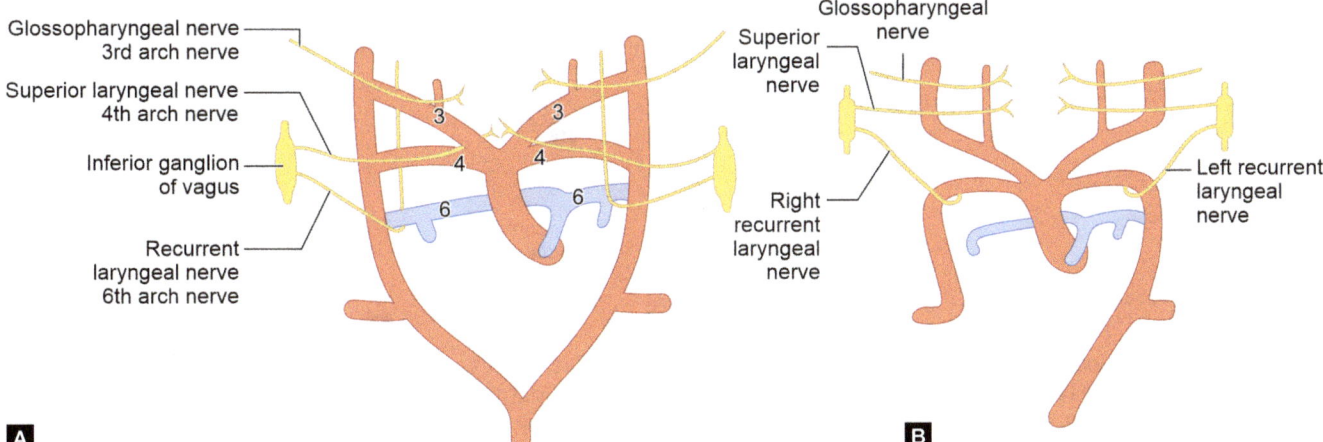

FIGS. 20.34A and B: Relationship of the vagus and recurrent laryngeal nerves to the aortic arches.

Clinical correlation

Anomalous Development of Pharyngeal Arch Arteries

We have seen that the development of the normal arterial pattern is dependent upon the disappearance of some parts of the pharyngeal arch arteries. Occasionally, this process is disturbed in that:
- Some parts that normally disappear may persist.
- Some parts that normally persist may disappear.

As a result, several anomalies may be produced. Some of these are as follows:
- **Double aortic arch (Fig. 20.35A):** Double aortic arch is a congenital vascular anomaly resulting from the persistence of both the right and left fourth embryonic aortic arches which form vascular ring and can compress the trachea and esophagus.
- **Right aortic arch (Fig. 20.35B):** A right aortic arch occurs when the embryonic right fourth aortic arch and right dorsal aorta persist, while the left fourth aortic arch and left dorsal aorta regress. This abnormal development leads to the formation of the aortic arch on the right side of the body instead of the left. Right aortic arch can be associated with other congenital heart defects and may form a vascular ring around the trachea and esophagus, potentially causing symptoms related to compression.
- The ductus arteriosus, which is normally occluded soon after birth, may remain patent *(patent ductus arteriosus)*. It is a most common congenital anomaly affecting great vessels resulting in shunting of blood from aorta to the pulmonary circulation. Some drugs have effects on these if taken during pregnancy results in patent ductus arteriosus, like prostaglandins E. NSAIDs like indomethacin promote closure of PDA.
- The *right subclavian artery* may arise as the last branch of the aortic arch **(Fig. 20.35C)**. Such an artery runs to the right behind the esophagus **(Fig. 20.36)**. Along with the aorta this artery forms an arterial ring enclosing the trachea and esophagus. The ring may press upon and obstruct these tubes. In this abnormality, the right recurrent laryngeal nerve does not hook around the subclavian artery. It passes directly to the larynx. An arterial ring can also be formed if the dorsal aorta persists on both sides.
- The *ductus caroticus* may persist. As a result, the left internal carotid arises directly from the aortic arch, and the right internal carotid from the subclavian **(Fig. 20.35D)**.
- **Interrupted aortic arch:** A segment of the aortic arch may be missing. The ascending aorta ends by supplying the left common carotid artery. The left subclavian artery arises from the distal segment which receives blood through a patent ductus arteriosus.
- The aorta may show a localized narrowing of its lumen, leading to partial or even complete obstruction to blood flow. This condition is called *coarctation of the aorta*.
  Coarctation is most frequently seen near the attachment of the ductus arteriosus to the aorta. It may be (1) proximal to the attachment *(preductal)* **(Fig. 20.35E)** or (2) distal to the attachment of the ductus *(postductal)* **(Fig. 20.35F)** in which case the right ventricle supplies the distal part of the body through the ductus arteriosus. When coarctation is postductal, numerous anastomoses are established between branches of the aorta taking origin above the constriction and those arising below this level. Coarctation is said to be a result of the process of obliteration of the ductus arteriosus extending into the aorta. It can also occur as an abnormality in the vessel wall.
- Some other anomalies and the mode of origin of the branches of arch of the aorta are illustrated in **Figure 20.35G**.

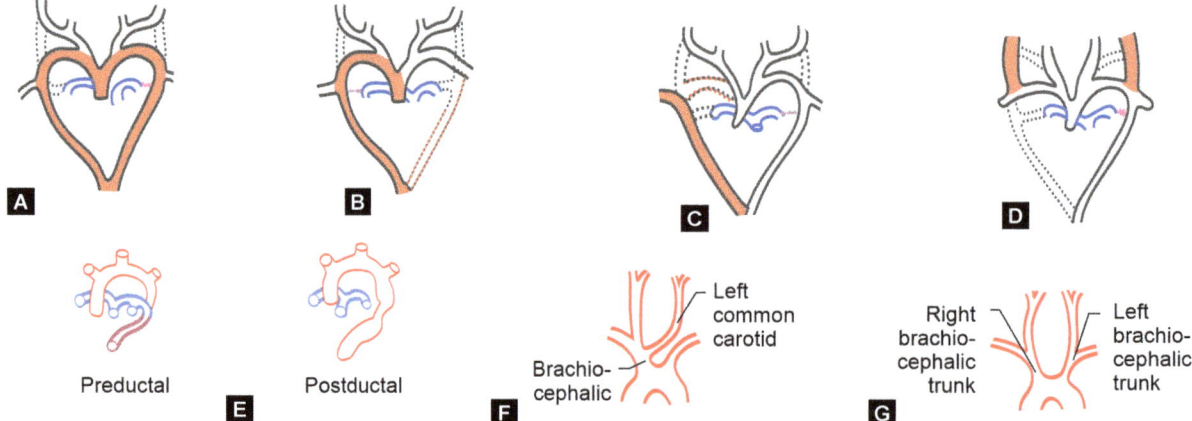

FIGS. 20.35A to G: Anomalies associated with the development of aortic arches. (A) Double aortic arch; (B) Right aortic arch; (C) Anomalous right subclavian artery; (D) Persistent ductus caroticus; (E) Coarctation of aorta (preductal); (F) Coarctation of aorta (postductal); (G) Anomalies in pattern of branches. Left common carotid artery arising from brachiocephalic artery. Left subclavian and left common carotid arising by a common stem (left brachiocephalic).

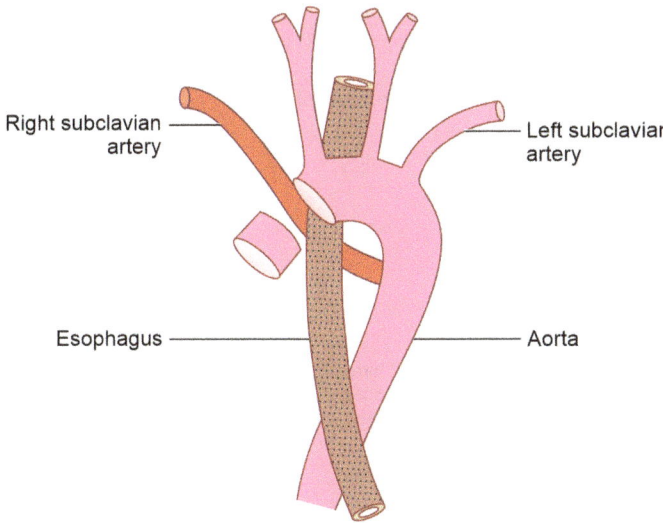

FIG. 20.36: Relationship of abnormal right subclavian artery to the esophagus and to the arch of the aorta.

Development of Other Arteries

The primitive dorsal aortae give off three groups of branches **(Fig. 20.37)**. These are as follows:

❖ The *ventral splanchnic arteries* supply the gut. Most of these arteries disappear but three arteries, the *celiac, superior mesenteric* and *inferior mesenteric* remain to supply the infradiaphragmatic part of the foregut, the midgut, and the hindgut respectively. Other remnants of these vessels are the *bronchial* and *esophageal arteries.*

❖ The *lateral or intermediate splanchnic arteries* supply structures developing from the intermediate mesoderm. These persist as the *renal, suprarenal, phrenic* and *spermatic or ovarian arteries.*

❖ The *dorsolateral (somatic intersegmental)* branches run between two adjacent segments. They retain their original intersegmental arrangement in the thoracic and lumbar regions where they can be recognized as the *intercostal* and *lumbar arteries.*

- Each dorsolateral artery divides into a dorsal and a ventral division. The ventral division gives off a lateral branch that is most conspicuous in the region of the limb buds. The dorsal division runs dorsally and supplies the muscles of the back. Each dorsal division gives off a spinal branch that runs medially to supply the spinal cord.
- The branches of the dorsolateral arteries of successive segments become interconnected by the formation of longitudinal anastomoses.
- In the neck, the dorsal branches are connected by anastomoses that are formed in three situations **(Fig. 20.38)**:
    - *Precostal*, in front of the necks of the ribs (or costal elements). The precostal anastomoses persist as *the thyrocervical trunk, ascending cervical* and *superior intercostal arteries.*
    - *Postcostal*, between the costal elements and the transverse processes. The postcostal anastomoses form the greater part of the *vertebral artery.*
    - *Post-transverse*, behind the transverse processes. The post-transverse anastomoses remain as the *deep cervical artery.*
- The ventral divisions of the somatic intersegmental arteries are interconnected by anastomoses that are formed on the ventral aspect of the body wall, near the midline **(Fig. 20.39)**. These form the *internal thoracic, superior epigastric* and *inferior epigastric* arteries.

❖ At this stage, special mention must be made of the *seventh cervical intersegmental artery*. The main stem of this artery becomes the *subclavian artery*. Like other dorsolateral arteries, it divides into dorsal, ventral and lateral divisions. The dorsal division forms the *stem of the vertebral artery*. The lateral division grows into the upper limb forming the *axillary and brachial arteries*. The ventral division forms the *stem of the internal thoracic (mammary) artery.*

Development of Vertebral Artery (Figs. 20.40A and B)

❖ The first part of the artery, from its origin to the point of entry into the foramen transversarium of the sixth cervical vertebra, is formed by the dorsal division of the seventh cervical intersegmental artery.

❖ The vertical part (second part), lying in the foramina transversaria, is formed from the postcostal anastomoses between the first to sixth cervical intersegmental arteries.

❖ The horizontal (third) part, running transversely on the arch of the atlas, is derived from the spinal branch of the first cervical intersegmental artery.

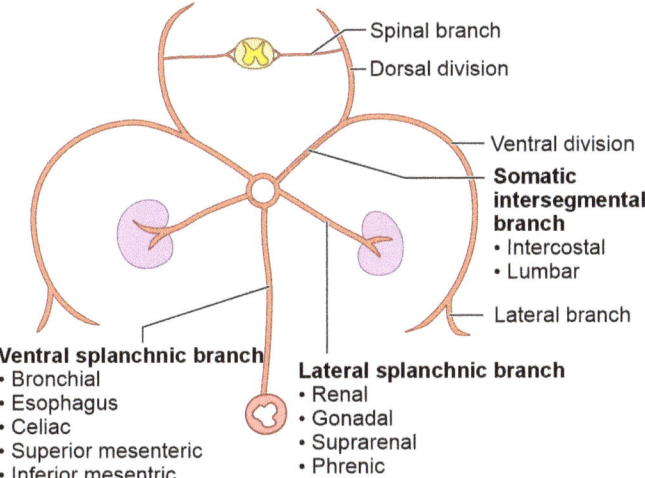

FIG. 20.37: Basic branching pattern of the embryonic dorsal aorta.

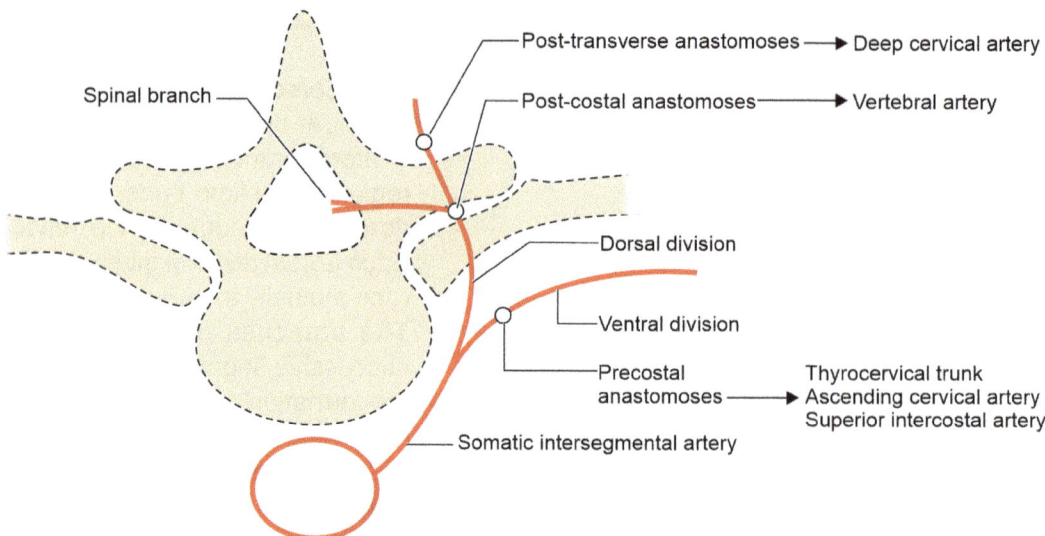

FIG. 20.38: Sites of vertical anastomoses between branches of dorsal aorta. The fate of the anastomoses is also shown.

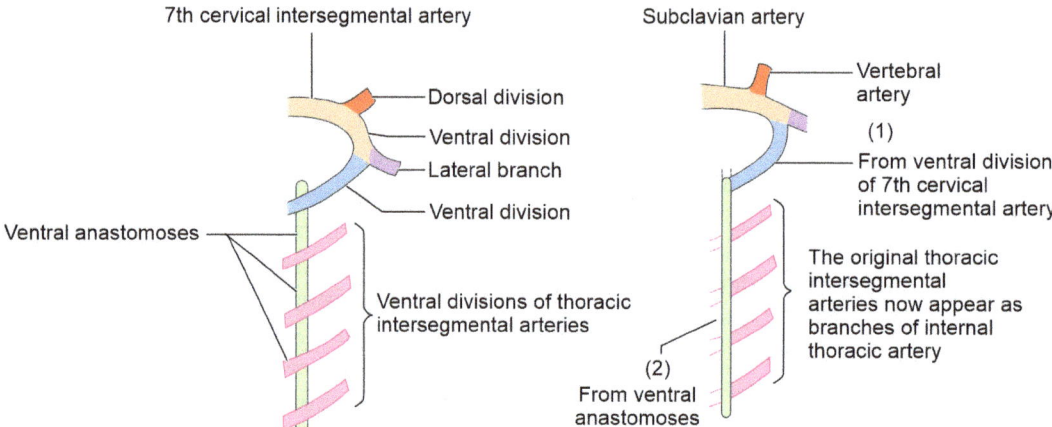

FIG. 20.39: Development of the internal thoracic artery.

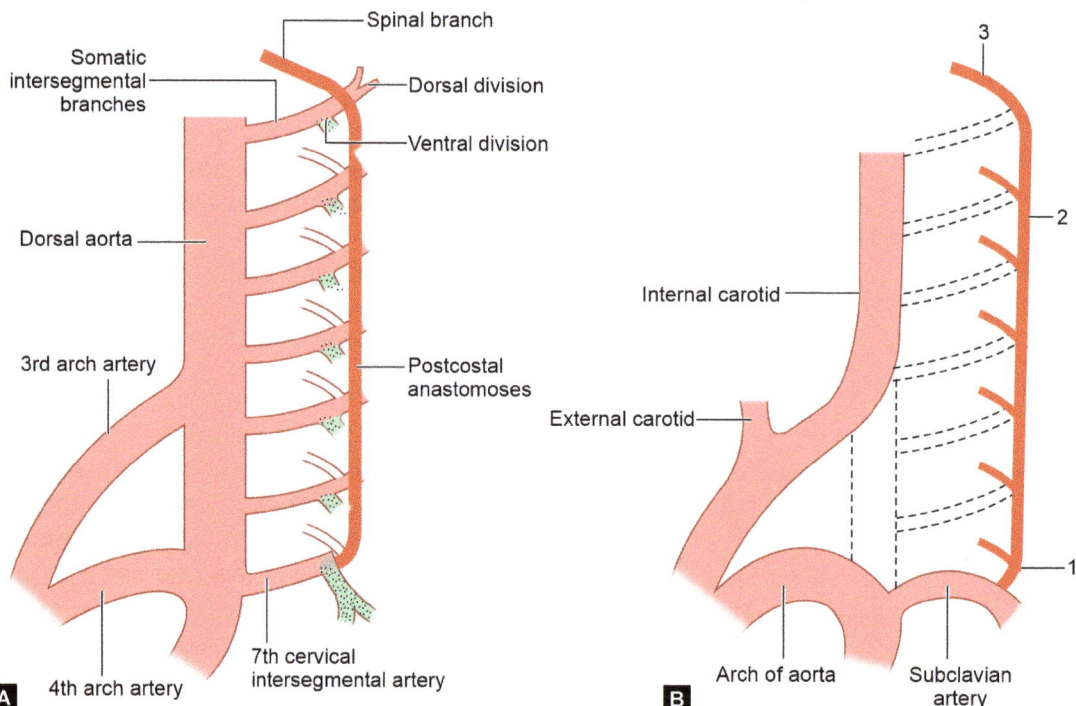

FIGS. 20.40A and B: Development of the vertebral artery. In (B) the part labeled 1 is derived from the dorsal division of the seventh cervical intersegmental artery; part 2 from the postcostal anastomoses; and part 3 from the spinal branch of the first cervical intersegmental artery.

Development of Internal Thoracic Artery (Fig. 20.39)

- The main stem of the artery is formed by the ventral division of the seventh cervical intersegmental artery.
- The vertical part of the artery (including its superior epigastric branch) is derived from the ventral anastomoses between the ventral divisions of the thoracic intersegmental arteries (intercostal arteries).

Umbilical Artery

- Before the fusion of the two dorsal aortae, the umbilical arteries appear as continuations of their distal ends **(Fig. 20.41A)**.
- After fusion of the dorsal aortae, they appear as lateral branches of the single dorsal aorta **(Fig. 20.41B)**.
- Subsequently, each umbilical artery gets linked up with that part of the fifth lumbar intersegmental artery which forms the *internal iliac artery* **(Fig. 20.41C)**.
- The part of the umbilical artery, between the aorta and the anastomosis with the internal iliac disappears so that the umbilical artery is now seen as a branch of the internal iliac artery **(Figs. 20.41D and E)**.
- In postnatal life, the proximal part of the umbilical artery becomes the *superior vesical artery*, while its distal part is obliterated to form the *medial umbilical ligament*.

Development of Arteries of Limbs

The limbs are supplied by lateral branches of the somatic intersegmental arteries that belong to the segments from which the limb buds take origin. These vessels form an *arterial plexus*.

However, each limb soon comes to have *one axis artery* that runs along the central axis of the limb. Other arteries that are formed as branches of the axis artery or as new formations later take over a considerable part of the arterial supply, due to which much of the original axis artery may disappear.

Axis Artery of the Upper Limb

- It is formed by the *seventh cervical intersegmental artery* **(Fig. 20.42)**.
- It runs along the ventral axial line and terminates in *palmar capillary plexus* in hand.
- It persists as the:
  - Axillary artery
  - Brachial artery
  - Anterior interosseous artery
  - Deep palmar arch
- A *median artery* develops from anterior interosseous artery and grows distally to communicate with palmar capillary plexus.
- The *digital arteries* of the hand develop from the palmar capillary plexus.
- The *radial* and *ulnar arteries* appear late in development.
- The *left subclavian artery* represents the main stem of the seventh cervical intersegmental artery, and the proximal part of its lateral division. This explains the origin of the vertebral (dorsal division) and internal thoracic (ventral division) arteries from it.
- The distal part of the *right subclavian artery* has a similar origin, but its proximal part is derived from the right fourth aortic arch.

Axis Artery of the Lower Limb

- It is derived from the *fifth lumbar intersegmental artery*.
- It is seen as a branch of *internal iliac artery* and runs on the dorsal aspect of the limb.

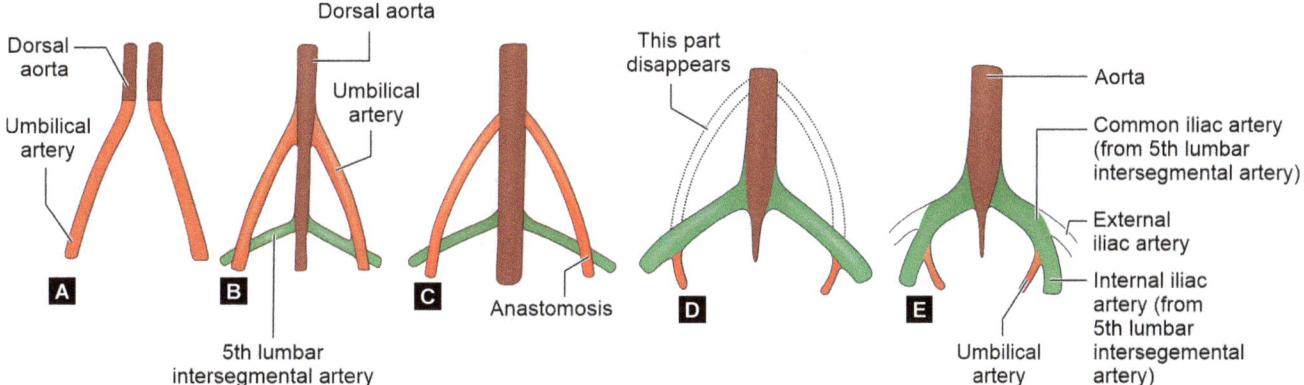

FIGS. 20.41A to E: Development of the umbilical artery. (A) Umbilical arteries are seen as continuations of the right and left dorsal aortae, before their fusion; (B) After fusion of dorsal aortae, the umbilical arteries appear as lateral branches of the aorta. They cross the 5th lumbar intersegmental artery; (C) Umbilical arteries establish anastomoses with the 5th lumbar intersegmental artery; (D) The part of the umbilical artery between the dorsal aorta and the 5th lumbar intersegmental artery disappears; and the umbilical artery is now seen as a branch of the 5th lumbar intersegmental artery; (E) The 5th lumbar intersegmental artery forms the common iliac and internal iliac arteries; and the umbilical is now seen as a branch of the internal iliac.

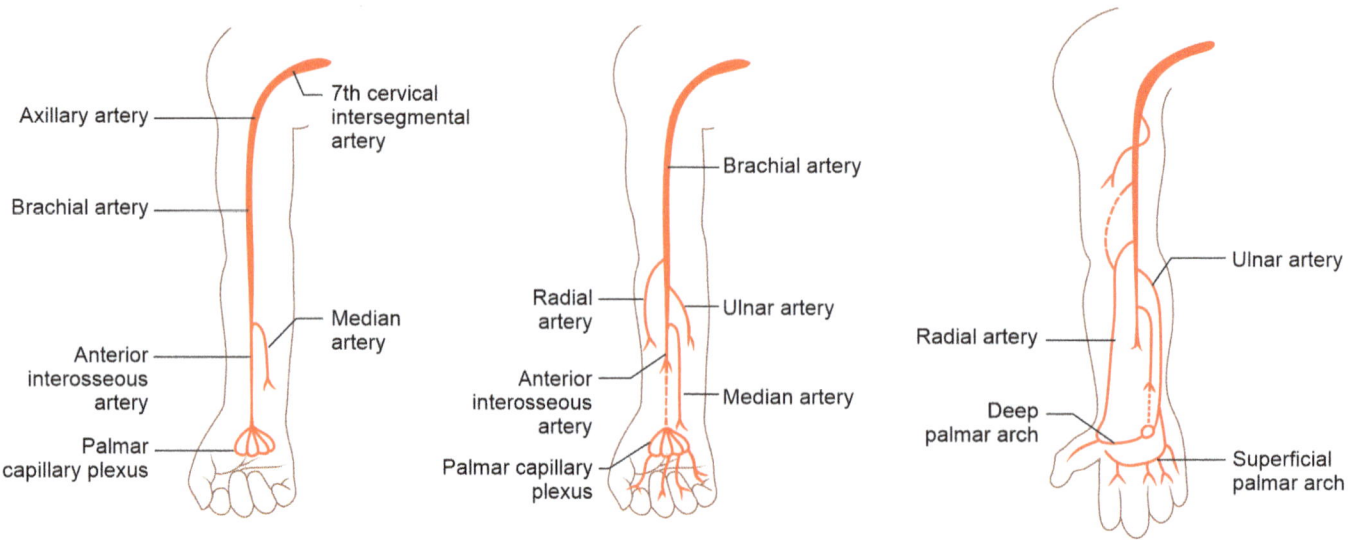

FIG. 20.42: Development of arteries of upper limb.

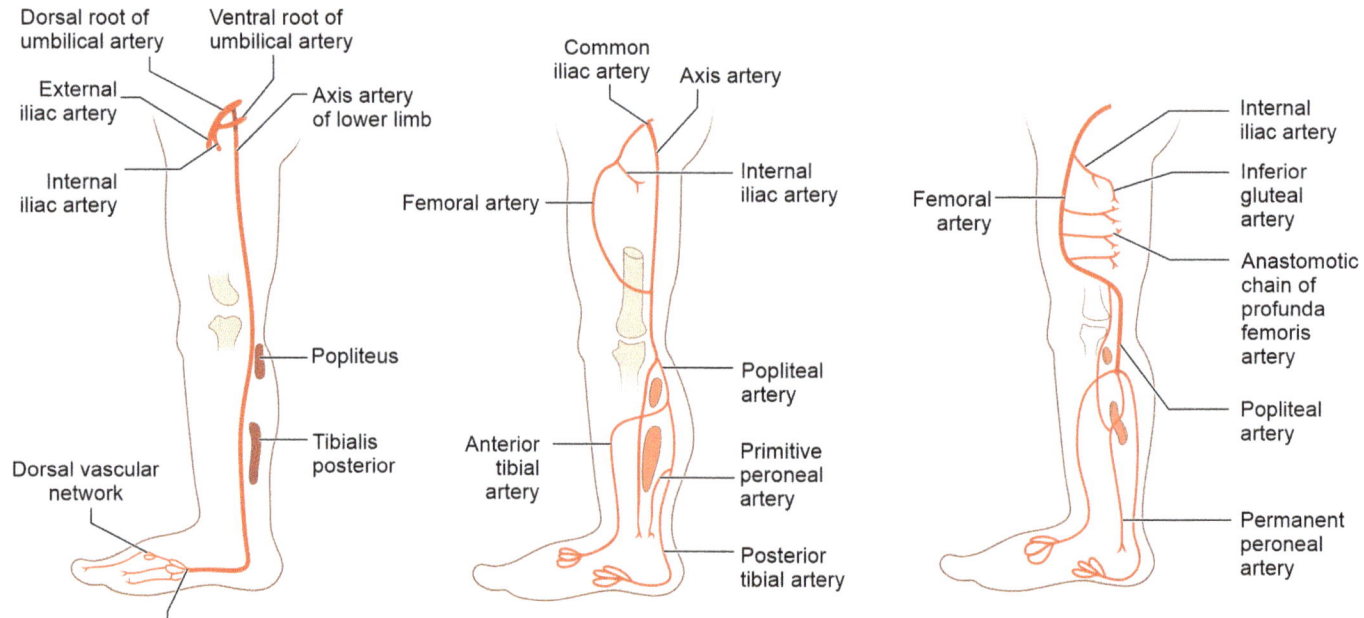

FIG. 20.43: Development of arteries of lower limb.

- The *femoral artery* is a new vessel formed on the ventral aspect of the thigh.
- Proximally it gets linked above with the *external iliac artery* (which is a branch of the axis artery), and below with the *popliteal artery*.
- In the adult, the original axis artery is represented by (Fig. 20.43):
  - Inferior gluteal artery
  - A small artery accompanying the sciatic nerve
  - Part of popliteal artery above the level of the popliteus muscle
  - Distal part of peroneal artery
  - Part of plantar arch

DEVELOPMENT OF VEINS

The main veins of the embryo are three sets/pairs of longitudinally directed veins—categorized into two groups, visceral and somatic (Fig. 20.44). All drain into sinus venosus.

- **Visceral veins:**
  - Vitelline/omphalomesenteric veins from yolk sac
  - Umbilical veins—carry oxygenated blood from placenta
- **Somatic veins:** Cardinal veins—these are the veins draining from the body wall.

Interconnections between the veins lead to establishment of shortest hemodynamic route by

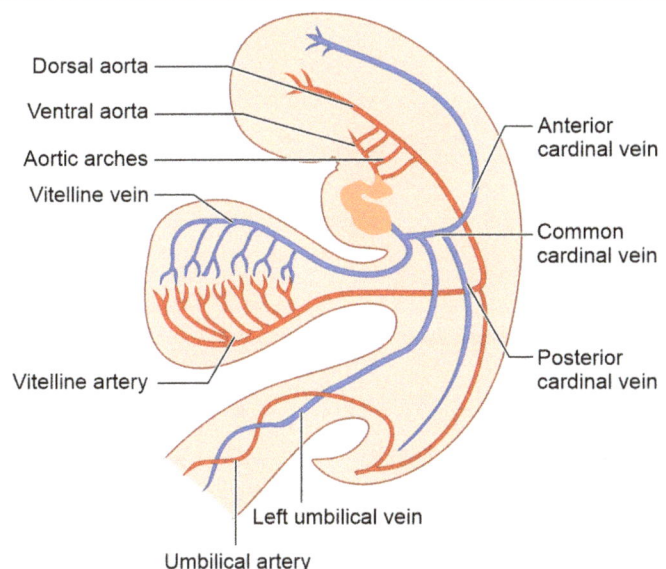

FIG. 20.44: Primitive veins of the embryo.

regression and/or enlargement of some veins. This results in the formation of three system of veins of adult.
1. Portal system
2. Caval system
3. Azygos system

Visceral Veins

These are as follows:
1. Right and left *vitelline veins* arise from the capillary plexus in the yolk sac. These are also called *omphalomesenteric veins*.
2. Right and left *umbilical veins* from the placenta.
The umbilical and vitelline veins open into the corresponding horn of the sinus venosus (**Fig. 20.45A**). The parts of these veins that are nearest to the heart are embedded in the septum transversum.

These veins undergo considerable changes as follows:
- With the appearance of hepatic bud in septum transversum, the *vitelline veins* can be divided into three parts:
  1. Infrahepatic part
  2. Intrahepatic part
  3. Suprahepatic part
  For easy understanding the intrahepatic and suprahepatic parts are described first followed by infrahepatic part.

Intrahepatic Part

With the development of the liver, in the septum transversum, the proximal parts of the vitelline and umbilical veins become broken up into numerous small channels that contribute to the sinusoids of the liver. These sinusoids drain into the sinus venosus, through the persisting terminal parts of the vitelline veins that are now called the right and left *hepatocardiac channels* (**Fig. 20.45B**). The proximal parts of the umbilical veins lose their communications with the sinus venosus.

Suprahepatic Part

- Meanwhile, the left horn of the sinus venosus undergoes retrogression and as result the left hepatocardiac channel disappears. All blood from the umbilical and vitelline veins now enters the sinus venosus through the right hepatocardiac channel (also called *common hepatic vein*). This vessel later forms the cranial most part of the inferior vena cava (**Fig. 20.45C**).
- The right umbilical vein disappears, and all blood from the placenta now reaches the developing liver through the left vein (*Note: The left vein is "left"*) (**Fig. 20.45D**). In order to facilitate the passage of this blood through the liver, some of the sinusoids enlarge to create a direct passage connecting the left umbilical vein to the right hepatocardiac channel. This passage is called the *ductus venosus*.
- At birth the ductus venosus gets obliterated and becomes the *ligamentum venosum*. The left umbilical vein becomes fibrosed and forms the *ligamentum teres hepatis*.

Infrahepatic Part

While these changes are occurring within the liver, the parts of the right and left vitelline veins that lie outside the substance of the liver undergo alterations leading to the formation of the *portal vein*.

Development of Portal Vein

- The proximal (infrahepatic) parts of the two vitelline veins lie on the right and left sides of the developing duodenum (**Fig. 20.46A**).
- The two vitelline veins soon become interconnected by three transverse anastomoses, two of which lie ventral to the duodenum. The third anastomosis lies dorsal to the duodenum and is between the two ventral anastomoses (**Fig. 20.46B**). These anastomoses form a *'figure of eight'*, around the Ushaped duodenum:
  - Cephalic ventral anastomosis
  - Middle dorsal anastomosis
  - Caudal ventral anastomosis
- The *superior mesenteric* and *splenic veins* (which develop independently) join the left vitelline vein, a short distance caudal to the dorsal anastomosis.
- Some parts of the vitelline veins now disappear. The portal vein and its right and left divisions are derived from the veins that remain (**Fig. 20.46C**).

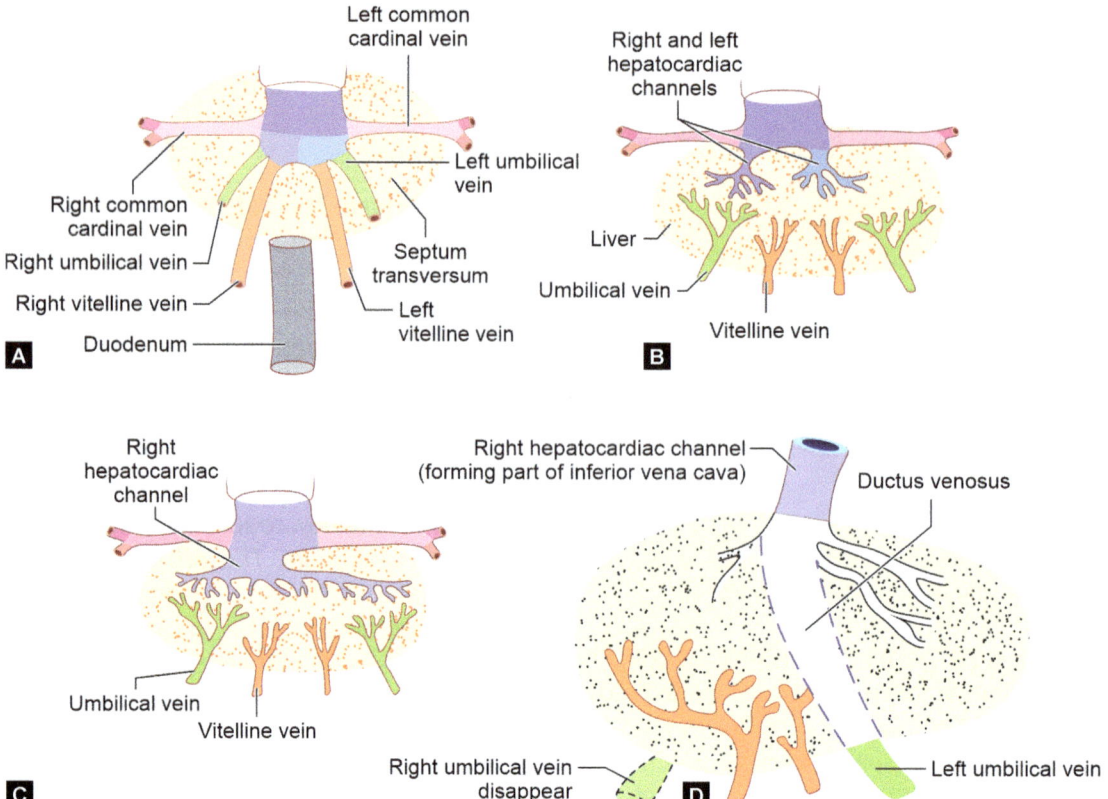

FIGS. 20.45A to D: Umbilical and vitelline veins. (A) Note the umbilical and vitelline veins passing through the septum transversum to reach the sinus venosus; (B) Growth of liver cells within the septum transversum breaks up part of the umbilical and vitelline veins into capillaries. Blood reaching the liver through the umbilical and vitelline veins now goes to the heart through the right and left hepatocardiac channels; (C) Left hepatocardiac channel disappears; (D) Right hepatocardiac channel (which later forms part of the inferior vena cava) now drains the liver. Right umbilical veins disappear. All blood from the placenta now reaches the liver through the left umbilical vein. Formation of ductus venosus short circuits, this blood to the right hepatocardiac channel.

The veins that disappear are:
- Part of right vitelline vein caudal to the dorsal anastomosis.
- Part of left vitelline vein caudal to the entry of the superior mesenteric and splenic veins.
- Caudal ventral anastomosis
- Left vitelline vein between dorsal anastomosis and cranial ventral anastomosis.

The veins that persist to form the *stem of the portal vein* are (**Fig. 20.46C**):
- Left vitelline vein between the entry of the superior mesenteric and splenic veins and the dorsal anastomosis (1, in **Fig. 20.46C**).
- Dorsal anastomosis itself (2, in **Fig. 20.46C**)
- Right vitelline vein between the dorsal anastomosis and the cranial ventral anastomosis (3, in **Fig. 20.46C**).

Left branch of portal vein is formed by:
- Cranial ventral anastomosis
- A part of left vitelline vein cranial to cranial ventral anastomosis (4, in **Fig. 20.46C**).

Right branch of portal vein is formed by:
Right vitelline vein cranial to cranial ventral anastomosis (5, in **Fig. 20.46C**).

The sinusoids that carry the blood of these branches to the liver substance constitute the *venae advehentes* (intrahepatic branches of portal vein). Those sinusoids that drain this blood to the inferior vena cava are called the *venae revehentes* (tributaries of the hepatic veins).

The left umbilical vein now ends in the left branch of the portal vein (left end of cephalic ventral anastomosis; **Fig. 20.46D**), while the ductus venosus connects the left branch of the portal vein to the inferior vena cava (right hepatocardiac channel).

Somatic Veins

The earliest somatic veins are:
- Right and left *anterior cardinal veins* that drain the cranial part (head, neck and upper limb) of the embryo, including the brain.
- Right and left *posterior cardinal veins* that drain the caudal part (lower limbs and pelvis) of the embryo.

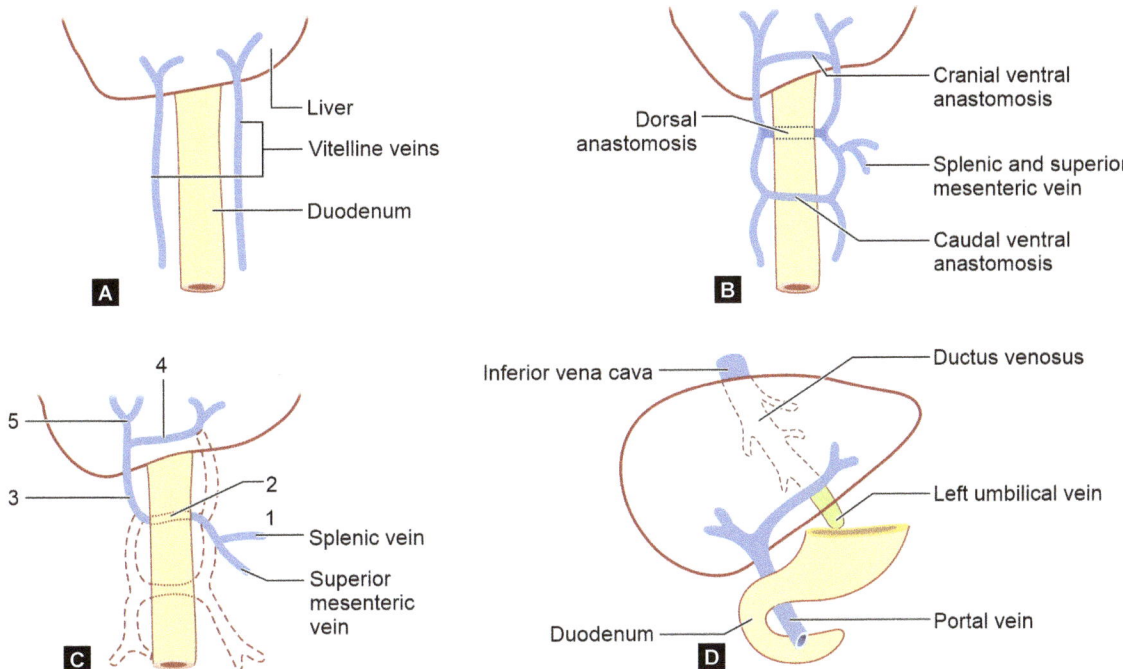

FIGS. 20.46A to D: Development of the portal vein. (A) Right and left vitelline veins; (B) Vitelline veins joined by three transverse anastomoses: cranial ventral, caudal ventral and middle dorsal; (C) Some of the veins disappear. The portal vein is formed from: (1) Part of left vitelline vein. (2) Dorsal anastomosis. (3) Part of right vitelline vein. (4) The cranial ventral anastomosis becomes the left branch of the portal vein. (5) Right vitelline cranial to cranial ventral anastomosis forms right branch; (D) The left umbilical vein ending in left branch of portal vein and the ductus venosus connecting it with inferior vena cava.

The anterior and posterior cardinal veins of each side join to form the corresponding *common cardinal vein* (or *duct of Cuvier*) which opens into the corresponding horns of the sinus venosus **(Fig. 20.47A)**.

Fate of Anterior Cardinal and Common Cardinal Veins

The anterior cardinal veins are joined by *subclavian veins* that drain the forelimbs **(Fig. 20.47B)**. Soon thereafter, the anterior cardinal veins become interconnected by a transverse anastomosis **(Fig. 20.47C)**, proximal to their junction with the subclavian veins. The part of the left anterior cardinal vein caudal to this anastomosis retrogresses, and so does the left common cardinal **(Fig. 20.47D)**.

Anterior Cardinal Veins

They are divided into a cranial part the primary head vein and the caudal cervicothracic part.

Veins of Cervicothoracic Region

These are the superior vena cava, brachiocephalic, jugular and subclavian veins and left superior intercostal vein.

Superior vena cava is derived from **(Fig. 20.47E)**:
- *Right anterior cardinal vein*, caudal to the transverse anastomosis with the left anterior cardinal vein.
- *Right common cardinal vein*: Note that the right horn of the sinus venosus forms part of the right atrium, and thus the superior vena cava comes to open into this chamber.

Right brachiocephalic vein is derived from the right anterior cardinal vein, between the point of its junction with the subclavian vein and the point of its junction with the transverse anastomosis **(Fig. 20.47F)**.

Left brachiocephalic vein is derived from **(Fig. 20.47G)**:
- The part of left anterior cardinal vein corresponding to the right brachiocephalic vein.
- The transverse intercardinal anastomosis.

Internal jugular veins develop from the parts of the anterior cardinal veins cranial to their junction with the subclavian veins **(Fig. 20.47H)**.

External jugular veins arise as secondary channels and are not derived from the anterior cardinal veins.

The anterior and posterior cardinal veins receive a series of *intersegmental veins* from the body wall (corresponding to the intersegmental branches) of the dorsal aortae. The *subclavian veins* are formed by

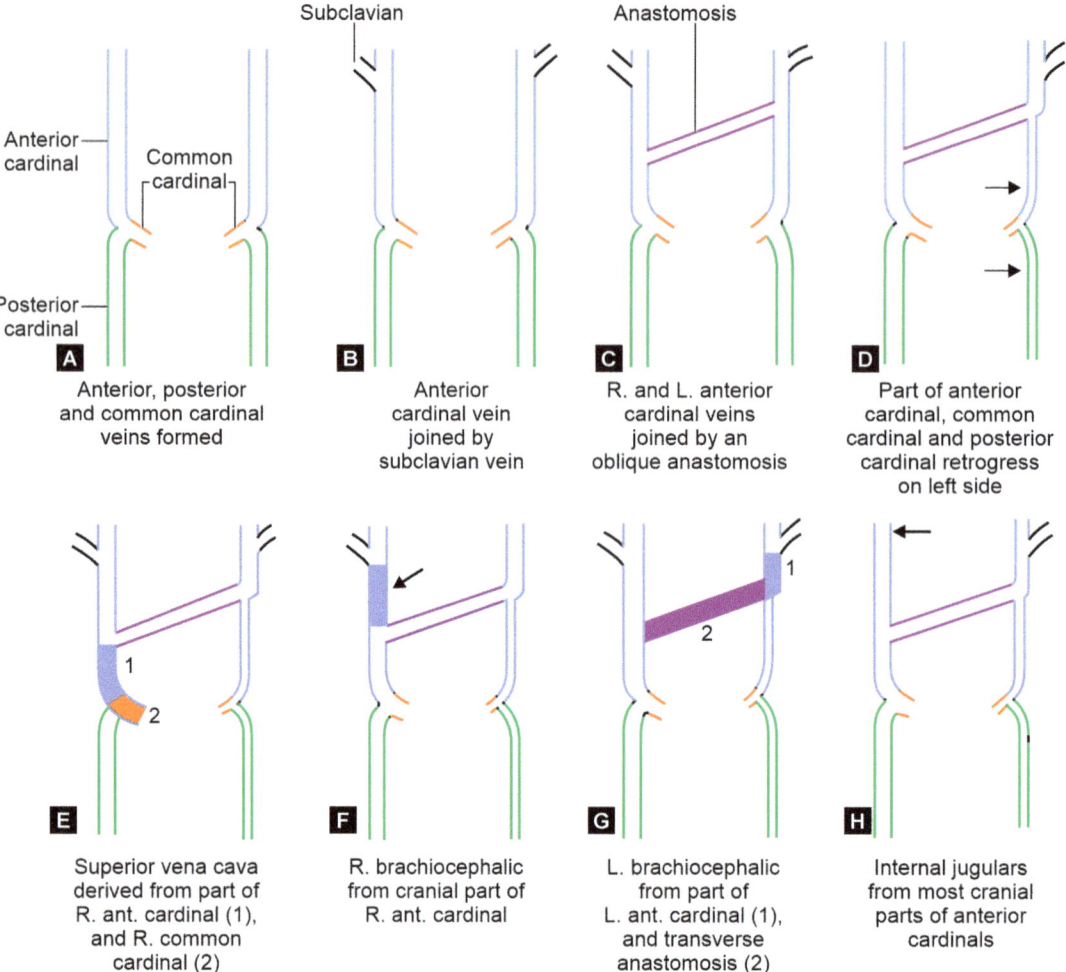

FIGS. 20.47A to H: Fates of anterior cardinal veins, and the development of major veins draining the upper part of the body.

considerable enlargement of one of these veins in the region of the upper limb bud (Figs. 20.48A and B).

Retrogressing Veins of Left Side

Caudal part of anterior cardinal vein and whole of the common cardinal vein of left side undergo retrogression. These retrogressing veins of the left side persist into adult life as the left superior intercostal vein and the coronary sinus which are derived as follows:

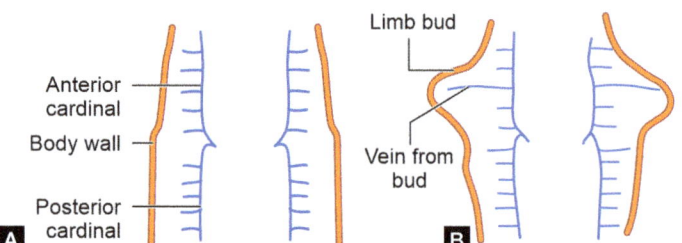

FIGS. 20.48A and B: Formation of the vein for the forelimb bud. In Figure (A), we see veins from the body wall draining into the anterior and posterior cardinal veins. In Figure (B), we see that one of these veins lying at the level of the limb bud enlarges to drain the limb.

Left Superior Intercostal Vein

It is formed by (Fig. 20.49):
- Left anterior cardinal vein caudal to the transverse anastomosis.
- Most cranial part of the left posterior cardinal vein. The second and third intercostal veins drain into this vein.

Coronary Sinus

The medial part of the *coronary sinus* is derived from the left horn of the sinus venosus (Figs. 20.50A and B). The lateral part of the coronary sinus is derived from the proximal part of the left common cardinal vein. The remaining part of the left common cardinal vein persists as the *oblique vein of the left atrium (oblique vein of Marshall)*.

Veins of Abdomen

The inferior vena cava, the veins of the kidneys, gonads and suprarenals, and the veins draining the walls of the thorax and abdomen, are derived from a series of

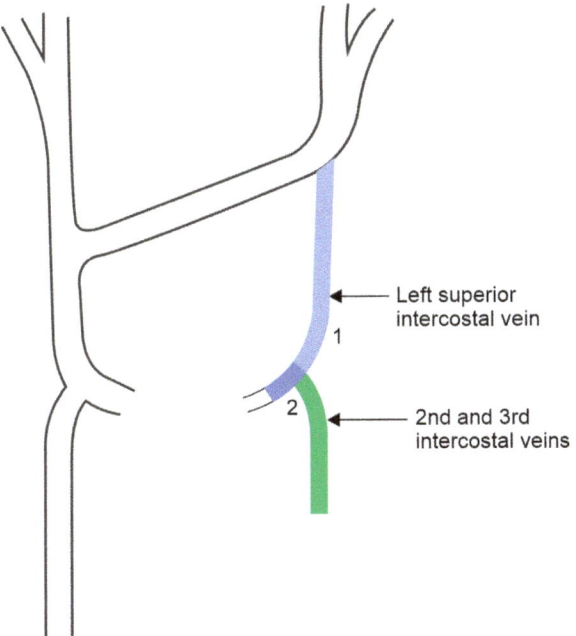

FIG. 20.49: Development of the left superior intercostal vein. The part labeled 1 is derived from the anterior cardinal vein; and part 2 from posterior cardinal vein. Note the intercostal veins draining into it.

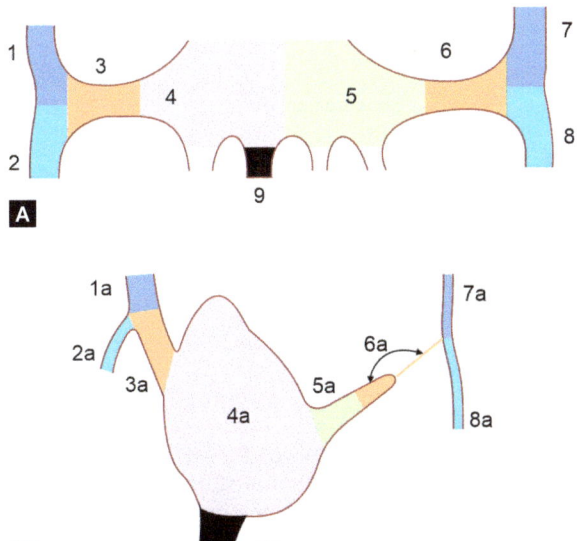

FIGS. 20.50A and B: (A) Derivation of the coronary sinus and related structures. 1 and 7 = right and left anterior cardinal veins; 2 and 8 = posterior cardinal veins; 3 and 6 = common cardinal veins; 4 and 5 = right and left horns of sinus venosus; 9 = right vitelline vein. The fate of these structures is shown in (B) 1a + 3a = superior vena cava; 2a = terminal part of the azygos vein; 4a = part of right atrium; 5a and proximal half of 6a = coronary sinus; distal half of 6a = oblique vein of left atrium; 7a + 8a = left superior intercostal vein; 9a = inferior vena cava.

longitudinal venous channels that appear in the embryo. Some of these are as follows:

- **Posterior cardinal veins:** At their cranial ends, these veins join the anterior cardinal veins to form the common cardinal veins. Near their caudal ends, they receive the veins of the lower limb bud (external iliac) and of the pelvis (internal iliac) **(Fig. 20.51A)**. The caudal ends of the two posterior cardinal veins become interconnected by a transverse anastomosis **(Fig. 20.51B)**.
- **Subcardinal veins** (green in **Figs. 20.51C and D**) are formed in relation to the mesonephros. Cranially and caudally they communicate with the posterior cardinal veins. The subcardinals receive the veins from the developing kidneys.
  - At the level of renal veins, the two subcardinals become connected by a transverse *intersubcardinal anastomosis* **(Figs. 20.51C and D)**. This is anterior to the aorta. Hence, also known as *preaortic anastomosis*.
  - The cranial part of right subcardinal vein also establishes an anastomosis with the right hepatocardiac channel **(Fig. 20.52A)**. This is known as the right subcardinal and right hepatocardiac channel anastomosis.
- **Supracardinal veins** (also called thoracolumbar veins) (orange in **Figs. 20.52A to D**) communicate cranially and caudally with posterior cardinal veins. They also communicate with the subcardinal veins through anastomoses which join the subcardinals just below the renal veins **(Fig. 20.52B)**.

Many parts of these longitudinal venous channels disappear **(Fig. 20.52C)**. The veins that remain give rise to the inferior vena cava, renal veins, veins of gonads and the suprarenal veins as discussed below.

Inferior Vena Cava

Inferior vena cava is derived from the following in caudal to cranial sequence **(Fig. 20.52D):**

Postrenal Part

- **Lowest part of the right posterior cardinal vein** (between its junction with the supracardinal, and the anastomosis between the two posterior cardinals).
- **Lower part of the right supracardinal vein** (between its junction with the posterior cardinal, and the supracardinal subcardinal anastomosis).
- **Right supracardinal-subcardinal anastomosis.**

Renal Segment

Right subcardinal vein (between the supracardinal subcardinal anastomosis and the anastomosis between the subcardinal vein and the right hepatocardiac channel).

Hepatic Segment

- **Subcardinal-hepatocardiac anastomosis**
- **Right hepatocardiac channel**

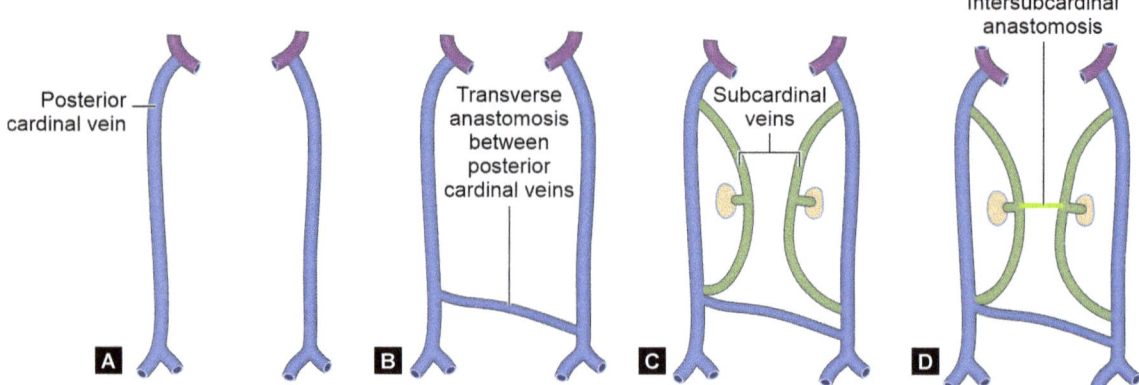

FIGS. 20.51A to D: (A) Posterior cardinal veins; (B) Formation of transverse anastomosis; (C) Formation of subcardinal veins. Note that they drain the developing kidney; (D) The two subcardinal veins become interconnected.

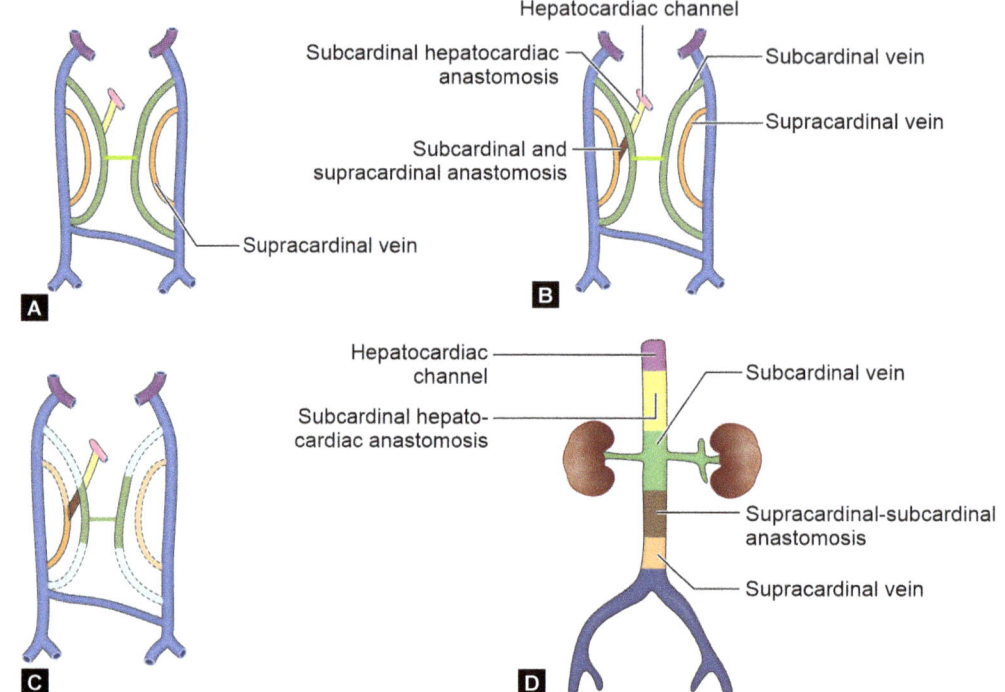

FIGS. 20.52A to D: Development of the inferior vena cava. Subcardinal veins are green; supracardinal veins are orange; the subcardinal-hepatocardiac anastomosis is yellow; the hepatocardiac channel itself is purple; and the supracardinal-subcardinal anastomosis is brown. The inferior vena cava receives contributions from each of these components as indicated by the color in (D).

Common Iliac Veins

* **Right common iliac vein** is derived from the most caudal part of the right posterior cardinal vein.
* **Left common iliac vein** represents the anastomosis between the two posterior cardinal veins.

Renal Veins

* The *right renal vein* is a mesonephric vein that originally drains into the subcardinal vein (**Fig. 20.53A**). It opens into that part of the vena cava that is derived from the subcardinal vein (**Fig. 20.53B**).
* The *left renal vein* is derived from:
  - Mesonephric vein that originally drains into the left subcardinal vein (**Fig. 20.53A**).
  - A small part of the left subcardinal vein.
  - Intersubcardinal anastomosis. As this anastomosis lies in front of the aorta, the left renal vein has a similar relationship (**Fig. 20.53B**).

The *suprarenal veins* are remnants of the part of subcardinal veins above the intersubcardinal anastomosis. It is clear from **Figure 20.47B** that the termination of the right suprarenal vein in the inferior vena cava, and that of the left suprarenal vein in the left renal vein, is because of their developmental origin.

The *testicular or ovarian veins* are remnants of parts of subcardinal veins below the intersubcardinal anastomosis. The reason for the difference in the manner of termination of the veins of the two sides is obvious from **Figure 20.53B**.

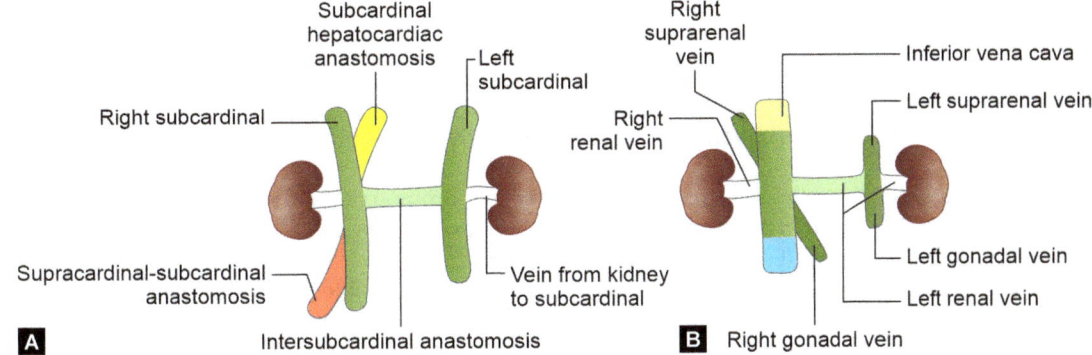

FIGS. 20.53A and B: Formation of renal, suprarenal and gonadal veins. The right renal vein is formed as a tributary of the right subcardinal vein. The left renal vein is derived from vein draining left kidney into left subcardinal vein; part of left subcardinal vein itself; and intersubcardinal anastomosis. On each side, the suprarenal veins and gonadal veins represent remnants of the subcardinal veins. From (B), it is seen why these veins drain, on the right side into the inferior vena cava; and on the left side into the left renal vein.

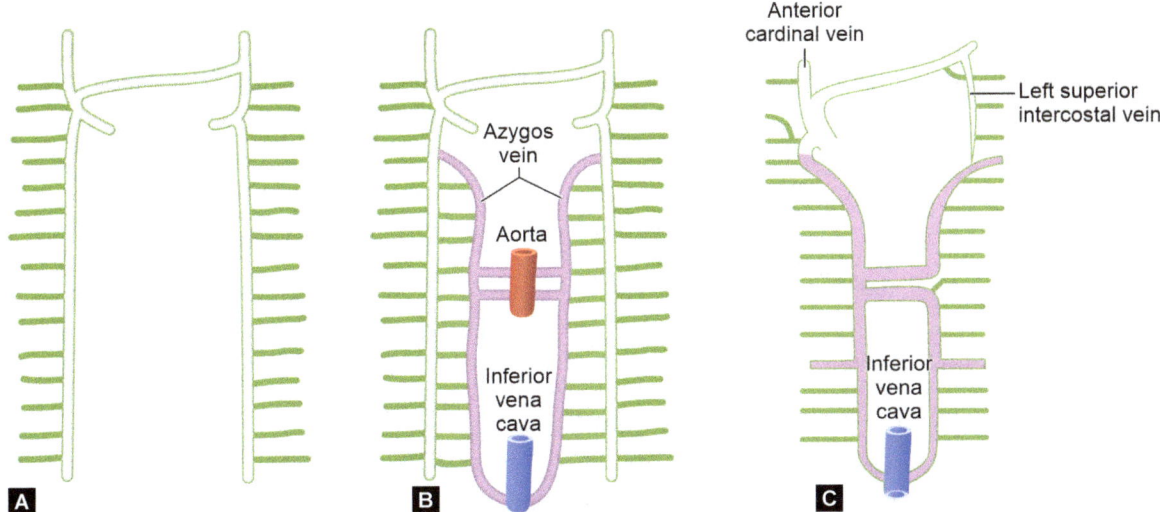

FIGS. 20.54A to C: (A) Veins from the body wall draining into anterior and posterior cardinal veins; (B) With the formation of the azygos venous channel, most of the veins of the body wall now drain into it; (C) Shows the ultimate arrangement. Note that veins from the 1st intercostal space drain into the innominate veins directly (anterior cardinal). The veins of the left 2nd and 3rd spaces drain into the left superior intercostal vein which is formed partly by the anterior cardinal and partly by the posterior cardinal veins. On the right side, the veins of these spaces drain into the part of the azygos vein representing the terminal part of the right posterior cardinal.

Azygos System of Veins

The veins draining the body wall at first drain into the posterior cardinal vein **(Fig. 20.54A)**. With the obliteration of major part of posterior cardinal veins their drainage is shifted to supracardinal veins.

Venous drainage from 4th to 11th intercostal spaces on the right side is into the right supracardinal vein (right azygos line) which together with a part of right posterior cardinal vein forms the *azygos vein*. On left side the 4th to 7th intercostal veins drain into the left supracardinal vein which is known as the *hemiazygos vein*. The intercostal spaces from 8th to 11th drain into *accessory hemiazygos vein*.

Hemiazygos and accessory hemiazygos veins empty into azygos, vein via postaortic anastomosis **(Fig. 20.54B)**.

Cranially these channels drain into the posterior cardinal veins. The channels of the two sides are brought into communication with each other by vessels that run dorsal to the aorta **(Fig. 20.54B)**.

The development of the azygos system of veins can now be summarized as follows **(Fig. 20.54C)**:

* The *azygos vein* is formed from:
  - The vein of the right azygos line; and
  - The most cranial part of the right posterior cardinal vein through which it opens into the superior vena cava (formed from the right common cardinal).
* The vertical parts of the *hemiazygos* and the *accessory hemiazygos* veins represent the left azygos line. Their horizontal parts are formed by the postaortic anastomoses between the azygos lines of the two sides.
* The second and third left intercostal veins retain their connection with the left posterior cardinal vein, and are drained through the left superior intercostal vein.
* The abdominal parts of the veins of the azygos line are represented by the ascending lumbar veins.

Clinical correlation

Anomalies of Veins

Minor anomalies in the mode of formation of various veins are extremely common. Anomalies of major veins are, however, rare. Some of these are as follows:
- **Left superior vena cava:** This is due to the failure of the left anterior and common cardinal veins to retrogress. The left superior vena cava opens into the right atrium through a large coronary sinus. In this condition, the normal (right) superior vena cava may be reduced in size or may even be absent (**Figs. 20.55A to D**).
- **Double inferior vena cava (Figs. 20.56A to D):** Generally, the vena cava is double only below the level of the renal veins. Both channels may be present on the right side (**Fig. 20.56B**). This is caused by persistence of both the subcardinal and supracardinal veins below the level of the kidneys. There may be an additional channel on the left side (**Figs. 20.56C and D**).
- **Left inferior vena cava:** The infrarenal part of the vena cava may be present on the left side only (**Fig. 20.56E**).
- **Azygos continuation of inferior vena cava:** The hepatic segment of the inferior vena cava may be absent. This is due to nondevelopment of the anastomosis between the right subcardinal vein and the right hepatocardiac channel. In such cases the upper part of the inferior vena cava follows the course of the azygos vein and opens into the superior vena cava. The hepatic veins open into the right atrium at the usual site of the inferior vena cava (**Figs. 20.56F and G**).
- **Preureteric vena cava:** The inferior vena cava normally lies posterior to the right ureter. Sometimes, it may be anterior to the right ureter. The ureter then hooks around the left side of the vena cava. This anomaly is caused when the infrarenal part of the vena cava develops from the subcardinal vein (which lies anterior to the ureter), instead of the supracardinal vein (which lies posterior to the ureter).

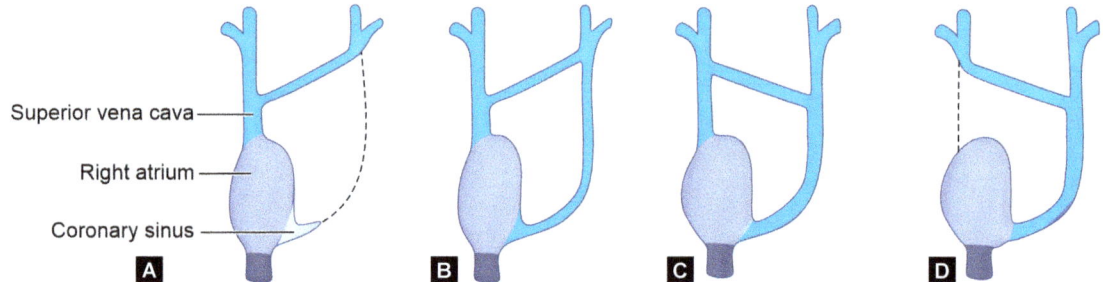

FIGS. 20.55A to D: Types of left superior vena cava. The normal pattern is shown in (A).

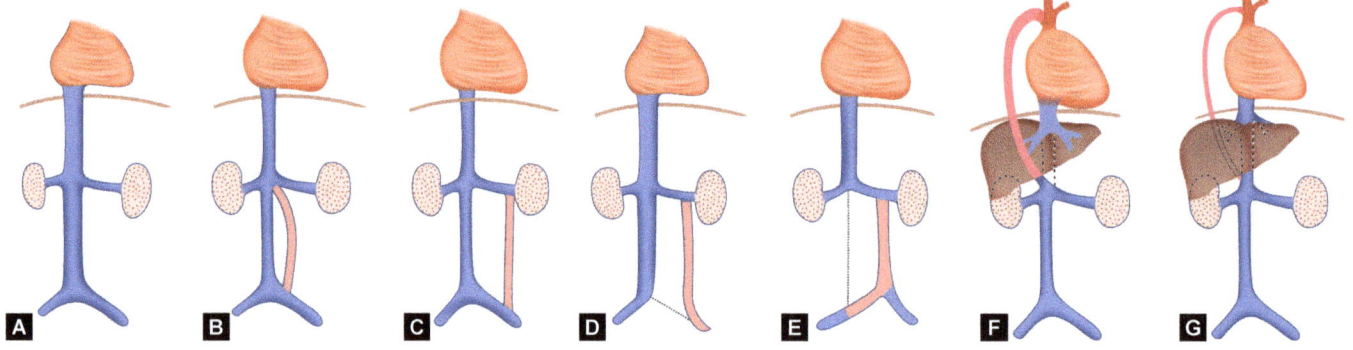

FIGS. 20.56A to G: Anomalies of the inferior vena cava. (A) Shows the normal pattern while (B to D) show various types of duplication of the infrarenal segment. In (E) the normal infrarenal segment is absent and is replaced by a vessel on the left side; (F) Shows absence of the hepatic segment of the vena cava, the blood flow taking place along a much enlarged vena azygos; (G) Shows the corresponding normal pattern.

FETAL CIRCULATION

The circulation in the fetus is essentially the same as in the adult except for the following (compare **Fig. 20.57** with **Fig. 20.58**).
- **Placenta:** The source of oxygenated blood is not the lung but the placenta. Gaseous exchange takes place here.
- **Umbilical vein:** Oxygenated blood from the placenta comes to the fetus through the umbilical vein, which joins the left branch of the portal vein. A small portion of this blood passes through the substance of the liver to the inferior vena cava, but the greater part passes direct to the inferior vena cava through the ductus venosus (**Fig. 20.45D**).

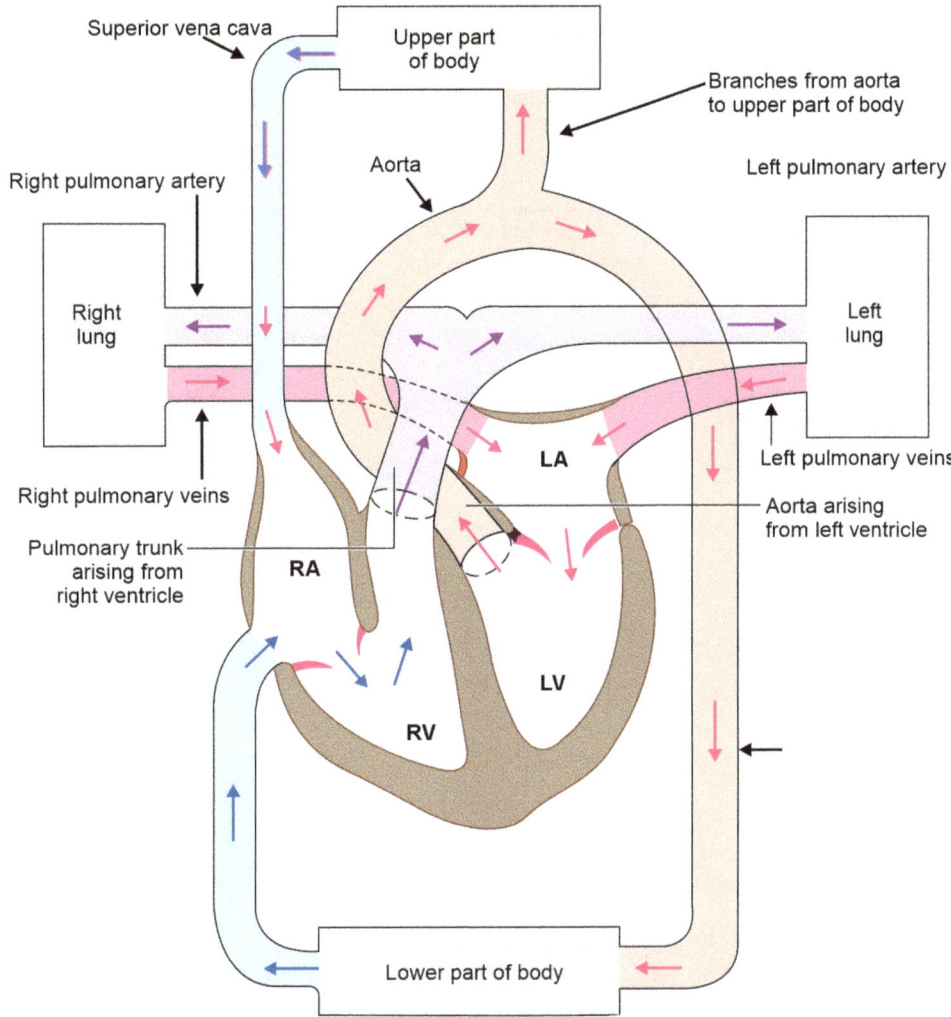

FIG. 20.57: Scheme of circulation in the human adult.

- ❖ **Ductus venosus:** It is for bypassing hepatic circulation. A sphincter mechanism in the ductus venosus controls blood flow.
- ❖ **Foramen ovale:** It connects the two atria. The oxygen rich blood reaching the right atrium through the inferior vena cava is directed by the valve of the inferior vena cava toward the foramen ovale. Here it is divided into two portions by the lower edge of the septum secundum *(crista dividens)*:
  - Most of it passes through the foramen ovale into the left atrium.
  - The rest of it gets mixed up with the blood returning to the right atrium through the superior vena cava, and passes into the right ventricle.
- ❖ **Ductus arteriosus:** It is for bypassing pulmonary circulation. From the right ventricle, the blood (mostly deoxygenated) enters the pulmonary trunk. Only a small portion of this blood reaches the lungs, and passes through it to the left atrium. The greater part is shortcircuited by the ductus arteriosus into the aorta.
- ❖ **Blood supply to fetus:**
  - We have seen that the left atrium receives blood from two sources the oxygenated blood from the right atrium and a small amount of deoxygenated blood from the lungs.
  - The blood in the left atrium is, therefore, fairly rich in oxygen. This blood passes into the left ventricle and then into the aorta. Some of this oxygen-rich blood passes into the carotid and subclavian arteries to supply the brain, the head and neck, and the upper extremities. The rest of it gets mixed up with poorly oxygenated blood from the ductus arteriosus.
  - The parts of the body that are supplied by branches of the aorta arising distal to its junction with the ductus arteriosus, therefore, receive blood with only moderate oxygen content.
- ❖ **Umbilical arteries:** They carry deoxygenated blood from fetus. Much of the blood of the aorta is carried by the umbilical arteries to the placenta where it is again oxygenated and returned to the heart.
- ❖ **Fetal circulation—peculiarities:**
  - Three times blood shunts along its course at:
    1. *Ductus venosus*—to direct blood to inferior vena cava by passing liver without losing oxygen content.

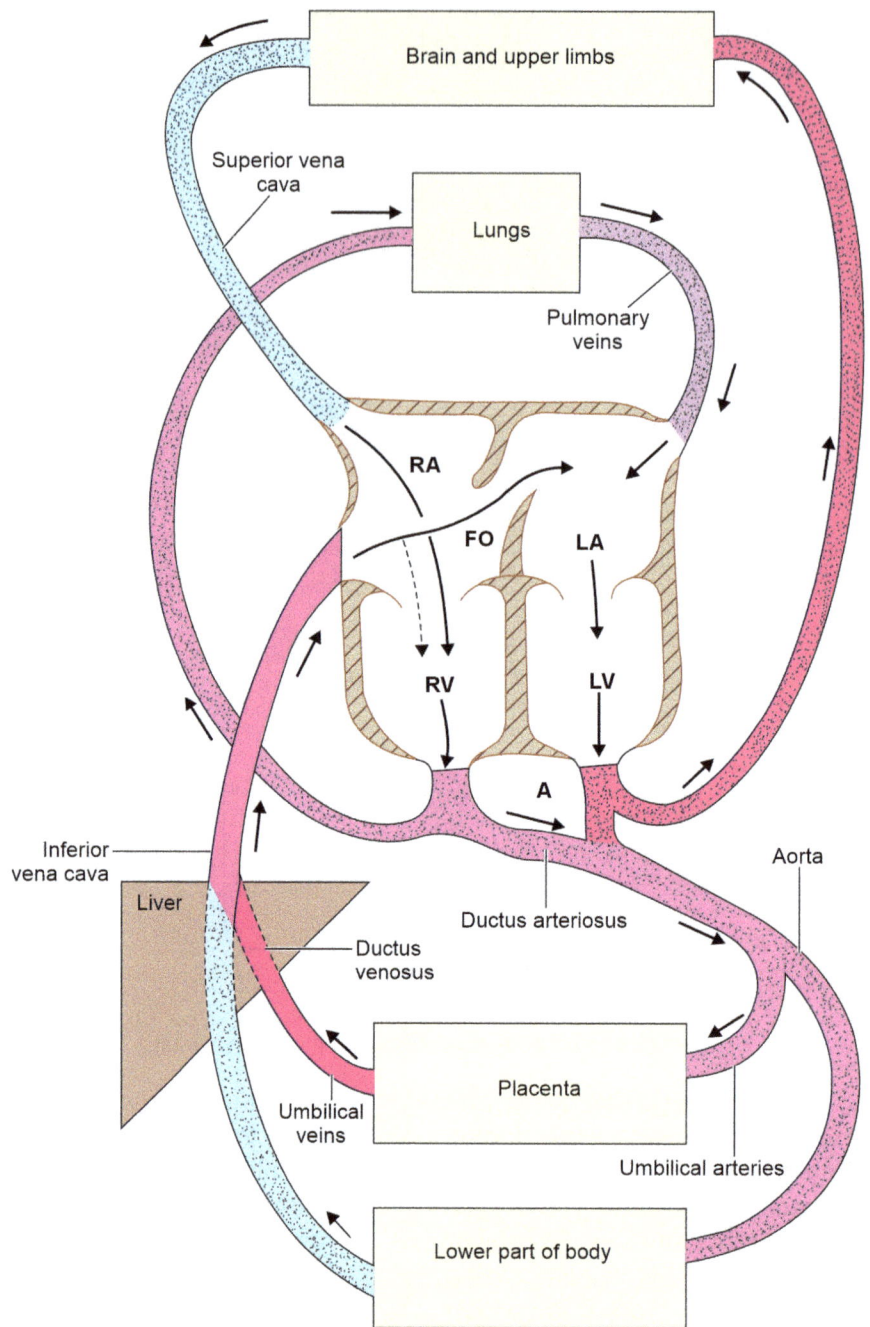

FIG. 20.58: Scheme of fetal circulation. The degree of deoxygenation is shown by the intensity of shading. (RA: right atrium; LA: left atrium; RV: right ventricle; LV: left ventricle; FO: foramen ovale)

2. *Foramen ovale*—to equalize distribution to each half of heart and more oxygenated blood to vital organs in the upper half of the body.
3. *Ductus arteriosus*—to direct blood to placenta for oxygenation by passing lungs.

- More oxygenated blood is provided for the upper limb. Hence, the length of upper limbs is more than lower limbs in the fetus.
- Sphincteric action at the junction of left umbilical vein and ductus venosus regulates oxygen content of inferior vena cava and excessive load on heart. Admixture of oxygenated and deoxygenated blood takes place in the liver, terminal part of inferior vena cava, both atria and distal part of arch of aorta.

❖ Transseptal blood flow throughout fetal life through ostium primum and foramen ovale.

CHANGES IN THE CIRCULATION AT BIRTH

Soon after birth, several changes take place in the fetal blood vessels. These lead to the establishment of the adult type of circulation. The changes are as follows:

❖ **Umbilical arteries:** The muscle in the wall of the umbilical arteries contracts immediately after birth,

and occludes their lumen. This prevents loss of fetal blood into the placenta.
- **Umbilical veins and ductus venosus:** The lumen of the umbilical veins and the ductus venosus is also occluded, but this takes place a few minutes after birth, so that all fetal blood that is in the placenta has time to drain back to the fetus.
- **Ductus arteriosus:** The ductus arteriosus is occluded, so that all blood from the right ventricle now goes to the lungs, where it is oxygenated. Initial closure of the ductus arteriosus is caused by contraction of muscle in the vessel wall. Later intimal proliferation obliterates the lumen.
- **Pulmonary vessels:** The pulmonary vessels increase in size and, consequently, a much larger volume of blood reaches the left atrium from the lungs. As a result, the pressure inside the left atrium is greatly increased. Simultaneously, the pressure in the right atrium is diminished because blood from the placenta no longer reaches it. The net result of these pressure changes is that the pressure in the left atrium now exceeds that in the right atrium causing the valve of the foramen ovale to close.

LYMPHATIC SYSTEM

- The first signs of the lymphatic system are seen in the form of a number of endothelium-lined *lymph sacs*. They are independent formations from mesenchyme.
- There are six major lymph sacs that can be recognized (Fig. 20.59). The right and left *jugular sacs* lie near the junction of the anterior cardinal and subclavian veins (i.e., at the junction between the future internal jugular and subclavian veins).
- The right and left *posterior (or iliac) sacs* lie around the corresponding common iliac vein. The *retroperitoneal sac* (unpaired) lies in relation to the root of the mesentery. The sixth sac (again unpaired) is the *cisterna chyli*. It lies in the midline some distance caudal to the retroperitoneal sac (Fig. 20.59).
- Lymphatic vessels are formed either by extension from the sacs or develop *de novo*, and extend into various tissues. Ultimately all the sacs except the cisterna chyli are invaded by connective tissue and

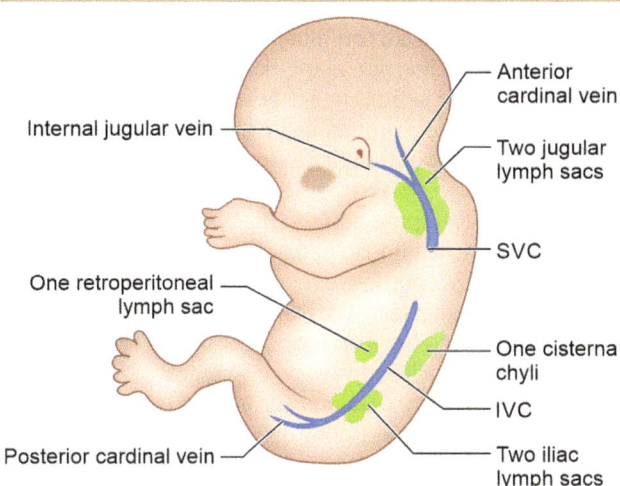

FIG. 20.59: Various lymph sacs.
(SVC: superior vena cava; IVC: inferior vena cava)

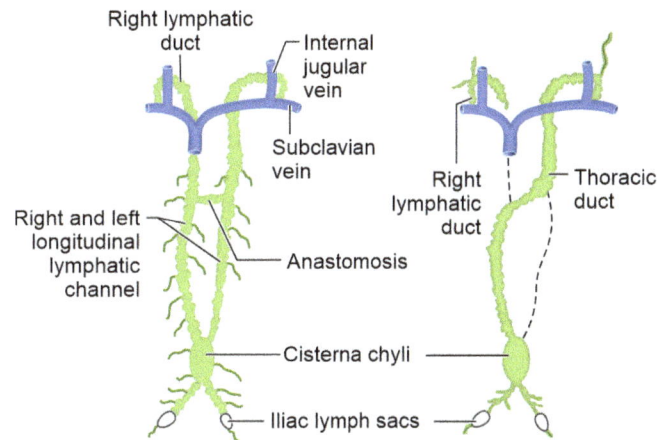

FIG. 20.60: Development of thoracic duct and right lymphatic duct.

lymphocytes, and are converted into groups of lymph nodes.
- The *thoracic duct* is derived from right and left channels that connect the cisterna chyli to the corresponding jugular sac. The two channels anastomose across the midline.
- The thoracic duct is formed from the caudal part of the right channel, the anastomosis between the right and left channels, and the cranial part of the left channel. The cranial part of the right channel becomes the *right lymphatic duct* (Fig. 20.60).

Case Based Learning

Case Scenario 1: Embryological Basis of Tetralogy of Fallot
A prenatal transabdominal fetal ultrasound presents an abnormal image of the fetal four-chambered heart showing a gap (marked with arrow) along with an overriding aorta as shown in Figure 20.61A. What could be the cause of this gap and the associated abnormalities? Give an embryological explanation.
- A four-chambered ultrasound view of the fetal heart is shown in **Figure 20.61A**.
- The four-chambered heart is formed by the development of the interatrial septum, interventricular septum, and AV endocardial cushions.

- In this fetus, there is a combination of four cardiac defects known as tetralogy of Fallot: ventricular septal defect (VSD), pulmonary stenosis, overriding aorta, and right ventricular hypertrophy.
- The ventricular septal defect arises from the failure of the membranous part of the interventricular septum to fuse properly.
- Pulmonary stenosis is due to the abnormal development of the pulmonary infundibulum, leading to narrowing of the right ventricular outflow tract.
- The overriding aorta results from improper alignment of the aorticopulmonary septum, causing the aorta to receive blood from both the right and left ventricles.
- Right ventricular hypertrophy develops as a consequence of increased workload on the right ventricle due to pulmonary stenosis.
- These defects collectively result from disruptions in the development and septation of the conotruncal region of the heart during embryogenesis.
- Postnatal X-ray shows boot shaped heart due to ventricular hypertrophy (Fig. 20.61B).

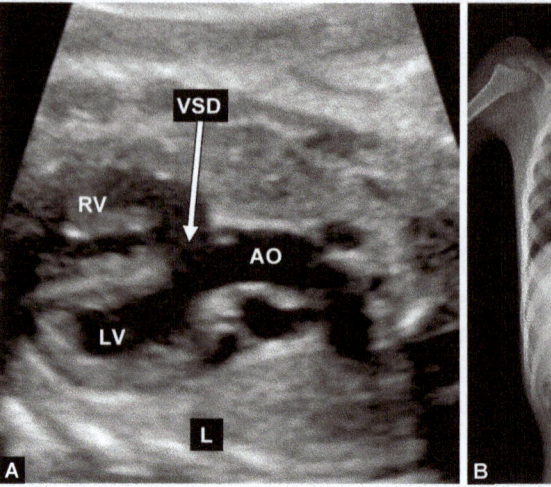
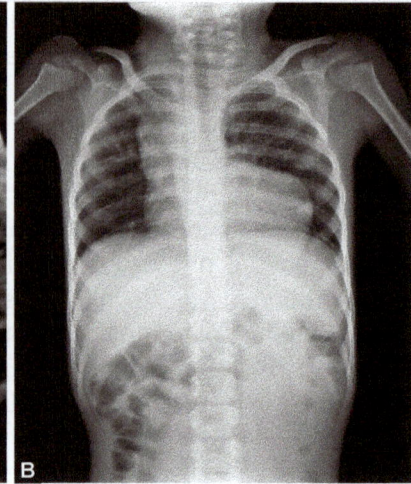

FIGS. 20.61A and B: (A) Fetal ultrasound showing ventricular septal defect in tetralogy of Fallot; (B) Postnatal X-ray showing boot shaped heart due to ventricular hypertrophy.

Case Scenario 1: Embryological Basis of Patent Ductus Arteriosus

A prenatal transabdominal fetal echocardiography presents an abnormal image of the fetal four-chambered heart with a persistent vessel (marked with arrow) connecting the pulmonary artery to the descending aorta, as shown in Figure 20.62. What could be the cause of this persistent vessel and the structures involved? Give an embryological explanation.

- A four-chambered ultrasound view of the fetal heart is shown in **Figure 20.62**.
- The abnormal persistent vessel is identified as a patent ductus arteriosus (PDA).
- During fetal development, the ductus arteriosus is a normal structure that connects the pulmonary artery to the descending aorta, allowing blood to bypass the nonfunctioning fetal lungs.
- Normally, the ductus arteriosus closes shortly after birth due to increased oxygen tension and decreased levels of prostaglandins, becoming the ligamentum arteriosum.
- In this fetus, the ductus arteriosus has failed to close, resulting in a patent ductus arteriosus (PDA).
- PDA can lead to abnormal blood flow between the aorta and pulmonary artery, causing complications such as pulmonary hypertension, heart failure, and increased risk of endocarditis.
- The persistence of the ductus arteriosus is due to a failure in the normal physiological mechanisms that induce its closure, which can be influenced by factors such as prematurity, genetic conditions, or maternal rubella infection during pregnancy.

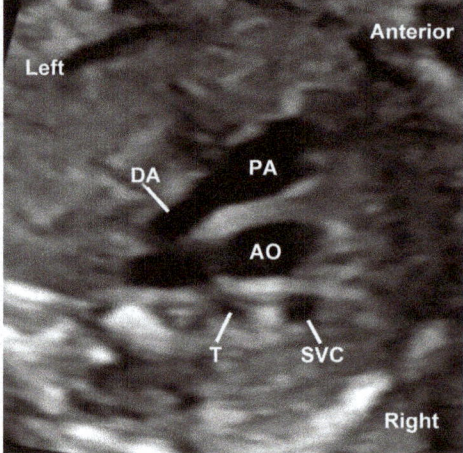

FIG. 20.62: Fetal echo showing patent ductus arteriosus.

TIMETABLE OF SOME EVENTS DESCRIBED IN THIS CHAPTER

Age	Developmental events
3rd week	- Blood and vessels forming cells (angioblastic islands) appear - The cardiogenic area, heart tubes and pericardium have formed
4th week	- Heart and pericardium lie ventral to foregut - Subdivisions of heart tube are visible - Heart begins to beat (becomes functional) - Heart septa begin to form - Aortic arches begin to establish in cranial to caudal sequence - Most of the first aortic arch disappears at the end of 4th week - Veins start forming
5th week	- The spiral septum is formed - Formation of aortic arches is complete - Lymphatic sacs form - The cardinal, umbilical and vitelline veins are formed - Conduction system of heart forms
6th week	- Coronary circulation is becoming established - Atrioventricular valves and papillary muscles are forming
7th week	Heart septa are completely formed

The heart is most susceptible to teratogens between three and six weeks. It can be affected up to the eighth week.

HIGHLIGHTS

- The *heart* develops from splanchnopleuric mesoderm related to that part of the intraembryonic coelom that forms the pericardial cavity. This mesoderm is the *cardiogenic area*.
- Two *endothelial heart tubes* (right and left) appear and fuse to form one tube. This tube has a venous end, and an arterial end.
- A series of dilatations appear in this tube. These are: (1) *bulbus cordis*, (2) *ventricle*, (3) *atrium* and (4) **sinus venosus**.
- Further subdivisions are named as follows. The bulbus cordis consists of a proximal one-third (which is dilated), a middle one-third called the *conus* and a distal one-third called the *truncus arteriosus*. The narrow part connecting atrium and ventricle is the *atrioventricular (AV) canal*. The sinus venosus has right and left horns.
- The right and left atria of the heart are formed by partition of the primitive atrium. This partition is formed by the *septum primum* and the *septum secundum*. A valvular passage, the *foramen ovale*, is present between these two septa. It allows flow of blood from right atrium to left atrium.
- The dilated proximal one-third of the bulbus cordis, the conus, and the primitive ventricle unite to form one chamber. This is partitioned to form right and left ventricles. This partition is made up of the following: (1) *Interventricular septum* that grows upward from the floor of the primitive ventricle; (2) A *bulbar septum* that divides the conus into two parts; (3) The gap left between these two is filled by proliferation of AV cushions that are formed in the AV canal.
- The truncus arteriosus is continuous with the *aortic sac*. This sac has right and left horns. Each horn is continuous with six *pharyngeal* (or *aortic*) *arch arteries*. These arteries join the dorsal aorta (right or left). The first, second and fifth arch arteries disappear. The caudal parts of the right and left dorsal aortae fuse to form one median vessel.
- The *ascending aorta* and *pulmonary trunk* are formed from the truncus arteriosus.
- The *arch of aorta* is formed by the aortic sac, its left horn and the left fourth arch artery.
- The *descending aorta* is formed partly from the left dorsal aorta, and partly from the fused median vessel.
- The *brachiocephalic artery* is formed from the right horn of the aortic sac.
- The *common carotid artery* is derived from part of the third arch artery.
- The *pulmonary artery* is derived from the sixth arch artery.
- The *arteries to the gut* are formed from ventral splanchnic branches of the dorsal aorta.
- The *renal, suprarenal* and *gonadal arteries* are formed from lateral splanchnic branches of the dorsal aorta.
- Arteries to the body wall and limbs are derived from dorsolateral (somatic intersegmental) branches of the aorta.
- The *left subclavian artery* is derived from part of the seventh cervical intersegmental artery.
- The *right subclavian artery* is formed from seventh cervical intersegmental artery and partly from the right fourth arch artery.
- The *portal vein* is derived from right and left vitelline veins and anastomoses between them.
- The *superior vena cava* is derived from part of the right anterior cardinal vein and from the right common cardinal vein.
- The *inferior vena cava* receives contributions from several veins (and anastomoses between them). These are the right posterior cardinal vein, right subcardinal vein, right supracardinal vein and right hepatocardiac channel.

Summary

- Development of atria (**Flowchart 20.1**).
- Derivatives of sinus venosus (**Table 20.1**).
- Development of major arteries (**Table 20.2**).
- Development of various veins (**Tables 20.3 to 20.6**).

FLOWCHART 20.1: Development of atria.

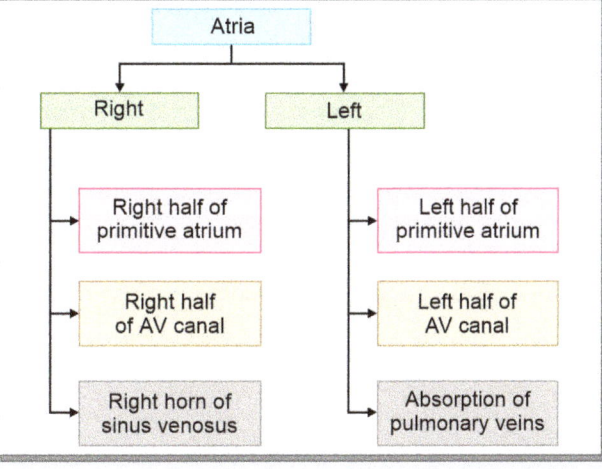

TABLE 20.1: Sinus venosus—embryonic parts and adult derivatives.

Embryonic part	Adult structure
Right horn	Sinus venarum
Left horn and body	Coronary sinus
Right duct of Cuvier/common cardinal vein	Superior vena cava (intrapericardial part)
Left duct of Cuvier/common cardinal vein	Oblique vein of left atrium
Cross communication between right and left anterior cardinal veins	Left brachiocephalic vein
Right anterior cardinal vein caudal to cross communication	Superior vena cava (extrapericardial part)
Left anterior cardinal vein caudal to cross communication	Left superior intercostal vein ligament of left vena cava
Suprahepatic part of right vitelline vein	Inferior vena cava (terminal part)
Cephalic part of right posterior cardinal vein	Arch of azygos vein

TABLE 20.2: Adult derivatives of truncus arteriosus, aortic sac and aortic arches.

Adult derivatives	Embryological structures
Ascending aorta	Truncus arteriosus
Arch of aorta	Aortic sac, left horn of aortic sac and left 4th arch artery
Descending aorta	Left dorsal aorta and fused dorsal aortae
Brachiocephalic artery	Right horn of aortic sac
Right subclavian artery	Right 4th arch artery, 7th cervical intersegmental artery and small part of right dorsal aorta between the two
Left subclavian artery	Left 7th cervical intersegmental artery
Common carotid artery	Proximal part of 3rd arch artery
Internal carotid artery	Distal part of 3rd arch artery and cervical part of dorsal aorta
External carotid artery	As a bud from 3rd arch artery
Pulmonary trunk	Truncus arteriosus
Pulmonary artery	Part of 6th arch artery
Ductus arteriosus	Part of left 6th arch artery between lung bud and aorta

TABLE 20.3: Development of major veins from cervicothoracic part of anterior cardinal and common cardinal veins.

Major veins	Developmental origin
Superior vena cava	• **Extrapericardial part:** Right anterior cardinal vein caudal to transverse anastomosis between two anterior cardinal veins • **Intrapericardial part:** Right common cardinal vein
Subclavian veins	Intersegmental veins draining the upper limb that join the anterior cardinal veins cranial to the oblique communication
Right brachiocephalic vein	Right anterior cardinal vein between oblique communication and the opening of right subclavian vein
Left brachiocephalic vein	• Oblique communication between anterior cardinal veins • Part of left anterior cardinal vein corresponding to right brachiocephalic vein
Internal jugular vein	Part of anterior cardinal vein cranial to the subclavian vein
External jugular vein	Secondary channels that develop in situ in the face
Left superior intercostal vein	• Left anterior cardinal vein caudal to oblique communication • Most cranial part of left posterior cardinal vein
Oblique vein of (Marshall) left atrium	Left common cardinal vein (distal part)

TABLE 20.4: Development of major veins of lower part of body.

Inferior vena cava	• Postrenal part
	  – Caudal part of right posterior cardinal vein
	  – Right supracardinal vein
	  – Right supracardinal and subcardinal anastomosis
	• Renal segment—right subcardinal vein
	• Hepatic segment
	  – Supracardinal and right hepatocardiac channel anastomosis
	  – Right hepatocardiac channel

Portal vein	• Stem
	  – Left vitelline vein between the entry of superior mesenteric and splenic veins and dorsal anastomosis
	  – Dorsal anastomosis between vitelline veins
	  – Right vitelline vein between dorsal anastomosis and cranial ventral anastomosis
	• Left branch
	  – Cranial ventral anastomosis between vitelline veins
	  – Left vitelline vein cranial to ventral anastomosis
	• Right branch—right vitelline vein cranial to cranial ventral anastomosis

External iliac veins	Veins developing in the lower limb bud that join common cardinal veins
Internal iliac veins	Veins developing in the pelvis that join the common cardinal veins
Common iliac veins	Right—caudal part of right posterior cardinal vein caudal to anastomosis between posterior cardinal veins. Left—anastomosis between the two posterior cardinal veins
Renal veins	Right—right mesonephric vein that drains into the IVC derived from right subcardinal vein Left—mesonephric vein, left subcardinal vein and inter-subcardinal anastomosis
Suprarenal veins	Parts of subcardinal veins above intersubcardinal anastomosis (right to IVC and left to left renal vein)
Gonadal veins	Parts of subcardinal veins below inter-subcardinal anastomosis (right to IVC and left to left renal vein)

TABLE 20.5: Embryonic veins and their adult derivatives.

Embryonic veins	Adult derivatives
Right and left vitelline veins	Portion of the IVC, hepatic sinusoids, hepatic vein, ductus venosus that becomes ligamentum venosum, portal vein, superior and inferior mesenteric veins and splenic vein
Right and left umbilical veins	Right vein disappears, left becomes ligamentum teres
Anterior cardinal veins	Superior vena cava, brachiocephalic veins, internal jugular veins, left superior intercostal vein
Posterior cardinal veins	Inferior vena cava, common iliac veins, azygos vein
Subcardinal veins	Inferior vena cava, renal veins, suprarenal veins, gonadal veins
Supracardinal veins	Inferior vena cava, intercostal, hemiazygos and azygos veins

TABLE 20.6: Postnatal occlusion of vessels and their remnants.

Vessel	Remnant
Umbilical arteries	• Proximal part—superior vesical artery • Distal part—fibrosed—medial umbilical ligament
Left umbilical vein	Ligamentum teres of the liver
Ductus venosus	Ligamentum venosum
Ductus arteriosus	Ligamentum arteriosum

TEST YOUR UNDERSTANDING

REVIEW OR PRACTICE QUESTIONS

1. Describe the sinus venosus.
2. Explain the development of right atrium.
3. Explain the development of left atrium.
4. Write notes on development of interatrial septum.
5. Write notes on development of interventricular septum.
6. Explain the development of pericardium.
7. Explain the development of arch of aorta.
8. Explain the development of subclavian artery.
9. Describe ductus arteriosus.
10. Explain the development of vertebral artery.
11. Explain the development of internal thoracic artery.
12. Describe axis artery of upper limb.
13. Describe axis artery of lower limb.
14. Explain the development of portal vein.
15. Describe coronary sinus.
16. Explain the development of inferior vena cava.
17. Describe fetal circulation.
18. Explain the development of thoracic duct.
19. Write short note on coarctation of aorta.
20. Write short note on patent ductus arteriosus.
21. Write short note on ventricular septal defect.

EXPLAIN WHY? (REASONING QUESTIONS)

1. Defect in the formation of the endocardial cushions can result in atrioventricular septal defects.
2. Persistence of the left superior vena cava can lead to an abnormal venous return to the heart.
3. Improper partitioning of the truncus arteriosus can result in transposition of the great arteries.
4. Failure of the ductus arteriosus to close after birth results in complications.

MULTIPLE CHOICE QUESTIONS

1. **Annulus ovalis represents the embryological:**
   A. Free upper edge of septum primum
   B. Free upper edge of septum secundum
   C. Free lower edge of septum secundum
   D. Septum primum

2. **Which one of the following does not take part in the formation of right subclavian artery?**
   A. Right 4th arch artery
   B. Right 7th cervical intersgmental artery
   C. Right dorsal aorta
   D. Right 2nd arch artery

3. **The most important contribution for the development of inferior vana cava is:**
   A. Supracardinal vein and subcardinal vein
   B. Umbilical vein
   C. Anterior cardinal vein
   D. Posterior cardinal vein

4. **Duct of Cuvier is the other name for:**
   A. Anterior cardinal vein
   B. Posterior cardinal vein
   C. Supracardinal vein
   D. Common cardinal vein

5. **Cardiac progenitor cells appear at:**
   A. 20–24 days
   B. 16–18 days
   C. 10–12 days
   D. 24–28 days

6. **Arch of azygos is formed from:**
   A. Left anterior cardinal vein
   B. Right anterior cardinal vein
   C. Right posterior cardinal vein
   D. Right vitelline vein

7. **A newborn presents with cyanosis, and imaging reveals a single large arterial trunk overriding a large ventricular septal defect. Which embryological defect is the most likely cause?**
   A. Failure of the endocardial cushions to fuse
   B. Incomplete septation of the truncus arteriosus
   C. Persistence of the ductus arteriosus
   D. Abnormal neural crest cell migration

8. **A 3-month-old infant has difficulty breathing and poor weight gain. Echocardiography shows a left-to-right shunt at the level of the atria. What embryological structure failed to close properly?**
   A. Foramen ovale
   B. Ductus arteriosus
   C. Ostium primum
   D. Sinus venosus

9. **A newborn with a harsh, holosystolic murmur at the lower left sternal border is found to have a ventricular septal defect. Which part of the interventricular septum is most likely affected?**
   A. Muscular part
   B. Membranous part
   C. Septum primum
   D. Septum secundum

10. **During a routine prenatal ultrasound, a fetus is found to have a persistent left superior vena cava. Which embryological structure failed to regress?**
    A. Right common cardinal vein
    B. Left common cardinal vein
    C. Left posterior cardinal vein
    D. Right anterior cardinal vein

11. A neonate presents with cyanosis and is diagnosed with transposition of the great arteries. Which embryological process is most likely defective?
    A. Septation of the atria
    B. Partitioning of the truncus arteriosus
    C. Formation of the endocardial cushions
    D. Development of the cardinal veins

12. A neonate presents with cyanosis and is found to have an overriding aorta, right ventricular hypertrophy, and a ventricular septal defect. Genetic testing reveals a deletion on chromosome 22q11.2. Which embryological process is most likely affected?
    A. Endocardial cushion formation
    B. Neural crest cell migration
    C. Septation of the primitive atrium
    D. Regression of the left sinus horn

Answers: 1. C   2. D   3. A   4. D   5. B
           6. C   7. B   8. A   9. B   10. B
          11. B   12. B

Urogenital System

CHAPTER 21

COMPETENCIES COVERED/LEARNING OUTCOMES

The student should be able to:

AN52.7	Describe the development of urinary system.
AN52.8	Describe the development of male and female reproductive system.

The urogenital system encompasses the urinary and genital structures, sharing a common developmental pathway initially. The urinary system includes the kidneys, ureters, bladder, and urethra, while the genital system involves the development of the gonads, internal reproductive tracts, and external genitalia, with differentiation directed by genetic and hormonal influences. The development of urinary system precedes genital system. The development of urinary starts at 4th week of intrauterine life (IUL) with formation of pronephric tubules while formation of urogenital membranes during 6th week initiates the genital system formation.

Two embryonic structures that play an important role in the development of the urogenital system are the *intermediate mesoderm* and the *cloaca*. These are briefly considered below.

INTERMEDIATE MESODERM

We have seen (*refer* Chapter 7) that the intraembryonic mesoderm is subdivided into:

1. The paraxial mesoderm which becomes segmented to form the somites.
2. The lateral plate mesoderm in which the intraembryonic coelom appears.
3. The intermediate mesoderm lying between the two **(Fig. 21.1)**.

Formation of Urogenital Ridge

- After the folding of the embryonic disc and the formation of the peritoneal cavity, the intermediate mesoderm forms a bulging on the posterior abdominal wall lateral to the attachment of the dorsal mesentery of the gut which is called *urogenital ridge* **(Fig. 21.2A)**.
- Its surface is covered by the epithelium lining the peritoneal cavity *(coelomic epithelium)*.
- The urogenital ridge is subdivided into parts, medial part of ridge gives rise to *genital ridge* which forms genital system. Lateral part of the ridge forms the *nephrogenic cord* that forms urinary system.

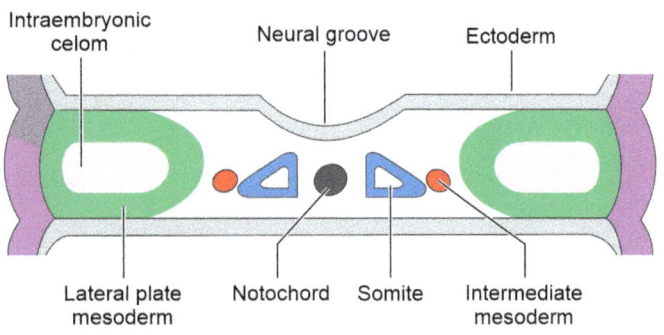

FIG. 21.1: Location of intermediate mesoderm.

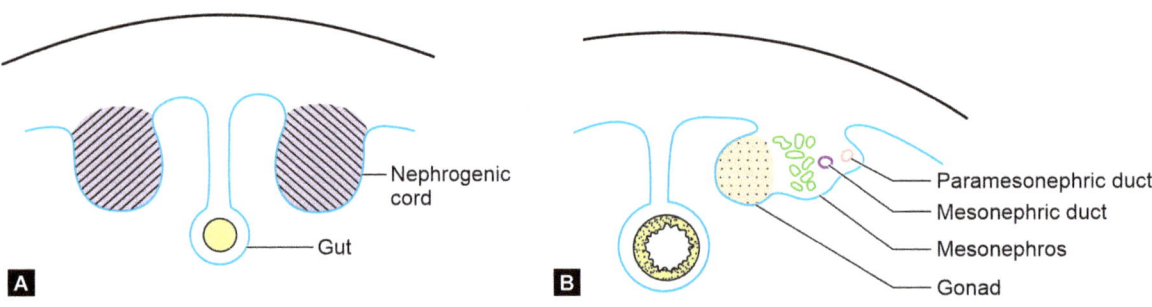

FIGS. 21.2A and B: Nephrogenic cord (A); and structures that develop in it (B).

Chapter 21: Urogenital System

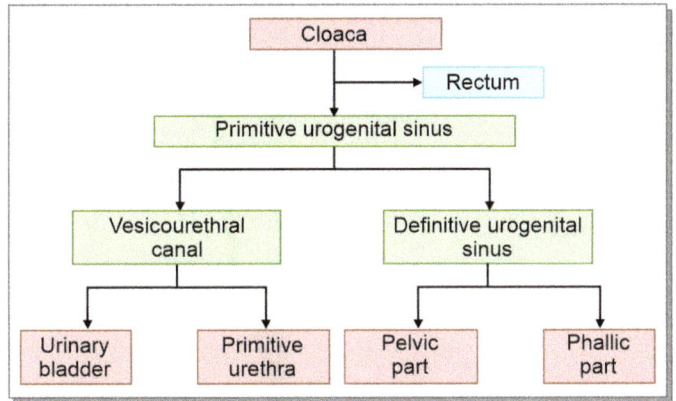

FIG. 21.3: Subdivisions of the cloaca. Also see **Figure 20.4**.

- This cord extends from the cervical region to the sacral region of the embryo.
- At varying stages of development, a number of important structures are formed in relation to the nephrogenic cord on each side. These are (**Fig. 21.2B**):
- *Excretory renal tubules* associated with the development of the kidney.
- The *nephric duct* which is formed in relation to the developing excretory tubules. At later stages, this becomes the *mesonephric duct*.
- The *paramesonephric duct*, which is formed lateral to the nephric duct.
- The *gonad (testis or ovary)*, which develops from the coelomic epithelium lining the medial side of the nephrogenic cord.

CLOACA

Cloaca is part of hindgut caudal to allantois, is divided into two subdivisions by the urorectal septum *primitive rectum* and primitive *urogenital sinus*. Refer Chapter 16 for detailed explanation.

- In further development, the primitive urogenital sinus is subdivided into a cranial part, called the *vesicourethral canal*, and a caudal part, called the *definitive urogenital sinus* (**Fig. 21.3**).
- The openings of the mesonephric ducts (see below) lie at the junction of these two subdivisions (**Fig. 21.4A**).
- Still later, the definitive urogenital sinus shows a division into a cranial *pelvic part*, and a caudal *phallic part* (**Fig. 21.4B**).
- The urogenital system is derived from the various structures that develop in the intermediate mesoderm, and from the various subdivisions of the cloaca.

URINARY SYSTEM

DEVELOPMENT OF KIDNEYS

The development of permanent kidneys initiates during 5th week of IUL. The definitive human kidney arises from two distinct sources.

- The *secretory part* comprising of excretory tubules (or *nephrons*) are derived from the lowest part of the nephrogenic cord. This part is the *metanephros*, the cells of which form the *metanephric blastema*.
- The *collecting part* of the kidney is derived from a diverticulum called the *ureteric bud* which arises from the lower part of the *mesonephric (Wolffian) duct* (**Fig. 21.5**).

Evolutionary History of Development of Kidneys

- Some of the features of the development of the kidney in the human embryo can be appreciated only if the evolutionary history of the organ is kept in mind. The vertebrate kidney has passed through three stages of evolution. The most primitive of these is called the *pronephros*. It is the functioning kidney in some cyclostomes and fishes. This has been succeeded in higher vertebrates by the *mesonephros* that is the functioning kidney of most anamniotes. The kidney of amniotes (including man) is called the *metanephros* (**Fig. 21.6**).

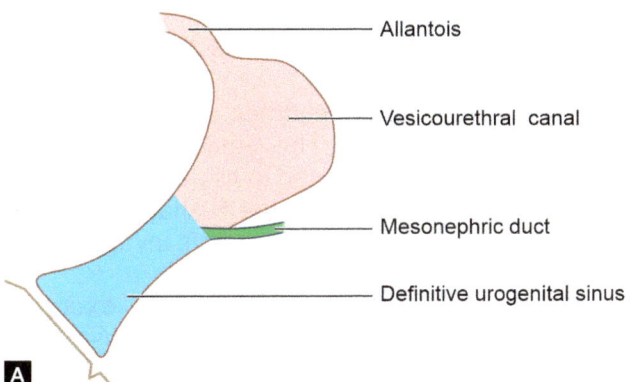
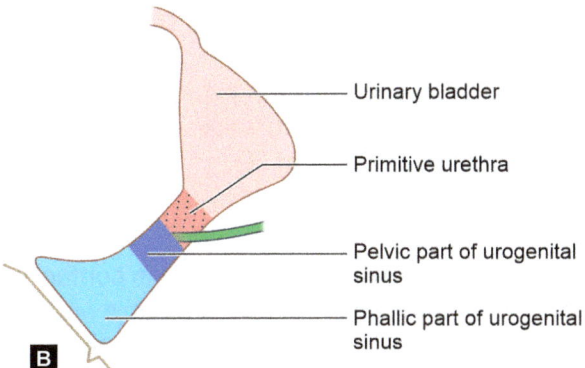

FIGS. 21.4A and B: Subdivisions of the primitive urogenital sinus. Also see **Figure 21.3**.

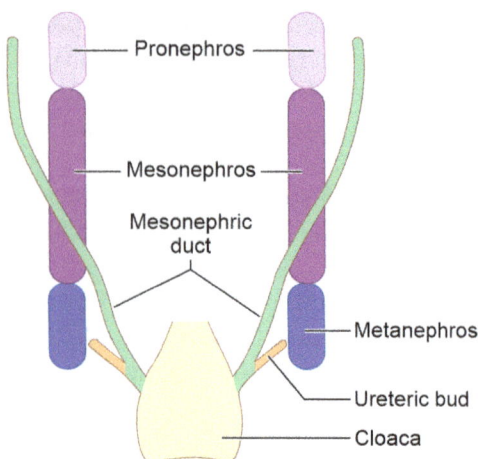

FIG. 21.5: Pronephros, mesonephros and metanephros. Note that the mesonephric duct opens into the cloaca; and gives off the ureteric bud.

- During the development of the human embryo, the evolutionary history of the kidney repeats itself being a classic example of the saying that *ontogeny repeats phylogeny*. The pronephros is formed in relation to the cervical region of the nephrogenic cord. This is followed by appearance of the mesonephros in the thoracolumbar region, and finally by formation of the metanephros in the sacral region **(Fig. 21.5)**.
- The human pronephros is nonfunctional and disappears soon after its formation. A *pronephric duct* formed in relation to the pronephros and ending in the cloaca, however, persists.
- The mesonephros consists of a series of excretory tubules that develop in the thoracolumbar region. These tubules drain into the nephric duct which may now be called the *mesonephric duct*. Most of the mesonephric tubules disappear, but some of them are modified and take part in forming the duct system of the testis forming *vasa efferentia*.

Formation of Collecting Tubules

❖ As the ureteric bud grows cranially towards the metanephric blastema, its growing end becomes dilated to form funnel shaped *ampulla*.
❖ The ampulla divides repeatedly up to 13 generations to form the collecting system. The first three to five generations of branches fuse to form the *pelvis* of the kidney. The next divisions become the *major calyces* while further divisions form the *minor calyces* and *collecting tubules* **(Figs. 21.7A to D)**.
❖ 1-3 million branches form the future *collecting ducts of Bellini*. Lobulation of fetal kidney occurs at 6th week with 2 lobes and at 16th week with 14–16 lobes. This persists up to 1 year of life.

Formation of Nephrons

❖ The cells of the metanephric blastema in contact with an ampulla undergo differentiation to form a *nephron*. This differentiation is induced by the ampulla.
❖ Loosely arranged cells of the metanephric blastema form solid clumps in relation to the ampullae, called

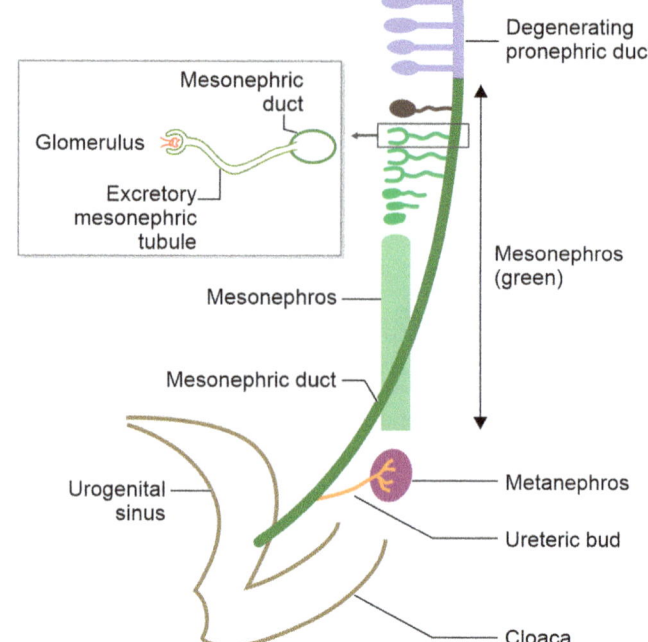

FIG. 21.6: Some details of developing pronephros, mesonephros and metanephros. The pronephros and pronephric duct degenerate soon after formation. The proximal part of the mesonephros shows segmentation (in craniocaudal sequence). The segments contain functional excretory tubules that drain into the mesonephric duct. Most of these tubules disappear by the time the metanephros forms the definitive kidney.

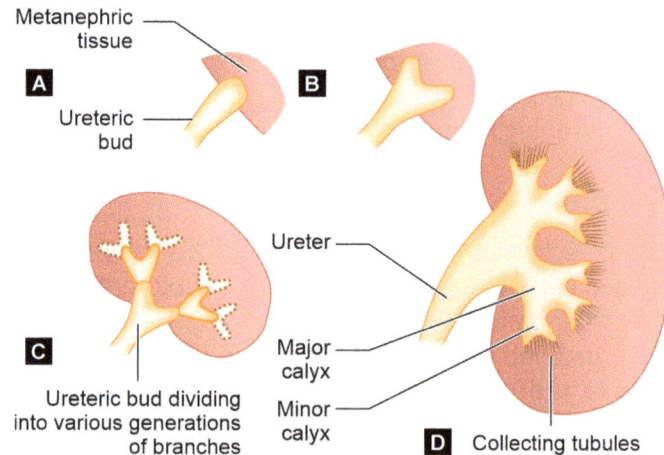

FIGS. 21.7A to D: Formation of the collecting system of the kidney, from ramifications of the ureteric bud.

mesonephric cap, which is soon converted into a *mesonephric vesicle*.
❖ The vesicle soon becomes pear-shaped and opens into the ampulla. The vesicle now becomes an S-shaped tube, referred to as *primitive renal tubule*. Its distal end comes of the S-shaped tube forms the *Bowman's capsule* which gets invaginated by a tuft of capillaries which form a *glomerulus*.
❖ Primitive renal tubules form the excretory unit, *nephron*, consisting of renal corpuscle, proximal convoluted tubule, loop of Henle and distal convoluted tubules. The latter joins the collecting tubules to form *uriniferous tubules*.

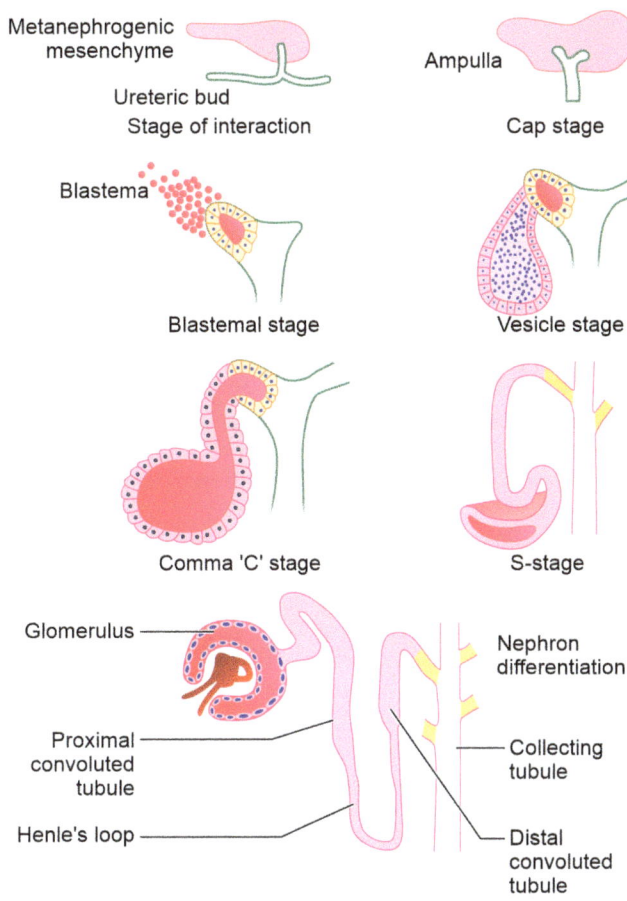

FIG. 21.8: Scheme to show stages in the development of the nephron.

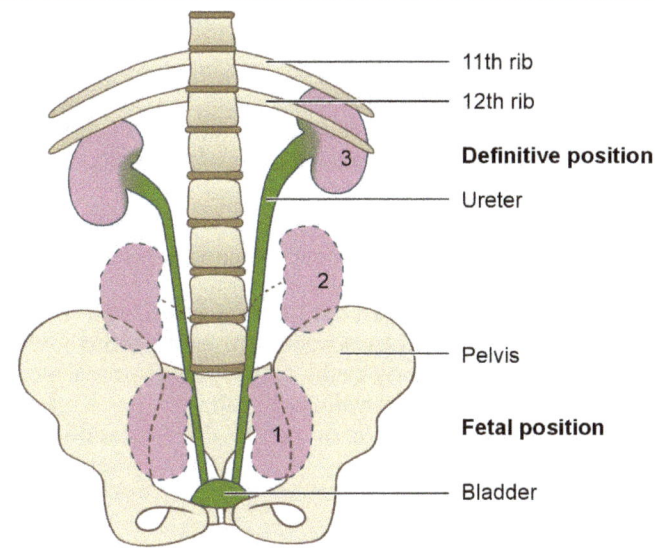

FIG. 21.9: Ascent of the kidney.

❖ The various parts of the nephron development is shown in **Figure 21.8**.

Ascent of the Kidney

The definitive human kidney is derived from the metanephros, which lies in the sacral region. In subsequent development of the embryo, differential growth of the abdominal wall causes the kidney to ascend to the *thoracolumbar region* by 9th week which is their final position **(Fig. 21.9)**. The ureter elongates with the ascent of the kidney.

Clinical correlation

Anomalies of Kidneys
- **Renal agenesis:** One or both kidneys may be absent, which occurs due to failure of development of ureteric bud which induces mesonephric tissue to form mesonephric blastema.
- This condition can be *unilateral*, which is common and usually sustainable with life. On other hand, *bilateral renal agenesis* is incompatible with life. It causes oligohydramnios resulting in *Potter syndrome* characterized by deformed limbs abnormal facial features and wrinkled skin.
  - The kidney may be underdeveloped *(hypoplasia)* or overdeveloped *(hyperplasia)*.
  - Adrenal tissue may be present within the substance of the kidney.
  - Distention of the pelvis with urine *(hydronephrosis)* may occur as a result of obstruction in the urinary passages.
- **Duplication:** There may be an extra kidney on one side. It may be separate, or may be fused to the normal kidney **(Fig. 21.12)** which occurs due to early division of ureteric bud.
- **Anomalies of shape:**
  - *Horseshoe kidney:* The lower poles of the two kidneys (or sometimes the upper poles) may be fused. The connecting isthmus may lie either in front of, or behind, the aorta and inferior vena cava **(Figs. 21.10G and H)**. A horseshoe kidney does not ascend higher than the level of the inferior mesenteric artery as the latter prevents its higher ascent. It occurs due to pushing of kidneys close together during ascent through fork of umbilical arteries.
  - *Pancake kidney:* The two kidneys may form one mass, lying in the midline or on one side **(Fig. 21.10I)**.
  - The two kidneys may lie on one side, one above the other, the adjacent poles being fused.
  - *Lobulated kidney:* The fetal kidney is normally lobulated. This lobulation may persist **(Fig. 21.10C)** beyond 1 year of life.
- **Anomalies of position:**
  - *Pelvic kidney:* The kidneys may fail to ascend. They then lie in the sacral/pelvic region.
  - The ascent of the kidneys may be incomplete as a result of which they may lie opposite the lower lumbar vertebrae.
  - The kidneys may ascend too far, and may even be present within the thoracic cavity.
  - Both kidneys may lie on one side of the midline. They may lie one above the other or side by side **(Figs. 21.10D and E)**. The ureter of the displaced kidney crosses to the opposite side across the midline.
  - Both kidneys may be displaced to the opposite side. The two ureters then cross each other in the midline **(Fig. 21.10F)**.

- **Abnormal rotation:**
  - *Non-rotation:* The hilum is directed forwards.
  - *Incomplete rotation:* The hilum is directed anteromedially.
  - *Reverse rotation:* The hilum is directed anterolaterally.
- **Congenital polycystic kidney:** Failure of the excretory tubules of the metanephros to establish contact with the collecting tubules, leads to the formation of cysts. Isolated cysts are commonly seen, but sometimes the whole kidney is a mass of such cysts **(Fig. 21.10A)**. The cysts press upon normal renal tissue and destroy it. This condition is usually bilateral and common hereditary disease.

  An alternative recent view about the formation of cysts in the kidney is that these urine filled cysts are due to abnormal dilatation of uriniferous tubules, mainly loop of Henle.
- **Aberrant renal arteries:** The kidney may receive its blood supply partially or entirely, from arteries arising at an abnormal level **(Fig. 21.10B)**. In the case of nonascent, or of incomplete ascent, the aberrant arteries may constitute the only supply to the organ. An aberrant artery may be the only source of arterial blood to a segment of the kidney. It may press upon the ureter and cause obstruction, leading to hydronephrosis.
- **Multiple anomalies:** Two or more of the above anomalies may coexist. Anomalies of position are frequently associated with those of rotation.

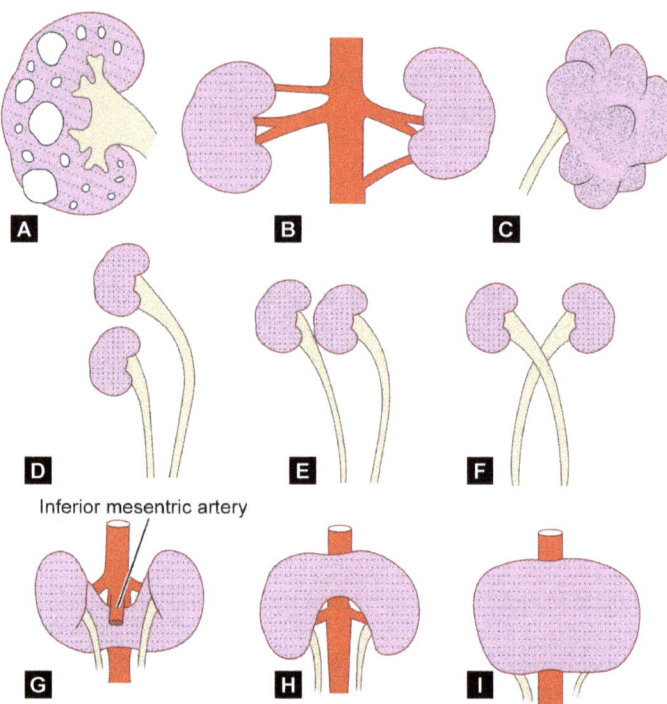

FIGS. 21.10A to I: Anomalies of the kidney: (A) Congenital polycystic kidney; (B) Aberrant renal arteries; (C) Lobulated kidney; (D to F) Transposition of kidney; (G and H) Horseshoe kidney; (I) Pancake kidney.

Arterial Supply

The metanephros, at first, receives its blood supply from the medial sacral and segmental arteries of pelvis aorta, but with its ascent, higher branches of the aorta take over the supply. The *definitive renal artery* represents the lateral splanchnic branch of the aorta at the level of the second lumbar segment.

During ascent, the kidneys pass through the fork like interval between the right and left umbilical arteries. If the arteries come in the way of ascent, the kidney may remain in the sacral region (*see* 'Anomalies of Kidneys').

Rotation of the Kidney

The hilum of the kidney, at first, faces anteriorly. The organ gradually rotates at 90° so that the hilum comes to face medially.

ABSORPTION OF LOWER PARTS OF MESONEPHRIC DUCTS INTO CLOACA

The lower ends of the mesonephric ducts open into that part of the cloaca that forms the urogenital sinus. It has also been seen that the ureteric buds arise from the mesonephric ducts, a little cranial to the cloaca **(Fig. 21.11A)**.

❖ The parts of the mesonephric ducts, caudal to the origin of the ureteric buds, are absorbed into the vesicourethral canal, with the result that the mesonephric ducts and the ureteric buds now have separate openings into the cloaca **(Fig. 21.11B)**. These openings are at first close together **(Fig. 21.11C)**.

❖ However, the openings of the ureteric buds move cranially and laterally due to continued absorption of the buds. The triangular area (on the dorsal wall of the vesicourethral canal) between the openings of the ureteric buds and those of the mesonephric ducts, is derived from the absorbed ducts and is, therefore, of mesodermal origin **(Fig. 21.11D)**.

DEVELOPMENT OF THE URETER

The ureter is derived from the part of the ureteric bud as a diverticulum from mesonephric duct that lies between the pelvis of the kidney, and the vesicourethral canal.

DEVELOPMENT OF THE URINARY BLADDER

The part above the mesonephric duct openings is called the *vesicourethral canal*, which has a wider upper part and a narrower lower part.

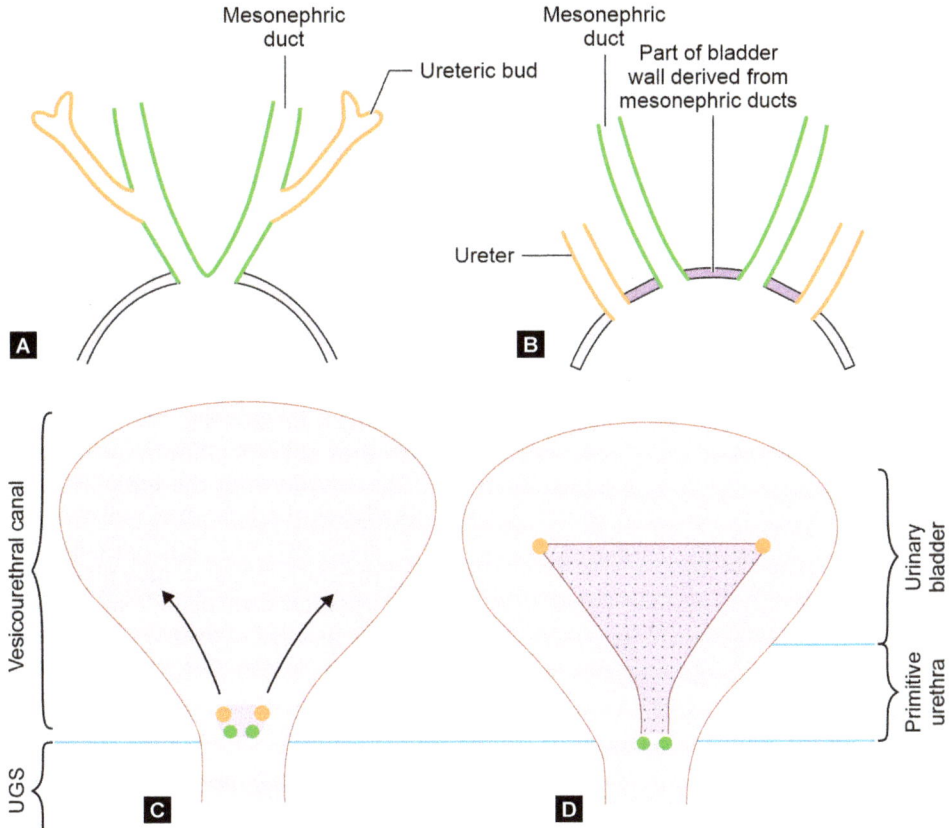

FIGS. 21.11A to D: (A) Mesonephric duct opens into primitive urogenital sinus (UGS); (B) As the sinus grows the proximal parts of mesonephric ducts are absorbed so that the mesonephric ducts and ureters now open separately; (C) The openings are at first close together; (D) Further absorption of ureters causes their opening to shift upwards and laterally. The shaded area is derived from absorbed parts of ureters and mesonephric ducts, and is mesodermal. It forms the trigone of the bladder and the posterior wall of part of the urethra.

- The part below is the *definitive urogenital sinus*. The allantois opens into the apex of the upper wider part of the vesicourethral canal and extends from the apex of the urinary bladder. The urinary bladder develops from this dilated part of the vesicourethral canal, including the proximal part of the allantois. The lower narrow part becomes the *primitive urethra*.
- With the absorption of the mesonephric ducts and ureteric buds into the posterior wall of the vesicourethral canal, the *trigone of the bladder* is formed. The trigone is mesodermal in origin.
- The epithelium of the urinary bladder develops from the cranial part of the vesicourethral canal (endoderm). The epithelium of the trigone of the bladder is derived from the absorbed mesonephric ducts (mesoderm), although it is later overgrown by surrounding endodermal cells.
- The muscular and serous walls of the bladder are derived from splanchnopleuric mesoderm.
- The developing bladder is continuous cranially with the allantois, which atrophies and forms the *urachus (median umbilical ligament)* in postnatal life, extending from the apex of the bladder to the umbilicus.

Clinical correlation

Anomalies of the Ureter
- **Double ureters and renal pelvis:** The ureter may be partially or completely duplicated **(Figs. 21.12A to C)**. This condition may, or may not, be associated with duplication of the kidney. Very rarely, there may be more than two ureters on one, or both, sides. Of the two ureters one may open into the urinary bladder while the other may open at an abnormal site (see below). This condition may cause urinary obstruction.
- **Abnormal site of opening:** Instead of opening into the urinary bladder, the ureter may end in the prostatic urethra, ductus deferens, seminal vesicles, or rectum, in the male **(Fig. 21.13B)**; and in the urethra, vagina, vestibule or rectum in the female **(Fig. 21.13A)**. This occurs due to incorporation of ureter in the trigone area.
- **Bifid ureter:** The upper end of the ureter may be blind, i.e., it is not connected to the kidney. In lower 1/3rd, two ureters can join to open in bladder through one orifice only.
- The ureter may be dilated *(hydroureter)* because of obstruction to urine flow.
- The ureter may have valves or diverticula.
- **Postcaval ureter:** The right ureter may pass behind the inferior vena cava. It then hooks around the left side of the vena cava; this may result in kinking and obstruction of the ureter. The real defect is in the development of the vena cava are described in **Chapter 20**.

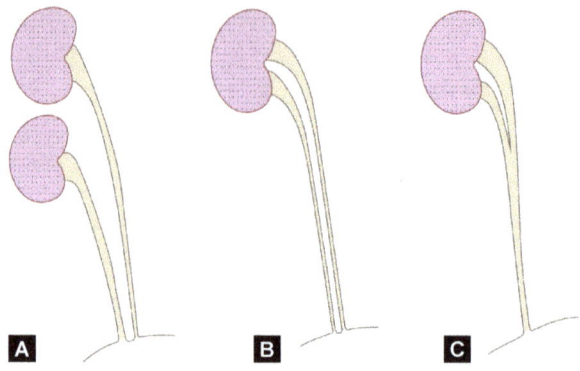

FIGS. 21.12A to C: Anomalies of ureters. Also see **Figure 20.10**.

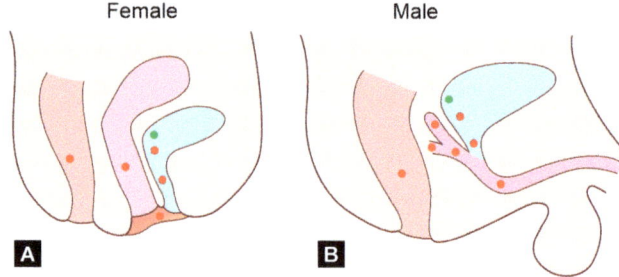

FIGS. 21.13A and B: Abnormal sites at which the ureter may open.

- **Urachal sinus:** If the distal part of the urachus near the umbilicus remains open while the rest of the urachus is obliterated, a urachal sinus can form, creating a tract that extends from the umbilicus but does not connect to the bladder. This anomaly arises from partial failure of the allantois to close.
- **Ectopia vesicae:** The lower part of the anterior abdominal wall, as well as the ventral wall of the bladder, may be missing. As a result, the cavity of the bladder showing ureteic orifices may be exposed on the surface of the body **(Fig. 21.14B)**. The urine can be seen dribbling from the orifices. This defect is usually associated with epispadias. Ectopia vesicae is caused by failure of mesoderm to migrate into the lower abdominal wall (between umbilicus and genital tubercle). Failure of migration may be due to excessive development of the cloacal membrane. The ectoderm of the anterior abdominal wall and the endoderm of the ventral wall of the urinary bladder remain unsupported and thin. Their rupture leads to the exposure of the cavity of the urinary bladder.
- **Congenital diverticula** may be present. These are found at the junction of the trigone with the rest of the bladder.

Clinical correlation

Anomalies of the Urinary Bladder
- The urinary bladder may be absent, or may be duplicated.
- The sphincter vesicae may be absent.
- The lumen of the urinary bladder may be divided into compartments by septa.
- The bladder may be divided into upper and lower compartments *(hourglass bladder)* because of a constriction in the middle of the organ **(Fig. 21.14A)**.
- The bladder may communicate with the rectum.

Congenital Urachus Anomalies
- **Patent urachus:** This occurs when the entire urachus remains open, forming a direct connection between the bladder and the umbilicus due to the failure of the allantois to obliterate during development.
- **Urachal cyst:** A localized area of the urachus may remain patent, resulting in a cyst formation.

DEVELOPMENT OF URETHRA

As we have discussed, caudal portion of the primitive urogenital sinus, located below the openings of the mesonephric ducts, becomes the *definitive urogenital sinus*. This structure is divided into an upper constricted *pelvic section* and a lower dilated *phallic section*.

The phallic part is in contact with the bilaminar urogenital membrane, which is the ventral aspect of the cloacal membrane. The dorsal wall of the pelvic part of the definitive urogenital sinus receives the terminal ends of the mesonephric ducts, which regress in females but persist as *ejaculatory ducts in males*.

Both the caudal section of the vesicourethral canal and the definitive urogenital sinus contribute to the development of the urethra.

Development of the Female Urethra

The female urethra is derived from the caudal part of the *vesicourethral canal* (endoderm). We have seen that the posterior wall of this canal is derived from

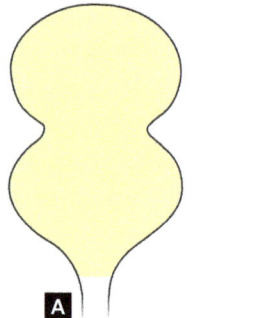
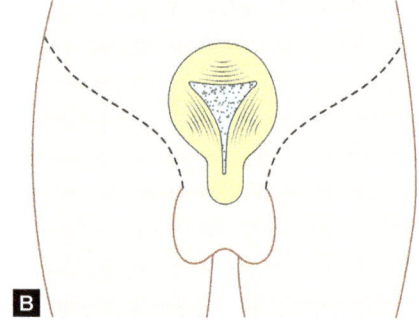
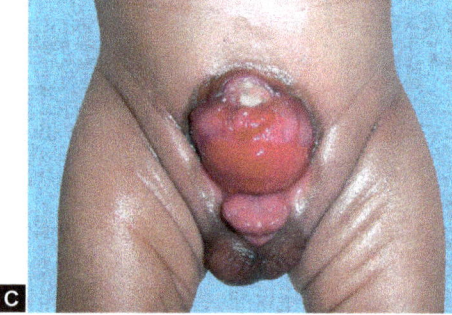

FIGS. 21.14A to C: Anomalies of the bladder: (A) Hourglass bladder; (B and C) Ectopia vesicae. The ureteric openings and the trigone are seen on the surface of the body, schematic presentation and clinical picture.
(Reproduced with permission from Dr Piyush Gupta. Source: Anup Mohta, Chapter 23. In: Gupta P, UG Textbook of Pediatrics, Jaypee Brothers Medical Publishers Pvt Ltd, 2023).

the mesonephric ducts and is, therefore, mesodermal in origin. The female urethra may receive a slight contribution from the pelvic part of the urogenital sinus (Figs. 21.15A to E).

Development of the Male Urethra

The male urethra is divided into four parts: Prostatic, membranous, penile and terminal (glans) urethra.

- **Prostatic urethra:** The part of the male urethra extending from the urinary bladder up to the openings of the ejaculatory ducts (original openings of mesonephric ducts), is derived from the caudal part of the vesicourethral canal (endoderm). The posterior wall of this part is derived from absorbed mesonephric ducts (mesoderm) (it may later be overgrown by endoderm).
- The rest of the prostatic urethra, and the *membranous urethra*, are derived from the pelvic part of the definitive urogenital sinus.
- The *penile part/spongy part* of the urethra (except the terminal part) is derived from the epithelium of the phallic part of the definitive urogenital sinus (see 'Development of Penis').
- The *terminal part* of the penile urethra, that lies in the glans, is derived from ectoderm (Figs. 21.15A to E).

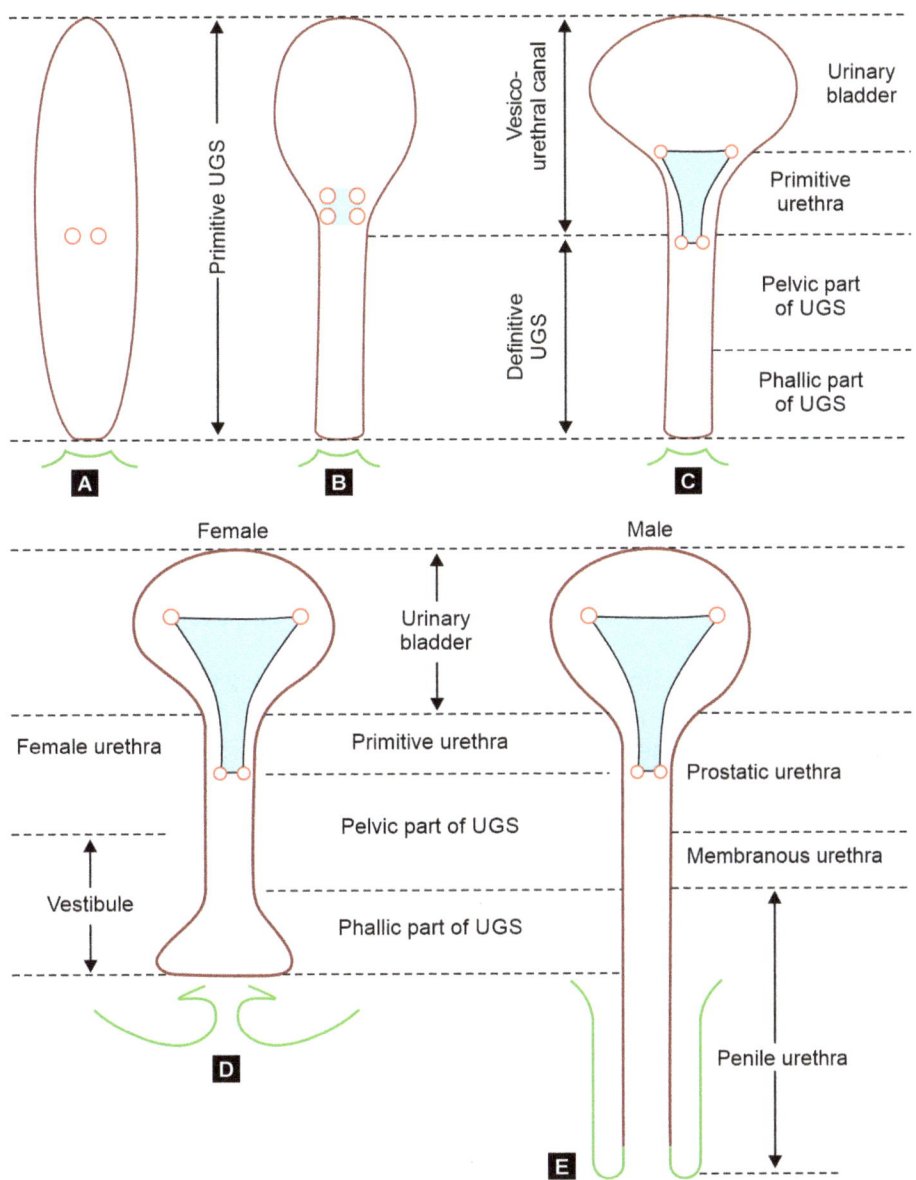

FIGS. 21.15A to E: Development of urethra: (A) Primitive urogenital sinus (UGS) showing opening of mesonephric ducts; (B) Primitive UGS divided into vesicourethral canal and definitive UGS. Mesonephric ducts and ureters open separately at the junction of the two parts; (C) Vesicourethral canal subdivided into urinary bladder and primitive urethra. The definitive UGS divides into pelvic and phallic parts; (D) The female urethra is formed from the primitive urethra and from part of the pelvic portion of UGS. The rest of the pelvic part of UGS forms the vestibule; (E) In the male the prostatic urethra is formed in the same way as the female urethra. The membranous urethra is derived from the pelvic part of UGS. The penile urethra is derived from the phallic part of UGS. Red circles = openings of mesonephric ducts and ureters. Blue = part derived from mesoderm. Green = ectoderm.

From the above it will be clear that the female urethra corresponds to the prostatic part of the male urethra.

Clinical correlation

Anomalies of the Urethra
- There may be *obstruction* to the urethra at its junction with the bladder.
- **Congenital stenosis** might be there due to failure of canalization of some points of urethral plate.
- The urethra may show *diverticula*.
- It may be *duplicated* in whole or in part.
- The urethra may have *abnormal communications* with the rectum (**Figs. 16.23B and C**), the vagina or the ureter (**Figs. 21.13A and B**).
- **Hypospadias** is a congenital condition where the urethral opening is located on the underside of the penis, while *epispadias* occurs when the urethral opening is on the upper surface.

DEVELOPMENT OF THE PROSTATE

This gland develops from a large number of buds that arise from the epithelium of the prostatic urethra, i.e., from the caudal part of the vesicourethral canal, and from the pelvic part of the definitive urogenital sinus. These buds form the secretory epithelium of the gland. The glandular part of prostate develops as solid *endodermal buds*. The buds that arise from the mesodermal part of the prostatic urethra (i.e., posterior wall, above the openings of the ejaculatory ducts) form the *inner glandular zone* of the prostate (**Figs. 21.16A and B**). Buds arising from the rest of the prostatic urethra (endoderm) form the *outer glandular zone*.

❖ The outer zone differentiates earlier than the inner zone. In later life the outer zone is frequently the site of carcinomatous change, while the inner zone is affected in senile hypertrophy of the organ.
❖ The muscle and connective tissue of the gland are derived from the surrounding mesenchyme which also forms the capsule of the gland.

❖ The secretory elements of the prostate are rudimentary at birth. They undergo considerable development at puberty. The organ undergoes progressive atrophy in old age, but in some men it undergoes *benign hypertrophy*. The prostate may, rarely, be absent.

Female Homologues of Prostate

Endodermal buds, similar to those that form the prostate in the male, are also seen in the female. The buds that arise from the caudal part of the vesicourethral canal give rise to the *urethral glands*, whereas the buds arising from the urogenital sinus form the *paraurethral glands of Skene*.

GENITAL SYSTEM

FEMALE GENITAL SYSTEM

Paramesonephric (Mullerian) Ducts

We have seen that these ducts are present in the intermediate mesoderm. They are formed by invagination of coelomic epithelium (**Figs. 21.17A to D**). They lie lateral to the mesonephric ducts in the cranial part of the nephrogenic cord (**Fig. 21.18A**).

❖ When traced caudally, they cross to the medial side of the mesonephric ducts. Here the ducts of the two sides meet and fuse in the middle line to form the *uterovaginal canal* (or *uterine canal*) (**Fig. 21.18B**).
❖ The caudal end of this canal comes in contact with the dorsal wall of, the definitive urogenital sinus. We have already seen that, in the female, this part of the sinus gives rise to the vestibule.
❖ In the female, the paramesonephric ducts give origin to the *uterine tubes, the uterus*, and *part of the vagina* (**Fig. 21.19A**).

Development of Uterus and Uterine Tubes

❖ The epithelium of the uterus develops from the fused paramesonephric (Müllerian ducts) ducts (uterovaginal canal: 1 in **Fig. 21.19A**). The *myometrium* is derived from surrounding mesoderm (3 in **Fig. 21.19A**).

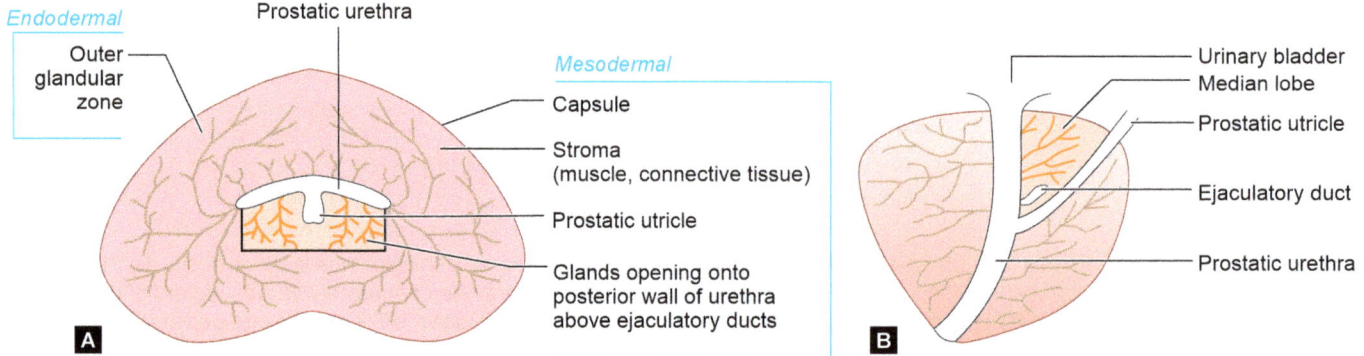

FIGS. 21.16A and B: Mesodermal and endodermal derivatives of the prostate. The glands of the median lobe, which open onto the posterior wall of the prostatic urethra (above the opening of the ejaculatory ducts), are mesodermal. (A) shows a transverse section above the level of the opening of ejaculatory ducts. (B) is a sagittal section.

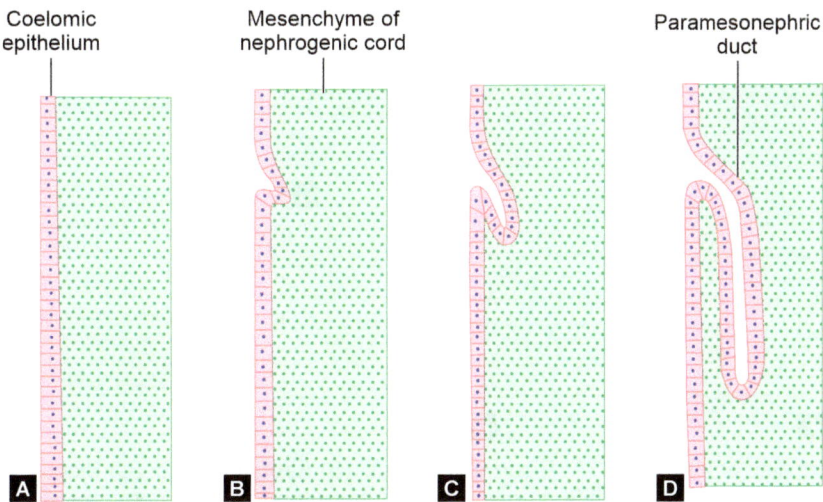

FIGS. 21.17A to D: Formation of paramesonephric ducts by invagination of coelomic epithelium.

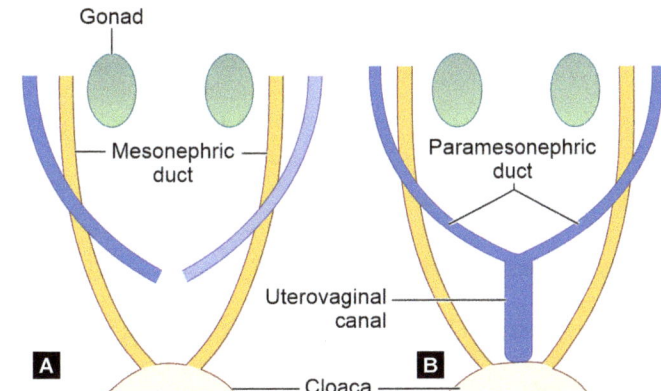

FIGS. 21.18A and B: Formation of uterovaginal canal by fusion of the caudal parts of paramesonephric ducts.

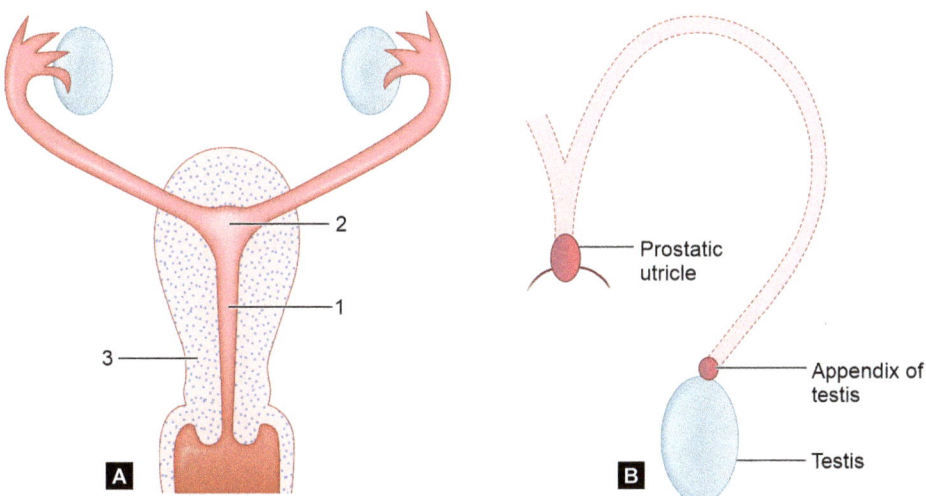

FIGS. 21.19A and B: Fate of paramesonephric ducts: (A) In the female they form the uterine tubes, the uterus, and part of the vagina:(1) uterovaginal canal, (2) fundus of uterus, (3) myometrium; (B) In the male most of the duct disappears. Remnants are seen as the appendix of the testis and the prostatic utricle.

- As the thickness of the myometrium increases, the unfused horizontal parts of the two paramesonephric ducts come to be partially embedded within its substance, and help to form the *fundus of the uterus* (2 in **Fig. 21.19A**).

- The *cervix* can soon be recognized as a separate region. In the fetus the cervical part is larger than the body of the uterus.

- The *uterine tubes* develop from the unfused parts of the paramesonephric ducts. The original points of

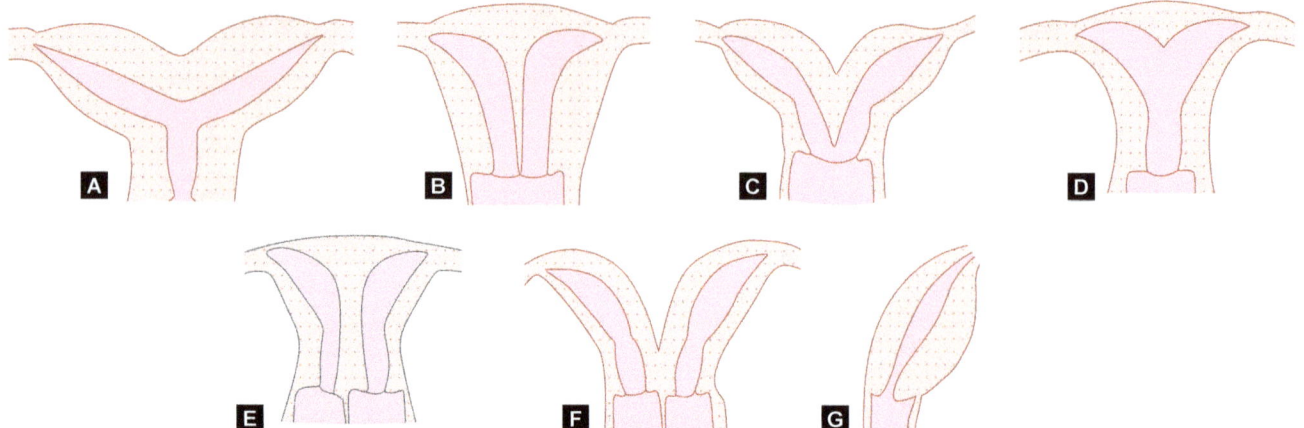

FIGS. 21.20A to G: Anomalies of the uterus: (A) Bicornuate uterus; (B) Septate uterus; (C) Bicornis bicollis uterus; (D) Uterus arcuatus; (E) Subseptate uterus; (F) Didelphys uterus; (G) Unicornuate uterus.

invagination of the ducts into the coelomic epithelium remain as the abdominal openings of the tubes forming *fimbriae* of the uterine tube.

Clinical correlation

Anomalies of the Uterus
Mullerian agenesis
- Failure of development of Müllerian ducts resulting in absence of uterus and varying degrees of vaginal hypoplasia.
- The uterus may be in the form of two horns (*bicornuate*, **Fig. 21.20A**) or completely or partially separated (*septate*, **Fig. 21.20B**). Complete duplication of uterus and cervix is referred to as *uterus didelphys* (**Fig. 21.20F**).
- The uterus is in two horns, the cervix is separated and the vagina is single and is known as *uterus bicornis* and *bicollis* (**Fig. 21.20C**).
- The entire uterus may be absent.
- Uterus may be slightly indented in the middle and is known as *arcuate uterus* (**Fig. 21.20D**).
- Uterus and vagina both may be separated into two and is known as *subseptate uterus* (**Fig. 21.20E**).
- The uterus may remain rudimentary.
- There may be atresia of the lumen either in the body or in the cervix.

- One half of uterus may be absent resulting in *unicornuate* uterus (**Fig. 21.20G**).

Anomalies of the Uterine Tubes
- The uterine tubes may be absent, on one or both sides.
- The tubes may be partially, or completely, duplicated on one or both sides.
- There may be atresia of the tubes.

Development of Vagina

❖ The lower end of the uterovaginal canal comes in close contact with the dorsal wall of the phallic part of the urogenital sinus (**Fig. 21.21A**).
❖ However, the uterovaginal canal and the urogenital sinus are soon separated from each other by the formation of a solid plate of cells called the *vaginal plate*. The vagina is formed by the development of a lumen within the vaginal plate (**Fig. 21.21D**).
❖ The vaginal plate is formed as follows:
  – Endodermal cells of the urogenital sinus proliferate to form two swellings called the sinovaginal bulbs (**Fig. 21.21B**). These bulbs soon fuse to form one mass.

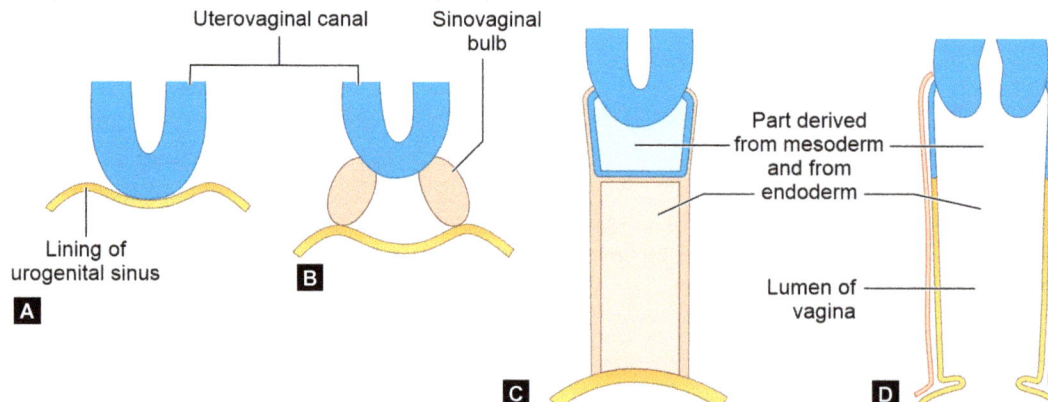

FIGS. 21.21A to D: (A) Uterovaginal canal (mesoderm) in contact with lining of UGS (endoderm); (B) Sinovaginal bulbs are formed by proliferation of endodermal lining; (C) Solid vaginal plate derived partly from mesoderm of uterovaginal canal and partly from endoderm of sinovaginal bulbs; (D) Vagina formed by canalization of vaginal plate.

- Most of the vaginal plate is formed from these sinovaginal bulbs **(Fig. 21.21C)**.
- The part of the vaginal plate near the future cervix is derived from mesodermal cells of the uterovaginal canal.
- The hymen is situated at the junction of the lower end of the vaginal plate with the urogenital sinus. Both surfaces of the hymen are lined by endoderm.

Paramesonephric Ducts in Male

The paramesonephric ducts remain rudimentary in the male. The greater part of each duct eventually disappears **(Fig. 21.19B)**. The cranial end of each duct persists as a small rounded body attached to the testis *(appendix of testis)* that may occasionally give rise to cysts. It has generally been considered that the prostatic utricle represents the uterovaginal canal and is, therefore, a homologue of the uterus. However, it is now believed to correspond mainly to the vagina (and possibly part of the uterus).

Clinical correlation

Anomalies of Vagina
- The vagina may be *duplicated*. This condition is usually associated with duplication of the uterus **(Fig. 21.20A)**.
- The lumen may be subdivided longitudinally, or transversely, by a *septum*.
- The vagina may be *absent*. This condition may or may not be associated with absence of the uterus.
- The hymen may be *imperforated*.
- The vagina may have abnormal communications with the rectum *(rectovaginal fistula)* or with the urinary bladder *(vesicovaginal fistula)* **(Fig. 21.22)**.

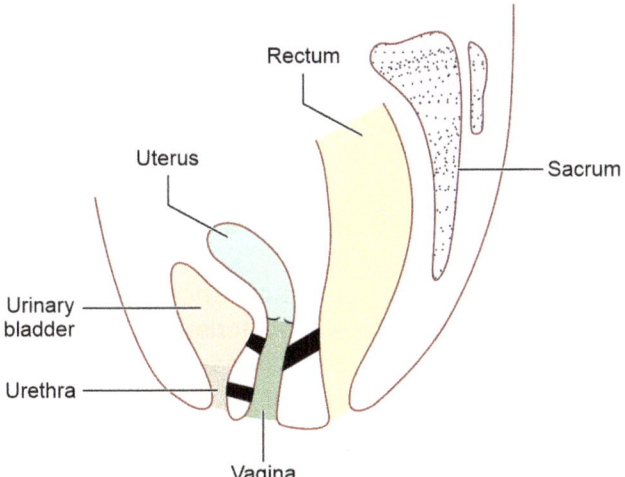

FIG. 21.22: Vaginal fistulae are abnormal communications between vagina and surrounding cavities. The fistulae are shown in solid black. They may connect the vagina to the rectum (rectovaginal fistula); to the urinary bladder (vesicovaginal fistula) or to the urethra (ureterovaginal fistula).

DEVELOPMENT OF EXTERNAL GENITALIA

With the formation of the urorectal septum, the cloacal membrane comes to be subdivided into a ventral, urogenital membrane, and a caudal anal membrane **(Figs. 21.23A and B)**. The urogenital membrane becomes elongated in a craniocaudal direction. The mesoderm on either side of it is soon heaped up to form two longitudinal elevations called the *primitive urethral folds* **(Figs. 21.23D and 21.24A)**. In addition to these folds, three other elevations of mesoderm are soon apparent. These are:

- The *genital tubercle* which is situated in the midline between the urogenital membrane and the lower part of the anterior abdominal wall.
- The right and left *genital swellings* **(Fig. 21.23C)**.

Development of Female External Genitalia (Figs. 21.23 and 21.24)

- The genital tubercle becomes cylindrical and forms the *clitoris*.
- The genital swellings enlarge to form the *labia majora*. Their posterior ends fuse across the midline to form the *posterior commissure*.
- The urogenital membrane breaks down, so that continuity is established between the urogenital sinus (which forms the vestibule) and the exterior. The primitive urethral folds now form the *labia minora*. It will be obvious that they are lined on the outside by ectoderm and on the inside by endoderm **(Figs. 21.24A and B)**.

Clinical correlation

Anomalies of Female External Genitalia
- The clitoris may be *absent*, may be *bifid*, or may be *double*. It may be enlarged in hermaphroditism.
- The labia minora may show partial fusion.
- The urethra may open on the anterior wall of the vagina; this is the female equivalent of male hypospadias.

Development of Male External Genitalia

- The genital tubercle becomes cylindrical and is now called the *phallus*. It undergoes great enlargement to form the *penis*. As the phallus grows, the *glans* becomes distinguishable by the appearance of a *coronary sulcus*. Still later, the *prepuce* is formed by reduplication of the ectoderm covering the distal part of the phallus **(Figs. 21.25A to C)**.
- We have seen that the urogenital membrane lies in a linear groove, flanked on either side by the primitive urethral folds **(Figs. 21.26A to C)**. As the phallus grows, this groove elongates and extends onto its

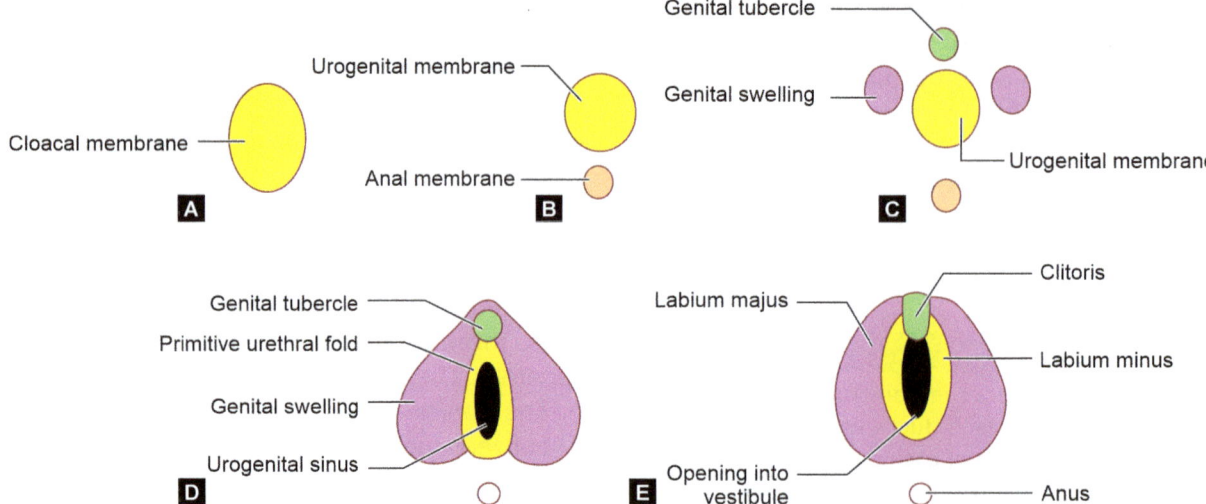

FIGS. 21.23A to E: (A) Cloacal membrane; (B) Cloacal membrane divides into urogenital membrane and anal membrane; (C) Right and left genital swellings, and a median genital tubercle appear; (D) Urogenital membrane breaks down. Its edges form the primitive urethral folds; (E) Genital tubercle becomes the clitoris. The genital swellings become the labia majora, and the primitive urethral folds become the labia minora.

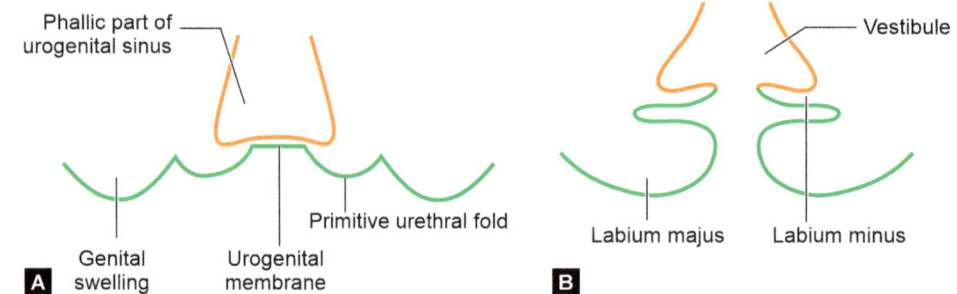

FIGS. 21.24A and B: Development of female external genitalia. Ectoderm shown in green and endoderm shown in orange line.

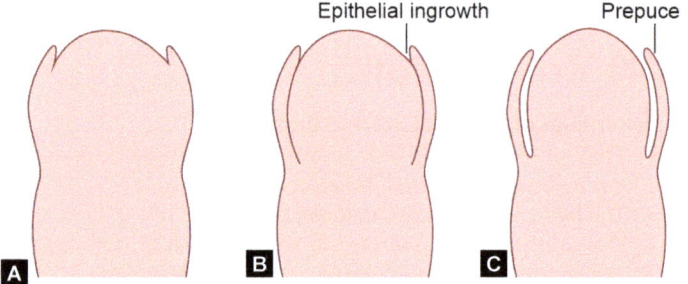

FIGS. 21.25A to C: Formation of the prepuce of the penis.

undersurface (Fig. 21.26B). This groove is lined by ectoderm and is called the *primitive urethral groove*.

❖ From **Figures 21.26C and D** it will be clear that the phallus is closely related to the endodermal lining of the phallic part of the urogenital sinus. The endodermal cells of this lining proliferate, and grow into the phallus, in the form of a solid plate of cells called the *urethral plate* (Fig. 21.26C). The cells of the urethral plate are in contact with the ectodermal cells lining the primitive urethral groove.

❖ The urogenital membrane soon breaks down, so that the urogenital sinus (phallic part) opens to the outside, in the caudal part of the primitive urethral groove (Fig. 21.26D).

❖ At the same time, the cells forming the core of the urethral plate degenerate, along with the ectodermal cells lining the primitive urethral groove. In this way, a deeper groove (called the *definitive urethral groove*) lined by endodermal cells, is now formed on the undersurface of the phallus (Fig. 21.26F).

❖ At the base of the phallus this groove is continuous with the cavity of the urogenital sinus (Fig. 21.26F). The margins of this groove are called the *definitive urethral folds*.

❖ These folds now approach and fuse with each other. The fusion begins posteriorly in the region of the urogenital sinus and extends forwards onto the phallus (Figs. 21.26G and H). The penile urethra is formed as a result of this fusion. It will now be apparent that the wall of the penile urethra is made up of:
- The original endodermal lining of the phallic part of the urogenital sinus, and
- The endodermal cells of the urethral plate.

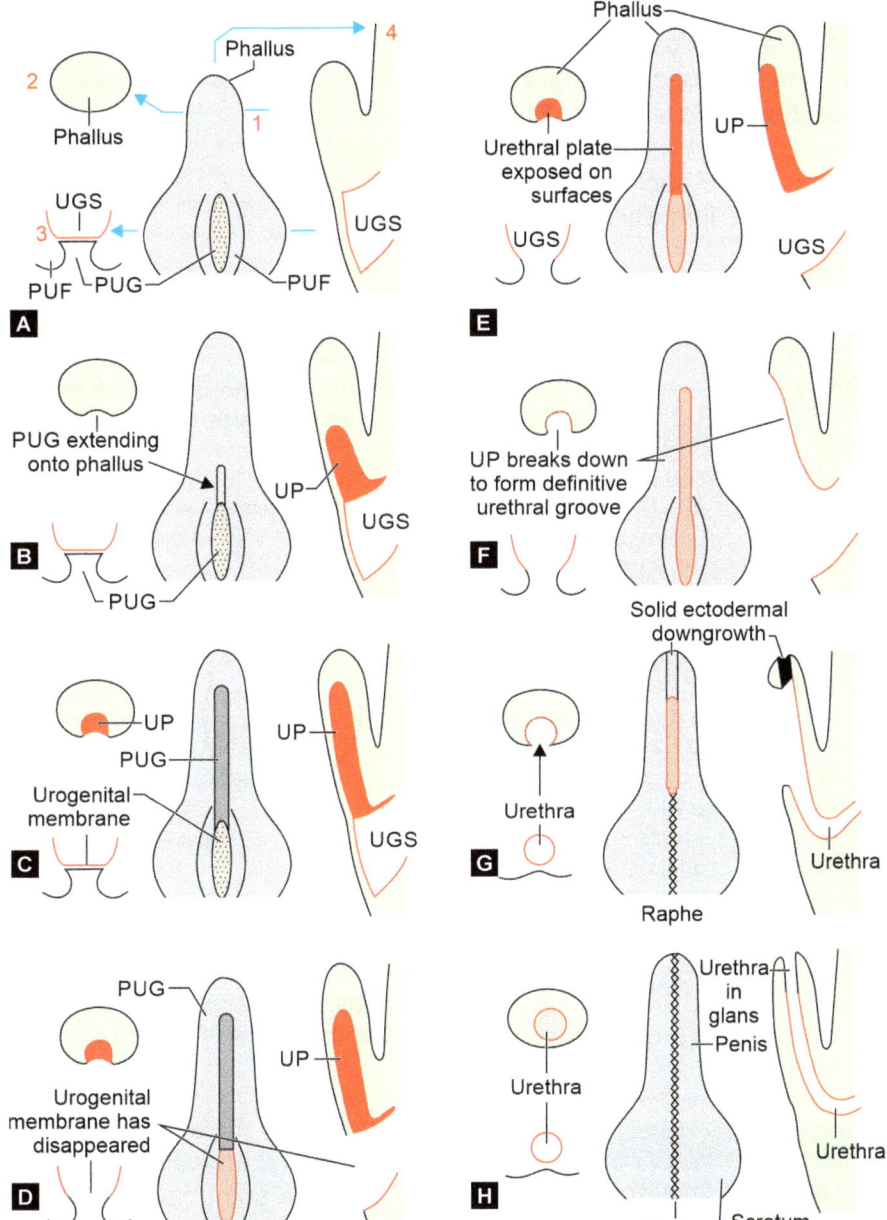

FIGS. 21.26 A to H: Stages in the development of male genitalia and of penile urethra. In each set (A to H), the central figure (1) shows the genital region from the ventral aspect; (2) and (3) are transverse sections at the levels indicated; and (4) is a median section through the region. In sections ectoderm is depicted in black line, and endoderm is red. Mesoderm is green.

A. Note the following. The phallus is formed by enlargement of the genital tubercle. Caudal to the phallus there is a median, longitudinal depression, the primitive urethral groove (PUG) bounded by primitive urethral folds (PUF). Lateral to these folds we see the genital swellings (GS). In the depth of the primitive urethral groove there is the urogenital membrane which separates the groove from the urogenital sinus.

B. The phallus has enlarged. The primitive urethral groove (PUG) is beginning to extend onto it. A solid mass of endodermal cells derived from the urogenital sinus, extends into the phallus. This mass is the urethral plate (UP).

C. The primitive urethral groove is now fully formed. The urethral plate has enlarged and extends deeper into the phallus.

D. The urogenital membrane has broken down so that endoderm of the urogenital sinus (UGS) can now be seen from outside.

E. Ectoderm overlying the urethral plate has disappeared. As a result endoderm of the plate is seen on the surface.

F. Cells in the center of the urethral plate now break down and convert the plate into a groove that is seen on the surface. This is the definitive urethral groove, and the folds forming its edges are the definitive urethral folds.

G. The definitive urethral folds grow towards each other and fuse to form a median raphe. In this way the definitive urethral groove is converted into a tube, which is the urethra. This process of fusion starts caudally and progresses cranially.

H. In this figure and in 'G' note that the urethra formed as described above does not extend into the glans. The part of the urethra lying in the glans is derived from ectoderm which first forms a solid cord that is later canalized.

- The penile urethra formed in this way extends only up to the glans penis. The distal-most part of the urethra is of ectodermal origin, and is formed by canalization of a solid mass of ectodermal cells **(Figs. 21.26G and H)**.
- The genital swellings fuse with each other, in the midline, to form the scrotal sac into which the testes later descend.

Clinical correlation

Anomalies of Male External Genitalia
- The entire penis may be absent. Alternatively, the corpora cavernosa, or the prepuce, may be missing. The opening of the prepuce may be too narrow to allow retraction *(phimosis)*.
- The penis may be *double or bifid*.
- Rarely, the penis may lie posterior to the scrotum.
- The urethral folds may fail to fuse, partially, or completely. When failure to fuse is complete the scrotum is in two halves and the genitals look like those of the female **(Fig. 21.27A)**. If the defect is confined to the anterior part of the phallus, the urethra opens on the undersurface of the penis. This condition is called *hypospadias* **(Fig. 21.27B)**.
- The urethra sometimes opens on the dorsal aspect of the penis. The condition is called *epispadias*, and is usually associated with ectopia vesicae. In such cases it is believed that the genital tubercle is formed caudal to the urogenital membrane instead of being ventral to it. When the membrane ruptures, the urogenital sinus opens cranial to the developing penis.

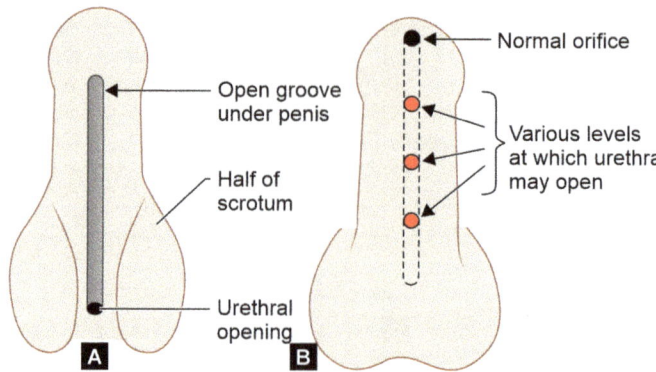

FIGS. 21.27A and B: (A) Cleft scrotum; (B) Hypospadias. The urethra opens onto the ventral aspect of the penis.

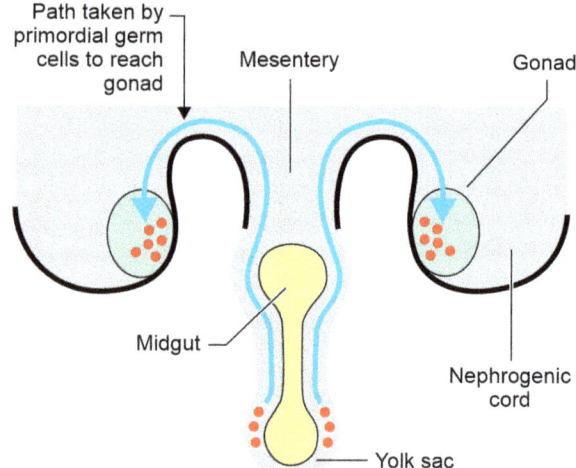

FIG. 21.28: Migration of primordial germ cells from the neighborhood of the yolk sac to the developing gonad.

DEVELOPMENT OF GAMETES PRODUCING ORGANS

Primordial Germ Cells (Fig. 21.28)

The cells of the ovaries and the testes, from which germ cells are formed, are believed to be segregated early in the life of the embryo. They probably differentiate in the wall of the yolk sac and migrate to the region of the developing gonads.

All spermatozoa and ova that are formed throughout the life of the individual are believed to arise from these primordial germ cells.

Migration of primordial germ cells into them is essential for development of the gonads. These cells have an inducing effect on the gonad.

Development of Testes

- Each testis develops from the coelomic epithelium, that covers the medial side of the mesonephros, of the corresponding side **(Figs. 21.29A to E)**. In the region where the testis is to develop, this germinal epithelium becomes thickened. This thickening is called the *genital ridge*.
- The cells of the germinal epithelium proliferate and form a number of solid *sex cords*, that grow into the underlying mesenchyme. They reach deep into the gonad and are called *medullary cords*.
- They are soon canalized to form the *seminiferous tubules*. Meanwhile, the primordial germ cells migrate to the region of the developing testis and get incorporated in the seminiferous tubules.
- The *interstitial cells* of the testis are derived from sex cords that are not canalized. Some of them are also derived from the surrounding mesenchyme.
- The mesenchymal cells, surrounding the developing testis, form a dense layer of fibrous tissue. This is the *tunica albuginea*. It completely separates the sex cords from the germinal epithelium and, thereafter, this epithelium can make no further contribution to testicular tissue.

Duct System of Testes

- We have seen, above, that the testis develops in close proximity to the mesonephros, and the mesonephric duct. We have also seen that most of the mesonephric tubules degenerate. Some of

Chapter 21: Urogenital System

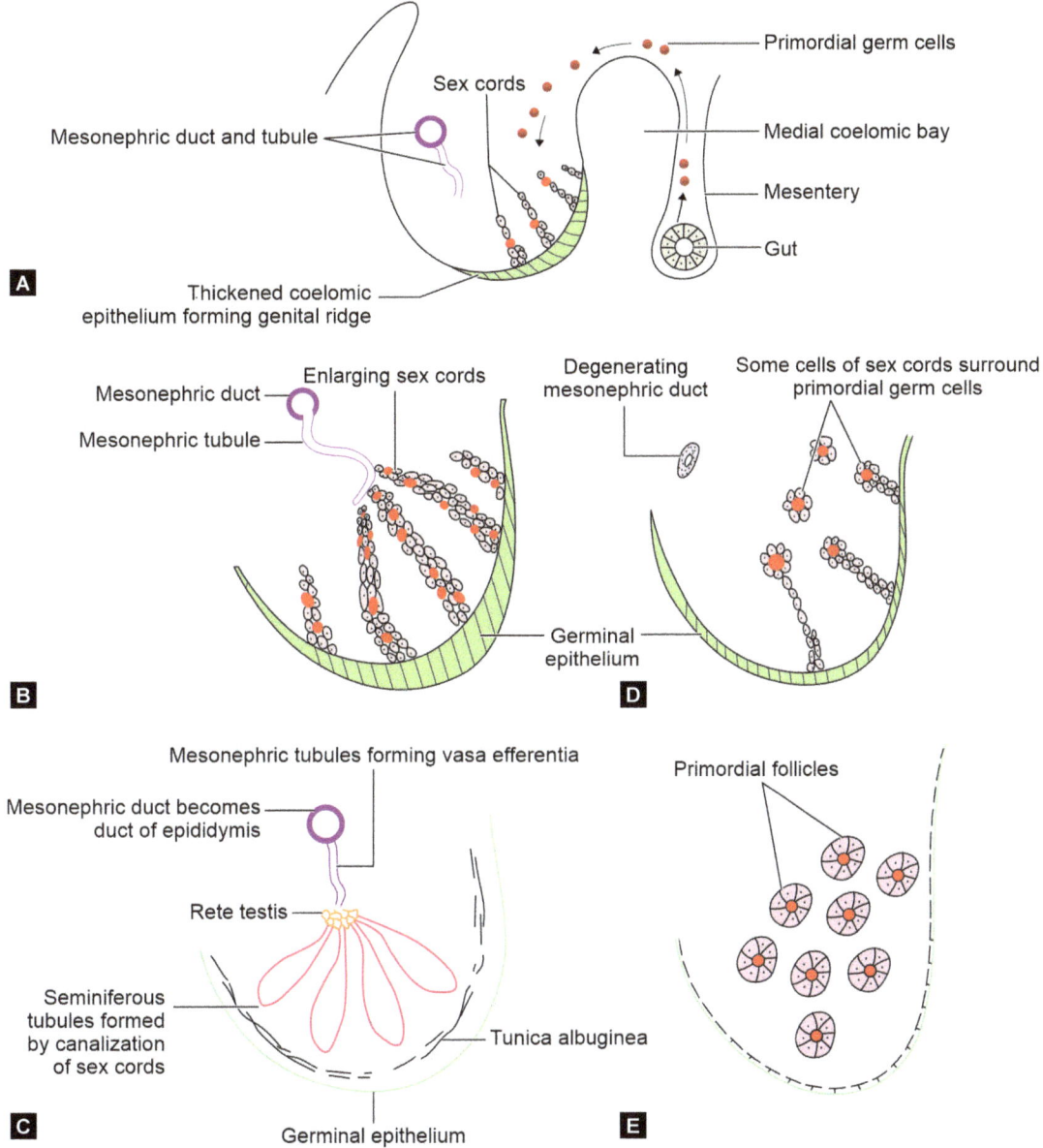

FIGS. 21.29A to E: Development of gonads: (A) Indifferent stage; (B and C) Testis; (D and E) Ovary.

them that lie near the testis persist and, along with the mesonephric duct, form the duct system of the testis **(Figs. 21.30A to C)**.

- The ends of the seminiferous tubules anastomose with one another to form the *rete-testes*. The rete-testes, in turn, establishes contact with persisting mesonephric tubules which form the *vasa efferentia*.
- The cranial part of the mesonephric duct becomes highly coiled on itself to form the *epididymis* while its distal part becomes the *ductus deferens*.
- The *seminal vesicle* arises, on either side, as a diverticulum from the lower end of the mesonephric duct.
- The part of the mesonephric duct between its opening into the prostatic urethra, and the origin of this diverticulum, forms the *ejaculatory duct*.

Descent of Testes

The testes develop in relation to the lumbar region of the posterior abdominal wall. During fetal life, they gradually descend to the scrotum. They reach the iliac fossa during the 3rd month, and lie at the site of the deep inguinal ring up to the 7th month of intrauterine life. They pass through the inguinal canal during the 7th month, and are normally in the scrotum by the end of the 9th month **(Fig. 21.31)**.

The descent of the testes is caused or assisted by several factors. These are:

- Differential growth of the body wall.
- **Formation of inguinal bursa:** About the sixth month of intrauterine life, the various layers of the abdominal wall, of each side, show an outpouching towards

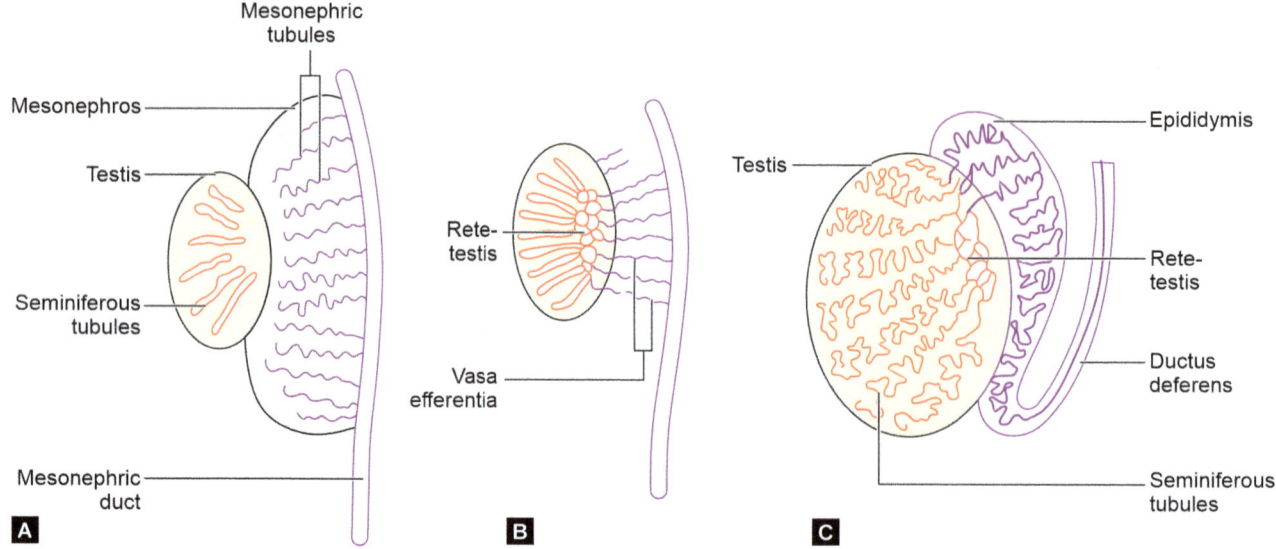

FIGS. 21.30A to C: Development of duct system of the testis.

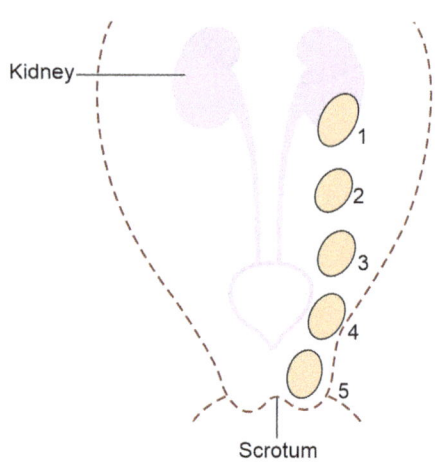

FIG. 21.31: Descent of the testis (from the lumbar region to the scrotum).

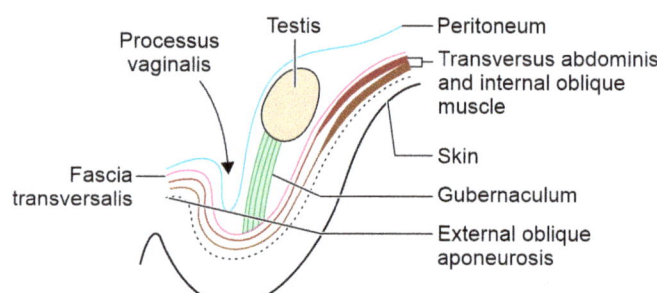

FIG. 21.32: The gubernaculum, which helps in descent of the testis.

the scrotum (Fig. 21.32). This pouch progressively increases in size, and depth, and eventually reaches the bottom of the scrotal sac. The descending testis enters this pouch to reach the scrotum. Note that the pouch is formed before the testis enters it. The cavity of the inguinal bursa becomes the *inguinal canal*, while the various layers of its wall form the coverings of the testis and spermatic cord.

- ❖ **The gubernaculum:** This is a band of mesenchyme which extends from the lower pole of the testis to the scrotum. For many years it was believed that descent of the testis was caused by shortening of the gubernaculum. However, we now know that this is not possible because the gubernaculum does not contain any contractile tissue. According to some authorities the gubernaculum does not reach the scrotum but reaches the bottom of the inguinal bursa. In spite of this, the gubernaculum does play an important part in the descent of the testis as follows:
  – When the embryo increases in size, the gubernaculum does not undergo a corresponding increase in length. There is thus a relative shortening of the gubernaculum and, as a result, the testis assumes a progressively lower position.
  – The gubernaculum helps to dilate the inguinal bursa.
  – It provides a continuous pathway for the descending testis.
- ❖ **Processus vaginalis:** This is a diverticulum of the peritoneal cavity. It actively grows into the gubernacular mesenchyme of the inguinal canal and of the scrotum (Fig. 21.32). As the testis descends, it invaginates the processus vaginalis from behind. After the descent of the testis is completed, the processus vaginalis loses all connection with the peritoneal cavity and becomes the *tunica vaginalis* (Figs. 21.33A to C).
- ❖ The descent of the testis is greatly influenced by hormones secreted by the pars anterior of the hypophysis cerebri.

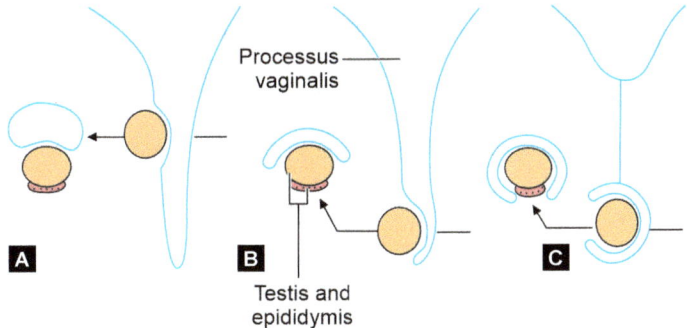

FIGS. 21.33A to C: Relation of descending testis to processus vaginalis. Note that as the testis descends it progressively invaginates the processus vaginalis.

Clinical correlation

Anomalies of Testis
- The testis may be absent, on one or both sides.
- The testis may be duplicated.
- The two testes may be fused together.
- **Anomalies of descent (cryptorchidism):** Descent of the testis may fail to occur, or may be incomplete. The organ may lie in the lumbar region, in the iliac fossa, in the inguinal canal, or in the upper part of the scrotum. This condition can be unilateral or bilateral **(Fig. 21.34)**. Some interesting facts about this condition are as follows:
  - The testis may complete its descent after birth.
  - Spermatogenesis often fails to occur in an undescended testis.
  - An undescended testis is more likely to develop a malignant tumor than a normal testis.
  - The condition can be surgically corrected.
- **Abnormal positions (ectopia):** The testis may lie **(Fig. 21.35)**:
  - Under the skin of the lower part of the abdomen.
  - Under the skin of the front of the thigh.
  - In the femoral canal.
  - Under the skin of the penis.
  - In the perineum behind the scrotum.
- Also see hermaphroditism.

Anomalies of Duct System of Testis
- The seminiferous tubules may fail to establish connection with the vasa efferentia.
- The ductus deferens may be absent, in whole or in part, on one or both sides.
- The ductus deferens may have no connection with the epididymis.

Anomalies of the Processus Vaginalis
We have seen that the part of the processus vaginalis, that extends from the deep inguinal ring up to the tunica vaginalis, normally disappears. This may persist in whole, or in part. Abdominal contents may enter it to produce various forms of *inguinal hernia*. Alternatively, fluid may accumulate in it producing the condition called *hydrocoele*. Various forms of hernia and of hydrocoele are shown in **Figures 21.36A to G**.

Seminoma
It is a type of testicular germ cell tumor arising from primordial germ cells. If the primordial germ cells fail to differentiate properly or undergo malignant transformation within the testes, they can give rise to seminomas. It is most commonly occur in young adult males.

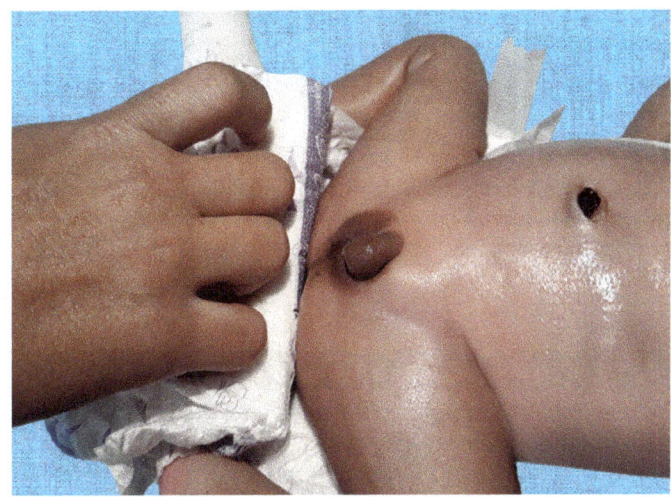

FIG. 21.34: Bilateral undescended testes. (Reproduced with permission from Dr Piyush Gupta. Source: Ruchi Rai and DK Singh, Chapter 15. In: Gupta P, UG Textbook of Pediatrics, Jaypee Brothers Medical Publishers Pvt Ltd, 2023).

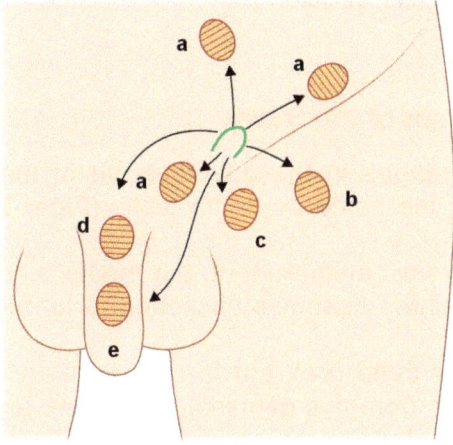

FIG. 21.35: Ectopic positions of the testis. a = under skin of the abdomen. b = over front of thigh. c = in femoral canal. d = under skin of penis. e = in perineum.

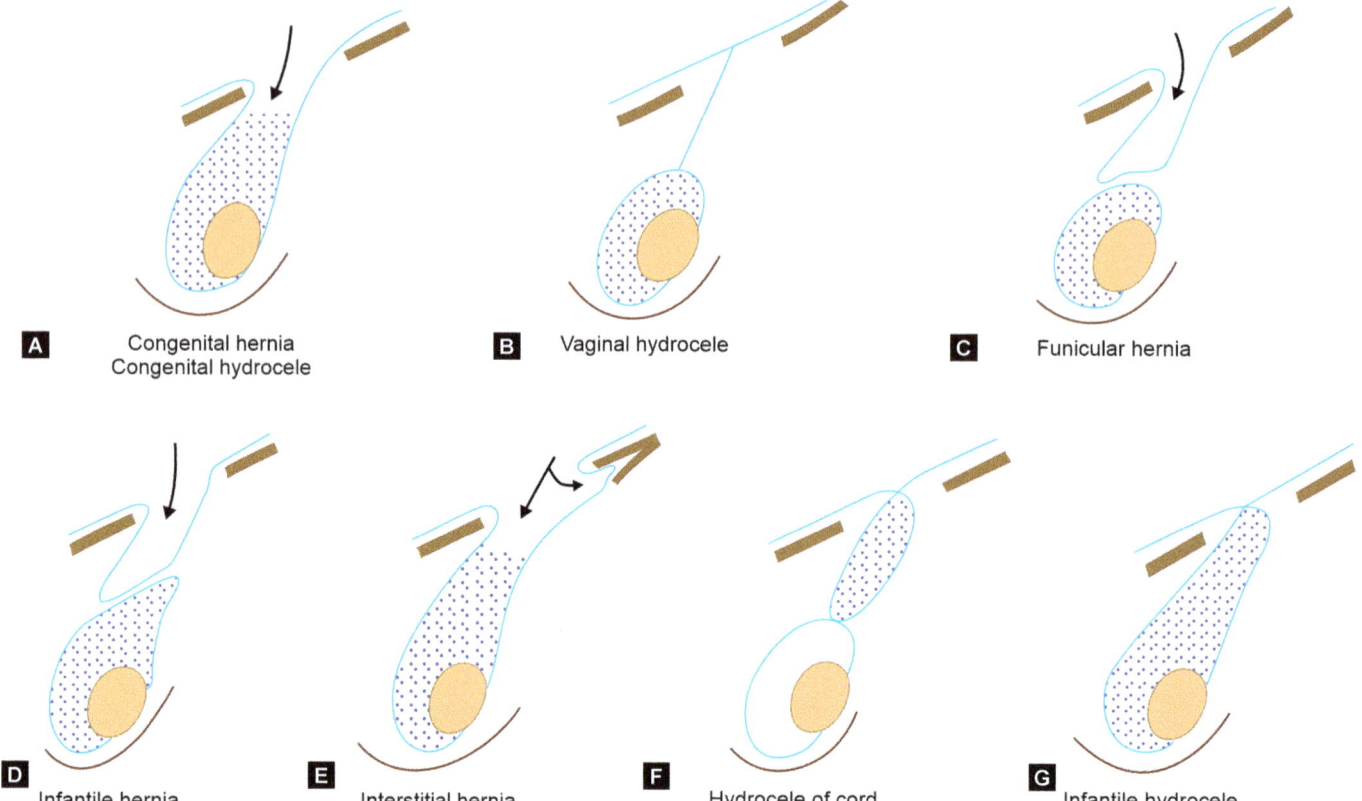

FIGS. 21.36A to G: Anomalies of processus vaginalis. Abnormal persistence of the processus vaginalis can lead to hernia (passage into it of abdominal contents, indicated by arrows); or hydrocele (collection of fluid, shown as dots). Various types of hernia and hydrocele are shown.

> **Vestigial Structures in the Region of the Testis**
>
> A number of vestigial structures are to be seen in the neighborhood of the testis. Their importance lies in the fact that any one of them may enlarge to form a cyst.
>
> These structures are:
> - Appendix of testis (also called hydatid of Morgagni)
> - Appendix of epididymis
> - Superior aberrant ductules
> - Inferior aberrant ductules
> - Paradidymis

Development of the Ovary

The early stages in the development of the ovary are exactly the same as in the testis **(Figs. 21.29A, C and E)**.

- The coelomic epithelium on the medial side of the mesonephros becomes thickened to form *genital ridges*.
- Cords of cells (sex cords or medullary cords) proliferate from this germinal epithelium, and grow into the underlying mesoderm.
- Primordial germ cells, that are formed in relation to the yolk sac, migrate to the region of the developing ovary, and give rise to *oocytes*.
- The sex cords become broken up into small masses. The cells of each mass surround one primordial germ cell, or oocyte, to form a *primordial follicle*.
- According to some authorities the original (medullary) sex cords undergo regression in the ovary, and are replaced by a new set of *cortical cords* arising from coelomic epithelium. Follicular cells are derived from these cortical cords.
- **Interstitial gland cells** differentiate from mesenchyme of the gonad.
- As no tunica albuginea is formed, the germinal epithelium may contribute to the ovary even in postnatal life.

Descent of the Ovary

- The ovary descends from the lumbar region, where it is first formed, to the true pelvis. A gubernaculum forms, as in the male, and extends from the ovary to the labium majus. It becomes attached to the developing uterus at its junction with the uterine tube.
- The part of the gubernaculum that persists between the ovary and the uterus, becomes the (round) *ligament of the ovary*. The part between the uterus and the labium majus, becomes the *round ligament of the uterus*.

Clinical correlation

Anomalies of Ovary
- The ovary may be absent on one or both sides.
- The ovary may be duplicated.
- The ovary may descend into the inguinal canal or even into the labium majus.
- Adrenal or thyroid tissue may be present in the ovary. The ovary sometimes contains cells that are capable of differentiating into various tissues like bone, cartilage, hair, etc., and the growth of these cell rests can give rise to a peculiar tumor called a *teratoma*.

FATE OF MESONEPHRIC DUCT

Fate of Mesonephric Duct and Tubules in the Male

The mesonephric ducts give rise to the following structures (Figs. 21.37 and 21.38):
- Ureteric buds from which the ureters, pelvis, calyces and collecting tubules of the kidneys are derived
- Trigone of the urinary bladder
- Posterior wall of the part of the prostatic urethra, cranial to the openings of the ejaculatory ducts
- Epididymis
- Ductus deferens
- Seminal vesicles
- Ejaculatory ducts
- Mesodermal part of prostate
- **Appendix of epididymis:** This is a small rounded structure attached to the head of the epididymis (Fig. 21.38A). It represents the cranial end of the mesonephric duct. Occasionally it may give rise to a cyst. This is not to be confused with the appendix of the testis, which is a remnant of the paramesonephric duct.

Remnants of Mesonephric Tubules

Most of the mesonephric tubules disappear. Some persist to form the *vasa efferentia*. Other mesonephric tubules persist to form some vestigial structures that are seen near the testes. Their only importance is that they sometimes give rise to cysts. These remnants are as follows:
- The *superior aberrant ductules* (or *epigenital tubules*) lie cranial to the vasa efferentia. They are connected to the testis but not to the epididymis.
- The *inferior aberrant ductules* lie caudal to the vasa efferentia. They are connected only to the epididymis.
- The *paradidymis* consists of tubules that lie between the testis and the epididymis *(paragenital tubules)* but are not connected to either of them.

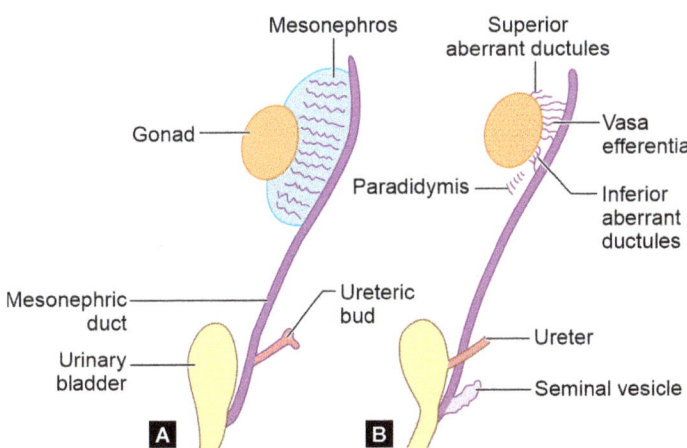

FIGS. 21.37A and B: (A) Mesonephric duct, early stage; (B) Mesonephric duct in the male, before descent of the testis

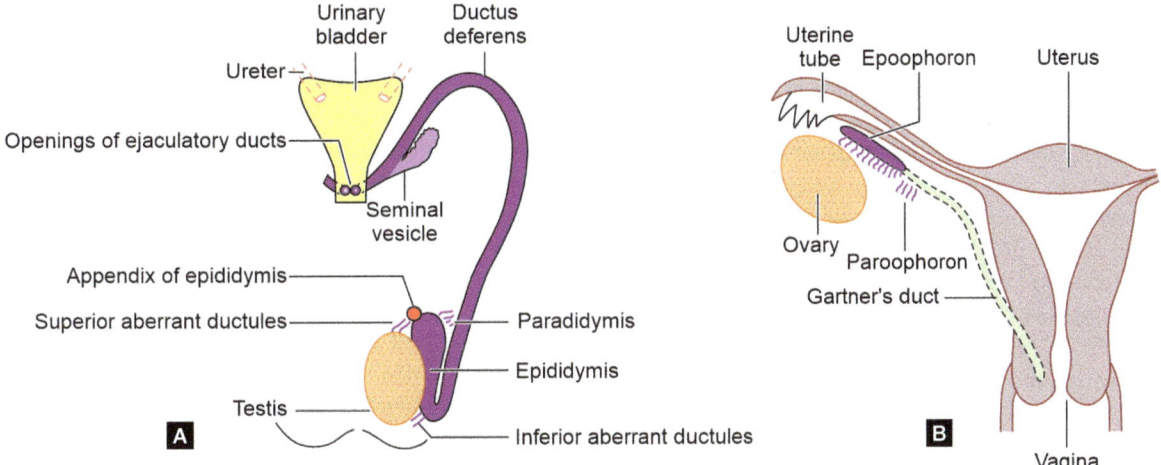

FIGS. 21.38A and B: Some structures derived from the mesonephric ducts: (A) In the male these are the epididymis, the ductus deferens, the seminal vesicles and ejaculatory ducts. The appendix of the epididymis is a vestigial remnant; (B) In the female most of the duct disappears, some remnants are seen as the epoophoron. For complete list of derivatives of the mesonephric ducts see text.

Fate of Mesonephric Ducts and Tubules in the Female

As in the male, the mesonephric ducts give rise to the ureteric bud from which the ureter, pelvis, calyces and collecting tubules of the kidneys are derived, and give rise to the trigone of the bladder. The posterior wall of the female urethra, is also derived from them.

The mesonephric ducts and tubules do not establish any connection with the developing ovary. However, they give rise to some vestigial structures seen in the broad ligament near the ovary. These are **(Fig. 21.38B)**:

- **Epoophoron:** This consists of a longitudinal duct running parallel to the uterine tube, and a number of transverse ductules that open into the longitudinal duct. It corresponds to the epididymis and vasa efferentia of the male (Note that the word 'epoophoron' means 'above egg basket': ep = above, oo = egg, and phoron = basket).

  In some cases the longitudinal duct is unusually long. It runs along the side of the uterus, and lower down, becomes embedded in the wall of the cervix. It, however, never opens into the uterine lumen. It is the equivalent of the male ductus deferens and is also called Gartner's duct.

- **Paroophoron:** This consists of small blind tubules lying between the ovary and the uterus, and is the female equivalent of the paradidymis. The word paroophoron means 'near egg basket'.

Male and female homologues derived from undifferentiated genital system are presented in **Table 21.1**.

Molecular Control of Gonadal Differentiation

- **Sry gene activation:** The Sry gene on the Y chromosome initiates male gonadal differentiation by triggering the development of testes from indifferent gonadal tissue.
- **Testes determining factor (TDF):** The protein product of the Sry gene, known as testes determining factor (TDF), is crucial for the formation of Sertoli cells, which are essential for male reproductive development.
- **Testosterone production:** Leydig cells in the developing testes produce testosterone, which promotes the development of male reproductive structures and inhibits female pathways.
- **Anti-Müllerian hormone (AMH):** Sertoli cells secrete AMH, causing the regression of Müllerian ducts, which would otherwise develop into female reproductive structures.
- **Wnt and β-catenin signaling:** In female gonadal development, the absence of Sry allows Wnt signaling pathways to promote ovarian differentiation and the formation of ovarian follicles.

TABLE 21.1: Summary of male and female homologues derived from undifferentiated genital system.

Embryonic structure	Male derivative	Female derivative
Gonad	Testis	Ovary
Sex cords	Sertoli cells (seminiferous tubules)	Granulose cells
Primordial germ cells	Spermatozoa	Ova
Paramesonephric duct	• Appendix of testis • Utricle of prostate	• Uterine tube, uterus • Upper vagina
Mesonephric duct	Appendix of epididymis, epididymis, ductus deferens, ejaculatory duct, seminal vesicle	• Appendix of ovary • Gartner's duct
Mesonephric tubules	• Vasa efferentia • Paradidymis	• Epoophoron • Paroophoron
Genital tubercle	Penis	Clitoris
Genital swellings	Scrotum	Labia majora
Urethral folds	Floor of penile urethra	Labia minora

Clinical correlation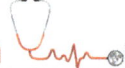

Hermaphroditism

Abnormal development of the gonad and the genitalia gives rise to various types of hermaphroditism. A hermaphrodite is really a person who is both a male and a female at the same time. Such a person has never been known to exist. However, persons having both testes and ovaries have been reported and such individuals are referred to as *true hermaphrodites*. The word *pseudohermaphrodite* is used for a person whose external genitalia look like those of one sex, whereas the gonad is of the other sex.

Some forms of hermaphroditism are as follows:

- **True hermaphroditism:** The person has at least one testis and one ovary in the body. The external genitalia may be male, or female, or midway between the two. The chromosomal sex may be either male or female.
- **Pseudohermaphroditism (ambiguous genitalia) (Fig. 21.39):** Gonads are of one sex, while genitalia (internal, external or both) are of opposite sex. A patient having a testis is described as a *male hermaphrodite*; and one having an ovary is described as a *female hermaphrodite*.

Female pseudohermaphroditism is caused by excess of androgens produced by the fetal suprarenal gland (adrenogenital syndrome). It may also be caused by administration of progestins to the mother during pregnancy.

Chapter 21: Urogenital System

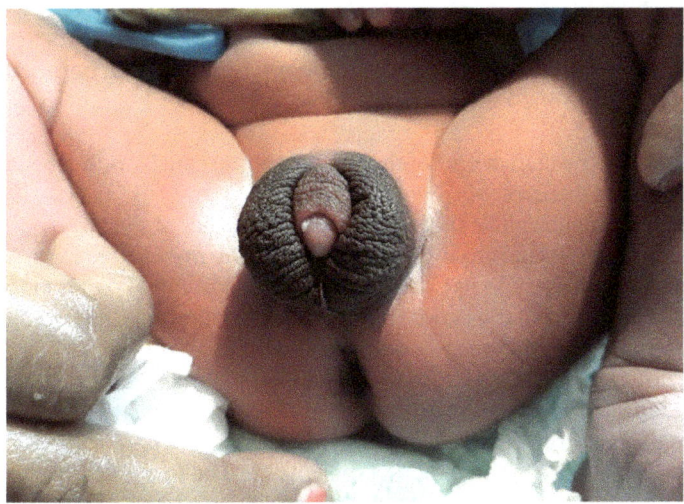

FIG. 21.39: Ambiguous genitalia.
(Reproduced with permission from Dr Piyush Gupta. Source: Ruchi Rai and DK Singh, Chapter 15. In: Gupta P, UG Textbook of Pediatrics, Jaypee Brothers Medical Publishers Pvt Ltd, 2023).

TIMETABLE OF SOME EVENTS DESCRIBED IN THIS CHAPTER

Age	Developmental events
3rd week	- Formation of intermediate mesoderm - External genitalia begin to form
4th week	- Pronephric tubules begin to form and have regressed by the end of the same week - Mesonephric tubules start forming. Urorectal septum begins to form - Genital organ begins to develop
5th week	The metanephros is formed
6th week	Mesonephros is well developed. The cloacal membrane divides into the urogenital and the anal membrane
7th week	- Urogenital sinus is established - Gonadal differentiation into ovaries and testes
9th week	Ascend of kidney to final position
12th week	The definitive kidney (metanephros) becomes functional
3rd month	- Urethral folds fuse with each other. At the end of the month, prostate begins to develop - Testes began to descend towards scrotum
5th month	Vagina gets canalized

The external genitalia are most susceptible to teratogens between the seventh and ninth weeks; but they can be affected later in pregnancy as well.

HIGHLIGHTS

- The *urogenital system* is derived from the *intermediate mesoderm*, and the *primitive urogenital sinus* (UGS) which is a part of the cloaca.
- The primitive UGS divides into the *vesicourethral canal* and the *definitive UGS* (**Fig. 21.3**).
- The vesicourethral canal divides into the *urinary bladder* and the *primitive urethra*.
- The definitive UGS has a *pelvic part* and a *phallic part*.

- The *kidneys* develop from two sources. The excretory tubules (nephrons) are derived from the *metanephros* (= lowest part of nephrogenic cord which is derived from intermediate mesoderm). The collecting part is formed by ramification of the *ureteric bud* (which arises from the mesonephric duct).
- The *ureter* arises from the ureteric bud.
- The *urinary bladder* is derived from the cranial part of the vesicourethral canal (endoderm). The epithelium of the trigone is derived from absorbed mesonephric ducts.
- The *female urethra* is derived from the primitive urethra and the pelvic part of the UGS.
- In the male, the *prostatic urethra* corresponds to the female urethra. The *membranous urethra* is derived from the pelvic part of UGS and the *penile urethra* from the phallic part of the UGS. The terminal part is ectodermal.
- The *prostate* is formed by buds arising from the caudal part of the vesicourethral canal and the pelvic part of the UGS.
- The *uterine tubes* are derived from *paramesonephric ducts* (mesoderm).
- The *uterus* is formed from the uterovaginal canal (fused right and left paramesonephric ducts).
- **External genitalia** are formed from swellings that appear around the urogenital membrane.
- **Gonads** (testis and ovary) are derived from coelomic epithelium covering the nephrogenic cord. Ova and spermatozoa arise from *primordial germ cells* that arise in the region of the yolk sac. The testis is formed in the lumbar region, and later descend to the scrotum.
- The *duct system of the testis* is derived from mesonephric tubules and from the mesonephric duct.

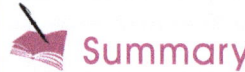
Summary

- Developmental contributions for urogenital system (**Flowcharts 21.1** and **21.2**)
- Development of kidney (**Flowchart 21.3** and **Table 21.2**)

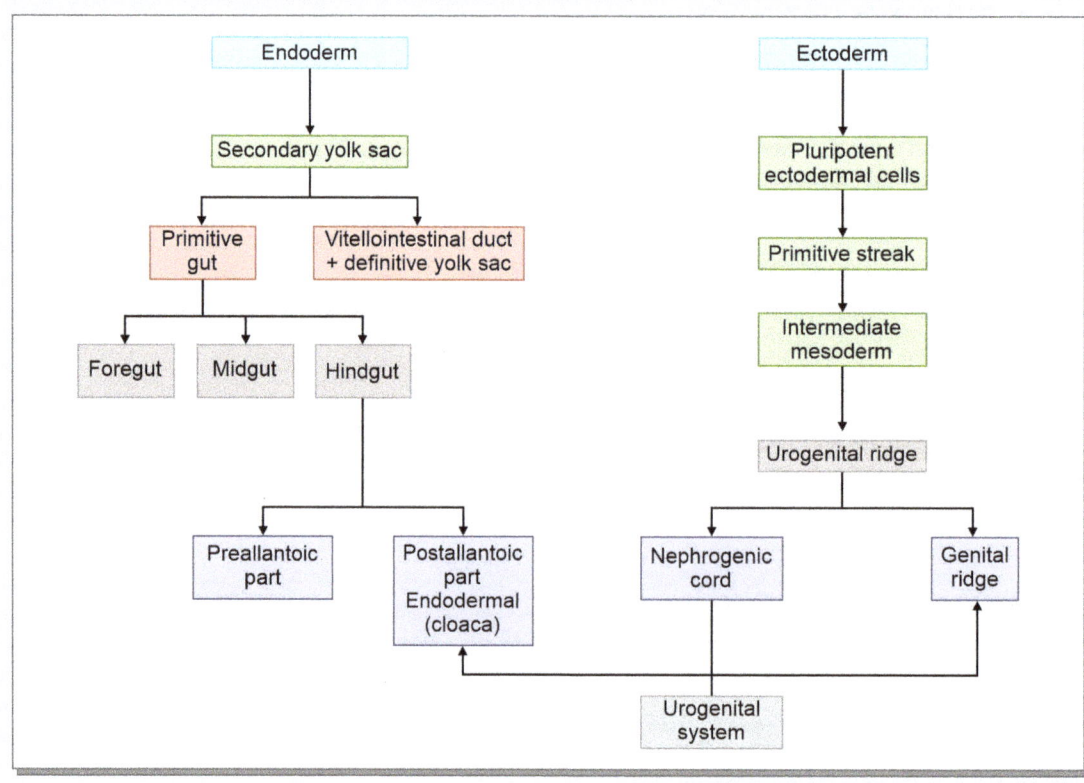

FLOWCHART 21.1: Developmental primordia of urogenital system.

Chapter 21: Urogenital System

FLOWCHART 21.2: Intermediate mesoderm—developmental subdivisions and contribution to urogenital system.

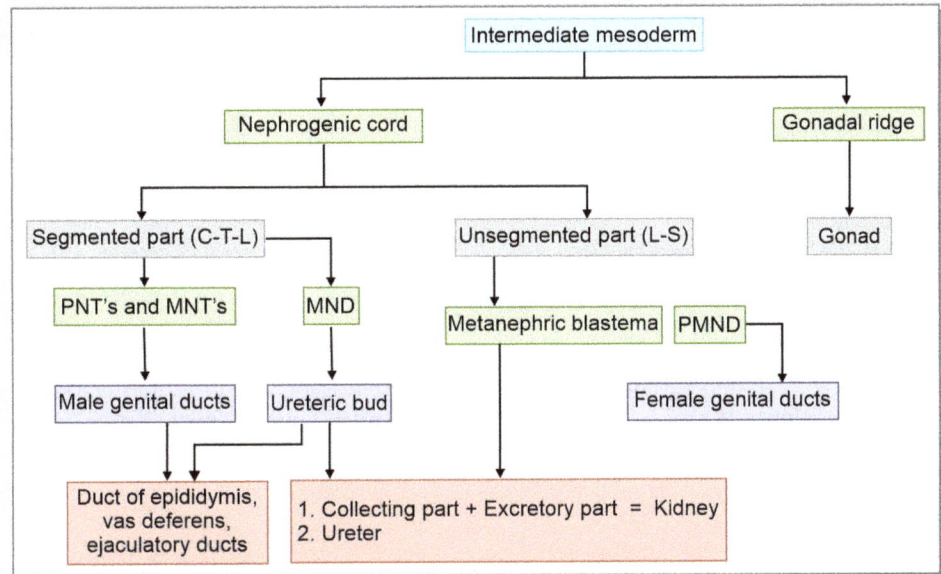

(C,T,L, S: cervical, thoracic, lumbar and sacral segments; PNT and MNT: pronephric and mesonephric tubules; MND and PMND: mesonephric and paramesonephric ducts)

FLOWCHART 21.3: Kidney—developmental components and their derivatives.

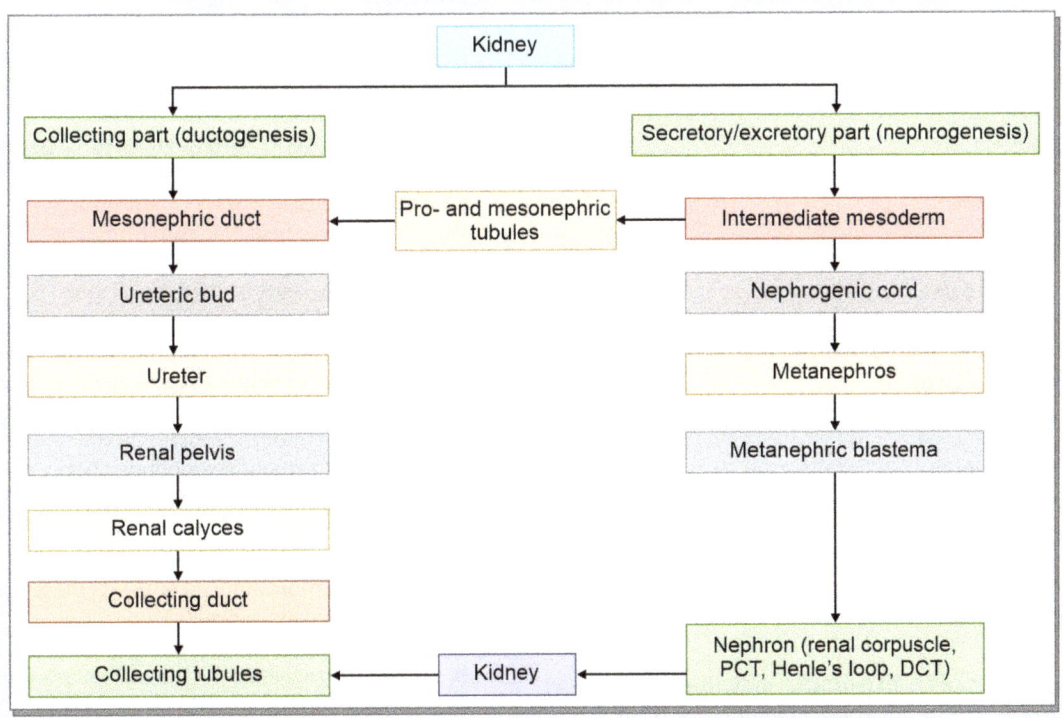

(DCT: distal convoluted tubule; PCT: proximal convoluted tubule)

TABLE 21.2: Kidney—developmental components.

Collecting part (ureteric bud)	Excretory part—nephrogenic (metanephric blastema)
Ureter	Bowman's capsule
Renal pelvis	Proximal convoluted tubule
Major and minor calyces	Loop of Henle
Collecting ducts and tubules	Distal convoluted tubule

Chapter 21: Urogenital System

TEST YOUR UNDERSTANDING

REVIEW QUESTIONS

1. Explain development of kidney.
2. Explain developmental anomalies of kidney.
3. Write a note on ectopia vesicae.
4. Explain development of testis.
5. Explain development of ovary.
6. Explain development of urethra in males and females.
7. Explain development of prostate.
8. Write a note on paramesonephric duct.
9. Write a note on mesonephric duct.
10. Write a note on urogenital sinus.
11. Write a note on primordial germ cells.
12. Describe descent of testis.
13. Describe the anomalies of testis.

EXPLAIN WHY? (REASONING QUESTIONS)

1. The horseshoe kidney typically gets trapped under the inferior mesenteric artery during development.
2. The urethral opening is located on the underside of the penis in newborn male infant.
3. A child is found to have unilateral renal agenesis.
4. A female patient presents with a bicornuate uterus.
5. An infant is diagnosed with polycystic kidney disease.

MULTIPLE CHOICE QUESTIONS

1. All the following are mesodermal, *except*:
   A. Trigone of urinary bladder
   B. Genital swellings
   C. Genital tubercle
   D. Vesicourethral canal

2. Attachment of gubernaculum is to:
   A. Cranial pole of testis
   B. Caudal pole of testis
   C. Epididymis
   D. Whole testis

3. During 7th month of intrauterine life testis lies at the following location:
   A. Scrotum   B. Abdomen
   C. Iliac fossa   D. Inguinal canal

4. Clitoris is derived from:
   A. Urogenital sinus   B. Genital swelling
   C. Genital tubercle   D. Urogenital membrane

5. Glans penis develops from:
   A. Urogenital sinus
   B. Vesicourethral canal
   C. Mesonephric ducts
   D. Surface ectoderm

6. Primordial germ cells are derived from:
   A. Mesoderm
   B. Yolk sac
   C. Neural crest cells
   D. Epiblast

7. A patient is diagnosed with a urachal cyst after experiencing recurrent urinary tract infections. What embryological remnant is likely involved in this condition?
   A. Allantois   B. Mesonephric duct
   C. Urogenital sinus   D. Cloaca

8. A child presents with urinary incontinence and a midline abdominal mass. Imaging shows a bladder exstrophy. Which developmental failure is most likely responsible for this anomaly?
   A. Improper closure of the ventral body wall
   B. Abnormal development of the urogenital sinus
   C. Failure of mesonephric duct regression
   D. Incomplete formation of the pelvic diaphragm

9. A 3-year-old boy is diagnosed with hypospadias. During development, which embryological process is likely disrupted?
   A. Fusion of the urogenital folds
   B. Development of the mesonephric ducts
   C. Formation of the urinary bladder
   D. Development of the metanephros

10. A newborn presents with bilateral renal agenesis, leading to severe oligohydramnios. What is the most likely embryological cause of this condition?
    A. Failure of nephrogenic cord formation
    B. Abnormal migration of primordial germ cells
    C. Incomplete regression of the allantois
    D. Improper development of the cloaca

11. A female infant is found to have an obstructed vagina and is diagnosed with vaginal agenesis. What embryological process is likely disrupted in this condition?
    A. Development of the urogenital sinus
    B. Fusion of the paramesonephric ducts
    C. Formation of the external genitalia
    D. Development of the mesonephric ducts

12. A 5-year-old boy presents with a noticeable undescended testis. Which embryological failure is most likely responsible for this anomaly?
    A. Failure of gubernaculum development
    B. Abnormal regression of the mesonephric ducts
    C. Impaired formation of the labioscrotal swellings
    D. Incomplete development of the paramesonephric ducts

13. A newborn is diagnosed with ambiguous genitalia and has both ovarian and testicular tissue present. What is the most likely embryological cause of this condition?
    A. Androgen insensitivity syndrome
    B. Congenital adrenal hyperplasia
    C. Intersex condition due to abnormal gonadal differentiation
    D. Turner syndrome

Answers: 1. D   2. B   3. D   4. C   5. D
           6. B   7. A   8. A   9. A   10. A
           11. B   12. A   13. C

Nervous System

CHAPTER 22

COMPETENCIES COVERED/LEARNING OUTCOMES

The student should be able to:

AN64.2	Development of neural tube, spinal cord, medulla oblongata, pons, midbrain, cerebral hemisphere and cerebellum.
AN64.3	Discuss various types of open neural tube defects with its embryological basis.
AN79.3	Describe the process of neurulation.
AN79.5	Explain the embryological basis of neural tube defects.

The nervous system is a complex network responsible for coordinating and controlling body activities. It consists of the central nervous system (CNS), which includes the brain and spinal cord, and the peripheral nervous system (PNS), comprising all neural elements outside the CNS, including sensory and motor neurons.

The formation of neural tissue has been discussed in Chapter 10, where we have seen that the ependymal (or neuroepithelial) cells of the neural tube give rise both to neurons and to neuroglia. We have also studied the formation of myelin sheath. We shall now consider the development of individual parts of the nervous system.

NEURAL TUBE AND ITS SUBDIVISIONS

Apart from its blood vessels and some neuroglial elements, the whole of the nervous system is derived from surface ectoderm. The part of the ectoderm that is destined to give origin to the brain and spinal cord, can be distinguished as a specialized part, called *neuroectoderm* while the embryo is still in the form of a three-layered embryonic disc.

Neurulation

It is the process of formation of neural plate from neuroectoderm and fording of neural plate to form neural tube. It extends from presomite to postsotime period of development as described below:

- During day 16th of IUL, neuroectoderm is situated on the dorsal (amniotic) aspect of the embryonic disc, in the midline, and overlies the notochordal process **(Figs. 22.1A and B)**. Due to induction from notochord, it soon becomes thickened to form the *neural plate* **(Figs. 22.1A and C)**.
- The neural plate becomes depressed along the midline as a result of which the *neural groove* is formed **(Fig. 22.1D)**.
- This groove becomes progressively deeper. At the same time, the two edges of the neural plate come nearer each other, and eventually fuse, thus converting the neural groove into the cylindrical *neural tube* **(Fig. 22.1E)**.
- These stages in the formation of the neural tube do not proceed simultaneously all over the length of the neural plate.
- The middle part is the first to become tubular, so that for some time the neural tube is open cranially and caudally. These openings are called the *anterior* and *posterior neuropores*, respectively.
- The fusion of the two edges of the neural plate extends cranially, and caudally, and eventually the neuropores disappear leaving a closed tube.
- Even before the neural tube has completely closed, it is divisible into an enlarged cranial part and a caudal tubular part **(Fig. 22.2 and Table 22.1)**.
- The enlarged cranial part forms the brain. The caudal tubular part forms the spinal cord: it is at first short, but gradually gains in length as the embryo grows.

DEVELOPMENT OF BRAIN

The cavity of the developing brain soon shows three dilatations **(Fig. 22.2B)**. Craniocaudally, these are the *prosencephalon*, *mesencephalon*, and *rhombencephalon*.

- The prosencephalon becomes subdivided into the *telencephalon* and the *diencephalon* **(Fig. 22.2C)**.
- The telencephalon consists of right and left *telencephalic vesicles*. The rhombencephalon

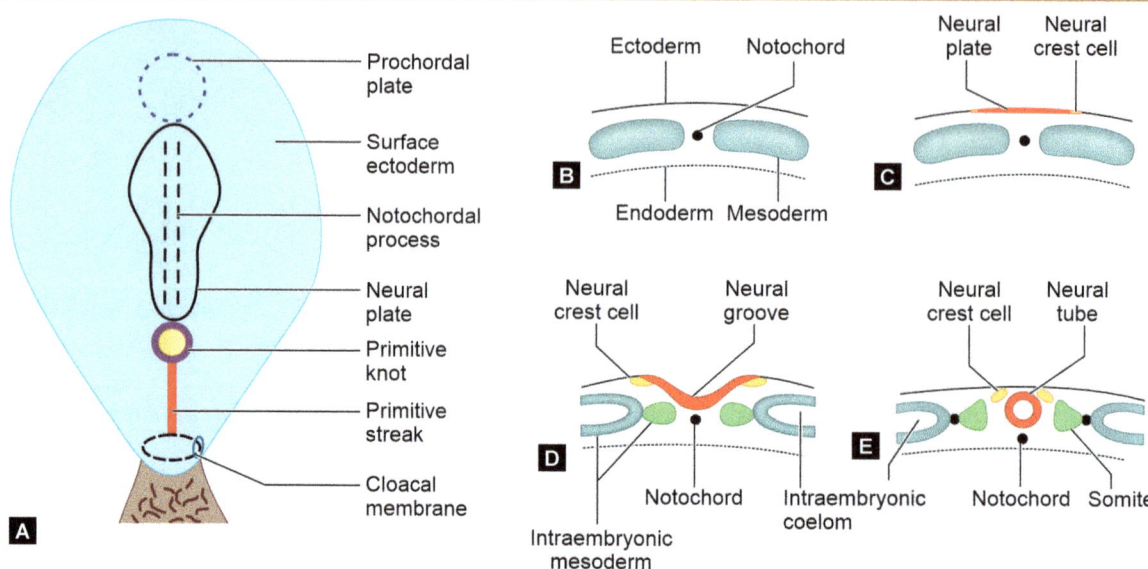

FIGS. 22.1A to E: Formation of neural tube (neurulation): (A) Dorsal view of pear-shaped embryonic disc with slipper-shaped neural plate; (B to E) Transverse sections of embryo showing various stages in the development of neural tube. (B) Embryonic disc before formation of neural plate; (C) Neural plate formed by thickening of ectoderm; (D) Neural plate is converted to a groove; (E) The groove is converted to a tube.

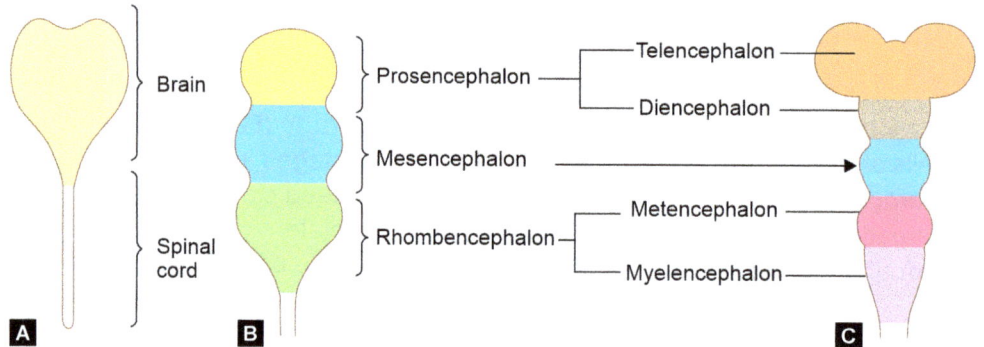

FIGS. 22.2A to C: Primary brain vesicles and their subdivisions.

TABLE 22.1: Subdivisions and adult derivatives of neural tube.

Neural tube subdivisions	Primary brain vesicles	Secondary brain vesicles	Parts of adult brain	Cavities
Brain	Prosencephalon (forebrain)	Telencephalon	• Cerebral hemispheres • Cerebral cortex • Corpus striatum • Caudate nucleus • Lentiform nucleus	Lateral ventricles
		Diencephalon	• Thalamus • Hypothalamus • Epithalamus	Third ventricle
	Mesencephalon (midbrain)	Mesencephalon	Midbrain	Cerebral aqueduct
	Rhombencephalon (hindbrain)	Metencephalon	• Pons • Cerebellum	Fourth ventricle
		Myelencephalon	Medulla oblongata	
Spinal cord	Spinal cord	Spinal cord	Spinal cord	Central canal

also becomes subdivided into a cranial part, the *metencephalon*, and a caudal part, the *myelencephalon*.
* The parts of the brain that are developed from each of these divisions of the neural tube are shown in **Figures 22.2A to C**.

Formation of Brain Flexures

The prosencephalon, mesencephalon and rhombencephalon are at first arranged craniocaudally **(Fig. 22.3A)**. Their relative position is greatly altered by the appearance of a number of flexures. These are:
* The *cervical flexure*, at the junction of the rhombencephalon and the spinal cord **(Fig. 22.3B)**.
* The *mesencephalic flexure* (or *cephalic flexure*), in the region of the midbrain **(Fig. 22.3C)**.
* The *pontine flexure*, at the middle of the rhombencephalon, dividing it into the metencephalon and myelencephalon **(Fig. 22.3D)**.
* The *telencephalic flexure*, that occurs much later, between the telencephalon and diencephalon.
* These flexures lead to the orientation of the various parts of the brain as in the adult **(Figs. 22.4A to D)**.

Formation of Ventricles

Each of the subdivisions of the developing brain encloses a part of the original cavity of the neural tube **(Fig. 22.5)**.
* The cavity of each telencephalic vesicle becomes the *lateral ventricle*, and that of the diencephalon (along with the central part of the telencephalon), becomes the *third ventricle.*
* The two lateral ventricles communicate with the third ventricle through *interventricular foramen of Monro.*
* The cavity of the mesencephalon remains narrow, and forms the *aqueduct of Sylvius*, while the cavity of the rhombencephalon forms the *fourth ventricle*. Its continuation in the spinal cord is the *central canal*. The central canal presents a terminal dilatation at its lower end called *terminal ventricle*.
* The *cerebrospinal fluid (CSF)* is formed in the ventricles; mainly in the lateral ventricle by choroid plexuses. CSF flows from lateral ventricles to third ventricle through *interventricular foramen* and from third ventricle to fourth ventricle through *cerebral aqueduct*. It leaves the ventricular system through three foramina (a median *foramen of Magendie* and two lateral *foramina of Luschka*) into the subarachnoid space around brain and spinal cord.

NEURAL CREST CELLS

At the time when the neural plate is being formed, some cells at the junction between the neural plate and the rest of the ectoderm become specialized (on either side) to form the primordia of the *neural crest* **(Figs. 22.1C and D)**.
* With the separation of the neural tube from the surface ectoderm, the cells of the neural crest appear as groups of cells lying along the dorsolateral sides of the neural tube **(Fig. 22.1E)**.
* The *neural crest cells* soon become free (by losing the property of cell-to-cell adhesiveness). They migrate to distance places throughout the body.
* In subsequent development, several important structures are derived from the neural crest. The cells are divided into a dorsal mass and a ventral mass. Various derivatives of neural crest cells are as shown in **Box 22.1 and Fig. 22.6**.

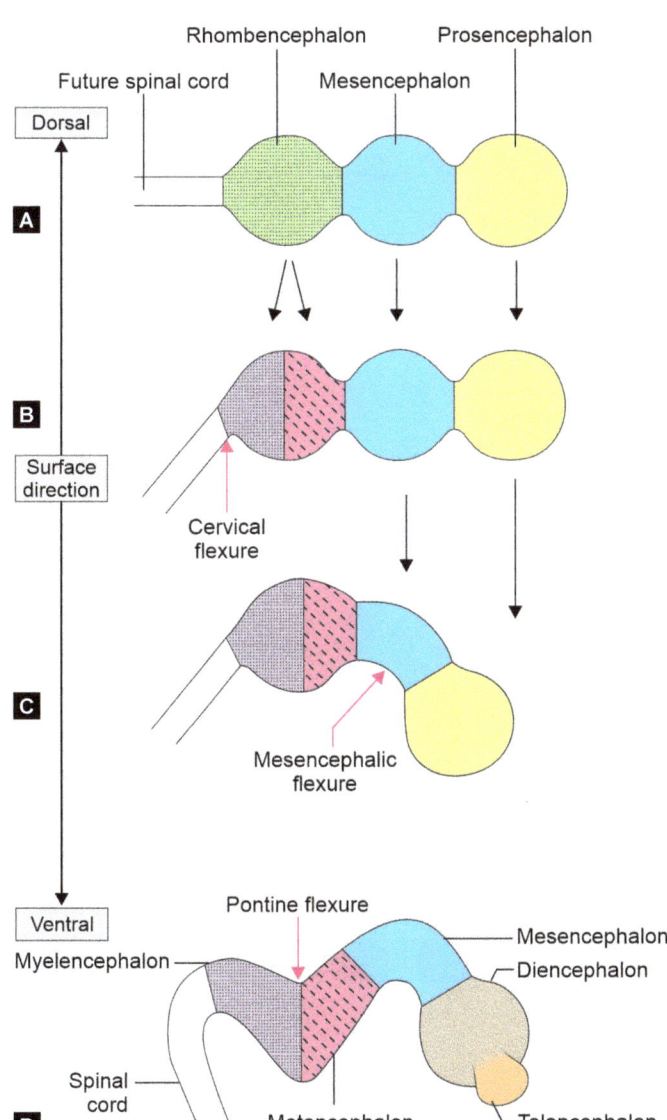

FIGS. 22.3A to D: (A) Neural tube before formation of flexures; (B) Cervical flexure formed; (C) Mesencephalic flexure formed; (D) Pontine flexure formed.

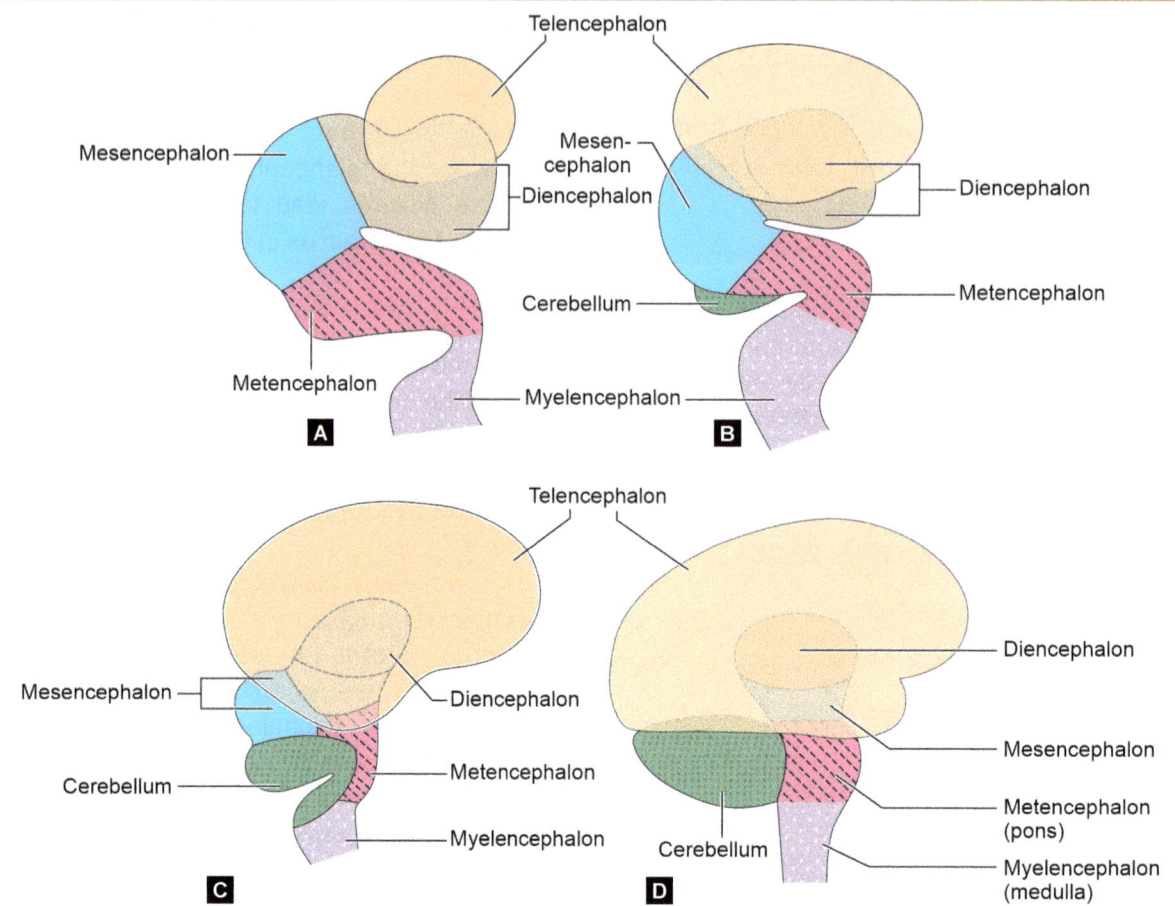

FIGS. 22.4A to D: Development of external form of the human brain. Note progressive overlapping of diencephalon and mesencephalon by the expanding telencephalon.

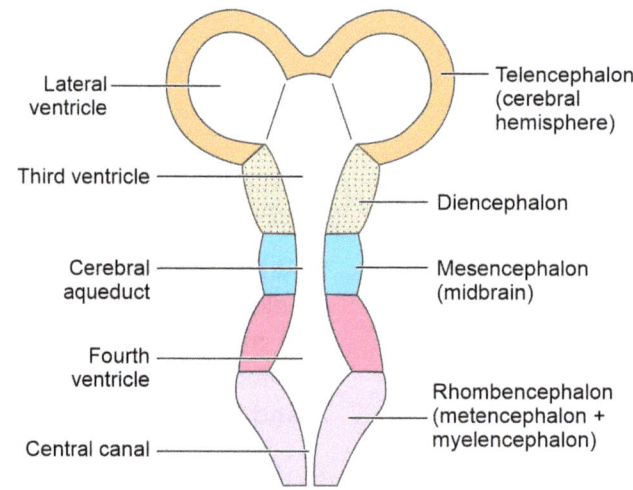

FIG. 22.5: Development of ventricles of the brain.

Box 22.1: Derivatives of neural crest cells.

Dorsal mass:
- **Neuroblasts:**
  - Pseudounipolar neurons of the posterior (dorsal) nerve root ganglia of spinal nerves
  - Neurons of the sensory ganglia of cranial nerves V, VII, VIII, IX, and X
- **Spongioblasts:**
  - Capsular/satellite cells of all sensory ganglia
  - Schwann cells that form the neurilemma and myelin sheaths of all peripheral nerves

- **Pluripotent cells:**
  - Mesenchyme of dental papilla, odontoblasts, and dentine
  - Melanoblasts: Pigment cells of the skin
  - Cartilage cells of branchial arches
  - Leptomeninges (pia mater and arachnoid mater)

Ventral mass:
- **Sympathoblasts (small cells):**
  - Neurons of the sympathetic ganglia
  - Neurons of peripheral parasympathetic ganglia of cranial nerves III, VII, IX, and X
- **Chromaffin cells (large cells):**
  - Suprarenal medulla
  - Para-aortic body
  - Argentaffin cells
  - Enterochromaffin cells/APUD cells

Other structures arising from the neural crest:
- Bones of the face and part of the skull vault (frontal, parietal, squamous temporal, part of the sphenoid, maxilla, zygomatic, nasal, vomer, palatine, and mandible)
- Dermis, smooth muscle, and fat of the face and ventral neck
- Muscles of the ciliary body
- Sclera and choroid of the eye
- Substantia propria and posterior epithelium of the cornea
- Connective tissues of the thyroid, parathyroid, thymus, and salivary glands
- Derivatives of the first, second, and third pharyngeal cartilages
- C cells of the thyroid gland
- Cardiac semilunar valves and conotruncal septum (spiral septum plus bulbar septum)
- Smooth muscle of blood vessels in the face and forebrain

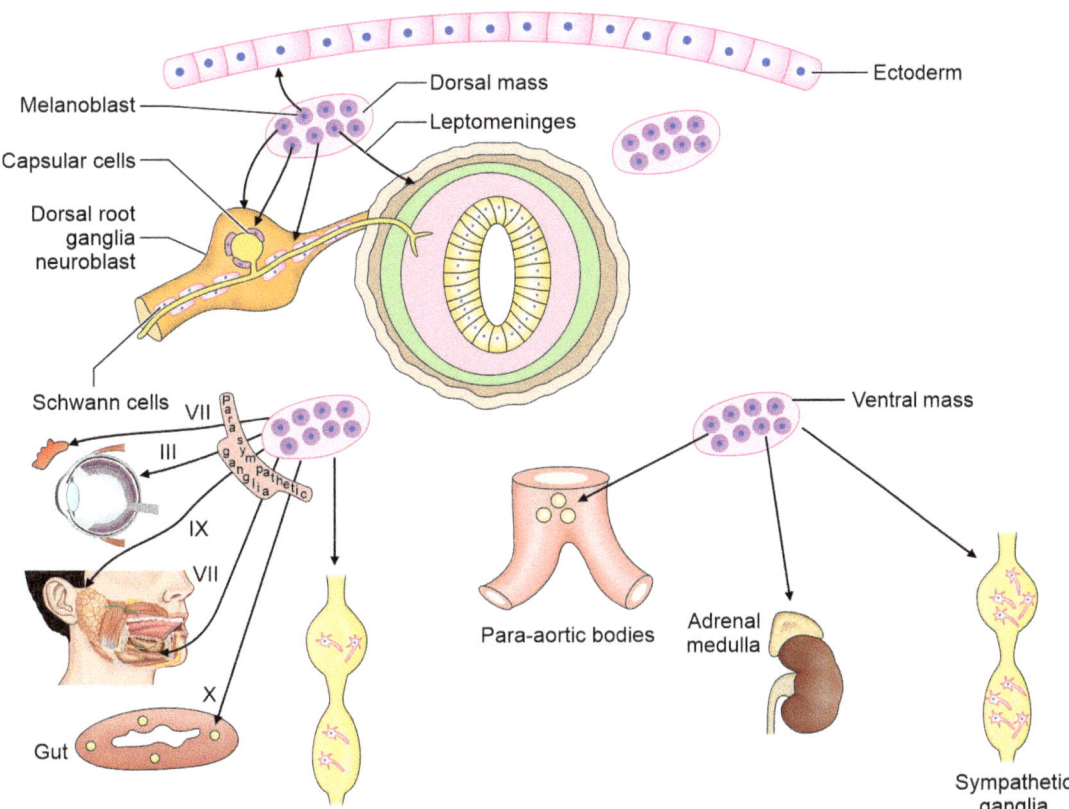

FIG. 22.6: Traditionally recognized derivatives of the neural crest. Some additional derivatives are now recognized (as mentioned in the text).

Clinical correlation

Several diseases and syndromes are associated with the disturbances of the neural crest, e.g., Hirschsprung's disease (aganglionic megacolon), aorticopulmonary septal defects of heart, cleft lip, cleft palate, frontonasal dysplasia, neurofibromatosis, tumor of adrenal medulla and albinism and others.

SPINAL CORD

The spinal cord is developed from the caudal cylindrical part of the neural tube.

When this part of the neural tube is first formed, its cavity is in the form of a dorsoventral cleft. The lateral walls are thick, but the roof (dorsal), and the floor (ventral), are thin **(Fig. 22.7A)**. The wall of the tube subdivides into the matrix cell or ependymal layer, the mantle layer and the marginal layer **(Fig. 22.7B)** as already described in Chapter 10.

* The mantle zone grows faster in the ventral part of the neural tube, and becomes thicker, than in the dorsal part. As a result, the ventral part of the lumen of the neural tube becomes compressed. The line separating the compressed ventral part, from the dorsal part, is called the *sulcus limitans* **(Fig. 22.7C)**.
* With its formation, the lateral wall of the developing spinal cord can be divided into a dorsal part, called the dorsal or *alar/dorsal lamina*, and a ventral part, called the ventral or *basal/ventral lamina*.
* This division is of considerable functional importance. The basal lamina develops into structures that are *motor* in function, and the alar lamina into those that are *sensory*. The alar and basal laminae are also called the *alar and basal plates* respectively.
* With continued growth in thickness of the mantle layer, the spinal cord gradually acquires its definitive form **(Figs. 22.7D and E)**.
* With growth of the alar lamina, the dorsal part of the cavity within the cord becomes obliterated: the *posterior median septum* is formed in this situation.
* The ventral part of the cavity remains as the *central canal*.
* Further enlargement of the basal lamina causes it to project forwards on either side of the midline, leaving a furrow, the *anterior median fissure*, between the projecting basal laminae of the two sides.
* The nerve cells that develop in the mantle zone of the basal lamina become the *neurons of the anterior gray column* **(Fig. 22.8)**. The axons of these cells grow out of the ventrolateral angle of the spinal cord to form the *anterior/ventral/motor nerve roots* of the spinal nerves.
* The nerve cells that develop in the mantle layer of the alar lamina form the *neurons of the posterior gray column*. These are sensory neurons of the second

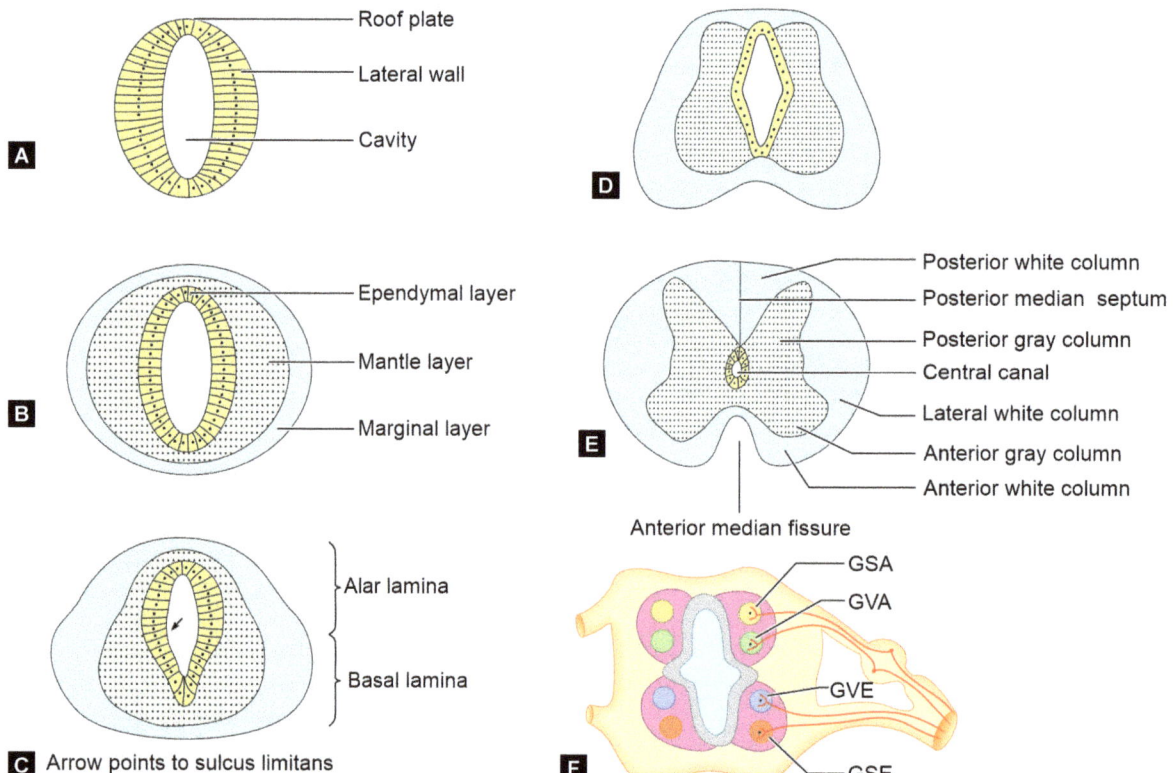

FIGS. 22.7A to F: Development of spinal cord: (A) Single layered neural tube; (B) Ependymal, mantle and marginal layers established; (C and D) Mantle layer divided into alar and basal laminae; (E) Ventral and dorsal gray columns established. The dorsal part of the cavity of the neural tube disappears. The ventral part persists as the central canal; (F) Functional columns of nuclei.

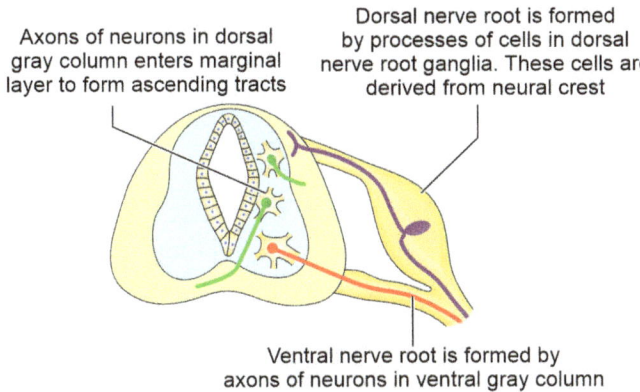

FIG. 22.8: Development of spinal nerve roots.

order. Their axons travel predominantly upwards in the marginal layer to form the *ascending tracts* of the spinal cord. Many of these cells form *interneurons*.

The *posterior/dorsal/sensory nerve roots* are formed by the axons of cells that develop from the neural crest **(Figs. 22.6 and 22.8)**. Groups of these cells collect on the dorsolateral aspect of the developing spinal cord to form the *dorsal nerve root ganglia* (or *spinal ganglia*).

- The axons of these cells divide into two. The *central processes* migrate towards the spinal cord, and establish contact with the dorsolateral aspect of the latter, thus forming the *dorsal nerve roots*. These axons finally synapse with neurons of the posterior gray column developing in the alar lamina. The *peripheral processes* of the cells of the dorsal nerve root ganglia grow outwards to form the sensory components of the spinal nerves.
- As stated above, the axons of neurons in the posterior gray column enter the marginal layer, to form the *ascending tracts* of the spinal cord. At the same time, axons of cells developing in various parts of the brain grow downwards to enter the marginal layer of the spinal cord and form its *descending tracts*.
- These ascending and descending tracts form the *white matter* of the spinal cord. As the mantle layer takes on the shape of the anterior and posterior *gray columns*, the white matter becomes subdivided into *anterior, lateral and posterior white columns*.

Functional Columns in the Gray Matter of the Spinal Cord

The cells of the basal and alar lamina are arranged as two longitudinal functional columns each, divided into somatic and visceral columns. Visceral columns are close to the *sulcus limitans* **(Fig. 22.7F)**. These four functional columns in the spinal cord are concerned with general sensations only.

Afferent columns in the alar lamina receive central processes of pseudounipolar neurons present in dorsal root ganglia.

Two functional columns in the alar lamina:
1. **General somatic afferent:** Extends throughout the spinal cord and receives exteroceptive and proprioceptive information.
2. **General visceral afferent:** Restricted to thoracolumbar and sacral regions of the spinal cord, receiving information from viscera and blood vessels.

Efferent columns in the basal lamina give origin to motor nerve fibers.

Two functional columns in the basal lamina:
1. **General visceral efferent:** Restricted to thoracolumbar and sacral regions of the spinal cord. Neurons provide preganglionic sympathetic fibers that synapse in the peripheral nervous system ganglia for supply to cardiac muscle, smooth muscle in the walls of viscera, glands, and blood vessels.
2. **General somatic efferent:** Extends throughout the spinal cord and provides fibers that innervate skeletal muscles.

Changes in Position of Spinal Cord

- At 3 months, the spinal cord at first extends throughout the length of the developing vertebral canal **(Fig. 22.9A)**. Initially, the length of the spinal cord and vertebral canal are equal, causing the spinal nerves to run horizontally from their segment of origin to exit through the corresponding intervertebral foramina.
- Subsequently, however, the vertebral column becomes much longer than the spinal cord with the result that at full term the lower end of the cord is at the level of the third lumbar vertebra at birth **(Figs. 22.9B and C)**.
- This process of *recession of the spinal cord* continues after birth as a result of which, in the adult, the cord usually ends at the level of the lower border of the first lumbar vertebra.

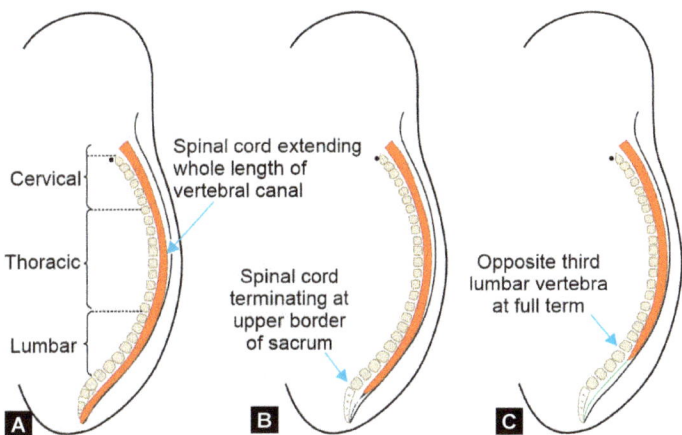

FIGS. 22.9A to C: Recession of spinal cord. Note that the lower end of the cord gradually move cranially, relative to the vertebrae.

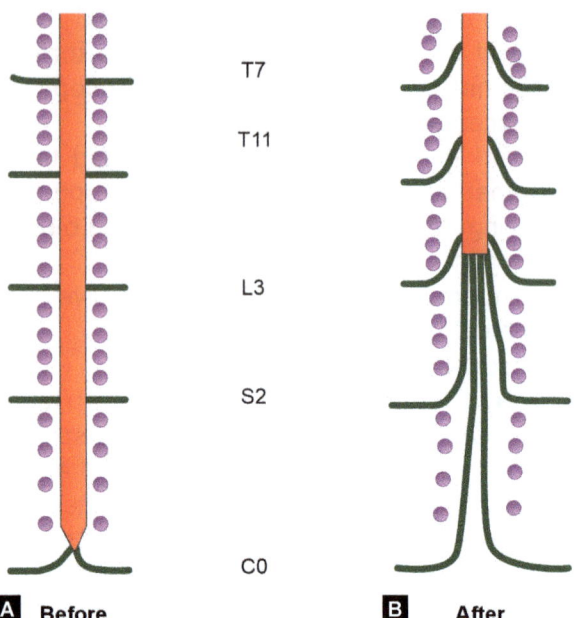

FIGS. 22.10A and B: Effect of recession of spinal cord on course of spinal nerves: (A) Shows the condition before recession begins. Spinal nerves pass horizontally from the spinal cord to their exit from the vertebral canal; (B) Shows the condition after recession has occurred. The nerves now have to run obliquely downwards to reach the points of exit. The obliquity is greatest in the case of the lowest nerves.

- One effect of this recession (of the cord) is that the intervertebral foramina no longer lie at the level at which the corresponding spinal nerves emerge from the spinal cord **(Figs. 22.10A and B)**.
- The nerves have, therefore, to follow an oblique downward course to reach the foramina. This obliquity is least for the cervical nerves, and greatest for the sacral and coccygeal nerves.

MEDULLA OBLONGATA

The medulla oblongata develops from the *myelencephalon*. The early development of the medulla is similar to that of the spinal cord. The appearance of the sulcus limitans divides each lateral wall into a dorsal or alar lamina, and a ventral or basal lamina **(Fig. 22.11A)**. Subsequently, the thin *roof plate* becomes greatly widened as a result of which the alar laminae come to lie dorsolateral to the basal laminae. Thus, both these laminae are now in the floor of the developing fourth ventricle **(Fig. 22.11B)**.

Cells developing in the lateral part of each alar lamina migrate ventrally, and reach the marginal layer overlying the ventrolateral aspect of the basal lamina. These cells constitute the caudal part of the *bulbopontine extension*, and develop into the *olivary nuclei* **(Figs. 22.11C and 22.12)**.

The remaining cells of the alar lamina develop into the sensory nuclei of the cranial nerves related to the

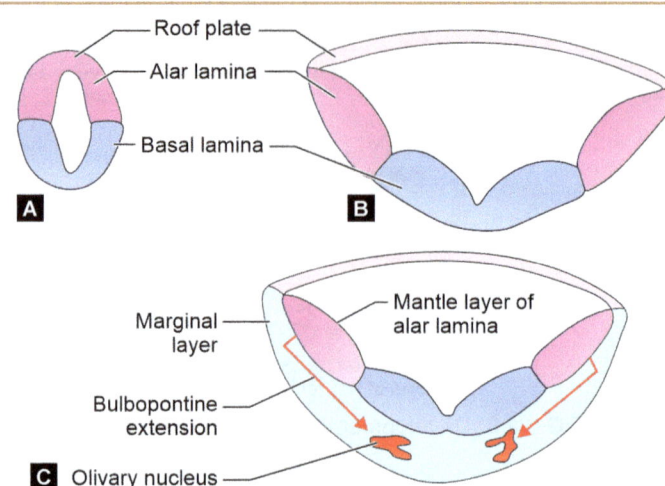

FIGS. 22.11A to C: Development of medulla oblongata. In 'B', note the great widening of the roof plate. In 'C', note the bulbopontine extension and the olivary nuclei.

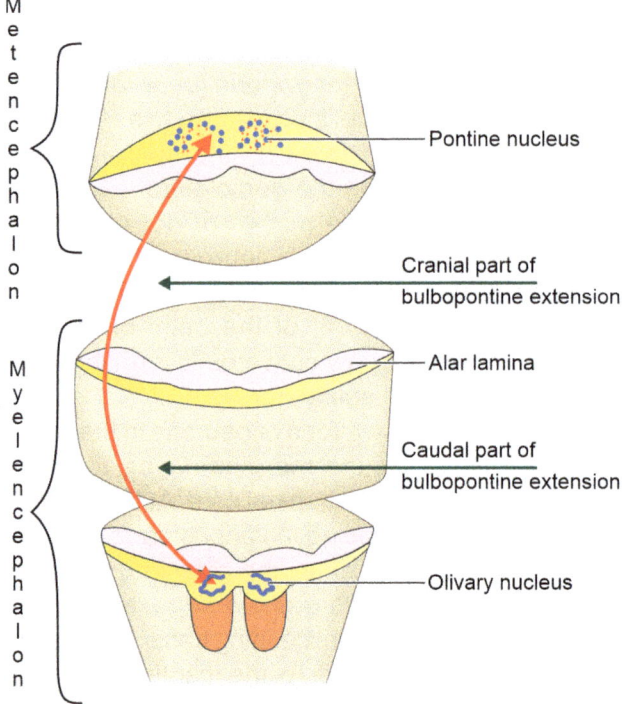

FIG. 22.12: Scheme to show the cranial and caudal parts of the bulbopontine extension. The caudal part lies in the medulla and forms the olivary nuclei, while the cranial part lies in the pons and forms the pontine nuclei.

medulla. The motor nuclei of these nerves are derived from the basal lamina **(Fig. 22.13)**.

The nerve cells of the alar and basal laminae are at first grouped in accordance with their function, and are arranged as illustrated in **Figure 22.13**. Subsequently, some of these nuclei migrate ventrally, from their primitive position in the floor of the fourth ventricle. Their ultimate position is indicated in **Figure 22.14**.

The *gracile and cuneate nuclei* are derived from the lowermost part of the somatic afferent column.

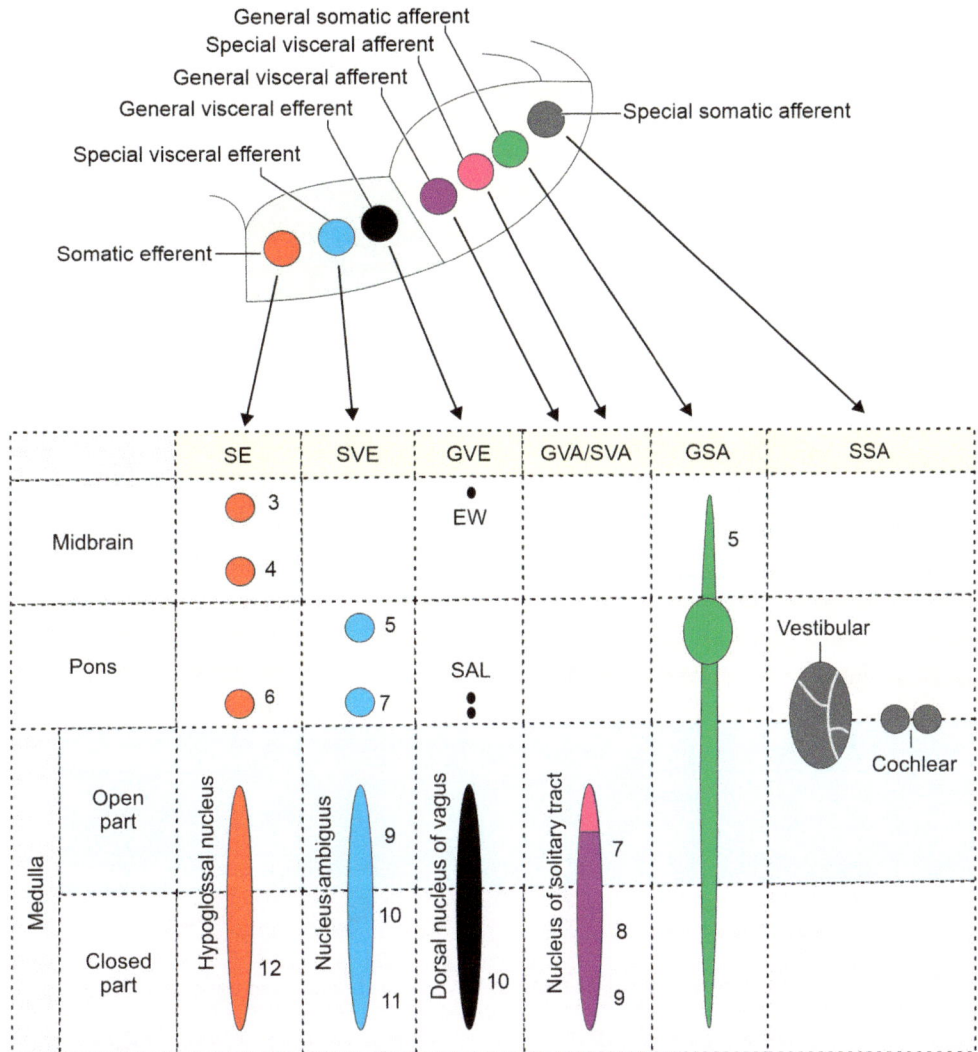

FIG. 22.13: Functional classification of cranial nerve nuclei. The upper figure shows the arrangement of nuclear columns in the brainstem of the embryo. The lower figure shows the nuclei derived from each column. Numbers indicate cranial nerves connected to the nuclei. (GSA: general somatic afferent; GSE: general somatic efferent; GVE: general visceral efferent; SSA: special somatic afferent; SVE: special visceral efferent; GVA: general visceral afferent; SVA: special visceral afferent)

The *white matter* of the medulla is predominantly extraneous in origin, being composed of fibers constituting the ascending and descending tracts that pass through the medulla.

Functional columns of nuclei in brainstem: The seven functional columns are represented in **Figure 22.13**.

PONS

The pons arises from the ventral part of the metencephalon. It also receives a contribution from the alar lamina of the myelencephalon, in the form of the cranial part of the bulbopontine extension **(Figs. 22.13 to 22.15)**. This extension comes to lie ventral to the metencephalon, and gives rise to the *pontine nuclei*. Axons of cells in these nuclei grow transversely to form the *middle cerebellar peduncle*.

As in the myelencephalon, the roof of the metencephalon becomes thin and broad **(Figs. 22.13 and 22.14)**.

The alar and basal laminae are thus orientated as in the medulla.

The lateral part of each alar lamina (often called the *rhombic lip*) becomes specialized to form the cerebellum. The ventral part of the alar lamina gives origin to the sensory cranial nerve nuclei, and the basal lamina to the motor cranial nerve nuclei, of the pons **(Figs. 22.13 and 22.14)**. Their derivation is illustrated in **Figures 22.13 and 22.14**.

The nuclei derived from the basal, and alar, laminae lie in the dorsal or tegmental part of the pons. The ventral part of the pons is constituted by:

❖ Cells of the bulbopontine extension (derived from the alar lamina of the myelencephalon), that form the pontine nuclei. Axons of the cells in these nuclei grow transversely and form the *middle cerebellar peduncle*.

❖ Corticospinal and corticobulbar fibers that descend from the cerebral cortex, and pass through this region

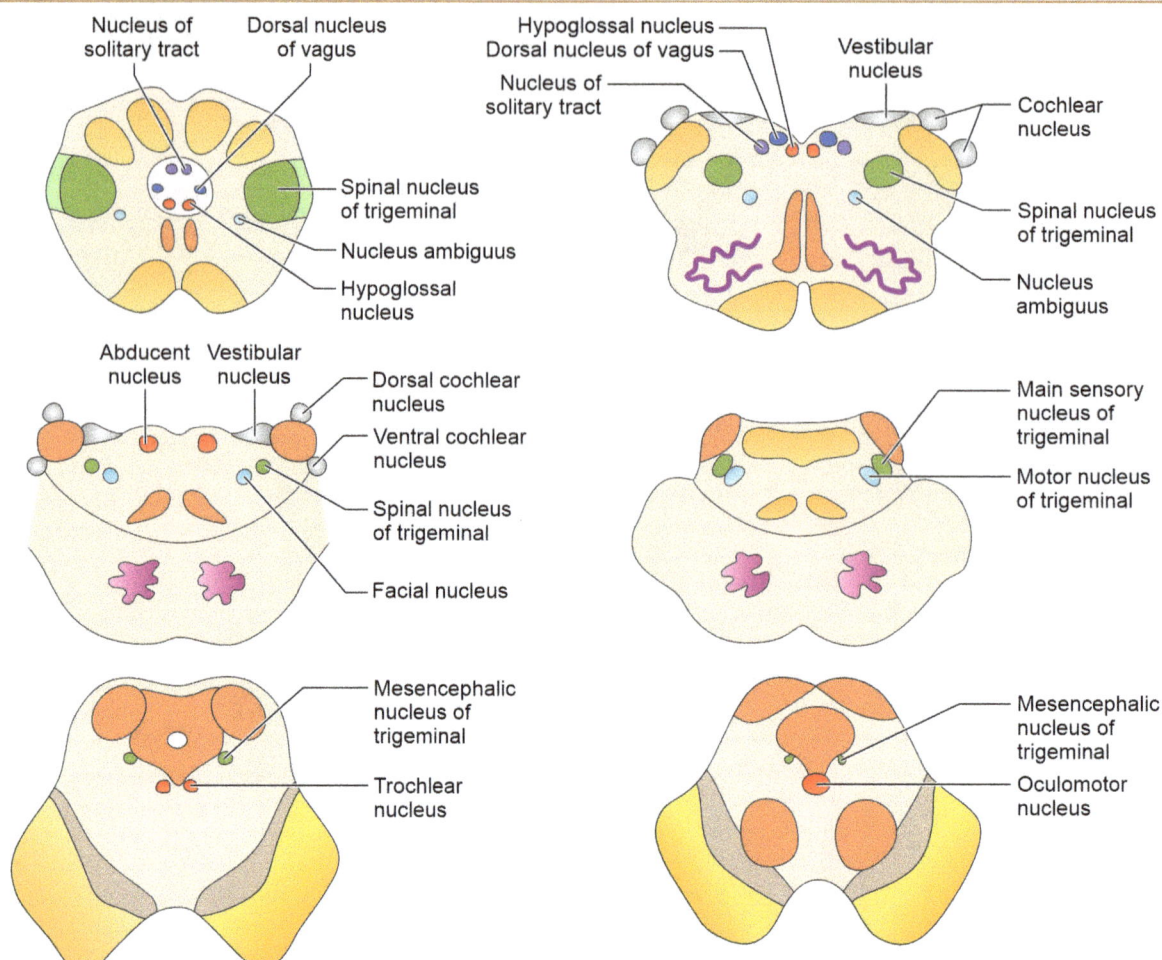

FIG. 22.14: Location of cranial nerve nuclei as seen in transverse sections at various levels of the brainstem.

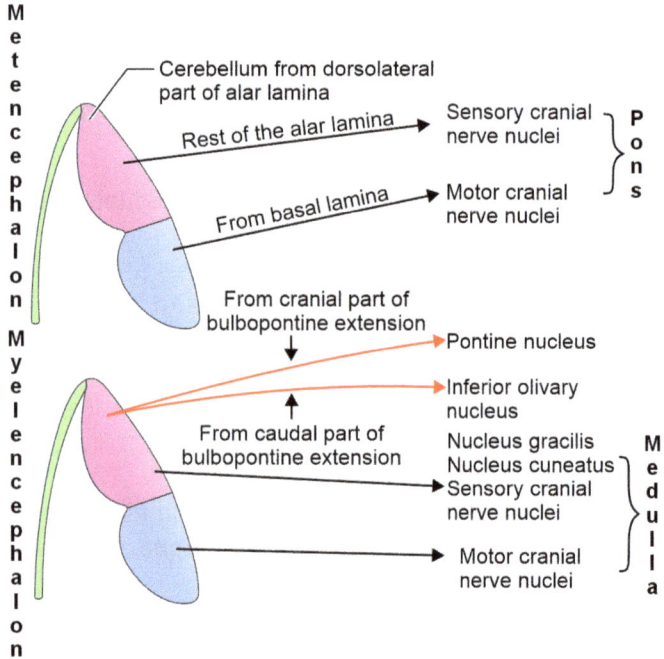

FIG. 22.15: Scheme of the development of medulla and pons.

on their way to the medulla and spinal cord. Some fibers from the cerebral cortex terminate in relation to the pontine nuclei. These are the corticopontine fibers.

MIDBRAIN

The midbrain is developed from the *mesencephalon*. The cavity of the mesencephalon remains narrow and forms the aqueduct. As described in the case of the spinal cord, the mantle layer becomes subdivided into a dorsal or alar lamina and a ventral or basal lamina by the appearance of the sulcus limitans **(Fig. 22.16)**. The nuclei which develop from the basal lamina are:

(1) the oculomotor nerve nucleus, (2) the trochlear nerve nucleus, and (3) the Edinger-Westphal nucleus (GVE).

The alar lamina gives rise to the cells of the colliculi. At first, these form one mass which later becomes subdivided by a transverse fissure. Some cells of the alar lamina migrate ventrally to form the *red nucleus* and the *substantia nigra* **(Fig. 22.16)**.

The marginal layer of the ventral part of the mesencephalon is invaded by downward growing fibers of the corticospinal, corticobulbar and corticopontine pathways. This region, thus, becomes greatly expanded, and forms the *basis pedunculi (crus cerebri)*.

	FROM ALAR LAMINA	FROM BASAL LAMINA
MIDBRAIN	Colliculi Substantia nigra Red nucleus Mesencephalic nucleus of trigeminal nerve	Oculomotor nucleus Edinger Westphal nucleus Trochlear nucleus
PONS	Pontine nucleus Vestibular nucleus Cochlear nucleus Main sensory nucleus of trigeminal nerve Nucleus of spinal tract of trigeminal nerve Nucleus of tractus solitarius	Motor nucleus of trigeminal nerve Motor nucleus of facial nerve Nucleus of abducent nerve Superior salivatory nucleus Lacrimatory nucleus
MEDULLA	Inferior olivary nucleus Vestibular nucleus Nucleus of spinal tract of trigeminal nerve Nucleus of tractus solitarius Part of dorsal nucleus of vagus nerve	Part of dorsal nucleus of vagus nerve Inferior salivatory nucleus Nucleus ambiguus Hypoglossal nerve

FIG. 22.16: Structures of the midbrain derived from alar and basal laminae.

CEREBELLUM

The cerebellum develops from the dorsolateral part of the alar lamina of the *metencephalon* **(Fig. 22.17A)**. Obviously, there are at first two primordia of the cerebellum, right and left. These extend medially in the roof plate of the metencephalon to eventually fuse across the midline **(Figs. 22.17B and C)**. As the cerebellum increases in size, *fissures* appear on its surface. The lateral lobes and vermis can soon be distinguished, as a result of differential growth.

The developing cerebellum can be divided into an *intraventricular part* that bulges into the cavity of the developing fourth ventricle, and an *extraventricular part* that is seen as a bulging on the surface **(Fig. 22.17C)**.

At first the intraventricular part is the larger of the two, but at a later stage, the extraventricular part becomes much larger than the intraventricular part and constitutes almost the whole of the organ **(Fig. 22.17D)**.

The cerebellum, at first, consists of the usual matrix cell, mantle and marginal layers. Some cells of the mantle layer migrate into the marginal layer to form the *cerebellar cortex*. The cells of the mantle layer that do not migrate into the cortex, develop into the *dentate, emboliform, globose* and *fastigial nuclei*.

The *superior cerebellar peduncle* is formed chiefly by the axons growing out of the dentate nucleus. The *middle cerebellar peduncle* is formed by axons growing into the cerebellum from the cells of the pontine nuclei, while the *inferior cerebellar peduncle* is formed by fibers that grow into the cerebellum from the spinal cord and medulla.

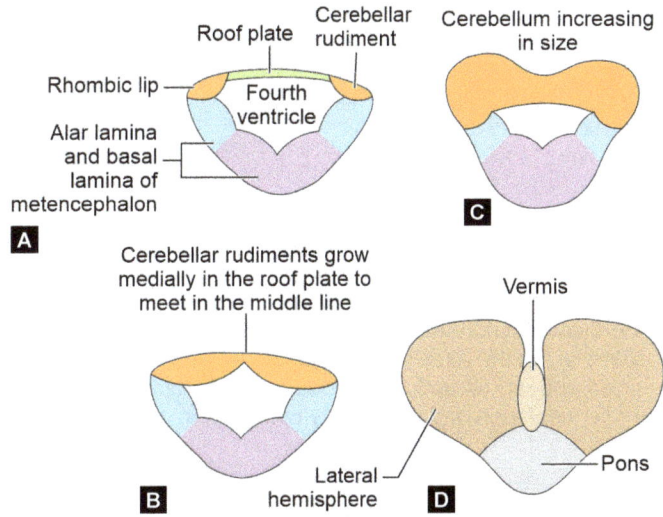

FIGS. 22.17A to D: Some stages in the development of the cerebellum: (A) Cerebellar rudiments appear from alar lamina of metencephalon; (B) They grow into the roof plate of the metencephalon to meet in the midline; (C) Cerebellum enlarges and bulges out of the fourth ventricle; (D) Lateral hemispheres and vermis can be distinguished.

CEREBRAL HEMISPHERE

The cerebrum is a derivative of the *prosencephalon*. We have seen that the prosencephalon is divisible into a median diencephalon and two lateral telencephalic vesicles **(Fig. 22.2C)**. The telencephalic vesicles give origin, on either side, to the *cerebral cortex* and the *corpus striatum*.

The diencephalon gives rise to the *thalamus*, *hypothalamus* and related structures. The telencephalic vesicles are at first small **(Figs. 22.18B and F)**, but

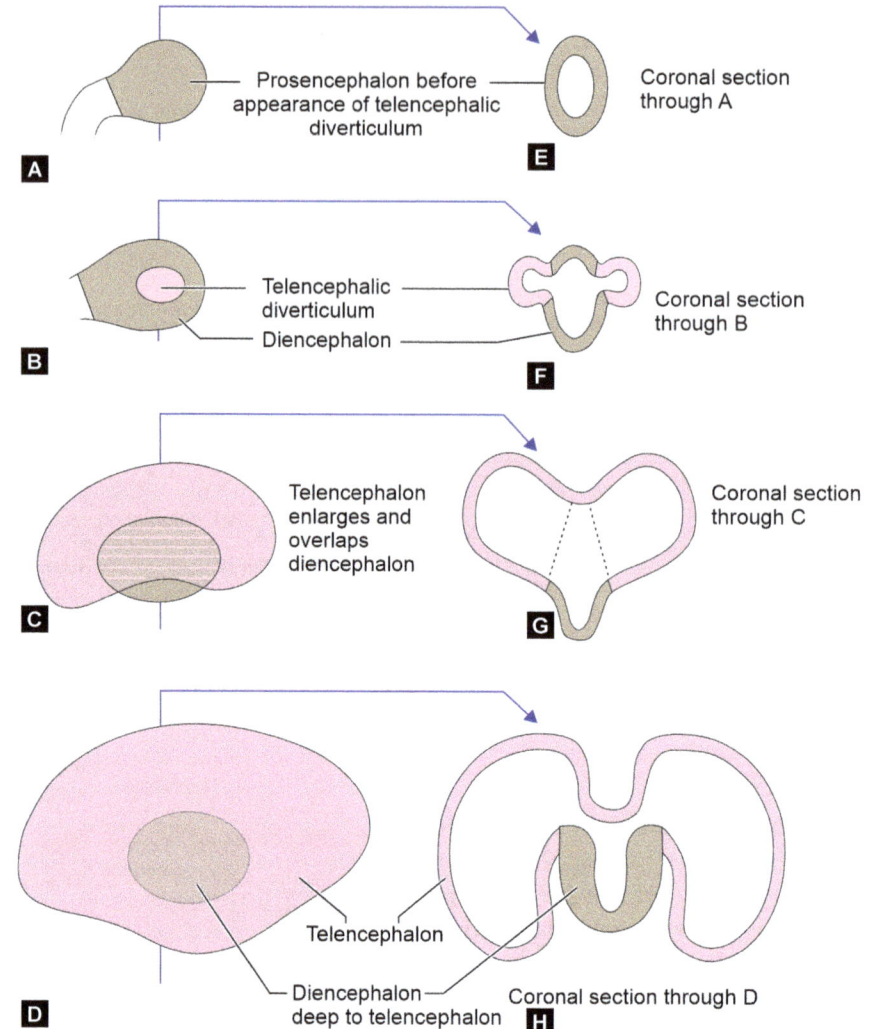

FIGS. 22.18A to H: Development of the cerebral hemisphere. This series of figures shows the changes in the relative size and position of the diencephalon and the telencephalic vesicles: Figures (A to D) are lateral views; Figures (E to H) are corresponding coronal sections along the axes indicated; (A and E) Prosencephalon before appearance of telencephalic vesicles; (B and F) Telencephalic vesicles appear; (C and G) Telencephalic vesicles enlarge and partially cover diencephalon; (D and H) Telencephalon much larger than diencephalon and completely overlapping it.

rapidly increase in size extending upwards, forwards and backwards **(Figs. 22.18 and 22.19)**.

As a result of this enlargement, the telencephalon comes to completely cover the lateral surface of the diencephalon **(Figs. 22.18D and H)** and eventually fuses with it **(Fig. 22.19)**. Thus, the cerebral cortex and corpus striatum come to lie lateral to the thalamus and hypothalamus.

With further upward, forward and backward extension of the telencephalic vesicles, the vesicles of the two sides come into apposition with each other above, in front of, and behind the diencephalon **(Figs. 22.18H and 22.19)**.

The cavity of the diencephalon forms the *third ventricle*, while the cavities of the two telencephalic vesicles form the *lateral ventricles* **(Fig. 22.5)**.

Development of Lateral Ventricles

❖ Each lateral ventricle is at first a spherical space within the telencephalic vesicle **(Fig. 22.20A)**. With

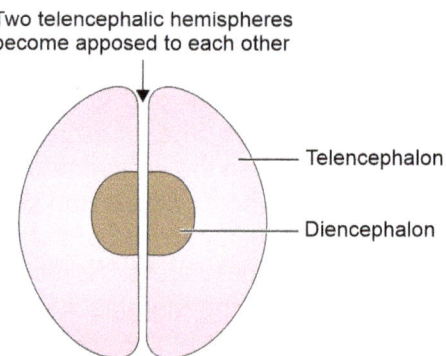

FIG. 22.19: Figure to show that the two telencephalic vesicles come to be apposed to each other in front of and behind the diencephalon.

the forward and backward growth of the vesicle, the ventricle becomes elongated anteroposteriorly **(Fig. 22.20B)**.

❖ The posterior end of the telencephalic vesicle now grows downwards and forwards, to form the temporal

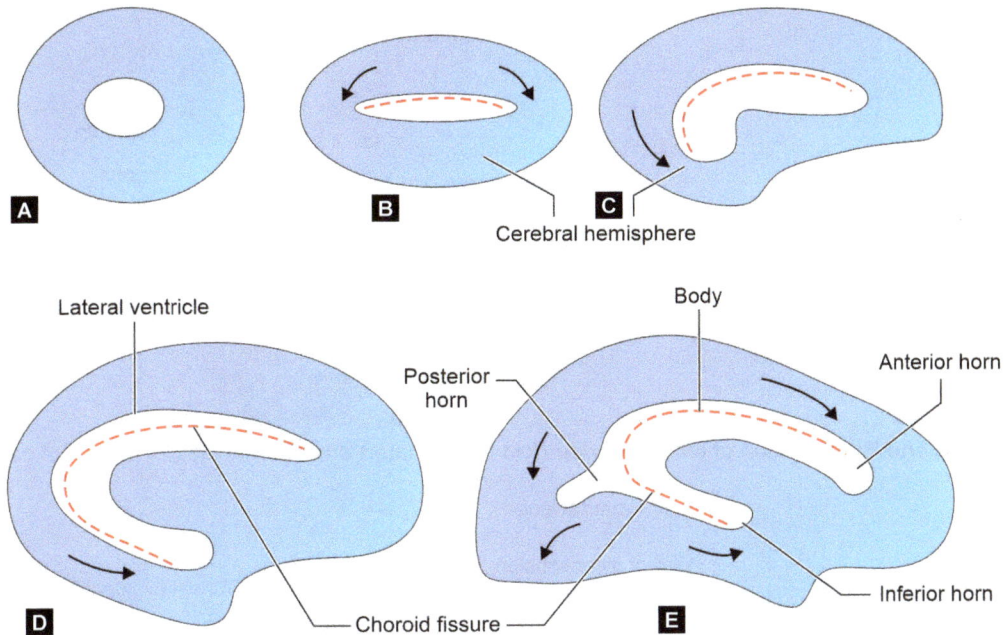

FIGS. 22.20A to E: Establishment of the form of the cerebral hemisphere and of the lateral ventricle. Arrows indicate direction of growth. The choroid fissure is shown in dotted line.

lobe, and the cavity within it becomes the *inferior horn* (Figs. 22.20C and D). The ventricle thus becomes C-shaped.

- Finally, as a result of backward growth, the occipital pole of the hemisphere becomes established, the part of the ventricle within it becoming the *posterior horn* (Fig. 22.20E).
- From **Figure 22.18H**, it will be seen that, with the enlargement of the telencephalic vesicles, their medial walls become apposed to each other. In this way a groove bounded by the two medial surfaces is formed, these surfaces being continuous with each other in the floor of the groove.
- Note that the floor of this groove forms the roof of the third ventricle. Just above the floor of this groove, the medial wall is invaginated laterally into the cavity of the lateral ventricle. The cavity of the invagination is the *choroid fissure* (Figs. 22.21A and B).
- A fold of pia mater extends into this fissure and forms the *tela choroidea*. A bunch of capillaries is formed within this fold and forms the *choroid plexus* (Figs. 22.22A and B). The original wall of the ventricle lining the choroid plexus, remains very thin and forms the ependymal covering of the plexus (Figs. 22.22A and B).
- Note that the *tela choroidea* is in intimate relationship to both lateral ventricles and also to the roof of the third ventricle (Figs. 22.22A and B).
- With the establishment of the temporal pole and the formation of the inferior horn of the lateral ventricle, the choroid fissure becomes C-shaped (Figs. 22.20A to E). The inferior part of the fissure now invaginates into the inferior horn of the lateral ventricle (Fig. 22.20E).

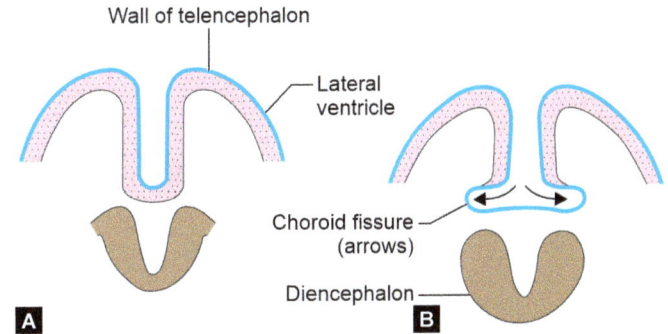

FIGS. 22.21A and B: Formation of the choroid fissure. The wall of the telencephalon remains thin at this site.

Thalamus and Hypothalamus

The thalamus and hypothalamus develop from the *diencephalon*. After the establishment of the telencephalon, the lateral wall of the diencephalon becomes thickened. It is soon subdivided into three regions by the appearance of two grooves, called the *epithalamic* and *hypothalamic sulci* (Fig. 22.23A).

The central part, lying between these two sulci, enlarges to form the *thalamus* (Figs. 22.23B and C). The part above the epithalamic sulcus remains relatively small and forms the *epithalamus*, which is represented by the *habenular nuclei* and the *pineal body*. The part below the hypothalamic sulcus forms the hypothalamus.

The various nuclei of the thalamus and hypothalamus are formed by multiplication of cells in the mantle layer of the wall of the diencephalon.

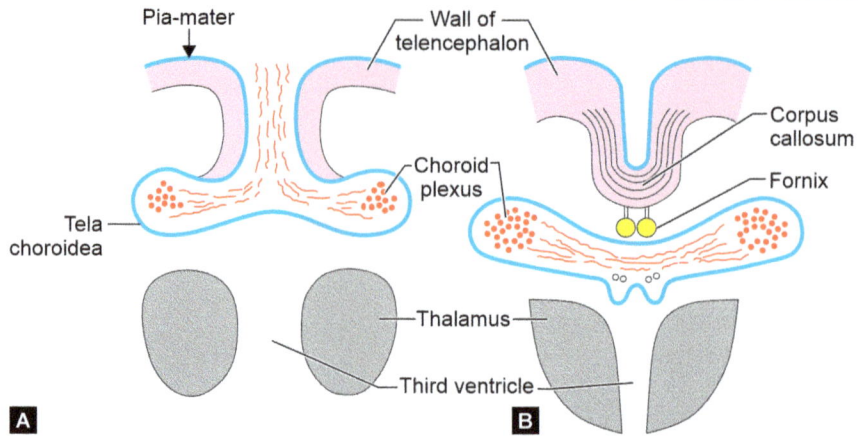

FIGS. 22.22A and B: Formation of tela choroidea (fold of pia mater) and choroid plexus (bunch of capillaries).

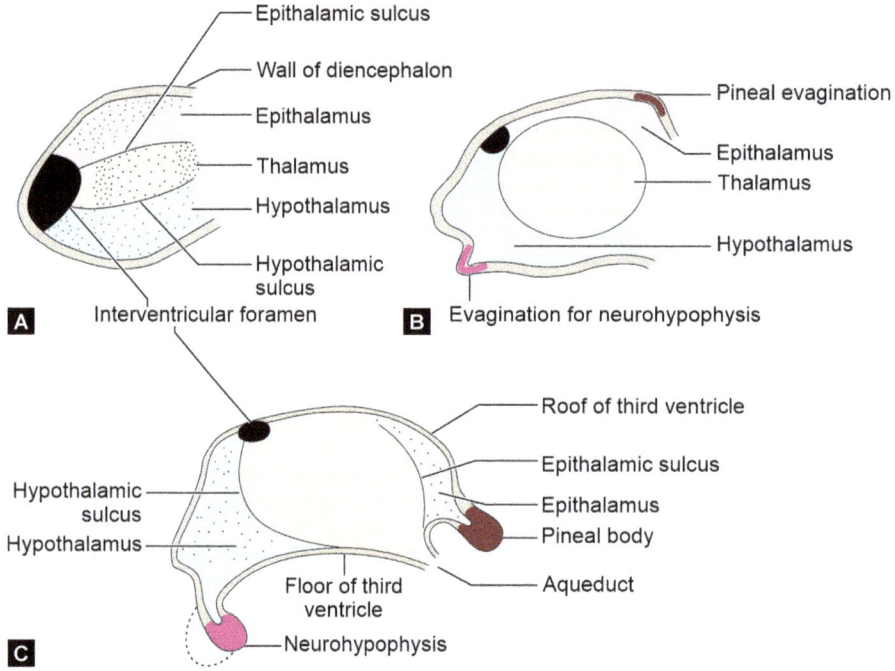

FIGS. 22.23A to C: Development of thalamus and hypothalamus. The appearance of the epithalamic and hypothalamic sulci divides the diencephalon into thalamus, epithalamus and hypothalamus. The pineal body is formed in relation to the epithalamus, and the neurohypophysis in relation to the hypothalamus.

Corpus Striatum

The corpus striatum is a derivative of the *telencephalon*. Early in its development each telencephalic vesicle can be subdivided into a basal part which is thick, and a superior part which is thin **(Figs. 22.24A and B)**. Some of the cells, in the mantle layer of the thick basal part, migrate into the overlying marginal layer to form part of the cerebral cortex. The remaining cells of the mantle layer of this region form the corpus striatum.

The developing corpus striatum soon becomes subdivided into *medial and lateral subdivisions*, which increase in thickness **(Fig. 22.24C)**.

Meanwhile, the cerebral cortex is developing and numerous axons, that are growing downwards from it, or are growing towards it, pass through the region of the corpus striatum and divide it into a deeper and a superficial part. These fibers constitute the *internal capsule* **(Fig. 22.25)**.

The part of the corpus striatum that comes to lie deep to the internal capsule, becomes the *caudate nucleus*, and the superficial part becomes the *lentiform nucleus* **(Fig. 22.26)**. The lentiform nucleus later becomes subdivided into the *putamen*, and the *globus pallidus* **(Fig. 22.27)**.

Cerebral Cortex

The cerebral cortex is formed by migration of cells from the mantle layer into the overlying marginal layer. These cells divide, and subdivide, leading to considerable thickening of the cortex. By full term, several layers of cells can be recognized.

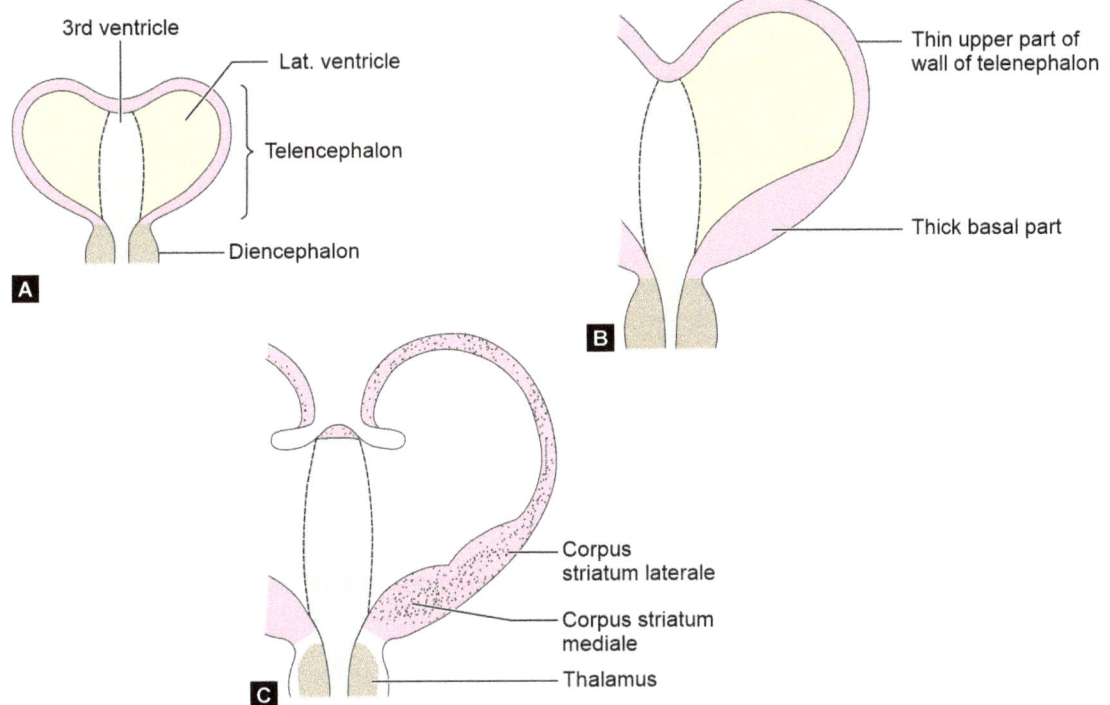

FIGS. 22.24A to C: Early development of corpus striatum as seen in coronal sections: (A) Telencephalon before appearance of corpus striatum; (B) Wall of basal part thickened; (C) Thickening divides into medial and lateral parts.

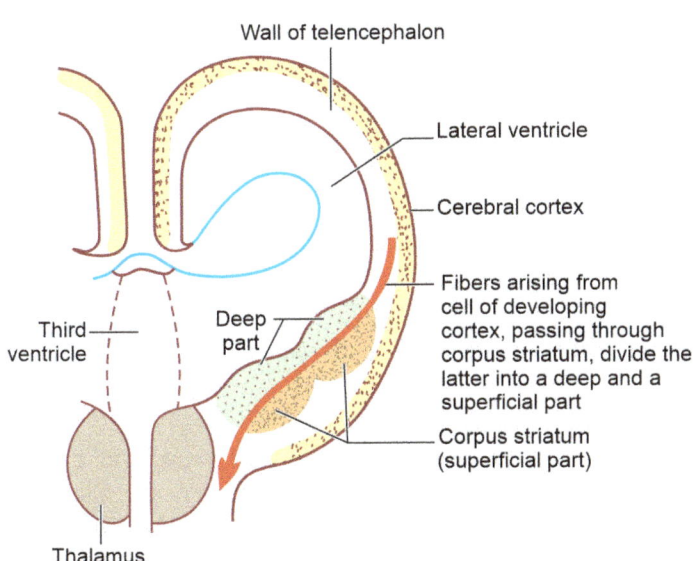

FIG. 22.25: Wall of telencephalon at a stage somewhat later than that shown in **Figure 22.31C**. The region of the developing corpus striatum is divided (longitudinally) into deep and superficial parts (by nerve fibers growing downwards through it).

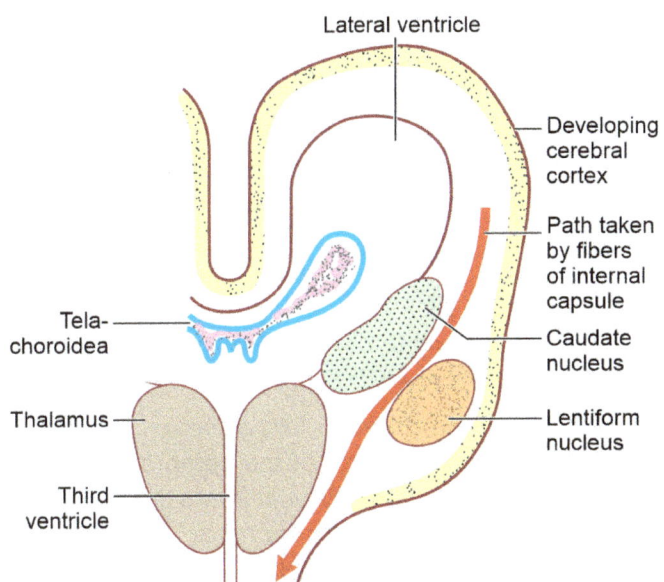

FIG. 22.26: Deep part of corpus striatum becomes the caudate nucleus. Superficial part becomes the lentiform nucleus. Note relation of these to the thalamus developing in the diencephalon.

Simultaneously, there is considerable side-to-side expansion of the cortex as a result of which its surface area is greatly increased. As the surface expansion is at a greater rate than that of the hemisphere as a whole, the cortex becomes folded on itself.

Sulci and gyri are formed as a result of this folding. The region of the insula is relatively slow in growth, and is gradually overgrown by adjacent areas, which form the *opercula of the insula*.

From a developmental point of view, the cerebral cortex consists of **(Figs. 22.28A and B)**: (a) the *hippocampal cortex*, (b) the *pyriform cortex*, and (c) the *neocortex*. The neocortex is the most important part. It undergoes very great expansion and forms the *whole of the cerebral cortex* seen on the superolateral and medial surfaces of the cerebral hemisphere, and the cortex of the inferior surface *excluding the pyriform area* (Fig. 22.28B). The hippocampal cortex forms the

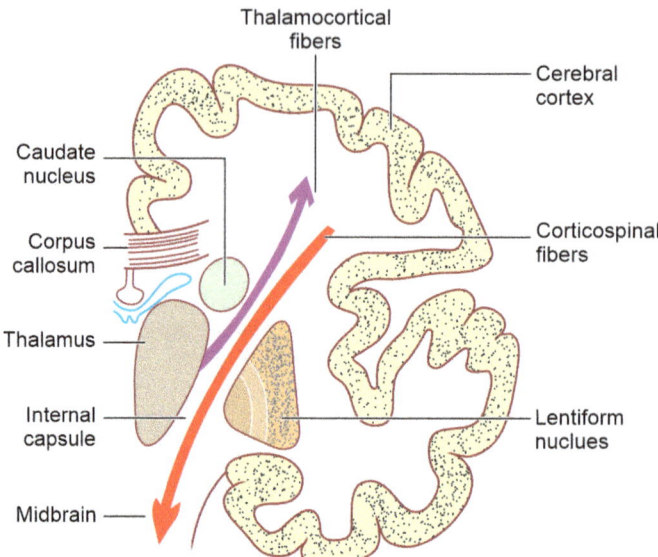

FIG. 22.27: With enlargement of the telencephalon the lentiform nucleus comes to lie lateral to the thalamus. The internal capsule passes through the interval between the lentiform nucleus laterally and the caudate nucleus and thalamus medially.

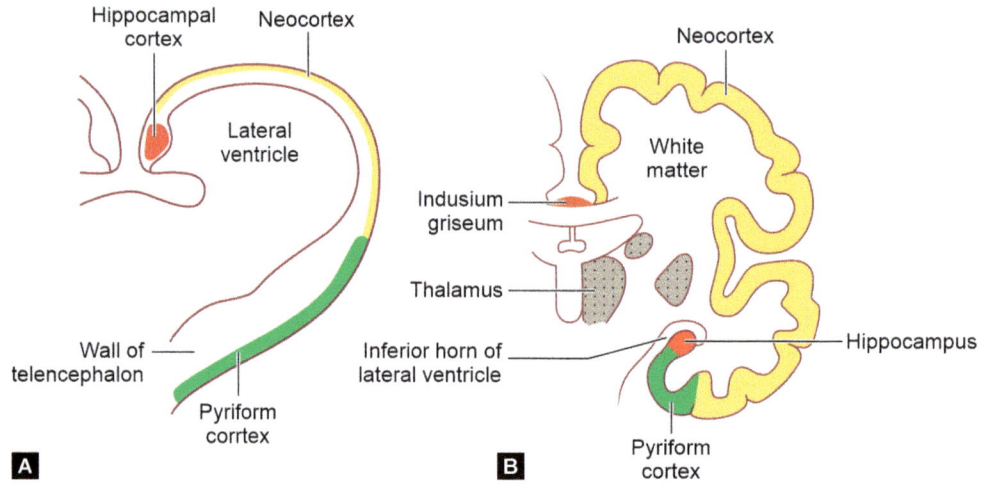

FIGS. 22.28A and B: Development of the cerebral cortex. Most of the cerebral cortex is derived from the neocortex. The hippocampal cortex forms the hippocampus and the indusium griseum. The piriform cortex forms part of the limbic system.

hippocampus, and the *indusium griseum*. The piriform cortex gives rise to the part of the cerebral cortex that receives *olfactory sensations*. It forms the *uncus*, the anterior part of the *parahippocampal gyrus*, and the *anterior perforated substance*.

White Matter of Cerebrum

The bulk of the cerebrum is constituted by its white matter. This is made up of:
- Axons of cortical cells that grow towards other areas of the cortex, either in the same or in the opposite hemisphere.
- Axons of cortical cells that grow downwards through the hemisphere, on their way to the brainstem and spinal cord.
- Axons that connect the thalamus, hypothalamus and basal ganglia to one another and to the cortex.
- Axons that grow into the hemisphere from the brainstem and spinal cord.

Cerebral Commissures

The part of the wall of the neural tube that closes the cranial end of the prosencephalon is called the *lamina terminalis* (Figs. 22.29 and 22.30A). After the appearance of the telencephalic vesicles, the lamina

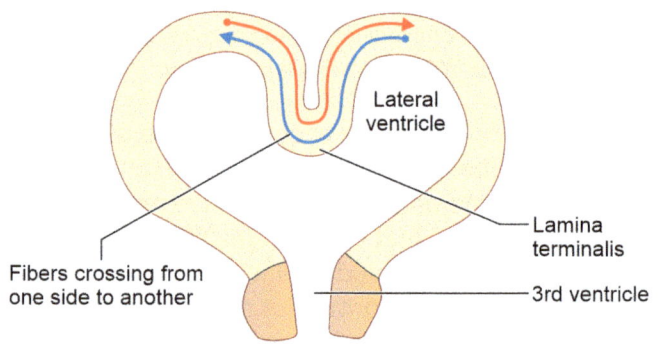

FIG. 22.29: Diagram to show how the lamina terminalis serves as a path for nerve fibers passing from one cerebral hemisphere to the other.

terminalis lies in the anterior wall of the third ventricle. Reference to **Figure 22.29** will show that any neuron growing from one hemisphere to the other must pass through this lamina. To facilitate this passage, the lamina terminalis becomes thickened to form the *commissural plate* **(Fig. 22.30B)**.

The first commissural fibers to develop form the *anterior commissure*. This is followed by the formation of the *hippocampal commissure*. The *corpus callosum* appears later. It, at first, lies anterior to the diencephalon, but because of rapid increase in its size it extends backwards and roofs over this region **(Fig. 22.30C)**.

Other commissures that appear are the *optic chiasma*, the *habenular commissure* and the *posterior commissure*.

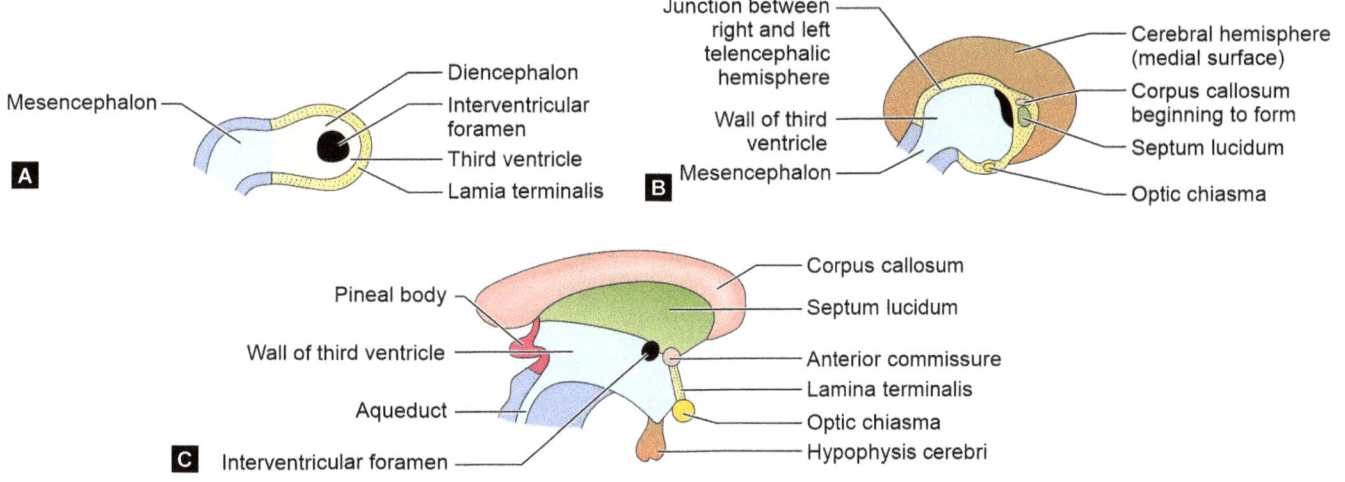

FIGS. 22.30A to C: Development of the corpus callosum and other commissures.

Clinical correlation

Anomalies of Brain and Spinal Cord
Neural tube defects (NTDs): These are a group of conditions where nonapproximation of neural folds results in an opening in the spinal cord or brain, or both, from early human development. There are two types of NTDs: open and closed.
1. **Open NTDs** are more common. They result when the brain and/or spinal cord are exposed at birth through a defect in the skull or vertebrae. Examples include anencephaly and spina bifida.
2. **Closed NTDs** are rare and occur when the spinal defect is covered by skin. They are due to malformation of fat, bone, or membranes.

Outward bulging of neural tube and covering membranes: As a result of nonfusion of the neural tube or the overlying bones (e.g., spina bifida), neural tissue may lie outside the cranial cavity or vertebral canal. When this happens in the brain region, it is called *encephalocele* **(Fig. 22.31A)**, and when it occurs in the spinal region, it is called *myelocele* **(Fig. 22.31B)**. Nonclosure of the neural tube exposes the nervous tissue on the surface. Failure of closure of the anterior and posterior neuropore results in conditions called *anencephaly* **(Figs. 22.32C)** and *spina bifida* **(Fig. 22.32D)**, respectively. Failure of closure of the entire neural tube results in a condition called *rachischisis*.

Anencephaly (Fig. 22.31C): Failure of closure of the anterior neuropore results in exposure of brain substance to the surface as an irregular degenerated mass. It is characterized by the absence of the vault of the skull, exposing the brain, which gets degenerated and malformed. There will be an absence of swallowing reflex in the fetus and hydramnios in the last trimester. Antenatal diagnosis is by ultrasonography and estimation of alpha-fetoproteins in amniotic fluid. Prevention is through the administration of folic acid before and during pregnancy.
- **Rachischisis (Figs. 22.32A):** Failure of closure of the neural groove results in exposure of neural tissue onto the surface.
- **Spina bifida (Figs. 22.32B to E):** When the neural tube has closed and the outward bulging of the spinal cord or its coverings is a result of a defect of the overlying bones. There are different types of spina bifida depending on the contents of the bulging.
  - *Spina bifida occulta*—where the spinal cord is normal **(Fig. 22.32B)**.
  - *Meningocele*—pia and arachnoid protrude through the gap in the bifid spine forming a cystic swelling covered with skin **(Fig. 22.32C)**.
  - *Meningomyelocele*—the cystic swelling includes the spinal cord **(Figs. 22.32D and 21.31E)**. Meningomyelocele is sometimes associated with the downward projection of some part of the cerebellum and medulla through the foramen magnum, leading to hydrocephalus. This combined malformation is called Arnold–Chiari malformation.
  - *Anterior spina bifida*—a rare anomaly where two halves of the vertebral body fail to fuse and the spinal meninges protrude ventrally through the gap **(Fig. 22.32E)**.

Chapter 22: Nervous System

Hydrocephalus (Fig. 22.33):
- This condition occurs due to the accumulation of an abnormal quantity of cerebrospinal fluid (CSF) in the ventricular system of the brain. This can be due to a blockage in the circulation of CSF or its excessive production. The pressure of the fluid causes degeneration of nervous tissue. The ventricles become very large, and the infant is born with a large head. The enlargement of the central canal and associated abnormal cavities near the central canal is called syringomyelia.
- **Dandy–Walker syndrome**—a form of hydrocephalus resulting from blockage of the median and lateral apertures of the fourth ventricle. Enlargement is predominantly in the posterior cranial fossa, and the cerebellum is abnormal.

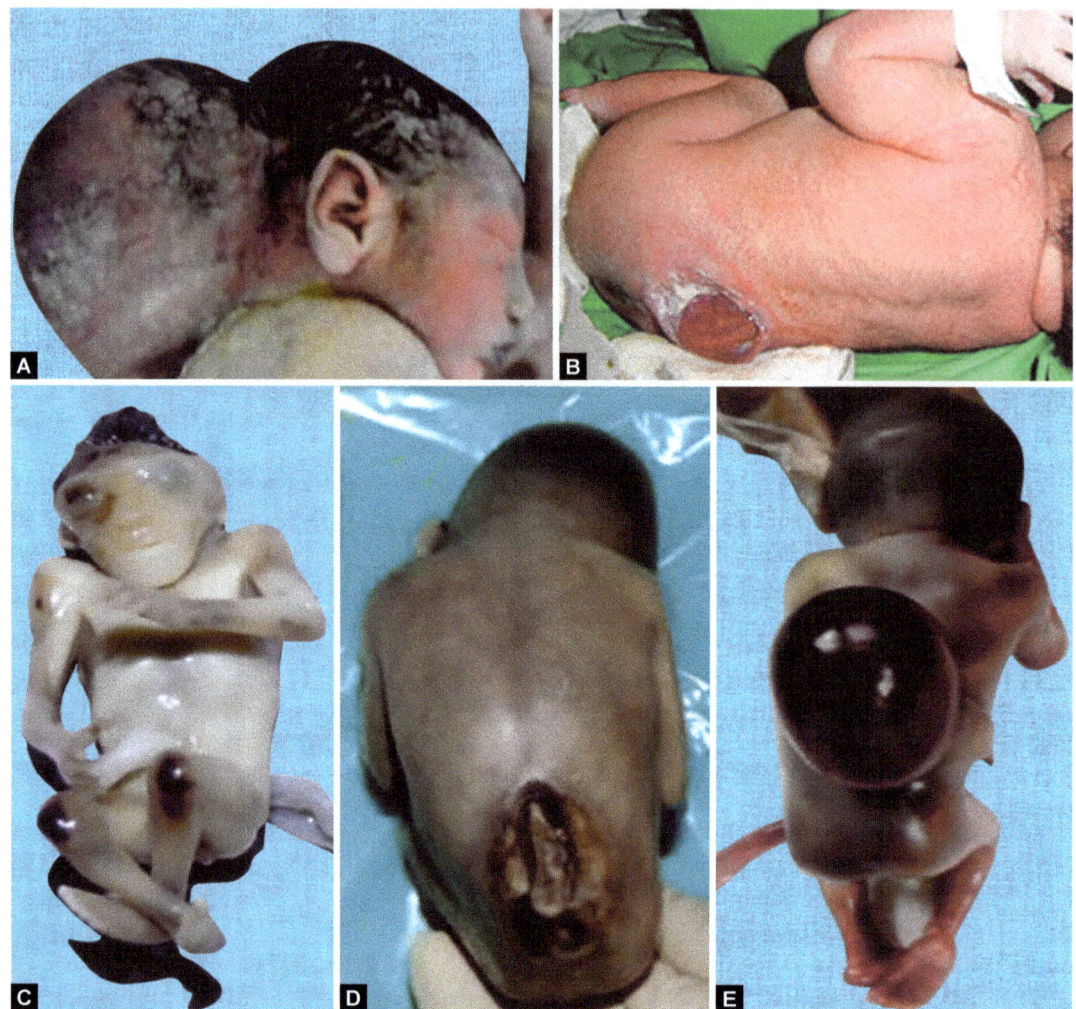

FIGS. 22.31A to E: Types of neural tube defects. (A) Encephalocele; (B) Myelocele; (C) Anencephaly; (D) Open spina bifida; (E) Meningomyelocele.
(Reproduced with permission from Dr Piyush Gupta. Source: Shubha R Phadke and Ranjana Mishra , Chapter 27. In: Gupta P, UG Textbook of Pediatrics, Jaypee Brothers Medical Publishers Pvt Ltd, 2023).

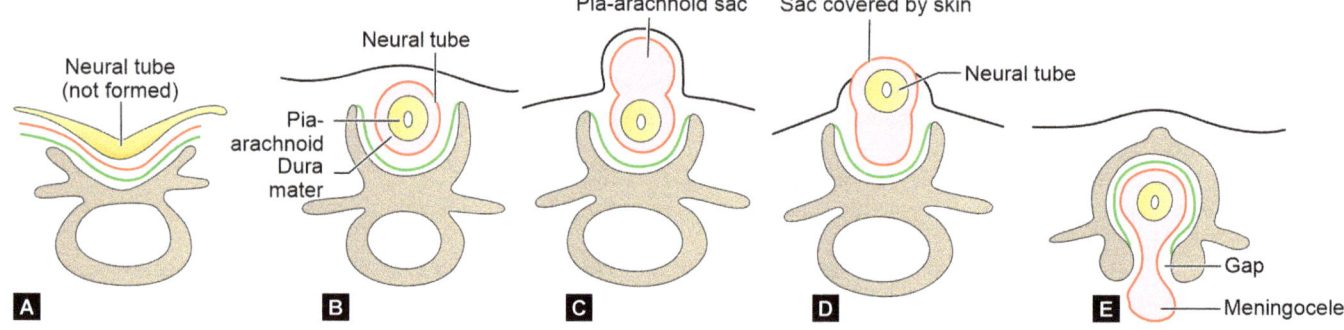

FIGS. 21.32A to E: Anomalies of neural tube due to defective formation of vertebra, i.e., spina bifida: (A) Rachischisis; (B) Spina bifida occulta; (C) Spina bifida with meningocele; (D) Spina bifida with meningomyelocele; (E) Anterior spina bifida.

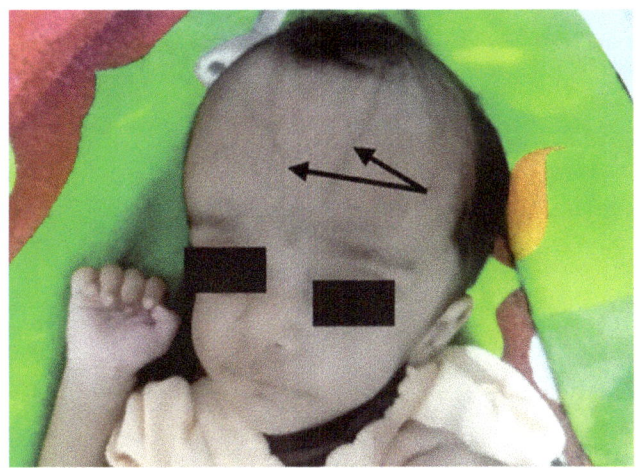

FIG. 21.33: Infant with hydrocephalus showing large skull with dilated superficial scalp veins (black arrows).
(Reproduced with permission from Dr Piyush Gupta. Source: Ranjith Kumar Manokaran and Jaya Shankar Kaushik, Chapter 27. In: Gupta P, UG Textbook of Pediatrics, Jaypee Brothers Medical Publishers Pvt Ltd, 2023).

AUTONOMIC NERVOUS SYSTEM

Sympathetic Neurons

Any sympathetic pathway consists of two neurons, i.e., a preganglionic and a postganglionic neuron.
1. The preganglionic neurons develop in the mantle layer of the thoraco-lumbar region of the spinal cord (segments T1 to L2 or L3). These cells are located near the sulcus limitans, and form the lateral horn of the cord **(Fig. 22.34)**. The axons growing out from them are myelinated. They pass into the ventral nerve roots to enter the spinal nerves. After a very short course through the spinal nerves, they leave them and grow towards the postganglionic neurons. The postganglionic neurons form the various ganglia of the sympathetic trunk. Some postganglionic neurons come to lie near the viscera, and form visceral sympathetic ganglia. The preganglionic fibers meant for them do not relay in the sympathetic trunk but pass through branches of the trunk to reach the visceral ganglia.
2. The axons of the postganglionic neurons grow towards the various viscera of the body, to innervate them. Some of them enter spinal nerves and are distributed through them to blood vessels, hair and sweat glands. Postganglionic neurons are generally believed to be derived from cells of the neural crest.

Parasympathetic Neurons

As in sympathetic pathways, parasympathetic pathways also consist of two neurons (preganglionic and postganglionic).

Preganglionic Neurons

The preganglionic neurons of the parasympathetic system are formed in two distinct situations.

Cranial Parasympathetic Outflow

These neurons are formed in relation to the general visceral efferent nuclear column of the brainstem **(Fig. 22.34A)**. They give rise to the Edinger-Westphal nucleus, salivatory and lacrimatory nuclei and the dorsal nucleus of the vagus. The preganglionic parasympathetic fibers taking origin from the Edinger-Westphal nucleus run in the oculomotor nerve to reach the ciliary ganglion. The superior salivatory and lacrimatory nuclei give origin to preganglionic fibers, which run in the facial nerve to reach the sphenopalatine and submandibular ganglia. The inferior salivatory nucleus give origin to the fibers which are related to the glossopharyngeal nerve and terminate in the otic ganglion. The dorsal nucleus of the vagus gives preganglionic parasympathetic fibers that terminate in various ganglia situated in the walls of viscera supplied by the vagus nerve.

Sacral Parasympathetic Outflow

The preganglionic neurons are formed in the mantle layer of the sacral part of the spinal cord (S2–S4). These cells lie near the sulcus limitans. Their axons constitute the preganglionic parasympathetic fibers, which terminate by synapsing with postganglionic neurons situated in the walls of pelvic viscera and hindgut.

Postganglionic Neurons

Postganglionic parasympathetic neurons are derived from the neural crest cells.

In the cranial region, the postganglionic parasympathetic neurons form the ciliary, otic, submandibular and sphenopalatine ganglia. Ganglia are also present in various viscera supplied by the vagus nerve.

Postganglionic parasympathetic neurons are also present in various ganglia that lie in relation to the hindgut and pelvic viscera. These neurons receive preganglionic fibers of the sacral outflow.

It should be noted that the entire length of the gut (from esophagus to anal canal) is populated by postganglionic parasympathetic neurons which are of neural crest origin. The neural crest cells within the gut form the *enteric nervous system*.

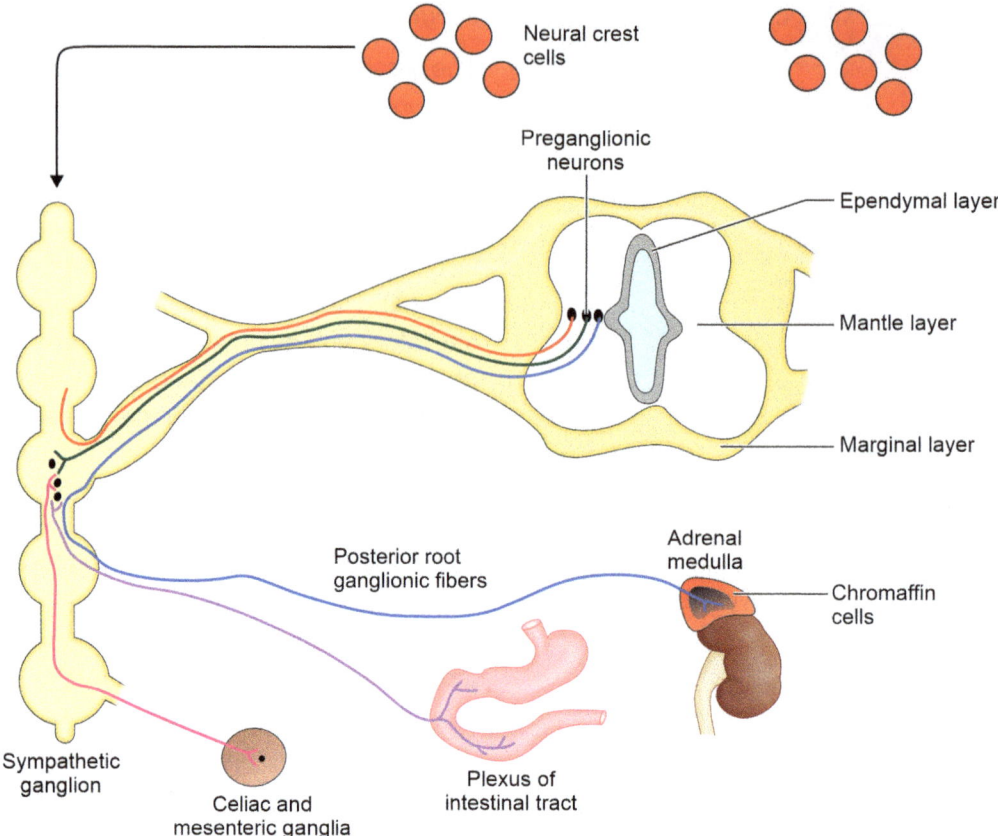

FIG. 22.34: Development of preganglionic and postganglionic sympathetic neurons.

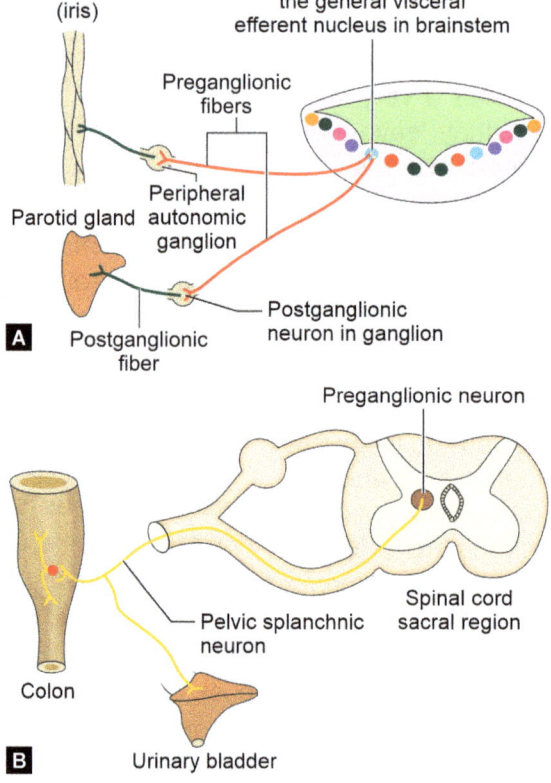

FIGS. 22.35A and B: Development of preganglionic and postganglionic parasympathetic neurons: (A) Cranial outflow; (B) Sacral outflow.

TIMETABLE OF SOME EVENTS DESCRIBED IN THIS CHAPTER

Age	Developmental events
3rd week	Neural tube begins to form
4th week	• Neural folds begin to fuse • Primordia of sensory ganglia (spinal and cranial) are formed • Formation of primary brain vesicle
25th day	Closure of anterior neuropore
27th day	Closure of posterior neuropore
28th day	The most cranial pair of cervical spinal ganglia develops
5th week	Formation of brain vesicle Sympathetic ganglia are formed. Cerebral hemispheres begin to form
8th week	Cerebellum starts forming
10th week	The corpus callosum forms
12th week	Cerebellar cortex and Purkinje cells are formed
15th week	The dentate nucleus is seen
4th month	Myelination of nerve fibers begin
Late fetal life	Sulci and gyri appear over cerebral hemispheres

Case Based Learning

Embryological Basis of Arnold–Chiari Malformation
Case Scenario
A neonate presents to the neonatologist with a soft bulging in the lumbosacral region and a large head, exhibiting symptoms of dyspnea, dysphagia, and noisy breathing. A diminished gag reflex is noted on examination. Based on physical examination and radiological investigations, a diagnosis of Arnold–Chiari malformation is made. Provide the embryological explanation for this condition.

- **Arnold–Chiari malformation** is a congenital deformity characterized by meningomyelocele, caudal displacement of the medulla and cerebellar tonsils through the foramen magnum, and hydrocephalus.
- **The soft bulging** is due to a posterior gap in the vertebrae resulting from the nonfusion of laminae to form the vertebral spine, known as spina bifida.
- **The bulging** may contain only meninges (meningocele) or both meninges and spinal cord (meningomyelocele). In this case, it is a meningomyelocele covered with skin.
- **The large head** is due to the accumulation of cerebrospinal fluid (CSF) in the brain's ventricles, known as hydrocephalus. Radiological investigations likely showed herniation of the cerebellar tonsils and medulla oblongata through the foramen magnum into the vertebral canal. This herniation leads to blockage of CSF flow due to obstruction at the foramen magnum, resulting in hydrocephalus.
- **Symptoms such as dyspnea, dysphagia, and diminished gag reflex** result from the compression of the medulla and stretching of cranial nerves IX, X, XI, and XII, which are attached to the medulla.
- These embryological defects disrupt the normal formation and separation of neural and skeletal tissues, leading to the clinical presentation observed in Arnold–Chiari malformation.

HIGHLIGHTS

- Nervous system develops from the specialized ectoderm overlying the notochord known as *neurectoderm*.
- Neurectoderm overlying the notochord becomes thickened to form the *neural plate*.
- Neural plate is converted to *neural groove*, and then to *neural tube*.
- Neural tube has an enlarged cranial part that forms the *brain*, and a narrow caudal part that becomes the *spinal cord*. Neural tube presents a *central cavity* (lumen) that contains cerebrospinal fluid and a *peripheral wall* that forms *nervous tissue*.
- The cranial part of neural tube shows three dilatations: *prosencephalon, mesencephalon* and *rhombencephalon*.
- The prosencephalon divides into diencephalon and telencephalon. The telencephalon forms most of the *cerebral hemisphere* including the *corpus striatum*. The *lateral ventricle* is the cavity of the telencephalon. The diencephalon forms the thalamus, hypothalamus and related structures. Its cavity is the *third ventricle*.

- The mesencephalon forms the *midbrain*. Its cavity forms the *cerebral aqueduct*.
- The rhombencephalon divides into *metencephalon* and *myelencephalon*. The metencephalon forms the *pons*. It also forms the *cerebellum*. The myelencephalon forms the *medulla oblongata*. The *fourth ventricle* is the cavity of the rhombencephalon.
- The *neural crest cells* are made up of specialized surface ectodermal cells that lie along the lateral edges of the neural plate and later along the dorsolateral aspect of neural tube. Its most important derivatives are cells of *sensory ganglia*, *parasympathetic ganglia* and of *sympathetic ganglia*. It also forms the cells of the *adrenal medulla* and *Schwann cells* that form *myelin* and *neurilemmal sheaths* for peripheral nerve fibers.
- The wall of neural tube at first has a single layer of cells. They multiply and form three layers/zones. They are ependymal/matrix, *mantle* and *marginal* from the lumen to periphery. *Neurons* develop in the mantle layer which forms the *gray matter* and the processes of neurons occupy the marginal layer that becomes the *white matter*. The mantle layer is divided into a ventral part, the *basal lamina/floor plate* and a dorsal part, the *alar lamina/roof plate*. These are separated by a groove, the *sulcus limitans*.
- In the spinal cord, the alar lamina forms the *posterior/dorsal gray column*, and the basal lamina forms the *anterior/ventral gray column*. The marginal layer becomes the *white matter*.
- In the medulla, pons and midbrain, *efferent cranial nerve nuclei* develop in the basal lamina and *afferent nuclei* in the alar lamina.
- The alar lamina of the myelencephalon also forms the *olivary nuclei* (which migrate ventrally), and the *pontine nuclei* (which migrate into the pons). The alar lamina of the metencephalon contributes for the development of *cerebellum*. The alar lamina of the mesencephalon forms the *colliculi*, the *red nucleus* and the *substantia nigra*.

Summary

- **Subdivisions and adult derivatives of neural tube (Figs 22.2 and 22.3).**
- **Flexures of neural tube:**
  - Cervical
  - Pontine
  - Mesencephalic
- **Neural crest cell derivatives (Fig. 22.6):**
  - *Dorsal mass:* Neurons of dorsal root ganglia and sensory ganglia of 5th, 7th, 8th, 9th and 10th cranial nerves; capsular and Schwann cells, melanoblasts and leptomeninges.
  - *Ventral mass:* Neurons of sympathetic ganglia and peripheral parasympathetic ganglia; suprarenal medulla and para-aortic bodies.
  - *Others:* Bones of face and vault of skull, sclera and choroid of eye, C cells of thyroid gland.

TEST YOUR UNDERSTANDING

REVIEW QUESTIONS

1. Describe neurulation in detail.
2. Write a short note on neural crest cells.
3. Tabulate the nuclei of pons, medulla and midbrain.
4. Discuss development of brain.
5. Enumerate structures derived from neural crest cells.
6. Explain the development of cerebellum.
7. Write a short note on spina bifida.
8. Write a short note on hydrocephalus and anencephaly.
9. Discuss neural tube defects.

MULTIPLE CHOICE QUESTIONS

1. Trochlear nucleus develops from:
   A. Alar lamina of midbrain
   B. Basal lamina of midbrain
   C. Alar lamina of medulla
   D. Basal lamina of pons
2. Lentiform nucleus develops from:
   A. Mesencephalon
   B. Rhombencephalon
   C. Telencephalon
   D. Metencephalon
3. Neural crest cells originate from:
   A. Mesenchyme
   B. Somite
   C. Surface ectoderm
   D. Mesoderm
4. Efferent cranial nerve nuclei develop in which part of brainstem:
   A. Alar lamina
   B. Basal lamina
   C. Neural crest cells
   D. Notochord

5. Alar lamina of mesencephalon forms all, *except*:
   A. Colliculi
   B. Red nucleus
   C. Substantia nigra
   D. Olivary nuclei

6. A newborn presents with a sac-like protrusion at the base of the skull. Imaging reveals that the protrusion contains both meninges and brain tissue. Which congenital anomaly does this describe?
   A. Spina bifida occulta
   B. Encephalocele
   C. Anencephaly
   D. Myelomeningocele

7. A prenatal ultrasound at 20 weeks gestation reveals a fetus with severe hydramnios and an absent cranial vault. What is the likely diagnosis?
   A. Meningocele
   B. Spina bifida
   C. Anencephaly
   D. Dandy-Walker syndrome

8. A newborn is diagnosed with a congenital defect where a cystic swelling contains both spinal cord and meninges. This defect is commonly associated with hydrocephalus and cerebellar herniation. What is the diagnosis?
   A. Spina bifida occulta
   B. Meningocele
   C. Myelomeningocele
   D. Rachischisis

9. A child presents with developmental delay and motor deficits. MRI shows enlargement of the fourth ventricle and agenesis of the cerebellar vermis. What congenital condition is most likely responsible?
   A. Dandy-Walker syndrome
   B. Arnold-Chiari malformation
   C. Syringomyelia
   D. Hydrocephalus

10. A newborn has a small dimple covered with a tuft of hair over the lumbosacral region. No neurological deficits are present, and the spinal cord is found to be intact on imaging. What is the diagnosis?
    A. Meningocele
    B. Myelomeningocele
    C. Spina bifida occulta
    D. Anencephaly

Answers:
1. B   2. C   3. C   4. B   5. D
6. B   7. C   8. C   9. A   10. C

Pituitary, Pineal and Adrenal Glands

COMPETENCIES COVERED/LEARNING OUTCOMES	
The student should be able to:	
AN43.4	Describe the development and developmental basis of congenital anomalies of pituitary gland and thyroid gland.
AN52.1	Microanatomical structure of suprarenal gland.

In this chapter, we will consider the development of three endocrine glands, pituitary gland (hypophysis cerebri), pineal gland and adrenal gland, the development of these closely connected with that of the nervous system.

HYPOPHYSIS CEREBRI/PITUITARY GLAND

The hypophysis cerebri, or pituitary gland, develops from two distinct sources: surface ectoderm and neuroectoderm.

- The *adenohypophysis (anterior pituitary)* originates from an ectodermal diverticulum that grows upward from the roof of the stomodeum (primitive mouth) just in front of the buccopharyngeal membrane, called *Rathke's pouch* **(Fig. 23.1A)**.
- Rathke's pouch appears in the 3rd week of intrauterine life, extends upward toward the developing diencephalic floor, loses contact with the surface epithelium by the 2nd month, and separates from the stomodeum **(Figs. 23.1B to D)**. The cavity of the pouch remains after birth as an intraglandular cleft.
- The *neurohypophysis (posterior pituitary)* develops from a downgrowth from the floor of the 3rd ventricle (diencephalon) in the infundibulum region **(Figs. 23.1B and C)** during the 6th week. This downgrowth (infundibular process) contacts and fuses with the posterior aspect of Rathke's pouch **(Figs. 23.1D and E)**, which is critical for pituitary development.
- The anterior wall of Rathke's pouch proliferates significantly to form the *pars anterior (pars distalis)* of the hypophysis, while the posterior wall remains thin and forms the pars intermedia. The original cleft of Rathke's pouch separates these two parts. Some cells of the anterior part grow upward along the infundibular stalk to form the *tuberal part (pars tuberalis)* of the hypophysis **(Fig. 23.1E)**.
- The infundibular process forms the *infundibular stalk and posterior lobe (pars nervosa)* of the neurohypophysis. The cavity of the infundibulum remains as the infundibular recess of the 3rd ventricle. Although the posterior lobe is neuroectodermal in origin, it does not contain nerve cells but mainly neuroglial cells and is penetrated by nerve fibers originating from hypothalamic nuclei.
- Rathke's pouch constricts at its base, separates from the stomodeum, and moves closer to the neurohypophysis. As the mouth and pharynx form, the original site of Rathke's pouch attachment to the stomodeum shifts to the roof of the nasopharynx, corresponding to the junction of the nasal septum and palate.
- **Acidophil cells** develop in the pars anterior during the 3rd month of intrauterine life, followed by other cells. During pituitary development, six different cell types develop from Rathke's pouch, forming the pars anterior and pars intermedia. Despite its neuroectodermal origin, the posterior lobe does not contain neurons; its cells are neuroglial (pituicytes) and are traversed by nerve fibers from the hypothalamus **(Fig. 23.1F)**.

Clinical correlation

Anomalies of Pituitary Gland
- **Craniopharyngiomas:** The original track of Rathke's pouch is known as the craniopharyngeal canal. Detachment of Rathke's pouch from the roof of the stomodeum forms the adenohypophysis. Remnants of Rathke's pouch can sometimes develop into brain tumors called craniopharyngiomas, which are found near the sphenoid bone and the roof of the nasopharynx. These tumors are most commonly seen in children but can also occur in adults in their 50s and 60s. The features are headache, excessive thirst, weight gain and blurring of vision.
- **Pharyngeal hypophysis:** Accessory anterior lobe tissue found in relation to the posterior wall of the pharynx.
- **Pituitary agenesis/hypoplasia:** In rare cases, the hypophysis may fail to develop (agenesis) or may be underdeveloped (hypoplasia).
- **Pharyngeal hypophysis:** The gland may be located in the roof of the nasopharynx.

Chapter 23: Pituitary, Pineal and Adrenal Glands

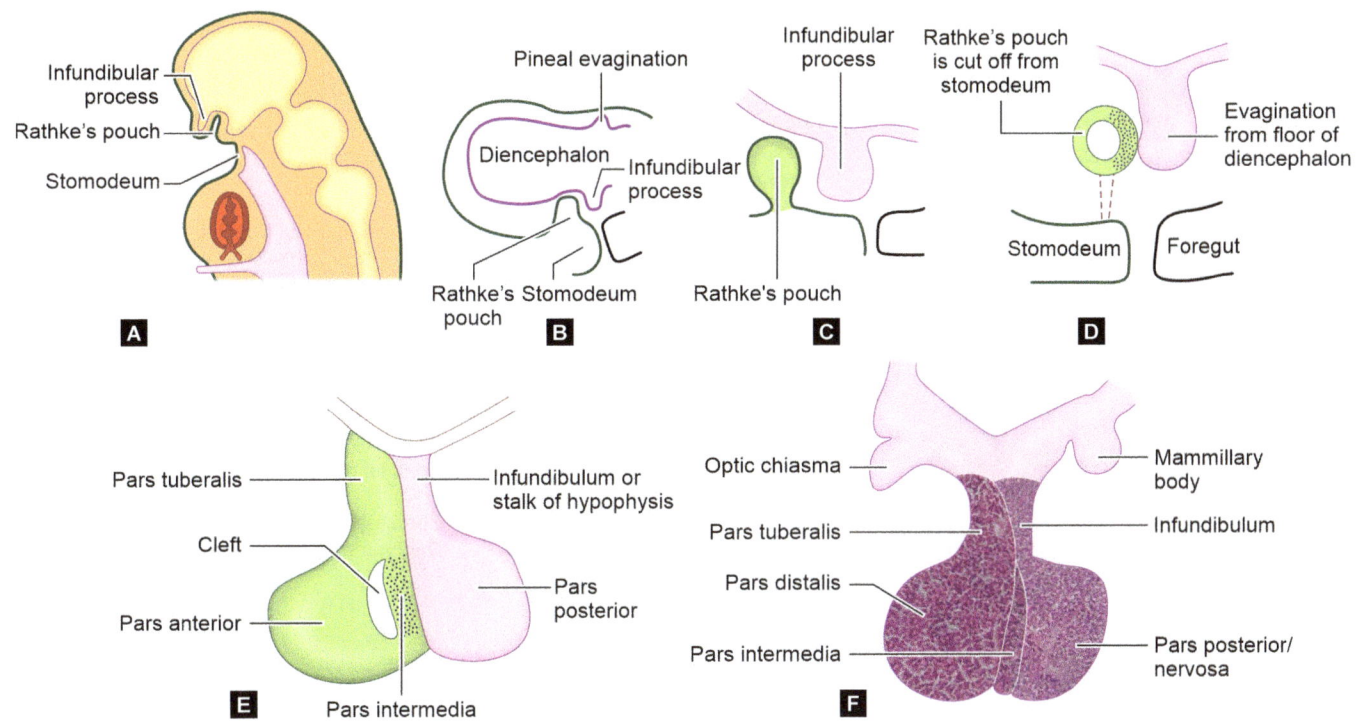

FIGS. 23.1A to F: Development of hypophysis cerebri. (A) Rathke's pouch and infundibular process; (B and C) Approximation of the two developmental components of pituitary gland; (D) Rathke's pouch separating from stomodeum; (E) Closely placed developmental components and their subdivisions; (F) Microscopic appearance of pars anterior, intermedia, and posterior.

PINEAL GLAND/EPIPHYSIS CEREBRI

The pineal gland (or pineal body) arises as an diverticulum from the roof of the diencephalon **(Figs. 23.1B and 23.2A)**. The outgrowth is at first hollow but later becomes solid **(Figs. 23.2B and C)**.

The specific cells of the pineal body are believed to be modified neuroglial cells. For long considered to be a vestigial structure of no importance, the pineal gland is now known to secrete a number of hormones that have a regulatory influence on many other endocrine glands.

ADRENAL GLAND/SUPRARENAL GLAND

The adrenal gland consists of a superficial cortex and a deeper medulla. The cells of the *cortex* arise from the coelomic epithelium (intermediate mesoderm). The cells of medulla are derived from the neural crest cells (ectoderm). The adrenal gland begins to develop in the 5th week of intrauterine life.

- The cells of the cortex arise from the coelomic epithelium that lies in the angle between the developing gonad and the attachment of the mesentery **(Fig. 23.3A)**. The cells arising from the coelomic epithelium may be divided into two groups:
  1. The cells that are formed first are large and are acidophils. They surround the cells of the medulla, and form the *fetal cortex* **(Figs. 23. 3B to D)**. The fetal cortex disappears after birth.
  2. Subsequently, the coelomic epithelium gives origin to smaller cells that surround the fetal cortex. These smaller cells form the *definitive cortex* **(Figs. 23.3C and D)**. According to some authorities, the cells of the fetal cortex are incorporated into the reticular zone of the definitive cortex.
- The differentiation of cortical zones **(Fig. 23.3D)** begins during the late fetal period. The zona glomerulosa and zona fasciculata are present at birth but the zona reticularis becomes recognizable at the end of the third year.
- The suprarenal of the human fetus is almost of the same size as that of the adult. It is quite large as compared to the fetal kidney. The size of the gland (particularly of fetal cortex) becomes smaller during the first year of postnatal life.

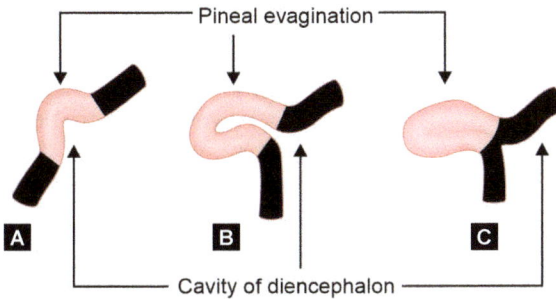

FIGS. 23.2A to C: Development of pineal gland.

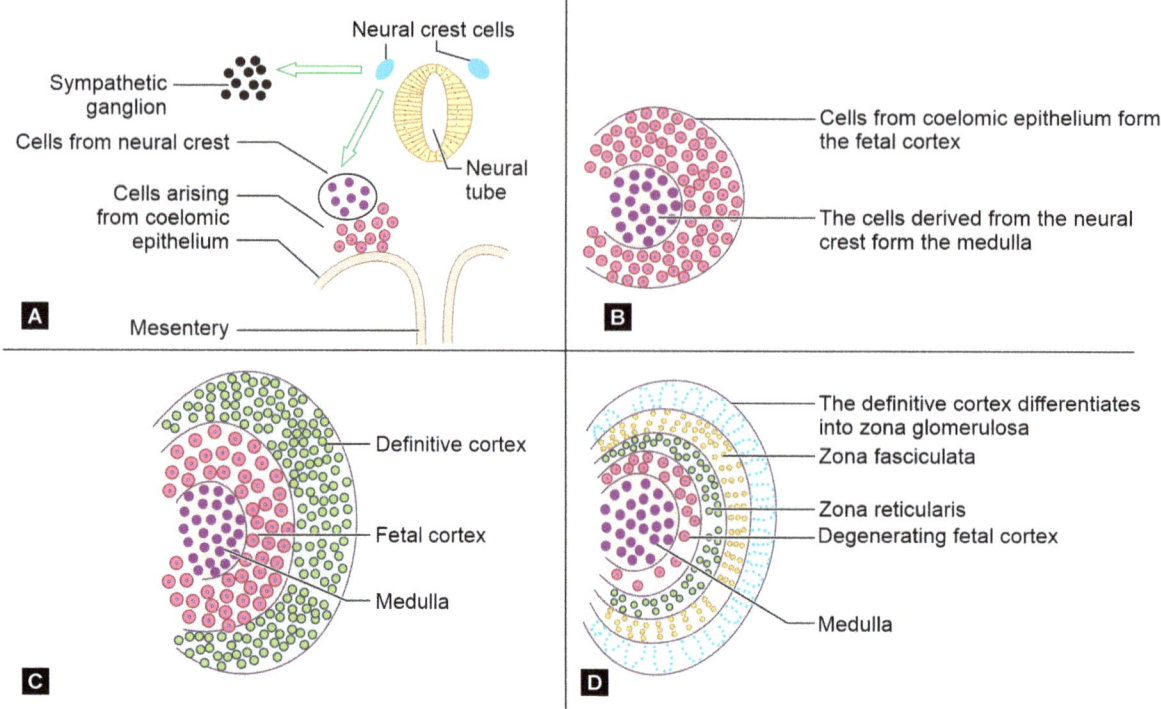

FIGS. 23.3A to D: Stages in the development of adrenal gland. (A) Contributions from coelomic epithelium and neural crest cells; (B) Formation of fetal cortex and medulla; (C) Formation of definitive cortex; (D) Differentiation of various zones of definitive cortex.

- The cells of the medulla are derived from the neural crest. They are similar to the postganglionic sympathetic neurons (cells of sympathetic ganglia). Preganglionic sympathetic neurons terminate in relation to them. These cells migrate to the region of the developing cortical cells and come to be surrounded by them.

Clinical correlation

Anomalies of Adrenal Gland
- **Ectopic adrenal gland:** Adrenal cortical tissue may be present at various ectopic sites. The entire adrenal may be ectopic and may lie deep in the capsule of the kidney. It may be fused to the liver or the kidney. This can lead to hormonal imbalances depending on the functional capacity of the ectopic tissue.
- **Congenital hyperplasia (over development) of the cortex:** CAH is a genetic disorder caused by enzyme deficiencies in the adrenal steroidogenesis pathway, leading to excessive production of androgens and insufficient cortisol.
- In the male, this leads to the *adrenogenital syndrome marked* by very early development of secondary sexual characters. In the female, it may cause enlargement of the clitoris and the child may be mistaken for a male *(pseudohermaphroditism)*.

Chromaffin Tissue

Chromaffin tissue is made up of cells similar to those of the adrenal medulla, and is derived from the cells of the neural crest. This tissue is to be seen in relation to the abdominal aorta where it forms the para-aortic bodies (*refer* **Fig. 22.6**). It is also seen in relation to sympathetic ganglia and plexuses and along the splanchnic nerves (*refer* **Fig. 22.6**).

Clinical correlation

Pheochromocytoma is a tumor of the adrenal medulla that arises from chromaffin cells, which are derived from neural crest cells during embryonic development. These tumors typically secrete catecholamines, leading to symptoms such as hypertension, palpitations, and anxiety. The embryological basis lies in the differentiation of neural crest cells into sympathoblasts, which form the adrenal medulla and sympathetic ganglia.

TIMETABLE OF THE EVENTS DESCRIBED IN THIS CHAPTER

Age	Developmental events
3rd week	Infundibular diverticulum develops in the floor of 3rd ventricle
4th week	Rathke's pouch projects from the roof of stomatodeum
5th week	Adrenal gland begins to develop
8th week	Rathke's pouch loses its connection with the oral cavity

Chapter 23: Pituitary, Pineal and Adrenal Glands

HIGHLIGHTS

- Endocrine gland is a ductless gland. Its cells secrete the substance called hormone, which is directly poured into the blood and transported to the target organ through circulation where it exerts its physiological function.
- The major endocrine glands of the body are *pituitary, pineal, adrenal, thyroid,* and *parathyroid*. The others are islets of *Langerhans* in pancreas, *gonads*, and *hypothalamus*.
- The endocrine glands develop from all three germ layers.
- They produce steroid hormones. Those developing from ectoderm or endoderm secrete amines.
- The pituitary gland develops from two different components. The *adenohypophysis* develops from a diverticulum extending upward from the roof of stomodeum called Rathke's pouch. The *neurohypophysis* develops from a downgrowth called infundibular process arising from the floor of the 3rd ventricle.
- The *pineal gland* develops as a diverticulum from the roof of the 3rd ventricle (diencephalon).
- The adrenal gland develops from two different sources. The *adrenal cortex* is derived from coelomic epithelium. The cells of the *adrenal medulla* are derived from the neural crest.

TEST YOUR UNDERSTANDING

REVIEW QUESTIONS

1. Explain the development of pituitary gland.
2. Explain the development of adrenal gland.
3. Write short note on craniopharyngioma.
4. Write short note on pheochromocytoma.
5. Write short note on congenital adrenal hyperplasia.

MULTIPLE CHOICE QUESTIONS

1. Which structure gives rise to the anterior pituitary gland during embryonic development?
   A. Infundibulum
   B. Rathke's pouch
   C. Neuroectoderm
   D. Surface ectoderm

2. The adrenal cortex develops from which embryological layer?
   A. Endoderm
   B. Ectoderm
   C. Mesoderm
   D. Neural crest

3. Chromaffin cells of the adrenal medulla are derived from which of the following embryonic origins?
   A. Neural crest cells
   B. Mesoderm
   C. Ectoderm
   D. Endoderm

4. During the development of the pituitary gland, the posterior pituitary (neurohypophysis) forms from a downgrowth of which structure?
   A. Rathke's pouch
   B. Third ventricle
   C. Diencephalon
   D. Stomodeum

5. What condition may arise from remnants of Rathke's pouch in the region of the sphenoid bone?
   A. Adrenal hyperplasia
   B. Pheochromocytoma
   C. Craniopharyngioma
   D. Ectopic adrenal gland

Answers: 1. B   2. C   3. A   4. C   5. C

24
The Eye and Ear

COMPETENCIES COVERED/LEARNING OUTCOMES

The student should be able to:

AN43.4 Describe the development and developmental basis of congenital anomalies of eye.

There are five sensory organs in the human body. We have studied about nose, tongue and skin in previous chapters.

Eyes and ears are essential for vision and hearing. The eyes develop from the optic vesicles, lens placode, and neural ectoderm, forming complex structures like the retina, lens, and optic nerve. The ears arise from the otic placodes and pharyngeal arches, giving rise to components such as the cochlea for hearing and the semicircular canals for balance.

DEVELOPMENT OF THE EYE

As stated above, eyes are the essential sense organ for vision. The various structures of eyes are eyeball, eyelids, muscles, retina, lens, lacrimal apparatus, optic nerve and refractive media.

The various components of the eyeball are derived from the following primordia:

1. Neuroectodermal outgrowth from the prosencephalon called the *optic vesicle*, from which retina, iris, optic nerve forms.
2. A specialized area of surface ectoderm called the *lens placode* that gives rise to the lens and corneal epithelium.
3. The mesoderm surrounding the optic vesicle which gives rise to fibrous and vascular coats of eye.
4. Neural crest cells that migrate in the region that forms choroid, sclera and corneal epithelium.

Formation of the Optic Vesicle

- During day 22 of IUL (8th somite stage), the region of the neural plate **(Figs. 24.1A to E)** destined to form the prosencephalon shows a linear thickened area on either side **(Fig. 24.1B)**.
- This area soon becomes depressed to form the *optic sulcus* **(Fig. 24.1C)**.
- Meanwhile, the neural plate becomes converted into the prosencephalic vesicle. As the optic sulcus deepens, the wall of the prosencephalon overlying the sulcus bulges outwards to form the *optic vesicle* **(Figs. 24.1D and E)**.
- The proximal part of the optic vesicle becomes constricted, and elongated, to form the *optic stalk* **(Figs. 24.2A to C)**.

Formation of the Lens Vesicle

- As the optic vesicle grows laterally, it comes into relation with the surface ectoderm. An area of

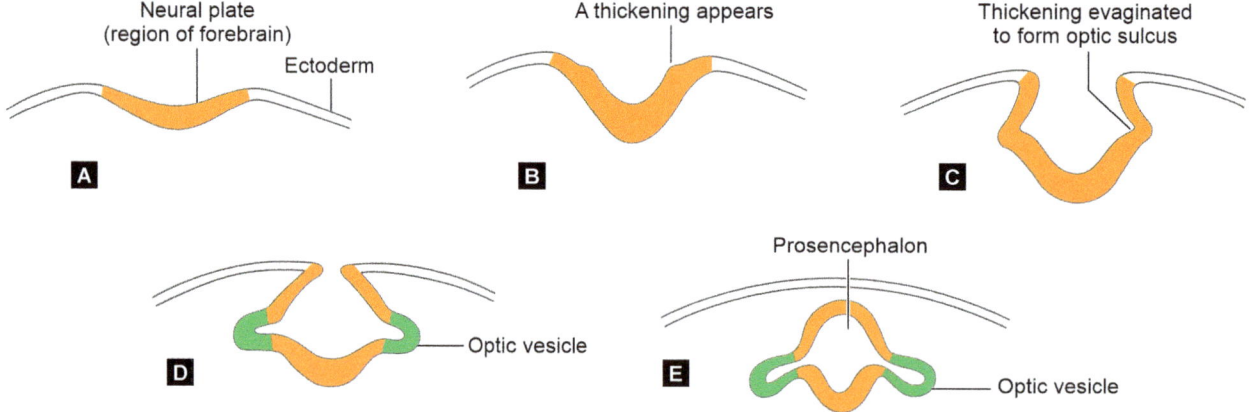

FIGS. 24.1A to E: Formation of the optic vesicle.

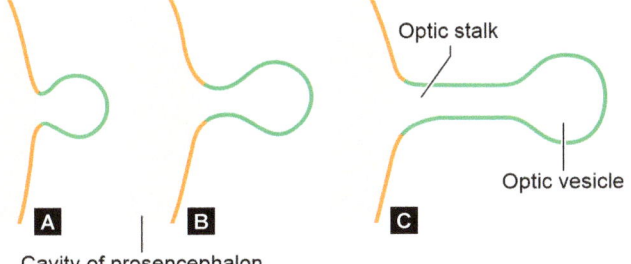

FIGS. 24.2A to C: Formation of the optic stalk.

this surface ectoderm, overlying the optic vesicle, becomes thickened to form the **lens placode** (Fig. 24.3A).

* The lens placode soon sinks below the surface to form **lens pit** and is gradually convened into the **lens vesicle** (Figs. 24.3A to D).
* At the 33rd day, the lens vesicle becomes completely separated from the surface ectoderm.

Formation of the Optic Cup

* While the lens vesicle is forming, the optic vesicle becomes converted into a double-layered **optic cup** (Figs. 24.3A to D).
* The optic cup is not formed by the invagination of the developing lens into the optic vesicle. Instead, the transformation of the optic vesicle into the optic cup results from the differential growth of the optic vesicle wall.
* The margins of the cup grow over the upper and lateral sides of the lens to enclose it. However, such overgrowth does not take place on the inferior aspect of the lens, as a result of which the wall of the cup shows a deficiency in this situation. This deficiency extends for some distance along the inferior surface of the optic stalk and is called the **choroidal or fetal fissure** (Fig. 24.4). This is also referred as **retinal or optic fissure**.
* Hyaloid vessels develops in choroid fissure supplying optic cup which later degenerate and only proximal part persists as central artery and vein of retina.
* The developing neural tube is surrounded by mesoderm, which subsequently condenses to form the meninges. An extension of this mesoderm covers the optic vesicle. Later, this mesoderm differentiates to form a **superficial fibrous layer** corresponding to the dura mater, and a **deeper vascular layer** corresponding to the pia-arachnoid.
* With the formation of the optic cup, part of the inner vascular layer is carried into the cup, through the choroidal fissure (Fig. 24.5A).
* With the closure of fissure during 7th week, the mesenchyme inside the optic cup gives rise to hyaloid vessels.
* The outer fibrous layer surrounding the anterior part of the optic cup forms the **cornea**. The corresponding vascular layer forms the iridopupillary membrane, which attaches to the anterior part of the optic cup and forms the **iris**.

Derivation of Parts of the Eyeball

The derivation of the various parts of the eyeball can now be summarized as follows **(Table 24.1)**:

Lens

* The **lens** is formed during 7th week from the lens vesicle.
* The vesicle is at first lined by a single layer of cubical cells (Fig. 24.6A).
* The cells in the anterior wall of the vesicle remain cubical. Those in the posterior wall gradually become

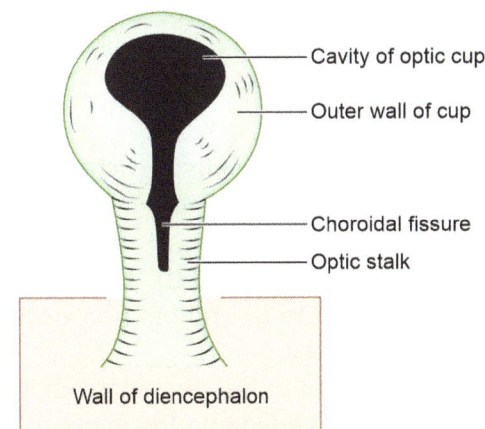

FIG. 24.4: Optic cup and stalk seen from below to show the choroidal fissure.

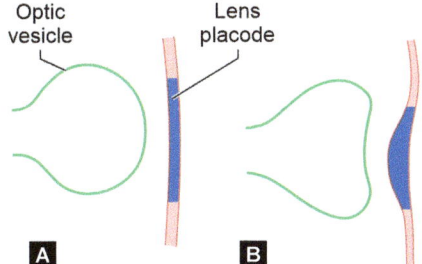
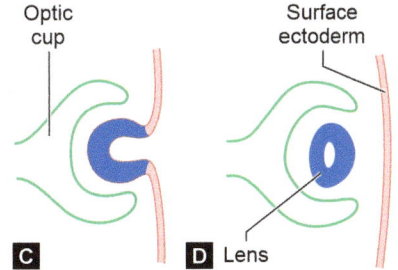

FIGS. 24.3A to D: Development of the lens vesicle and its invagination into the optic cup.

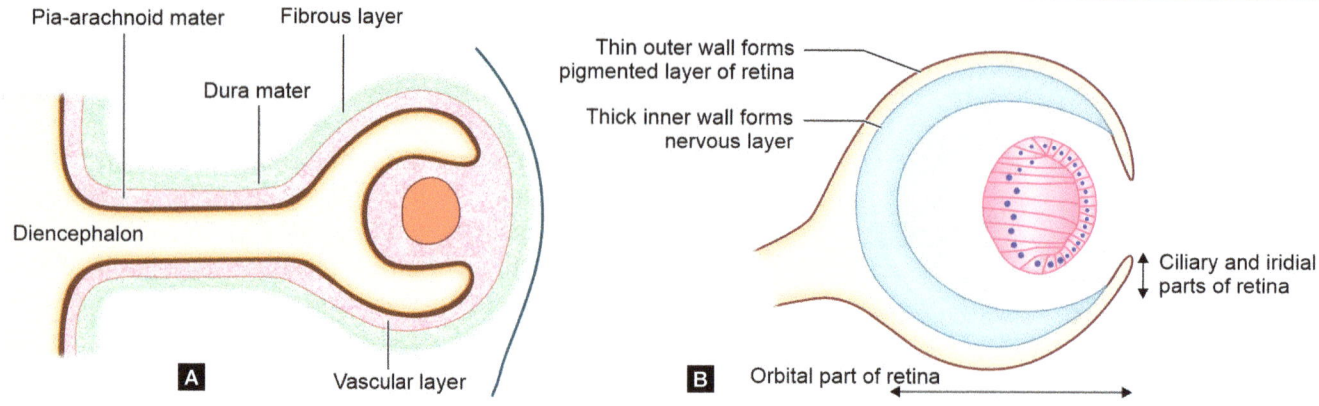

FIGS. 24.5A and B: (A) Developing optic cup surrounded by extensions of pia-arachnoid and dura mater; (B) Subdivisions of the optic cup.

TABLE 24.1: Summary of derivation of various part of the eye ball.

Part	Derived from
Lens	Surface ectoderm
Retina	Neuroectoderm (optic cup)
Vitreous	Mesoderm
Choroid	Mesoderm (infiltrated by neural crest cells?)
Ciliary body	Mesoderm
Ciliary muscles	Mesenchymal cells covering the developing ciliary body (neural crest?)
Iris	Mesoderm
Muscles of iris	Neuroectoderm (from optic cup)
Sclera	Mesoderm (infiltrated by neural crest cells?)
Cornea	Surface epithelium by ectoderm, substantia propria and inner epithelium by neural crest
Conjunctiva	Surface ectoderm
Blood vessels	Mesoderm
Optic nerve	Neuroectoderm. Its coverings (pia, arachnoid and dura) are derived from mesoderm

elongated **(Figs. 24.6B and C)**. As they do so the cavity of the vesicle is encroached upon and is eventually obliterated.

- The elongated cells of the posterior wall lose their nuclei and are converted into the fibers of the lens. The anterior layer remains as the epithelium covering this aspect of the lens.

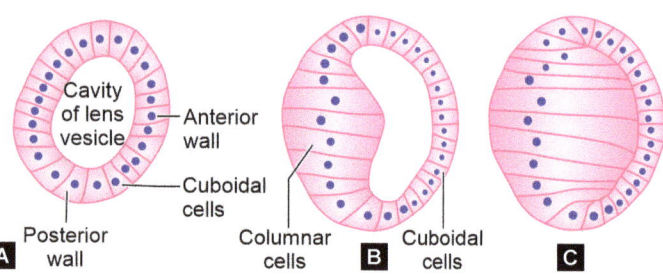

FIGS. 24.6A to C: Stages in the formation of the lens of the eye.

- Cells in the equatorial region of the lens form secondary lens fibers, increasing the lens's diameter during childhood, while the primary lens fibers become harder.
- Initially supplied by the hyaloid artery, the lens becomes an avascular structure after the distal part of the artery degenerates.

Retina

- The *retina* is derived from the layers of the optic cup.
- The optic cup is divisible into anterior and posterior parts.
    - The larger posterior part, becomes thick, and forms the retina proper *(optical part of retina)*.
    - The anterior part remains thin, and forms an epithelial covering for the ciliary body and iris *(ciliary and iridial parts of retina* **(Fig. 24.5B)**.
- The outer wall of the posterior part of the optic cup remains thin. Its cells form the *pigmented layer* of the retina **(Figs. 24.7A and B)**.
- The inner wall of the cup is called the *nervous layer* and differentiates into matrix cell, mantle and marginal layers as in the neural tube.
    - After giving origin to the cells of the mantle layer, the cells of the matrix layer form the *rods and cones*.
    - The cells of the mantle layer form the *bipolar cells*, the *ganglion cells*, and other neurons of the retina, and also the supporting elements.
    - The axons of the ganglion cells grow into the marginal layer to form the *layer of nerve fibers*.
    - These fibers grow into the optic stalk by passing through the choroidal fissure. The optic stalk, is thus, convened into the *optic nerve* **(Figs. 24.7A and B)**.
- The space between the pigmented and nervous layers is called the intraretinal space, representing the original cavity of the optic cup **(Figs. 24.6A and B)**.

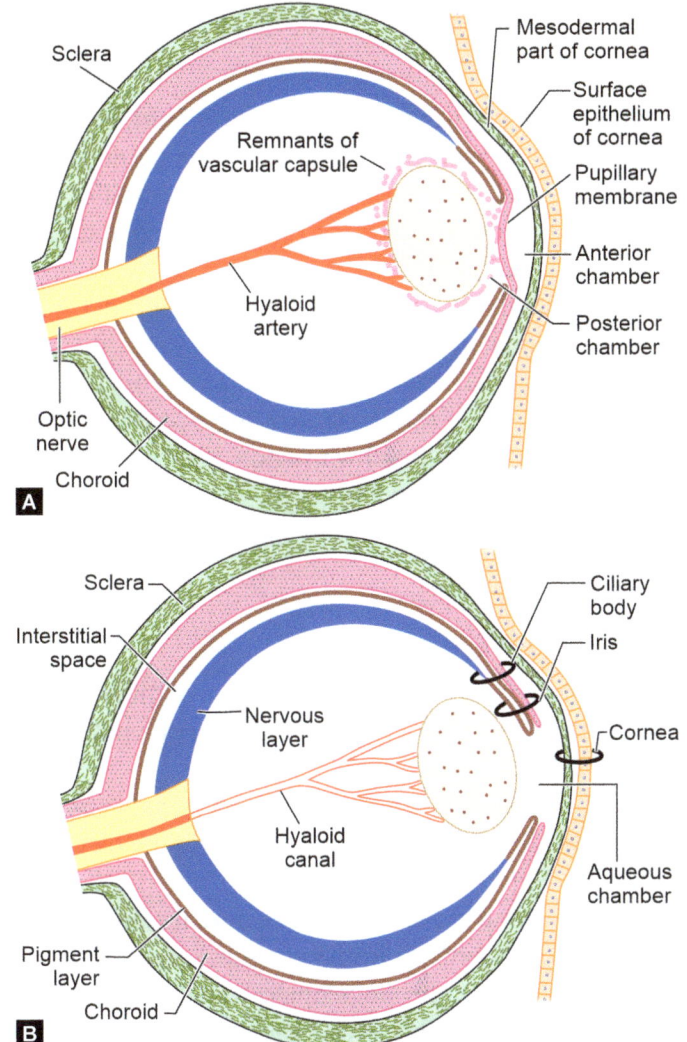

FIGS. 24.7A and B: (A) Derivation of coats of the eyeball. Note pupillary membrane and hyaloid artery. See the layers of retina, remnants of vascular capsule; (B) The hyaloid artery and pupillary membrane have disappeared. Position of artery can be seen as the hyaloid canal.

- Before birth, this space is obliterated by the proliferation of cells of the inner layer, bringing rod and cone cells into contact with the pigment epithelium.

Vitreous Humor

- The *primary vitreous humor* is formed by neural crest mesoderm of optic cup.
- Later, gelatinous *secondary vitreous humor* replaces it, which is derived mainly from ectoderm of optic cup but the lens vesicle may also contribute to it.
- The mesodermal component comes into the optic cup through the choroidal fissure.

Choroid

- The *choroid* is formed from the inner vascular layer of mesoderm that surrounds the optic cup **(Figs. 24.5A and 24.7)**.

- According to some authorities this mesoderm contains cells derived from the neural crest.
- The choroid is continuous with ciliary body anteriorly and with pia-arachnoid around optic nerve posteriorly.

Ciliary Body and Iris

- The mesodermal basis of the *ciliary body and iris* is derived from a forward prolongation of the mesoderm forming the choroid.
- The inner surface of this mesoderm comes to be lined by two layers of pigmented epithelium derived from the ciliary and iridial parts of the retina. The two layers of epithelium correspond to the two layers of the optic cup **(Figs. 24.7A and B)**.
  The *musculature of the iris* (sphincter and dilator pupillae) is of ectodermal origin (neuroectodermal cells of optic cup). The *ciliary muscles* have been generally regarded as mesodermal but the present view is that they are of neural crest origin. The connective tissue of ciliary body is derived from mesoderm.
- The iris, characterized by its color and structure, features a central opening called the *pupil*. Pigment distribution within iris *chromatophores* determines its color: concentrated melanin on the posterior iris surface results in a blue hue, whereas dispersed melanin in the stroma produces a brown coloration.

Sclera

The *sclera* is formed from the posterior part of the outer fibrous layer of mesoderm surrounding the optic cup, and corresponding to the dura **(Figs. 24.5A and 24.7)**. Some researchers believe that (like the choroid) the mesoderm forming the sclera is infiltrated by cells from the neural crest.

Cornea

- The Bowman's layer, substantia propria, Descemet's membrane and inner epithelium of the *cornea* are derived from the neural crest and are formed by the same layer that forms the sclera.
- The superficial surface epithelium of the cornea is derived from the surface ectoderm **(Figs. 24.7A and B)**.

Anterior and Posterior Chambers of Eye

- The *anterior and posterior chambers* of the eye (aqueous chamber) are formed by a splitting of the mesoderm in the region, and correspond to the subarachnoid space of the brain.

- The cavity of the anterior chamber is formed by vacuolization of mesoderm present anterior to the lens.
- Vacuolization splits the mesenchyme into outer (anterior) and inner (posterior) layers.
- The outer layer becomes continuous with the sclera and with the substantia propria of the cornea.
- The inner layer lies in front of lens and iris and is termed the *pupillary membrane* (Fig. 24.7A).
- The mesodermal cells lining the cavity give origin to a flattened mesothelium.

Blood Vessels

- The *blood vessels of the eyeball* are formed in the mesodermal layer that is a continuation of the pia-arachnoid.
- Part of this mesoderm, that gets invaginated into the optic cup, forms the *retinal vessels*. The central artery and vein of the retina at first lie in the choroidal fissure, but come to be buried in the fibers of the developing optic nerve. As the choroidal fissure extends for some distance along the optic stalk, the central artery of the retina runs through the substance of distal part of the optic nerve.
- Initially, the lens is completely surrounded by a vascular capsule. The posterior part of the capsule is supplied by the hyaloid artery (Fig. 24.7A). This artery is a continuation of the central artery of the retina and passes through the vitreous. Later in fetal life, the vascular capsule and the hyaloid artery disappear, but the hyaloid canal in the vitreous (through which the artery passes) persists.
- The anterior part of the vascular capsule of the lens, comes to be lined posteriorly by the iridial part of the retina, and forms the iris (Figs. 24.7A and B). The pupil is for some time closed by a part of this vascular tissue, which is termed the *iridopupillary membrane*. This membrane normally disappears before birth.

Accessory Structures of Eyeball

Eyelids

- The *eyelids* are formed by reduplication of the surface ectoderm above and below the cornea (Figs. 24.8A to D). The ectodermal folds formed contain some mesoderm that gives rise to muscle and to the tarsal plates.
- As the folds enlarge, their margins approach each other. Ultimately, they meet and fuse together.
- The lids thus cut off a space called the *conjunctival sac*. The conjunctiva is, thus, of ectodermal origin.
- The lids remain united with each other until the 7th month of intrauterine life.
- The eyelashes and glands in the eyelids develop from surface ectoderm.

Lacrimal Apparatus

- The *lacrimal gland* is formed from a number of buds that arise from the upper angle of the conjunctival sac (Fig. 24.8D).
- The *lacrimal sac* and *nasolacrimal duct* are derived from the ectoderm of the naso-optic (or nasolacrimal) furrow (Fig. 24.9). This furrow lies along the line of junction of the maxillary process and the lateral nasal process, and extends from the medial angle of the eye to the region of the developing mouth (Fig. 24.10). The ectoderm of the furrow becomes buried to form a solid cord that is subsequently canalized (Figs. 24.11A to C).
- The upper part of this cord forms the *lacrimal sac*. The lower part, acquires a secondary connection to the nasal cavity, and forms the *nasolacrimal duct*.
- The *lacrimal canaliculi* are formed by canalization of ectodermal buds that arise from the margin of each eyelid near its medial end and grow to the lacrimal sac.

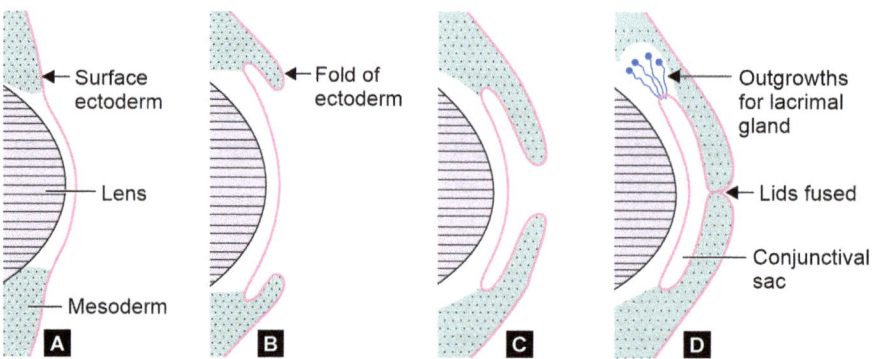

FIGS. 24.8A to D: Formation of eyelids, conjunctival sac and lacrimal gland.

Chapter 24: The Eye and Ear

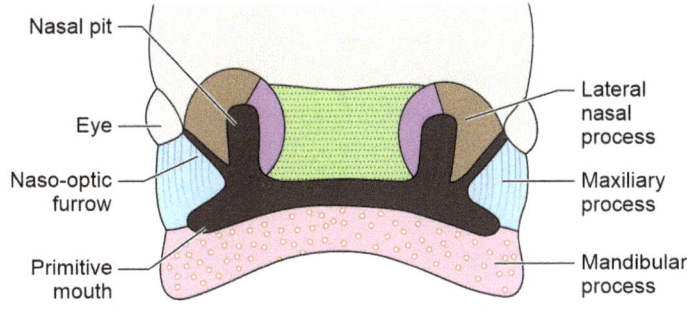

FIG. 24.9: Nasolacrimal (naso-optic) furrow.

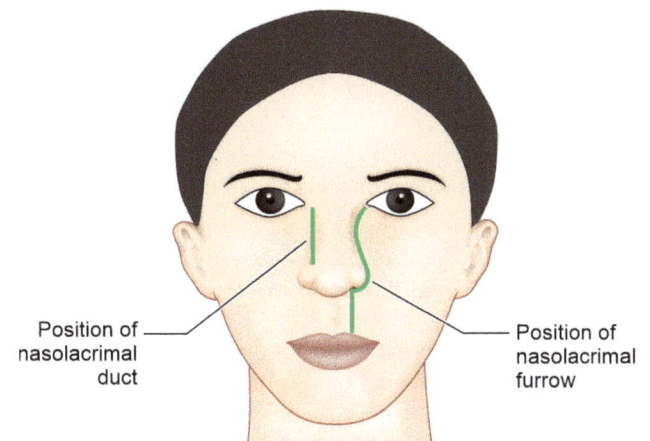

FIG. 24.10: Position of nasolacrimal furrow and of nasolacrimal duct projected on to an adult human face.

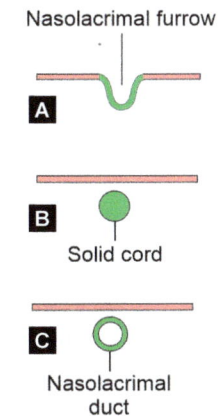

FIGS. 24.11A to C: Formation of nasolacrimal duct.

Extraocular Muscles of Eyeball

They are derived from preoccipital myotomes that are supplied by 3rd, 4th and 6th cranial nerves.

Molecular Regulation of Development of Eye

- The proteins Wnt, BMP, TGF-β, and FGF are responsible for optic vesicle formation, while PAX6 is crucial for lens vesicle differentiation.
- Inhibition of sonic hedgehog (Shh) and expansion of PAX2 expression can lead to cyclopia, a condition where the eyes fail to separate.
- Overexpression of Shh results in the loss of eye structures.
- Vitamin A deficiency during embryonic development can cause anterior segment defects in the cornea and eyelid.

Clinical correlation

Anomalies of Eyeball
- **Anophthalmos:** The entire eyeball may fail to develop due to failure of formation of optic vesicle.
- **Microphthalmos:** The entire eyeball may remain very small. It is generally associated with intrauterine infections.
- **Cyclopia:** The two eyes may fuse completely to form one median eye **(Figs. 24.12A and C)**. This is the recessive inheritance and severely uncommon condition of face.
- **Synophthalmos:** The two eyes may fuse partially **(Fig. 24.12B)**. There will be associated under development of prosencephalon *(holoprosencephaly)* and frontonasal process *(proboscis)* as tubular appendage above median eye.
- The optic vesicle may not be invaginated by the lens and may remain as *a cyst*.
- The various layers of the eye may show anomalies of pigmentation. There may either be too little pigment as in *albinism*, or too much.

Anomalies of Lens
- **Congenital aphakia:** The lens may, very rarely, be absent due to failure of development of lens placode.
- Lens may be very small. It may be abnormal in position or shape.
- **Congenital cataract:** It may show congenital opacities (cataract), may be due to parathyroid deficiency, to avitaminosis or to the infection, German measles (acquired during early pregnancy). Cataract may be genetically determined.

Anomalies of Iris, Sclera, Pupil and Cornea
- The cornea may be absent. It may show anomalies of size and shape, and may also show congenital opacities.
- **Coloboma:** It results from failure of the choroidal fissure to obliterate completely. It may lead to deficiencies (clefts) in various layers of the eyeball including the iris, ciliary body, and choroid **(Fig. 24.13B)**.
- The sclera may be thin with the result that the pigment of the choroid can be seen through it *(blue sclera)*.
- In addition to various types of coloboma, the iris may show anomalies of its histological structure. Very rarely, the sphincter or dilator pupillae muscle may be absent. The pupil may be abnormal in position, shape or size.
- **Congenital aniridia:** This is the complete absence of iris which occurs due to failure of development of rim of optic cup.
- **Persistent pupillary membrane:** The hyaloid artery and the vascular capsule of the lens, or their remnants, may persist. When the capsule persists on the anterior aspect of the lens, it may completely occlude the pupil.

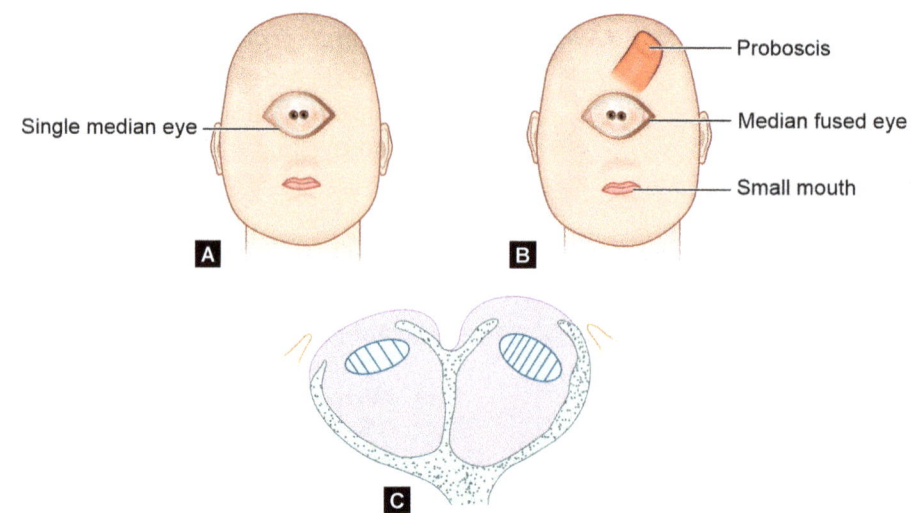

FIGS. 24.12A to C: (A) Synophthalmos (fused median eye); (B) Synophthalmos with proboscis above the median eye; (C) A section through synophthalmos.

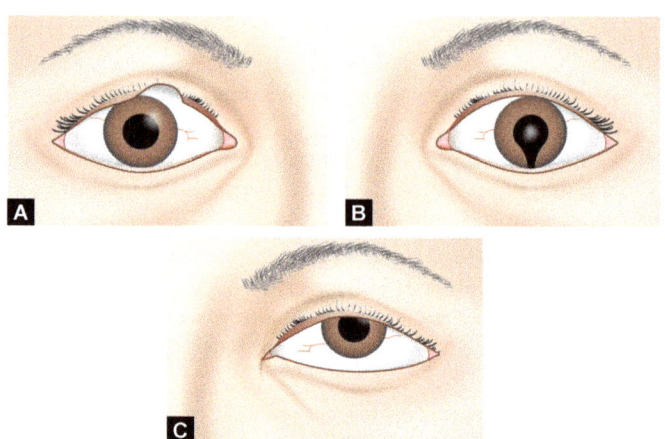

FIGS. 24.13A to C: (A) Coloboma of upper eyelid; (B) Coloboma of iris; (C) Epicanthal fold (Mongolian eye slant).

- **Congenital glaucoma:** It is a rare eye condition present at birth, resulting from abnormal development of the eye's drainage system. This abnormality leads to increased intraocular pressure, which can damage the optic nerve and result in vision loss. This occurs due to the improper development of the trabecular meshwork and anterior chamber angle, hindering aqueous humor drainage and increasing intraocular pressure.

Anomalies of Retina
- The retina may show various congenital anomalies in its structure. These may involve the macula, and may result in visual defects, including those of color vision.
- **Retinal detachment** takes place along the intraretinal space, which is the plane of cleavage between pigment epithelium and nervous layers of retina. This separation, rooted in the incomplete obliteration of the intraretinal space, disrupts the contact between the rod and cone cells and the pigment epithelium, leading to visual impairment.

Anomalies Accessory Structures
- The eyelids may very rarely be absent. In these cases, there is no conjunctival sac. The conjunctiva and the cornea are replaced by skin.

- **Coloboma of eyelid:** Part of the eyelid may be missing (Fig. 24.13A).
- The palpebral fissure may be abnormally wide or narrow. It may be abnormal in orientation and shape. The two lids may be completely, or partially, fused with each other.
- There may be abnormal folds of skin in relation to the lids. Similar folds, e.g., *epicanthus* (Fig. 24.13C) may be a normal feature in certain races.
- The lid margins may be turned inwards *(entropion)* (Fig. 24.14B) or outwards *(ectropion)* (Fig. 24.14C) and rarely, the whole lid may be everted. Normal lid margins are shown in **Figure 24.14A**.
- The levator palpebrae superioris may fail to develop. This leads to drooping of the lids *(ptosis)*.
- The eyelashes, and eyebrows, may be missing, or may be duplicated. The eyelashes may be abnormal in direction.

Anomalies of the Lacrimal Apparatus
- The lacrimal gland may be absent or nonfunctional. The gland may be ectopic in position.
- The lacrimal passages may be absent in whole or in part, or there may be atresia of some part.
- The lacrimal duct may be represented by an open furrow on the face, due to nonobliteration of the naso-optic furrow (*refer oblique facial cleft*, Fig. 14.12A).
- There may be supernumerary puncta, or canaliculi.

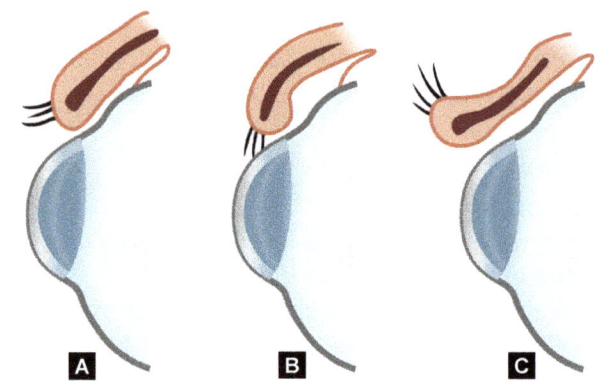

FIGS. 24.14A to C: (A) Normal lid; (B) Entropion; (C) Ectropion.

DEVELOPMENT OF THE EAR

The ear is essential organ for hearing and balance. The three morphological subdivisions of the ear (namely the external, middle and internal ear), each have a separate developmental origin.

Internal Ear

The internal ear is the first part to develop among the three parts of the ear. The developmental components of internal ear are membranous labyrinth and bony labyrinth.

Membranous Labyrinth

- It is derived from a specialized area of surface ectoderm on either side of the developing rhombencephalon. This area is first apparent as a thickening called the *otic placode* (Fig. 24.15A).
- The otic placode soon becomes depressed below the surface to form the *otic pit* (Fig. 24.15B).
- The otic pit then becomes rounded to form the *otic vesicle/otocyst* which separates from the surface ectoderm (Fig. 24.15C).
  The otic vesicle is at first an oval structure. By differential growth of various parts of its wall, it gives rise to the structures comprising the *membranous labyrinth*.
- The otic vesicle divides into *vestibular (dorsal)* and *cochlear (ventral)* components.
- The ventral cochlear part forms the *saccule, cochlear duct (organ of Corti)*, and connects with the *spiral ganglion* of the vestibulocochlear nerve derived from neural crest cells (Figs. 24.16 and 24.17).
- The dorsal part forms the *utricle, semicircular ducts, endolymphatic duct, and sac*, and connects with the *vestibular ganglion* of the vestibulocochlear nerve derived from neural crest cells (Figs. 24.16 and 24.17).
- Localized areas of the epithelium of the membranous labyrinth undergo differentiation to form specialized sensory end organs of hearing, and of equilibrium.
- The equilibrium sensory organs include the *cristae of semicircular ducts* and the *macula of the utricle*.

For hearing, the sensory organs are the *macula of the saccule* and the *organ of Corti* in the cochlea.

- These structures are innervated by peripheral processes from cells in the vestibular and cochlear ganglia, respectively, which originate from neural crest cells. Notably, these ganglion cells retain a bipolar morphology throughout life (Fig. 24.17).

Bony Labyrinth

- The *bony labyrinth* is formed from the mesenchyme surrounding the membranous labyrinth (Fig. 24.18A). This mesenchyme becomes condensed to form the *otic capsule*. The mesenchymal condensation is soon converted into cartilage.
- Between this cartilage and the membranous labyrinth, there is a layer of loose periotic tissue (Fig. 24.18B).
- The spaces of the bony labyrinth are created by the disappearance of this periotic tissue (Fig. 24.18C). The membranous labyrinth is filled with a fluid called *endolymph*, while the periotic spaces surrounding it are filled with *perilymph*.
- The periotic tissue, around the utricle and saccule, disappears to form a space called the *vestibule* (Fig. 24.19). The periotic tissue, around the semicircular ducts also disappears to form the *semicircular canals*.
- Two distinct spaces are formed, one on either side of the cochlear duct. These are the *scala tympani* and the *scala vestibuli*. The scala vestibuli communicates with the vestibule while the scala tympani grows towards the tympanic cavity, from which it remains separated by a membrane (Fig. 24.19).
- The cartilaginous labyrinth is subsequently, ossified to form the bony labyrinth (Fig. 24.18D).

Middle Ear

- The epithelial lining of the middle ear and of the pharyngotympanic tube is derived from the *tubotympanic recess*. This recess develops from

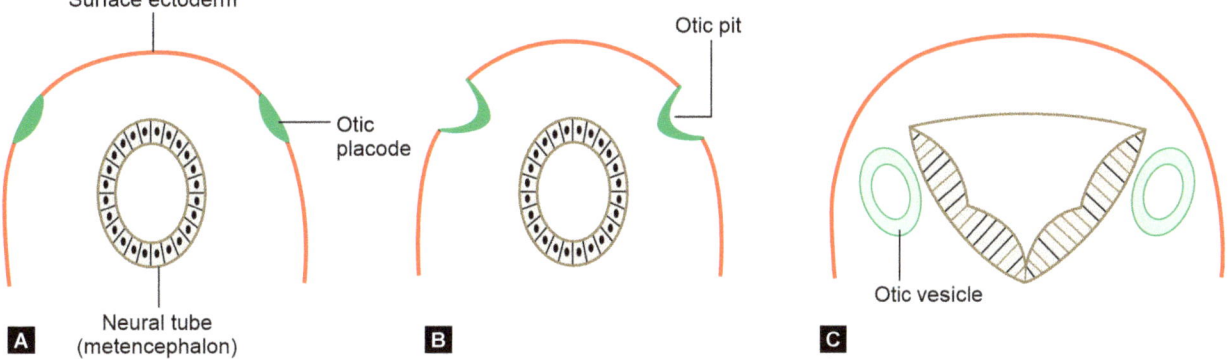

FIGS. 24.15A to C: Three stages in the formation of the otic vesicle.

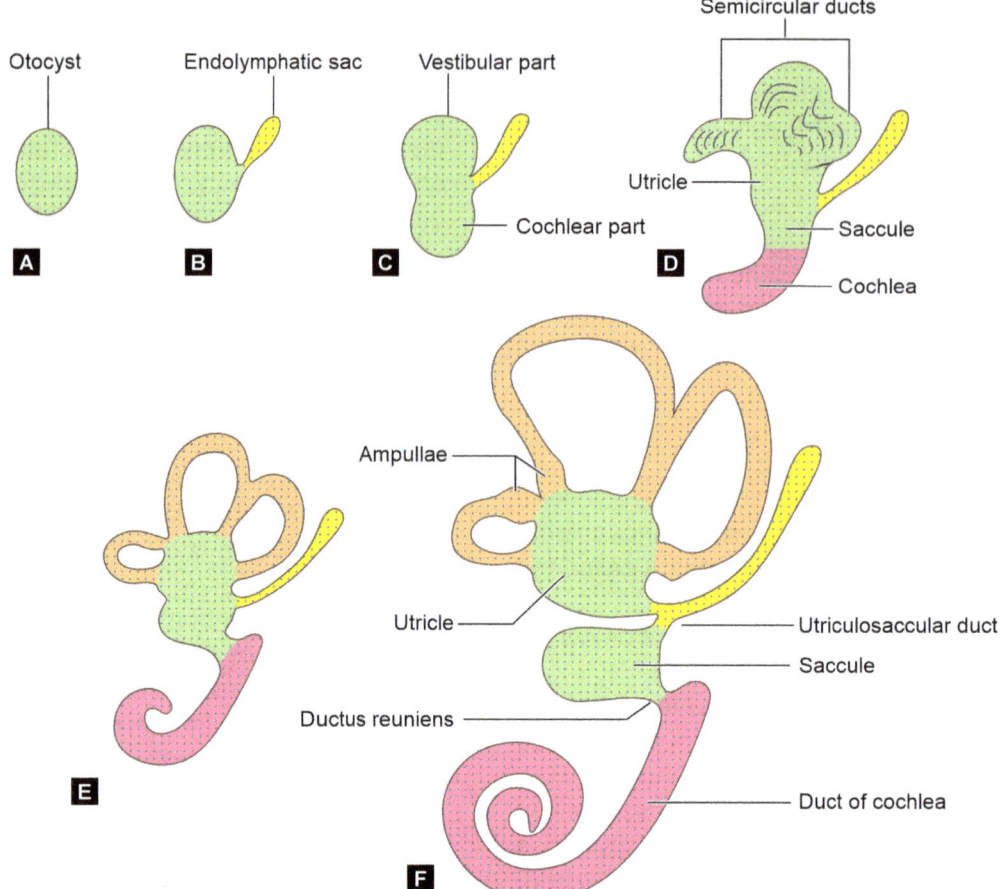

FIGS. 24.16A to F: Gradual transformation of a rounded otic vesicle to the highly complicated form of the membranous labyrinth. (A) Otocyst; (B) Formation of endolymphatic sac; (C) Division of otocyst into vestibular and cochlear parts; (D) Division of vestibular part into utricle and semicircular ducts and cochlear part into saccule and cochlear duct; (E and F) Further differentiation of components.

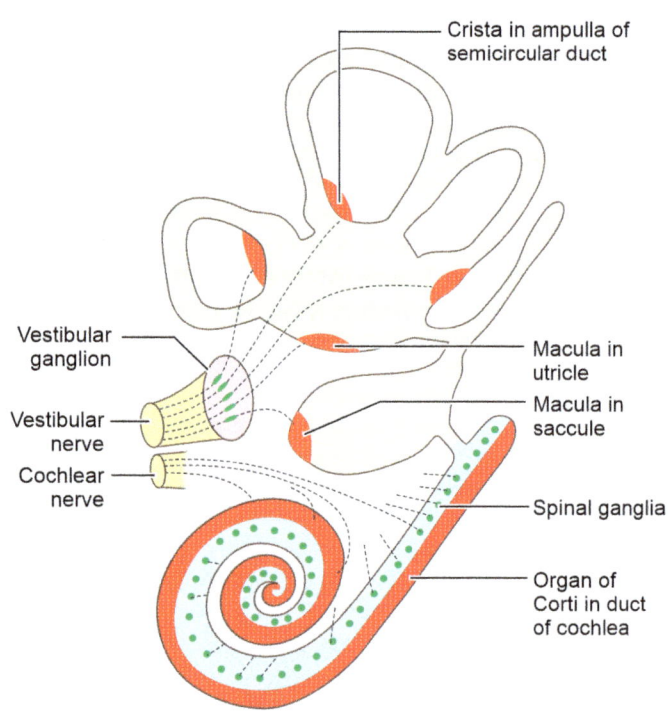

FIG. 24.17: Specialized sensory areas developing in the internal ear and their nerve supply.

the dorsal part of the first pharyngeal pouch, and also receives a contribution from the second pouch **(Figs. 24.20A and B)**.

- The *tympanic antrum*, and *mastoid air cells* are formed by extensions from the middle ear.
- The *malleus* and *incus* are derived from the dorsal end of Meckel's cartilage, while the *stapes* is formed from the dorsal end of the cartilage of the second pharyngeal arch (Reichert's cartilage) **(Figs. 24.21A and B)**.
- The ossicles are at first outside the mucous membrane of the developing middle ear. They invaginate the mucous membrane, which covers them throughout life **(Figs. 24.22A to C)**.
- The ossicles of the ear fully ossify in the 4th month of intrauterine life. They are the first bones in the body to do so.
- The *tensor tympani* is derived from the mesoderm of the first pharyngeal arch and the *stapedius* from that of the second arch.

External Ear

- The *external acoustic meatus* is derived from the dorsal part of the first ectodermal cleft **(Fig. 24.23A)**.

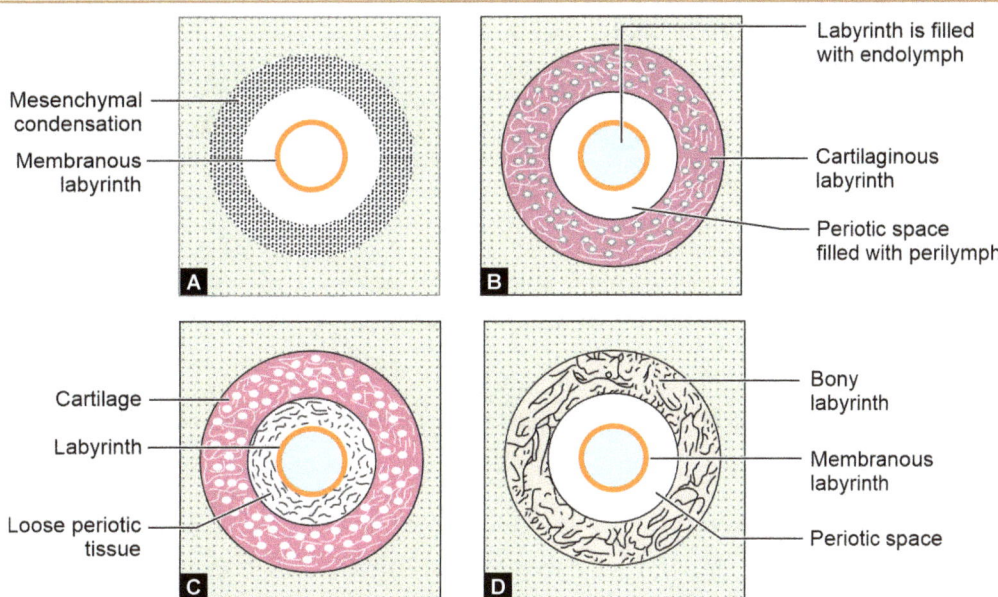

FIGS. 24.18A to D: Establishment of the basic structure of the bony labyrinth.

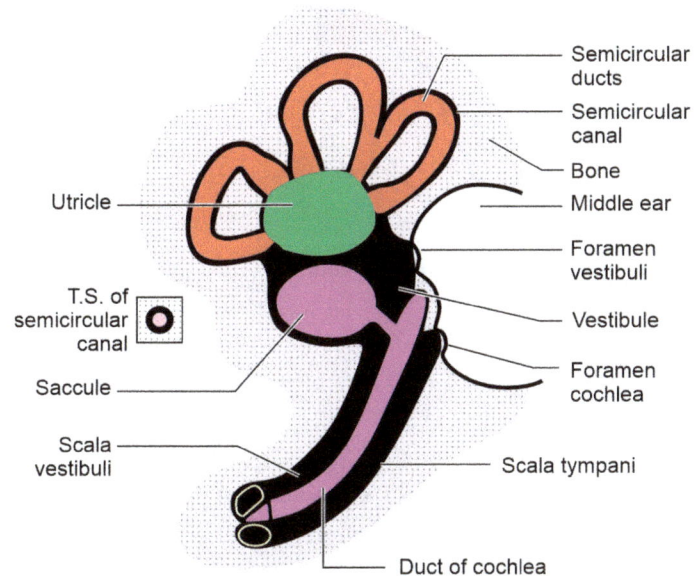

FIG. 24.19: Some parts of bony labyrinth (black) and of membranous labyrinth (red, green and purple).

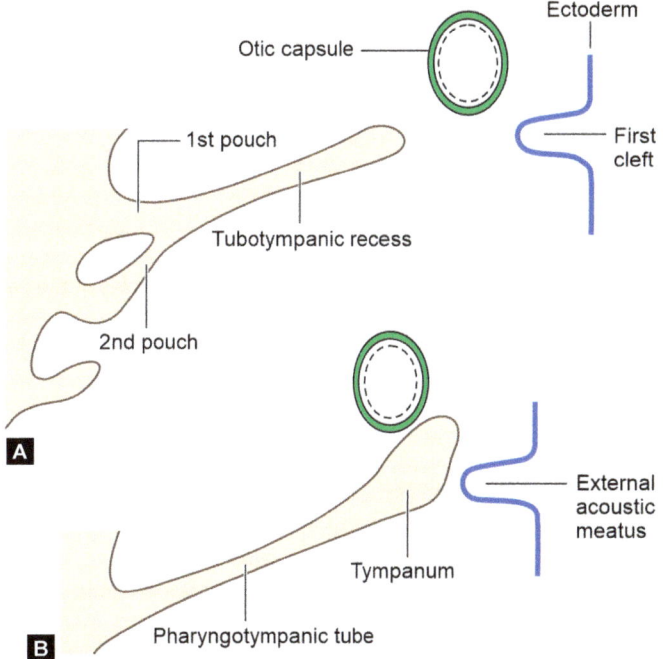

FIGS. 24.20A and B: Development of the middle ear (tympanum). Formation of tubotympanic recess (A), and its subdivision into the tympanum and the Pharyngotympanic tube (B).

- However, its deeper part is formed by proliferation of its lining epithelium, which grows towards the middle ear **(Fig. 24.23B)**.
- This proliferation is at first solid *(meatal plug)*, but is later canalized **(Fig. 24.23C)**.
- The auricle, or *pinna*, is formed from about six mesodermal thickenings (called *tubercles* or *hillocks*) that appear on the mandibular and hyoid arches, around the opening of the dorsal part of the first ectodermal cleft (i.e., around the opening of the external acoustic meatus) **(Figs. 24.24A to D)**.
- The mandibular arch forms only the tragus and a small area around it, the rest of the auricle being formed from the hyoid arch. This is consistent with the fact that the auricular muscles are supplied by the facial nerve.

Tympanic Membrane

This is formed by apposition of the tubotympanic recess and the first ectodermal cleft, these two forming the inner (endodermal) and outer (ectodermal) epithelial linings of the membrane **(Fig. 24.25)**. The intervening mesoderm forms the connective tissue basis.

Two points worth noting are as follows:
1. The handle of the malleus grows into the connective tissue from above.
2. The chorda tympani nerve is at first outside the membrane but comes to lie within its layers, because of upward extension of the membrane.

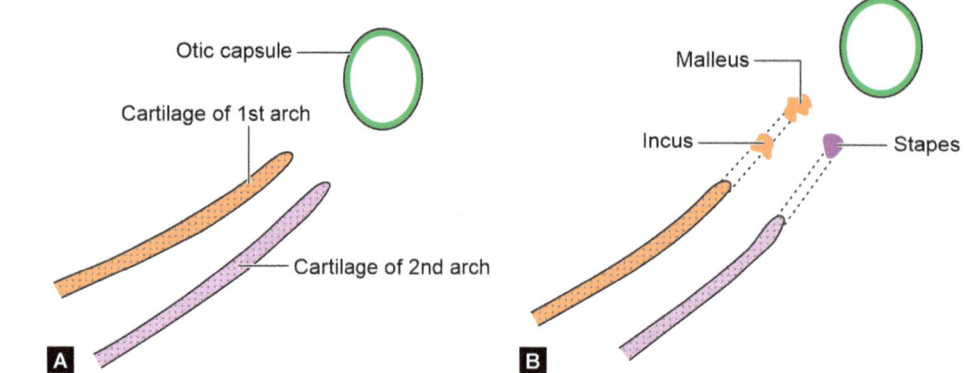

FIGS. 24.21A and B: The ossicles of the middle ear develop from the first and second pharyngeal arches.

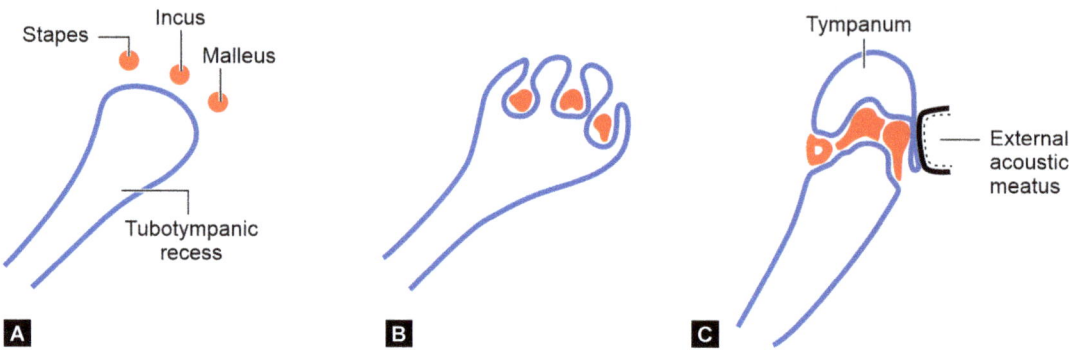

FIGS. 24.22A to C: Ossicles of the ear gradually invaginate into the tympanum.

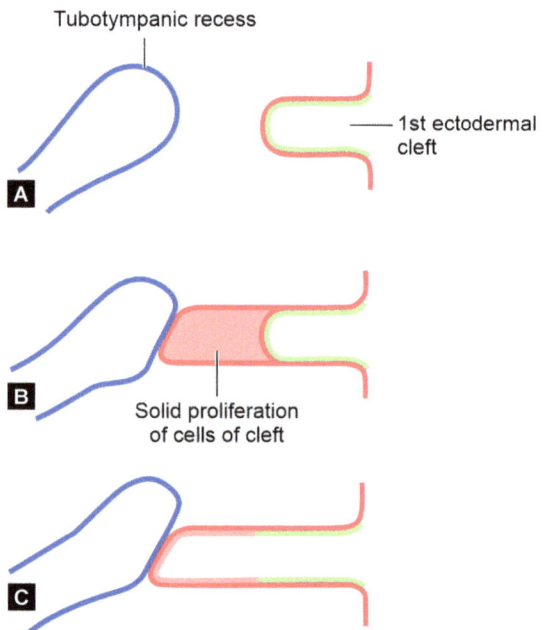

FIGS. 24.23A to C: Development of external acoustic meatus. The solid mass of ectodermal cells seen in (B) has been canalized as seen in (C).

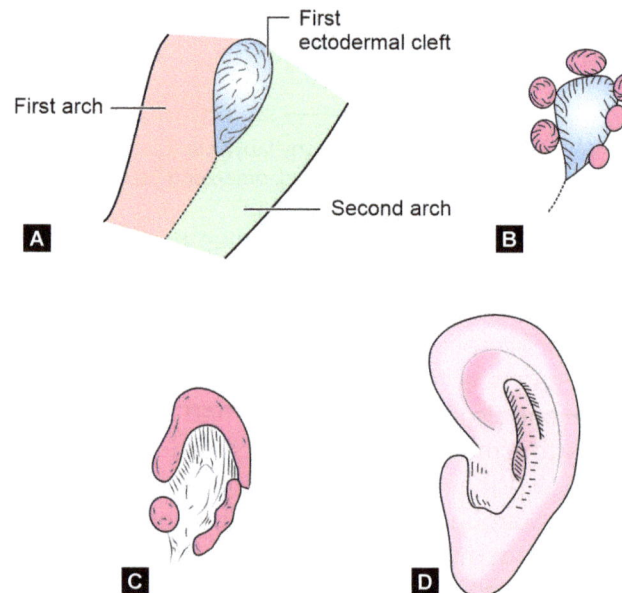

FIGS. 24.24A to D: Development of the auricle: (A) First ectodermal cleft around which the auricle develops; (B) Small swellings or hillocks appear; (C and D) Hillocks gradually fuse with one another to form the auricle.

Molecular Regulation of Development of Ear

- Wnt and BMP are crucial for otic placode formation.
- Retinoic acid influences anteroposterior differentiation of the otic vesicle.
- Wnt and Shh contribute to the development of semicircular canals and cochlear duct.
- Noggin and *PAX2* gene defects are implicated in sensory neural deafness affecting cochlear development.

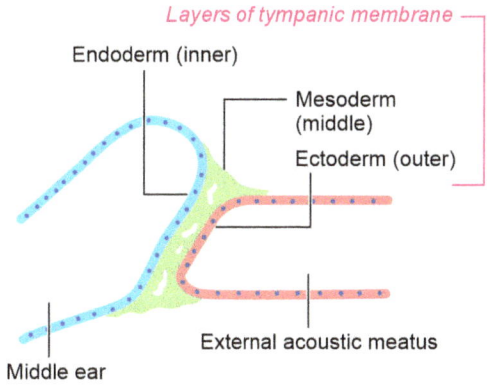

FIG. 24.25: Layers of tympanic membrane.

Clinical correlation

Anomalies of the Auricle
- **Anotia:** The development of the auricle may get arrested at any stage. As a result of this, it may be totally, or partially, absent.
- It may be represented by isolated nodules; or it may be very small. Alternatively, it may be very large.
- **Preauricular appendages:** These are skin tags mostly in preauricular area due to formation of accessory hillocks.
- The migration of the auricle from its primitive caudoventral position may remain incomplete. This migration occurs because of the growth of the maxillary and mandibular processes. This explains the association of caudoventral displacement of the auricle with *mandibulofacial dysostosis*.

Anomalies of the External Auditory Meatus
- There may be *stenosis or atresia* of the meatus over its whole length, or over part of it. The lumen may be closed by fibrous tissue, by cartilage, or by bone. This causes conduction deafness.
- The normal curvature of the meatus may be accentuated as a result of which the tympanic membrane cannot be fully seen from the outside.

Anomalies of the Middle Ear
- The ossicles may be malformed. They may show abnormal fusion to one another or to the wall of the middle ear. The stapes may be fused to the margins of the fenestra vestibuli.
- The facial nerve may bulge into the middle ear and may follow an abnormal course. The stapedial artery may persist.

Anomalies of the Internal Ear
Various parts of the membranous labyrinth may remain underdeveloped. In some cases, the cochlea alone is affected. These anomalies lead to congenital deafness.

TIMETABLE OF SOME EVENTS DESCRIBED IN THIS CHAPTER

Age	Developmental event
Eye	
22nd day	Appearance of optic sulcus (over the neural plate)
4th week	• Optic vesicle comes in contact with surface ectoderm • Lens placode is forming
5th week	Eye primordium is completely surrounded by loose mesenchyme
6th week	• Choroid fissure is formed • Lens vesicle is seen
7th week	A solid lens is formed
The eyeball is most susceptible to teratogens during the 4th to 8th week, and can get affected till the end of pregnancy	
Ear	
22nd day	Otic placode is seen
5th week	Tubotympanic recess develops
6th week	Auricle starts forming. The cochlea and semicircular canals starts forming
7th week	The mesenchymal condensations for three ossicles appear
8th week	The cochlea and semicircular canal assume their definitive external form
10th week	Scala vestibuli and scala tympani appear
7th month	External acoustic meatus gets canalized
The ear is most sensitive to teratogens during the 4th to 9th weeks, and can be affected up to the 12th week	

Case Based Learning

Embryological Basis of Anotia and Atresia of External Auditory Canal

Case Scenario

A female baby presented with a small peanut-like tag of soft tissue representing the right auricle **(Fig. 24.26)** and a normal left auricle. Upon conducting a computed tomography (CT) scan of the fetal head, the following findings were observed:
- Normal auricle and external auditory canal on the left side.
- Absence of auricle and external auditory canal on the right side.
- Bilateral absence of middle ear cavity and ossicles.
- Normal internal auditory canal, cochlea, semicircular canals, mastoid air cells, and VII and VIII nerve complexes on both sides.

Diagnosis: Bilateral middle ear atresia with right-sided microtia.

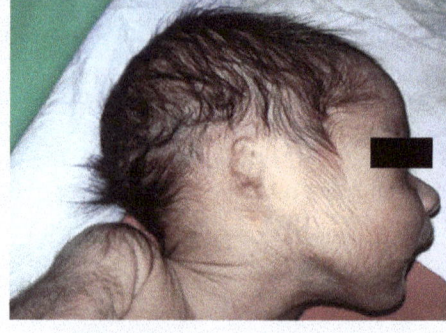

FIG. 24.26: Anotia of right ear.

Explanation

Microtia and atresia: Microtia refers to a congenital deformity where the auricle (external ear) is small and malformed. Atresia refers to the absence or closure of the external auditory canal.

Embryological Basis
- The external acoustic meatus forms from the canalization of ectodermal cells of the first ectodermal cleft.
- The middle ear cavity arises from the tubotympanic recess, which derives from the dorsal part of the first and part of the second pharyngeal pouches.
- The ear ossicles (malleus, incus, stapes) develop from mesodermal tissue located between the ends of the first ectodermal cleft and the tubotympanic recess.

Causes

Genetic factors: Mutations or genetic abnormalities can disrupt the normal development of ear structures.
Environmental factors: Exposure to teratogenic agents such as radiation, infections, or certain medications during pregnancy can interfere with fetal development.

Specific Findings

Right side: Absence of ectodermal, endodermal, and mesodermal components of the first and second pharyngeal arches resulted in microtia, atresia of the external auditory canal, and absence of ear ossicles and middle ear cavity.
Left side: Absence of endodermal and mesodermal components of the first and second pharyngeal arches resulted in absence of the middle ear cavity and ossicles.

HIGHLIGHTS

EYES
- The *visual system* consists of eyeball, eyelids, extraocular muscles of eyeball and lacrimal apparatus. It includes walls/layers, refractive media and optic nerve.
- Developmental primordia of eyeball are *optic vesicle, lens placode* and the *mesoderm* surrounding the optic vesicle.
- *Optic vesicle* is an outgrowth of the prosencephalon. The optic vesicle is converted into the optic cup. Retina, the nervous layer of eyeball develops from the optic cup.
- *Lens placode* is a thickening of surface ectoderm close to optic vesicle from which the *lens* develops. Lens placode is converted to lens vesicle.
- Other coats of the eyeball *(choroid, sclera)* are derived from mesoderm surrounding the optic vesicle. The epithelium covering the superficial surface of the cornea is derived from surface ectoderm.
- The *eyelids* are formed by reduplication of surface ectoderm above and below the cornea.
- The *lacrimal sac* and *nasolacrimal duct* are derived from ectoderm buried in the naso-optic furrow.

EARS
- **Membranous labyrinth (internal ear)** is derived from a thickening of surface ectoderm called the *otic placode*. The otic placode is converted into the otic vesicle and then to different parts of the labyrinth.
- **Bony labyrinth** is formed from mesenchyme surrounding the membranous labyrinth.
- **Middle ear** and **auditory tube** develop from the tubotympanic recess (from 1st and 2nd pharyngeal pouches).
- **Ear ossicles:** The *malleus* and *incus* are derived from Meckel's cartilage. The stapes is derived from the cartilage of the 2nd pharyngeal arch.
- **External acoustic meatus** is derived from the first ectodermal cleft.
- **Auricle** is formed from swellings that appear around the cleft.

Chapter 24: The Eye and Ear

Summary
- Development of eye **(Flowchart 24.1)**.
- Development of ear **(Flowchart 24.2)**.

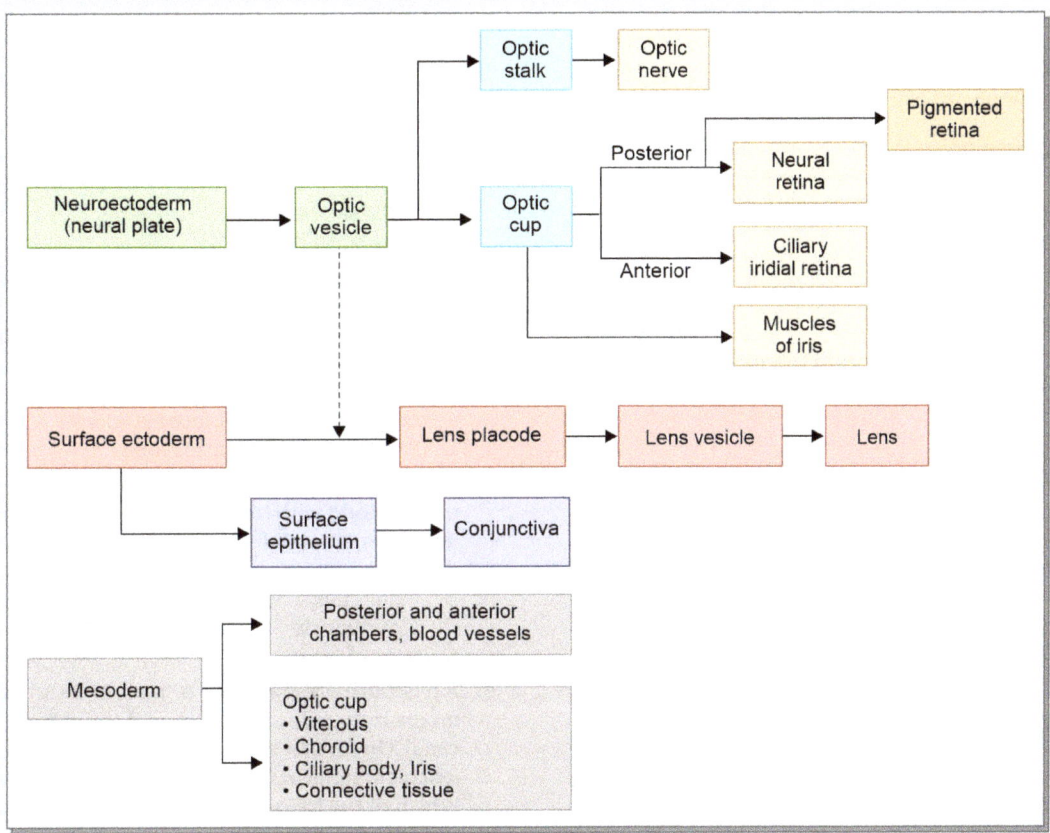

FLOWCHART 24.1: Development of eye.

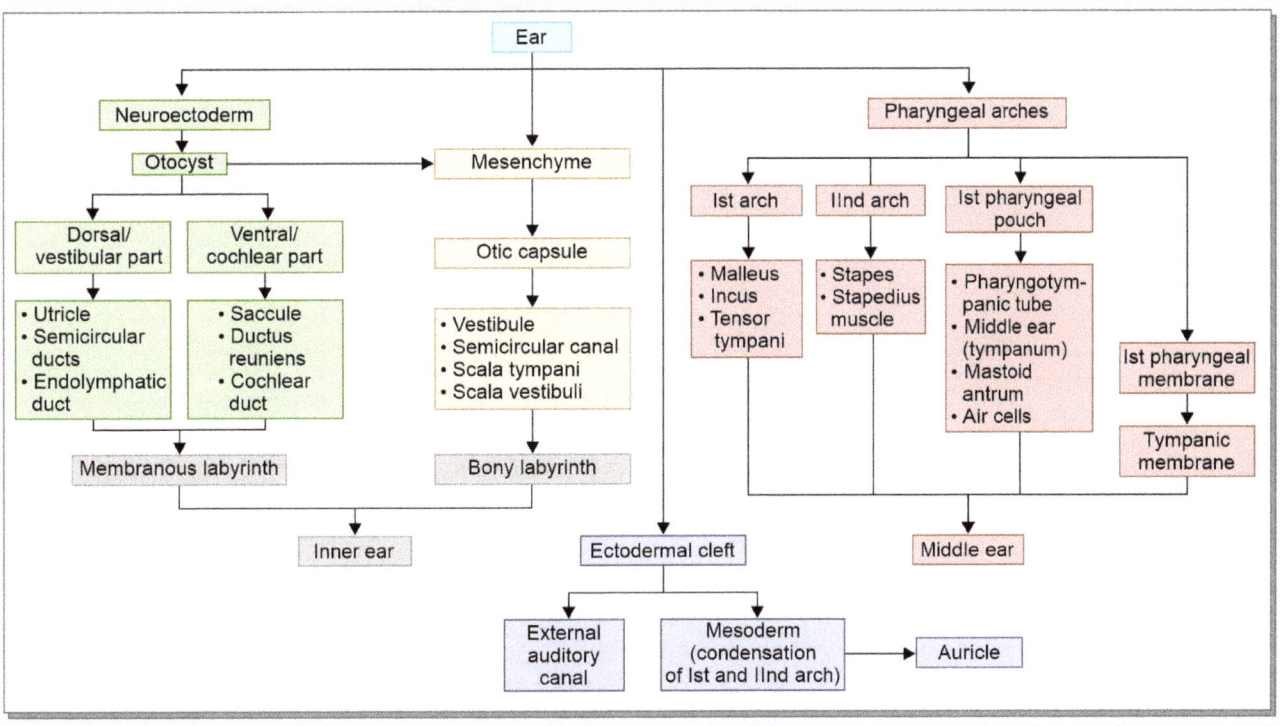

FLOWCHART 24.2: Development of ear.

TEST YOUR UNDERSTANDING

REVIEW QUESTIONS

1. Describe briefly the development of eyeball and its accessory structures.
2. Write short note on congenital anomalies affecting eyes.
3. Write short note on optic cup.
4. Explain development of lens.
5. Explain development of iris.
6. Explain development of retina.
7. Describe development of external ear with its congenital anomalies.
8. Describe development of internal ear.
9. Write short note on development of ear ossicles.

MULTIPLE CHOICE QUESTIONS

1. Sclera originates from:
   A. Ectoderm
   B. Mesoderm
   C. Endoderm
   D. Neural crest cell
2. Lens vesicle gets separated from the surface ectoderm by:
   A. 34th day
   B. 33rd day
   C. 36th day
   D. 40th day
3. Cochlear ganglion is related to:
   A. Equilibrium
   B. Static position
   C. Hearing
   D. Stereognosis
4. Inner ear develops from:
   A. Otic placode
   B. Pharyngeal pouches
   C. Ectodermal cleft
   D. Pharyngeal arches
5. An infant is born with bilateral absence of the eyeballs (anophthalmia). This congenital anomaly is associated with abnormal development of which embryonic structure?
   A. Optic cup
   B. Optic stalk
   C. Optic vesicle
   D. Lens placode
6. A newborn presents with a small, malformed external ear and absence of the external auditory canal. This condition is most likely due to a disruption in which embryonic process?
   A. Formation of the first pharyngeal arch
   B. Migration of neural crest cells
   C. Differentiation of surface ectoderm
   D. Formation of the otic placode
7. A child is born with bilateral coloboma of the iris and retina, along with hearing loss. This condition is due to a developmental defect in which embryonic structure?
   A. Optic cup
   B. Optic stalk
   C. Optic vesicle
   D. Lens placode
8. A newborn presents with a small, malformed external ear on the right side and absence of the external auditory canal. On further examination, the internal ear structures (cochlea, semicircular canals) are found to be normal. Which of the following embryonic processes is most likely disrupted in this case?
   A. Migration of neural crest cells
   B. Formation of the first pharyngeal pouch
   C. Differentiation of mesoderm
   D. Development of the otic placode

Answers: 1. B   2. B   3. C   4. A   5. C
          6. C   7. A   8. D

Chapter 25

Chromosomal and Genetic Abnormalities

COMPETENCIES COVERED/LEARNING OUTCOMES

The student should be able to:

AN74.1	Describe the various modes of inheritance with examples.
AN74.2	Draw pedigree charts for the various types of inheritance and give examples of diseases of each mode of inheritance.
AN74.3	Describe multifactorial inheritance with examples.
AN74.4	Describe the genetic basis and clinical features of achondroplasia, cystic fibrosis, vitamin D resistant rickets, hemophilia, Duchenne muscular dystrophy and sickle cell anemia.
AN75.1	Describe the structural and numerical chromosomal aberrations.
AN75.2	Explain the terms mosaics and chimeras with example.
AN75.3	Describe the genetic basis and clinical features of Prader Willi syndrome, Edward syndrome and Patau syndrome.
AN75.4	Describe genetic basis of variation: Polymorphism and mutation.
AN75.5	Describe the principles of genetic counseling.

In chapter 2, we discussed about the structures of chromosomes and genes, which are important for the development of individual as it contain all the genetic material. We have also been through the different periods of embryology that how zygote develops into full human after fertilization of gametes.

We should now focus on the abnormalities and pattern of inheritance of various disorders. Studying chromosomal abnormalities, genetics, and inheritance in medical embryology is of great importance for understanding the developmental origins of congenital disorders and genetic diseases. This knowledge aids in early diagnosis, prevention, and the development of targeted therapies, ultimately improving patient outcomes and enabling informed reproductive choices though genetic counseling.

CHROMOSOMAL ABNORMALITIES

Chromosomal abnormalities are broadly classified into two main categories: numerical and structural abnormalities. Each category can involve either autosomes (non-sex chromosomes) or sex chromosomes.

Structural Abnormalities (Table 25.1)

Structural abnormalities involve changes in the structure of chromosomes. These can include deletions, duplications, inversions, translocations, and other rearrangements. Structural abnormalities can also affect both autosomes and sex chromosomes.

Numerical Abnormalities (Table 25.2)

Numerical abnormalities refer to an atypical number of chromosomes, either an excess or a deficiency, relative to the normal diploid number (46 in humans). These abnormalities can affect either autosomes or sex chromosomes.

Patau's Syndrome (Trisomy 13)

It is an autosomal genetic disorder caused by the presence of an extra copy of *chromosome 13*.

Clinical Features

- Severe intellectual disability
- Holoprosencephaly (failure of the brain to divide properly)
- Microcephaly
- Polydactyly
- Cleft lip and palate
- Congenital heart defects
- Renal abnormalities
- Life expectancy: Most affected individuals die within the first year of life.

Chromosomal and Genetic Basis

- Trisomy 13 (47, XX, +13 or 47, XY, +13)
- Can occur due to nondisjunction during meiosis

TABLE 25.1: Structural abnormalities in chromosomes and associated clinical conditions.

Structural abnormality	Description	Associated clinical conditions
Deletion	Loss of a chromosome segment	Cri-du-chat syndrome (5p deletion)
Microdeletion	A small chromosomal deletion often too small to be detected by conventional cytogenetics	• DiGeorge syndrome (22q11.2 deletion) • Williams syndrome (7q11.23 deletion) • Prader-Willi syndrome (15q11-q13 deletion) • Angelman syndrome (15q11-q13 deletion)
Duplication	Repetition of a chromosome segment	Charcot-Marie-Tooth disease (17p duplication)
Inversion	Reversal of a chromosome segment	Often asymptomatic; can cause issues if breakpoint occurs within a gene
Translocation	Exchange of segments between non-homologous chromosomes	• Chronic myelogenous leukemia (CML) [Philadelphia chromosome t(9;22)] • Burkitt lymphoma [t(8;14)]
Insertion	Addition of a segment from one chromosome into another nonhomologous chromosome	Can lead to various syndromes depending on genes involved
Ring chromosome	A chromosome that forms a ring due to deletions at both ends and end-to-end fusion	Turner syndrome (ring chromosome X)
Isochromosome	A chromosome with identical arms due to division perpendicular to the usual axis	Turner syndrome (isochromosome Xq)
Marker chromosome	An abnormal chromosome that cannot be identified by standard cytogenetic techniques	Associated with various malignancies and developmental disorders
Robertsonian translocation	A type of translocation where two acrocentric chromosomes fuse near the centromere region	Down syndrome [translocation type, e.g., t(14;21)]

TABLE 25.2: Numerical abnormalities in chromosomes and associated clinical conditions.

Numerical abnormality	Type	Description	Associated clinical conditions
Trisomy 21	Autosomal	Presence of an extra copy of chromosome 21	Down syndrome
Trisomy 18	Autosomal	Presence of an extra copy of chromosome 18	Edwards syndrome
Trisomy 13	Autosomal	Presence of an extra copy of chromosome 13	Patau syndrome
XXY	Sex chromosomal	Presence of an extra X chromosome in males	Klinefelter syndrome
XYY	Sex chromosomal	Presence of an extra Y chromosome in males	XYY syndrome
Turner syndrome	Sex chromosomal	Presence of only one X chromosome in females (45, X)	Turner syndrome

Diagnostic Tests

- Prenatal screening (ultrasound, maternal serum screening)
- Noninvasive prenatal testing (NIPT)
- Amniocentesis and chorionic villus sampling (CVS)

Treatment Options

- Supportive care
- Surgical interventions for congenital defects
- Palliative care for severe cases

Edward's Syndrome (Trisomy 18)

It is an autosomal genetic disorder caused by the presence of an extra copy of *chromosome 18*.

Clinical Features

- Severe intellectual disability
- Microcephaly
- Clenched fists with overlapping fingers
- Rocker-bottom feet
- Congenital heart defects
- Growth retardation
- Life expectancy: Most affected individuals die within the first year of life.

Chromosomal and Genetic Basis

- Trisomy 18 (47,XX,+18 or 47,XY,+18)
- Can occur due to nondisjunction during meiosis

Treatment Options

- Supportive care
- Surgical interventions for congenital defects
- Palliative care for severe cases

Down's Syndrome (Trisomy 21)

It is a autosomal genetic disorder caused by the presence of an extra copy of *chromosome 21*. It is also known

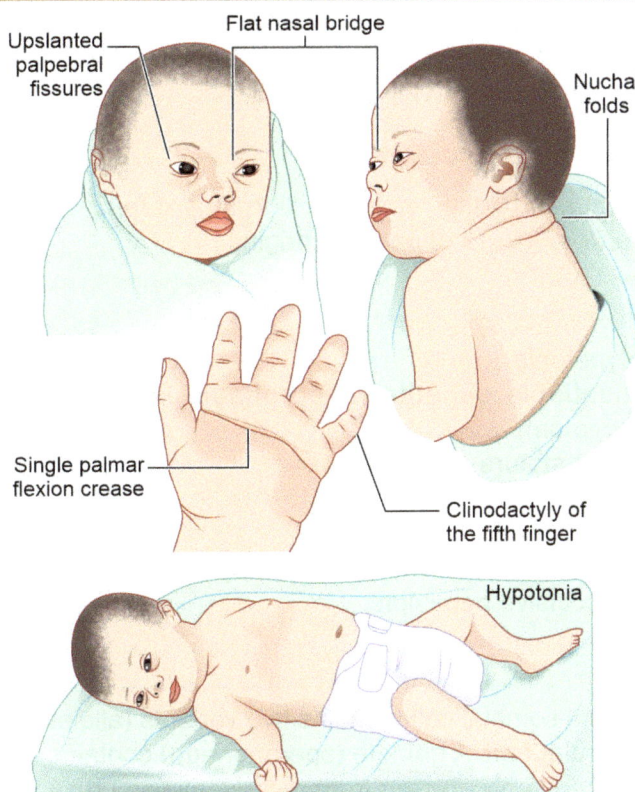

FIG. 25.1: Clinical features of Down syndrome.

as *mongolism* because of the facial features of a Mongolian. It is most common numerical chromosomal abnormality.

Clinical Features (Fig 25.1)

- Intellectual disability (mild to moderate)
- Characteristic facial features (flat facial profile, epicanthal folds, protruding tongue, small ears, sloping palpebral fissure)
- Congenital heart defects
- Hypotonia (reduced muscle tone)
- Short stature
- Increased risk of leukemia, Alzheimer's disease
- Hands—short and broad, and single palmar crease (Simian crease)
- Widely spaced great toe

Chromosomal and Genetic Basis

- Trisomy 21 (47,XX,+21 or 47,XY,+21)
- Can occur due to nondisjunction during meiosis
- Defect in the DSCR1 (Down Syndrome Critical Region 1) on chromosome 21 is responsible for this condition.

Diagnostic Tests

- **Prenatal screening:** Triple test at 16 weeks gestation.
  - Alfa-fetoproteins—reduced
  - Estriol—reduced
  - Human chorionic gonadotropin—increased
- Noninvasive prenatal testing (NIPT)
- Inhibin A—increased
- Amniocentesis and chorionic villus sampling (CVS)

Treatment Options

- Early intervention programs (physical, occupational, and speech therapy)
- Medical management of associated conditions (e.g., heart defects)
- Educational support

Turner Syndrome (45, X)

It is a genetic disorder affecting females, characterized by the partial or complete *absence of one X chromosome*.

Clinical Features (Fig. 25.2)

- Short stature
- Webbed neck
- Cubitus valgus
- Low set ears
- Rudimentary ovaries or streak gonads
- Amenorrhea
- Normal or slightly retarded intelligence
- Broad chest with widely spaced nipples
- Congenital heart defects (e.g., coarctation of the aorta)
- Lymphedema

Chromosomal and Genetic Basis

45, X karyotype (complete or partial absence of one X chromosome)

Diagnostic Tests

Buccal smear: Barr body absent due to nondisjunction in gametogenesis.

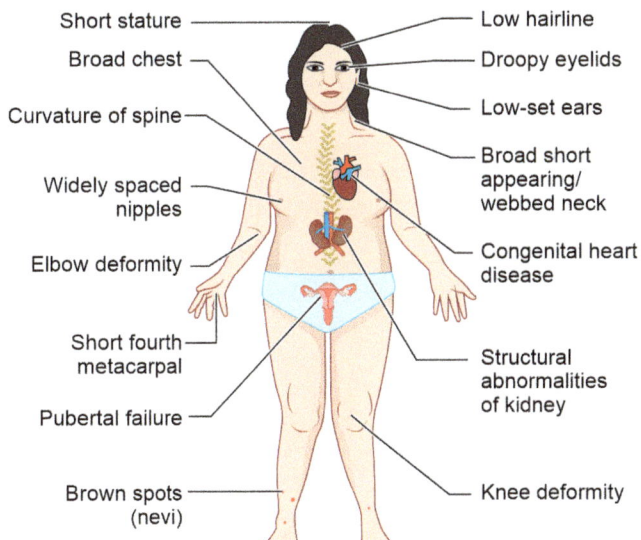

FIG. 25.2: Clinical features of Turner syndrome.

Treatment Options

* Growth hormone therapy to increase height
* Estrogen replacement therapy for the development of secondary sexual characteristics
* Management of associated medical conditions (e.g., cardiac monitoring)

Klinefelter Syndrome (47, XXY)

It is a genetic disorder affecting males, characterized by the presence of an *extra X chromosome*. It is also called *XXY syndrome*.

Clinical Features (Fig. 25.3)

* Tall stature with some degree of mental retardation
* Small testes leading to reduced fertility
* Gynecomastia (breast development in males)
* Reduced facial and pubic hair
* Learning difficulties
* Increased risk of osteoporosis and breast cancer

Chromosomal and Genetic Basis

* 47, XXY karyotype (presence of an extra X chromosome)
* Can occur due to nondisjunction during meiosis II

Diagnostic Tests

Buccal smear: Barr body positive

Karyotyping

Confirms the presence of an extra X chromosome (47,XXY)

Treatment Options

* Testosterone replacement therapy to address symptoms of testosterone deficiency
* Educational support for learning difficulties
* Fertility treatment options [e.g., assisted reproductive technologies (ART)]

Prader-Willi Syndrome

It is caused by the *microdeletion in the long arm of chromosome 15* of paternal origin.

Clinical Features

* Hypotonia
* Insatiable appetite (hyperphagia is a hallmark symptom)
* Short stature
* Small hands and feet
* Hypogonadism
* Behavioral problems like temper tantrums and compulsive behaviors

ALLELE

A normal somatic cell contains two variants (alleles) for a particular trait. A gamete (sperm or egg) contains one allele, randomly chosen from the two alleles present in the somatic cells. For example, if an individual has one allele for brown eyes (B) and one for blue eyes (b), their somatic cells will have both alleles (Bb), but each gamete will carry only one allele (either B or b).

When the two alleles are different (heterozygous, e.g., Bb), the trait associated with the dominant allele (B) will be expressed, while the trait associated with the recessive allele (b) will be hidden. If the two alleles are the same (homozygous), whether dominant (BB) or recessive (bb), the corresponding trait will be expressed.

GENE POLYMORPHISM AND MUTATION

Polymorphism

* A gene is considered polymorphic if more than one allele occupies a specific locus within a population, with each allele occurring in at least 1% of the population.
* Polymorphisms involve the inheritance of different forms of a gene, known as *alleles*, which have varying DNA sequences.
* Polymorphic variants of a gene can lead to abnormal protein expression and may be associated with diseases. For instance, a polymorphic variant of the *CYP4A11* gene is linked to hypertension, ischemic stroke, and coronary artery disease due to reduced enzyme activity in blood pressure regulation. Another example is the genes coding for the major histocompatibility complex (MHC).
* Polymorphisms can be identified in the laboratory using polymerase chain reaction (PCR) to amplify the gene sequence followed by DNA sequencing.

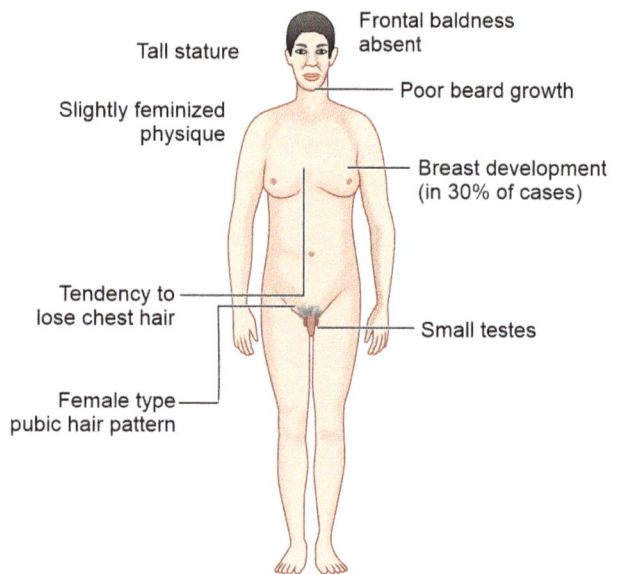

Fig. 25.3: Clinical features of Klinefelter syndrome.

- Clinical relevance of polymorphism is seen in conditions like lung cancer and asthma.
- Gene polymorphism also plays a crucial role in drug design (pharmacogenetics).

Mutation

- A gene mutation is a *permanent alteration in the DNA sequence*, ranging from a single base pair change to large segments involving multiple genes.
- Mutations can be germline (inherited from fertilization) or somatic (acquired during an individual's life).
- Germline mutations occur during fertilization and are present in all cells of the resulting individual.
- Somatic mutations are caused by environmental factors (e.g., UV radiation) and affect only specific cells, not passed to offspring.
- Mutagens, such as radiation and chemicals, cause mutations.
- Types of mutations include duplications, insertions, and deletions affecting chromosomes.

For a detailed understanding of polymorphism and mutation, *refer* to a genetics textbook.

Mosaicism

Mosaicism is a condition where somatic cells of the body contain more than one genotype. This occurs due to nondisjunction during early mitosis, resulting in the loss of a chromosome in some trisomic cells.

Examples:
- **Down syndrome mosaicism:** Some individuals have a mixture of cells, some with the normal 46 chromosomes and others with an extra copy of chromosome 21.
- **Turner syndrome mosaicism:** Some cells have the normal two sex chromosomes (XX), while others have only one X chromosome (X0).
- **Mosaic Klinefelter syndrome:** Individuals have some cells with the usual male XY chromosomes and others with the extra X chromosome (XXY).
- **McCune-Albright syndrome:** Affects bone, skin pigmentation, and hormonal problems due to mosaic mutations in the GNAS gene.

Chimerism

Chimerism is the presence of two or more genetically distinct cell lines derived from more than one zygote. There are two types:
- **Dispermic chimeras:** Result from fertilization of two ova by genetically different X and Y bearing sperms, forming two zygotes that fuse to create a single embryo, leading to distinct blood types, skin pigmentation, or organ structures.

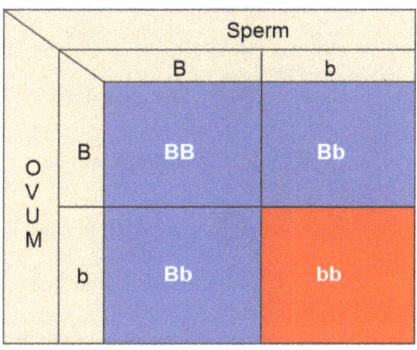

FIG. 25.4: Punnett square diagram.

- **Blood chimeras:** Occur when nonidentical twins exchange cells through the placental barrier in utero. For instance, one twin may have a karyotype of XY and blood group B, while the other twin has a karyotype of XX and blood group A.

The difference between chimerism and mosaicism is that mosaicism involves cell lines derived from a single zygote, whereas chimerism involves cell lines from different zygotes.

PUNNETT SQUARE

A Punnett square is a diagram used to predict the outcome of a genetic cross. It determines the probability of an offspring having a particular genotype **(Fig. 25.4)**.
- **Genotype:** The state of the two alleles at one or more loci associated with a trait.
- **Phenotype:** The observable state of a trait.

For example, consider the genotype and phenotype for eye color:

Genotype	Phenotype
BB	Brown eyes
Bb	Brown eyes
bb	Blue eyes

This table shows the genotype and phenotype relationship for brown and blue eyes.

INHERITANCE OF GENETIC DISORDERS

The pattern of inheritance of genetic disorders plays a crucial role in diagnosing the disorder, calculating the risk for present and future offspring, and counseling the parents. By obtaining a detailed family history, a pedigree chart can be prepared to understand the pattern of occurrence (inheritance) of the disease within the family. This chart helps to visualize how the disorder is passed down through generations. Additionally, by drawing a Punnett square, the percentage risk of the disorder can be interpreted, providing valuable information for genetic counseling and risk assessment.

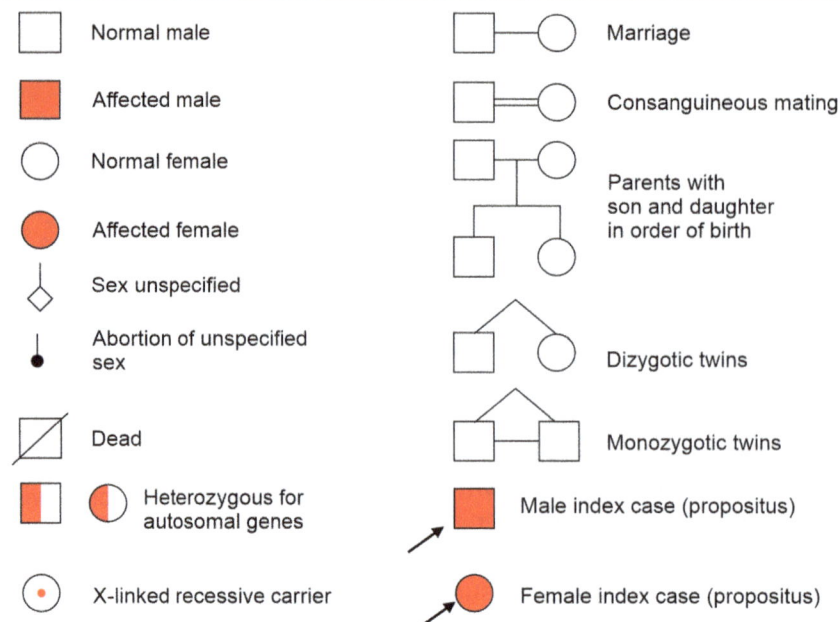

FIG. 25.5: Symbols used in pedigree chart.

Pedigree Chart

A pedigree chart is a pictorial representation of the generations of a family, showing detailed information about family members, their relationships, marriages (including consanguineous unions), and records of live births, stillbirths, and abortions. This chart visually illustrates genetic connections among individuals using standardized symbols.

For drawing pedigree charts, certain standard symbols are used **(Fig. 25.5)**. Understanding the probability and Mendelian patterns of inheritance is essential for interpreting these charts. Conclusions about the inheritance of a trait are most accurate when drawn from a large number of pedigrees (generations). A sample pedigree chart is presented in **Figure 25.6**, demonstrating how these symbols and patterns can be used to track genetic traits across generations.

Importance of understanding the pattern of inheritance of genetic disorders is—it facilitates:

- Diagnosis of genetic disorders
- Calculation of the risk of getting a genetic disease in the present and future offspring
- **Genetic counseling:** Suggest the preventive methods for genetic disorders.

According to the *mode of transmission the genetic disorders* can be classified as follows:

- Autosomal dominant inheritance
- Autosomal recessive inheritance
- X-linked dominant inheritance
- X-linked recessive inheritance
- Y-linked inheritance
- Multifactorial inheritance

Autosomal Dominant Inheritance (Fig. 25.7)

- Transmission occurs vertically from affected parent to child.
- There is a 50% chance of the dominant trait being passed on to offspring.
- Both males and females are equally affected.

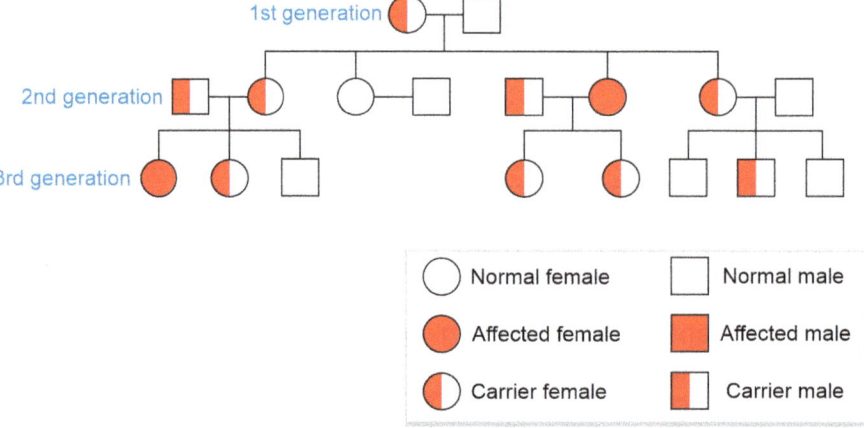

FIG. 25.6: Sample pedigree chart.

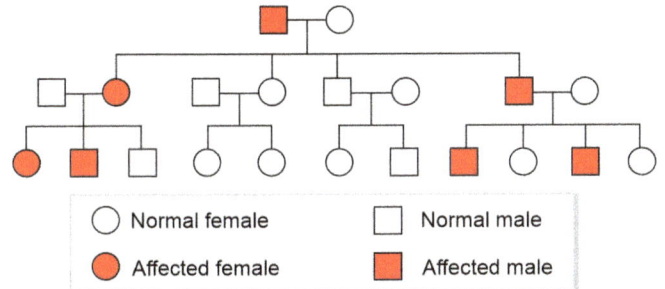

FIG. 25.7: Pedigree chart of autosomal dominant inheritance.

- The dominant gene is expressed in heterozygotes.
- Onset of symptoms typically occurs later in life.
- The trait appears in every generation without skipping.
- An unaffected offspring does not transmit the disease.
- **Examples:** Achondroplasia, angioneurotic edema, Huntington's chorea, multiple neurofibromatosis, and osteogenesis imperfecta.

Autosomal Recessive Inheritance (Fig. 25.8)

- Transmission is horizontal, appearing in siblings with normal parents.
- Occurs more frequently in populations with a history of consanguineous marriage.
- There is a 25% chance of having an affected child if both parents are carriers.
- Onset of symptoms usually occurs early in life.
- Both males and females have an equal chance of being affected.
- *Examples:* Cystic fibrosis, albinism, phenylketonuria, sickle cell anemia, and thalassemia.

X-linked Dominant Inheritance (Fig. 25.9A)

- The trait is more common in females than males.
- Affected males pass the trait to all their daughters but not their sons.
- Affected females, if homozygous, pass the trait to all their children.

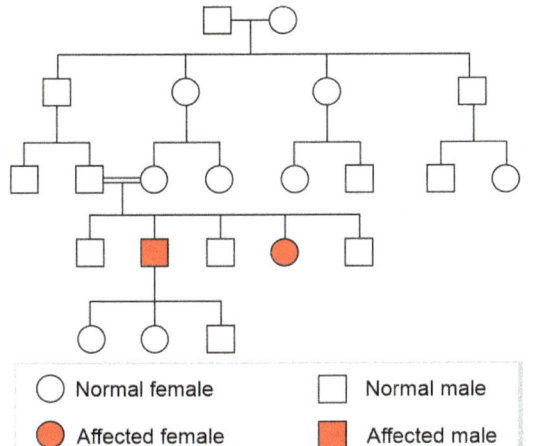

FIG. 25.8: Pedigree chart of autosomal recessive inheritance.

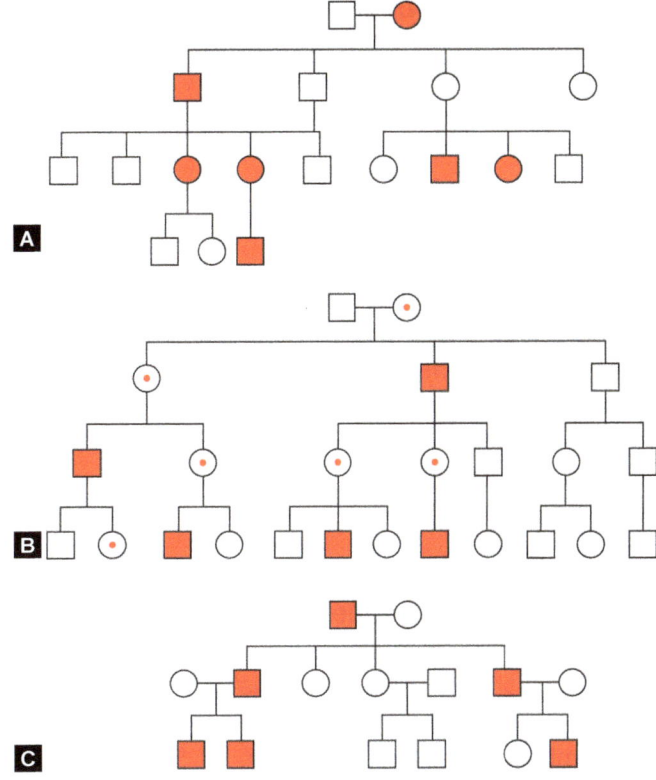

FIGS. 25.9A to C: Pedigree chart of sex-linked inheritance. (A) X-linked dominant inheritance; (B) X-linked recessive inheritance; (C) Y-linked inheritance.

- If heterozygous, affected females pass the trait to half of their children, regardless of sex.
- **Examples:** Vitamin D-resistant rickets and Xg blood groups.

X-linked Recessive Inheritance (Fig. 25.9B)

- Females are carriers (XX) with one X chromosome carrying the abnormal gene.
- Males (XY) are affected when the abnormal gene is present on their single X chromosome.
- If a mother is a carrier and the father is healthy, there is a 50% chance their sons will be affected and 50% chance their daughters will be carriers.
- **Examples:** Hemophilia, color blindness, glucose-6-phosphate dehydrogenase deficiency, and Duchenne muscular dystrophy.

Y-linked Inheritance (Fig. 25.9C)

- Y-linked traits are present in all male descendants of an affected male.
- Traits on the Y chromosome are called holandric genes.
- **Examples:** Hairy pinna.

Multifactorial Inheritance

- It involves the combined influence of multiple genes and environmental factors in determining traits or diseases.

- Traits influenced by multifactorial inheritance often show a spectrum of severity and do not follow simple Mendelian inheritance patterns.
- Teratogens are involved in these types of inheritance.
- **Examples:** Cleft lip and palate, clubfoot, congenital heart disease, and neural tube defects like anencephaly and spina bifida.
- Genetic counseling is essential for assessing recurrence risks in families with multifactorial conditions, considering both familial history and environmental factors.

Disorders of Inheritance

Achondroplasia

- Achondroplasia, also known as congenital osteosclerosis, occurs at an incidence of 1 in 15,000 to 40,000 births. It is characterized by:
    - Short stature (disproportionate)
    - Rhizomelic shortening (shortening of the proximal limbs)
    - Mid-face hypoplasia
    - Frontal bossing
- The genetic basis of achondroplasia involves a mutation in the fibroblast growth factor receptor 3 (FGFR3) gene located on chromosome 4p.
- It follows an autosomal dominant pattern of inheritance, where a person carrying the mutated gene has a 50% chance of passing it on to their children, who may develop dwarfism. If both parents carry the defective gene, the condition can be fatal in offspring.
- Prenatal ultrasound examination can detect features associated with achondroplasia in utero.

Cystic Fibrosis

- It is an autosomal recessive genetic disorder with an incidence of 1 in 2,500 people in the population.
- It is caused by mutations in the cystic fibrosis transmembrane conductance regulator (CFTR) gene on chromosome 7, which regulates salt and fluid movement across cell membranes.
- This gene affects cells that produce mucus, sweat, and digestive juices, leading to the accumulation of thick, sticky mucus primarily in the lungs and pancreas.
- Individuals with this condition experience breathing difficulties and frequent respiratory infections.

Sickle Cell Anemia

- It is a hemoglobinopathy caused by a mutation in the gene responsible for coding the beta polypeptide chain of hemoglobin, located on the short arm of chromosome 11.
- Changes in the hemoglobin structure lead to sickling of red blood cells (RBCs).
- Cells become deformed and rigid, impairing their ability to carry oxygen, which causes hemolytic anemia.
- It is an autosomal recessive inheritance thus affected person has 2 copies of recessive alleles, one from mother and one from father.

Vitamin D Rickets

- This condition is a X-linked dominant condition and hereditary form of hypophosphatemic rickets resulting from low phosphate levels in the blood, essential for normal bone and teeth formation.
- Manifestations vary but commonly include:
    - Slow growth leading to shorter stature compared to peers.
    - Movement difficulties and bone pain.
    - Physical characteristics like bowed legs or knock knees.
    - Craniosynostosis, the premature fusion of skull bones.
    - Dental abnormalities.
    - Enthesopathy, abnormal bone growth affecting ligament and tendon attachments to joints.

Hemophilia

- Hemophilia is an inherited clotting disorder, predominantly X-linked recessive.
- It is caused by deficiencies in clotting factors VIII (hemophilia A) or IX (hemophilia B).
- Hemophilia A affects approximately 1 in 5,000 males, while hemophilia B affects about 1 in 40,000 males.
- Clinical features include prolonged clotting times with normal bleeding times, leading to excessive bleeding following injury or surgery, as well as spontaneous bleeding into joints and muscles.
- The genetic basis lies in mutations on the X chromosome, affecting genes crucial for blood coagulation.
- Treatment typically involves replacement therapy with factor VIII or IX derived from plasma to manage bleeding episodes effectively.

Duchenne Muscular Dystrophy

- Duchenne muscular dystrophy (DMD) is a progressive muscular disorder primarily affecting males caused due to X-linked recessive inheritance, with an incidence of approximately 1 in 3,500 births.
- It involves gradual and irreversible muscle weakness and wasting, typically beginning around the age of 3.
- By adolescence, individuals often require a wheelchair for mobility.
- Diagnosis is confirmed through elevated creatinine kinase levels, muscle biopsy revealing muscle tissue replaced by fat and connective tissue.
- Genetic testing detects microdeletions on the Xp21 region, particularly affecting the DMD gene.
- This gene's absence leads to the degeneration of muscle cells due to disrupted dystrophin protein function, which links extracellular laminin to intracellular actin.

Color Blindness

- Color blindness, particularly red-green color blindness, is an X-linked recessive disorder that primarily affects males, given the presence of a single X chromosome.
- This condition results from mutations in the genes responsible for encoding photopigments in the retina, crucial for color vision resulting in impeding the ability to distinguish between red and green hues.
- Since males have only one X chromosome, a single mutated gene will manifest as color blindness.
- In contrast, females, with two X chromosomes, are typically carriers unless they inherit the mutation on both chromosomes.
- Diagnosis can be confirmed through color vision tests, and while there is no cure, adaptive strategies and tools, such as color-corrective lenses and digital aids, can help manage the condition.

GENETIC COUNSELING

Genetic counseling is a process by which individuals affected by or at risk for genetic disorders receive detailed information regarding their condition.

Key Information Provided

- **Consequences of the disorder:** Understanding the impact and progression of the disorder.
- **Probability of occurrence:**
  - *Personal risk:* The likelihood of the individual developing the disorder.
  - *Transmission risk:* The chances of passing the disorder to offspring.
- **Treatment options:** Information on available treatments and management strategies.
- **Prevention strategies:** Ways to avoid the occurrence of the disorder or related malformations.

Providers of Genetic Counseling

- **Family doctor:** For common genetic disorders.
- **Pediatrician:** Specialized knowledge in childhood genetic conditions.
- **Obstetrician:** Focus on prenatal genetic issues.
- **Genetic counselor:** Expertise in all aspects of genetic disorders and counseling.

Aspects of Genetic Counseling

- **Risk estimation:** Assessing the risk of developing or transmitting a disorder.
- **Diagnostic tests:**
  - *Prenatal tests:* Procedures to detect genetic disorders before birth.
  - *Other diagnostic tests:* Tests to identify genetic conditions at different life stages.
- **Psychological support:** Providing emotional and psychological support to the individual and their family.
- **Specialized services information:** Guidance on services such as speech therapy, educational therapy, and other supportive measures.

Candidates for Genetic Counseling

- **Maternal age over 35:** Increased risk of genetic abnormalities.
- **History of recurrent miscarriages:** Potential underlying genetic causes.
- **Birth of a fetus with anomalies:** Need for understanding genetic implications and risks.
- **Family history of genetic abnormalities:** Assessing the risk of inherited conditions.

Benefits of Genetic Counseling

- **Informed decision-making:** Empowering individuals with knowledge to make informed healthcare and family planning decisions.
- **Early detection and management:** Facilitating early intervention and management of genetic disorders.
- **Psychological well-being:** Offering support to cope with the emotional aspects of genetic conditions.

Chapter 25: Chromosomal and Genetic Abnormalities

HIGHLIGHTS

- **Genetics** is a branch of biology that deals with the transmission of *inherited characters (traits)* from parent to offspring at the time of fertilization. Some of the characters/traits are *dominant* and some are *recessive*.
- Characters of parents are transmitted to offspring through codes borne on strands of *DNA*. *Genes* are mades of such strands of DNA. They are located on *chromosomes*. Different forms of each gene are called *alleles*.
- **Gene mutation versus gene polymorphism:** Gene mutation is change in DNA sequence from normal. Gene polymorphism is occurrence of multiple alleles at a locus.
- **Mosaicism and chimerism:** Cell lines are derived from single zygote in *mosaicism*. Different cell lines result from fusion of different zygotes in *chimerism*.
- **Punnett square and pedigree chart:** *Punnett square* is a diagram to predict the results of genetic cross for predicting the probability of a particular genotype. *Pedigree chart* is a pictorial representation of genetic connections among individuals of different generations for understanding the basis for a trait.

TEST YOUR UNDERSTANDING

REVIEW QUESTIONS

1. Write short note on allele.
2. Describe patterns of inheritance.
3. Describe autosomal dominant inheritance
4. Describe autosomal recessive inheritance.
5. Discuss the numerical chromosomal abnormalities.
6. Discuss structural chromosomal abnormalities.
7. What is mosaicism and chimerism?
8. Write a short note on pedigree chart.

MULTIPLE CHOICE QUESTIONS

1. Which genetic disorder is characterized by an extra chromosome 18?
   A. Down syndrome
   B. Patau syndrome
   C. Edwards syndrome
   D. Turner syndrome
2. What condition is characterized by microdeletion of chromosome 22q11.2?
   A. Angelman syndrome
   B. DiGeorge syndrome
   C. Prader-Willi syndrome
   D. Williams syndrome
3. Which condition is associated with a karyotype of 47, XXY?
   A. Turner syndrome
   B. Klinefelter syndrome
   C. Down syndrome
   D. Edwards syndrome
4. A 32-year-old pregnant woman undergoes an ultrasound which reveals a fetus with multiple congenital anomalies including a cleft palate, heart defects, and polydactyly. Amniocentesis shows an extra chromosome 13. Which of the following syndromes is most likely?
   A. Down syndrome
   B. Turner syndrome
   C. Patau syndrome
   D. Edwards syndrome
5. A newborn exhibits severe hypotonia, poor feeding, and undescended testes. Genetic testing reveals deletion of paternal chromosome 15. What is the likely diagnosis?
   A. Angelman syndrome
   B. Prader-Willi syndrome
   C. Williams syndrome
   D. DiGeorge syndrome
6. A 45-year-old woman gives birth to a baby with prominent epicanthal folds, a single palmar crease, and hypotonia. What chromosomal abnormality is most likely?
   A. Trisomy 18
   B. Trisomy 13
   C. Trisomy 21
   D. Monosomy X
7. A family pedigree shows that a genetic disorder affects every generation and is seen in both males and females. Which inheritance pattern is most likely?
   A. Autosomal dominant
   B. Autosomal recessive
   C. X-linked recessive
   D. Mitochondrial
8. In a pedigree chart, a genetic trait appears in males more frequently than in females and is never passed from father to son. Which inheritance pattern does this indicate?
   A. Autosomal dominant
   B. Autosomal recessive
   C. X-linked recessive
   D. Mitochondrial

Answers: 1. C   2. B   3. B   4. C   5. B
          6. C   7. A   8. C

Index

Page numbers followed by *f* refer to figure, *fc* refer to flowchart, and *t* refer to table

A

Abdomen
  fetal 79*f*
  muscles of 116
  veins of 244
  wall 180*f*
Abembryonic pole 40
Aberrant renal arteries 262, 262*f*
Abortion 43
  induced 43
  spontaneous 43
Acardiac fetus 96
Acephalic fetus 96
Achalasia cardia 175
Achondroplasia 112, 145, 331, 332
Acidophil cells 306
Acrocephaly 143
Acrosome 19, 32
  reaction 21, 36, 37
Acrosomic cap 19
Actin 111
Adenine 8
Adenohypophysis 306, 309
Adrenal cortex 309
Adrenal gland 306, 307
  anomalies of 308
  development of 308*f*
  ectopic 308
Adrenal medulla 304, 309
Adrenogenital syndrome 278, 308
Afferent nuclei 304
Agenesis 196, 216
Agnathia 154
Alar lamina 288, 293*f*, 304
Albinism 120, 315, 331
Alcohol 80
Alimentary system 73, 161, 171
Alkaline phosphatase 106
Allantois 85, 87, 97, 99
  parts of 263
Allele 328
Alopecia, congenital 120
Alphafetoprotein assay 81
Alveolabial sulcus 161
Alveolar ducts 214
Alveolar process 162, 163*f*
Alveolar sacs 214
Alveoli 122, 214
  primordia of 121
Alveolingual sulcus 161
Alzheimer's disease 327
Amastia 123
Amelia 145
Ameloblasts 163, 164*f*, 169
Amelogenesis imperfecta 165
Amenorrhea 28
  primary 28
  secondary 28
Amniocentesis 80, 81*f*, 86
Amniogenic cells 48, 86
Amnioinfusion 82
Amnion 49, 85, 97, 99
  formation of 49
Amnioreduction 82
Amniotic bands 86
Amniotic cavity 48, 48*f*, 62, 70, 93, 94*f*, 97
  expansion of 85
  formation of 48, 85
Amniotic fluid 85, 86
  abnormal production of 86
  amount of 81
  functions of 86
Amniotic sac 50*f*, 87*f*
  number of 99
Ampulla 260
Amputations, congenital 145
Anal canal 181
  parts of 182*f*
  stenosis of 182*f*
Anal membrane 173, 182*f*
Anal valves 181
Anaphase 13
Anchoring villi 53, 53*f*, 66
Anencephaly 143, 299, 300*f*
  embryological basis of 146
Angioblasts 104
Angiogenesis 104, 233
Aniridia, congenital 315
Ankyloglossia 167
Annulus 20
  ovalis 224
Anodontia 165
Anonychia 120
Anophthalmos 315
Anotia 321, 322*f*
  embryological basis of 322
Anterior abdominal wall 205
  development of 205
Anterior cardinal vein 242, 243, 245*f*
  fate of 244*f*
Anterior median fissure 288
Anticodon 9
Anti-Müllerian hormone 45, 278
Antral follicle 23, 23*f*
  count 44
Anus, ectopic 182*f*
Aorta 233
  arch of 235*f*, 237*f*, 253
  ascending 225, 228*f*
  coarctation of 236, 236*f*, 327
  descending 253
  gonad-mesonephros 104
Aortic arch 233*f*, 235*f*, 236, 236*f*, 254*t*
  artery 233
  development of 236*f*
  double 236, 236*f*
  fate of 234*f*
  interrupted 236
Aortic sac 220, 233, 235*f*, 253, 254*f*
Aortic stenosis 231
  types of 231*f*
Aortic valves 230
  formation of 231*f*
Aortic vestibule 225
Aphakia, congenital 315
Apical ectodermal ridge 143, 144
Aplasia 119
Apocrine sweat glands 122
Apolar neuroblast 114
Appendicular skeleton 138, 143
Appendix 179, 180, 267*f*, 269, 277
  development of 179*f*
Aqueous chamber 313
Arachnodactyly 145
Arachnoid mater 115
Arch 130
  brachial 126
  muscles of 128, 130
  nerve of 128, 130
Areolae
  formation of 108*f*
  primary 107
  secondary 107
Arnold-Chiari malformation 303
  embryological basis of 303
Arrector pili 120
Arterial arch 128, 135
Arterial plexus 239
Artery 139*f*, 173, 253
  brachial 237
  brachiocephalic 234, 235*f*, 236*f*, 253
  bronchial 237
  development of 233, 237, 239
  intercostal 237
  mesenteric 185*f*
  pulmonary 235, 253
  suprarenal 253
Arytenoid 212
  cartilages 212
Assisted reproductive technique 39

Astroblasts 114
Astrocytes 114
Athelia 123
Atlas, occipitalization of 140
Atresia 192, 213, 231, 321, 322
   tracheal 213
Atria
   development of 253fc
   formation of 220
Atrial septal defects 224, 225f
Atrichia 120
Atrioventricular canal 220, 223, 253
   defect 227
   division of 223f
Atrioventricular orifice 225f
Auditory tube 131, 135, 322
Auricle 153, 322
   anomalies of 321
   development of 320f
Autonomic nervous system 301
Autosomal dominant inheritance, pedigree chart of 331f
Autosomal recessive inheritance 330, 331
   pedigree chart of 331f
Autosomes 7, 325
Axial filament 20
Axial skeleton 138
Axillary arteries 237
Axons 113
Azygos vein 216f, 245f, 247
   channel, formation of 247f

B

Barr body 11, 12, 20
Basal laminae 293f, 304
Basal plate 90, 288
Bell stage 164
Bellini, collecting ducts of 260
Bicuspid valve 230
Bifid ureter 263
Bifid uvula 157, 158f
Bilaminar germ disc 3, 48
   formation of 48
Bile canaliculi 190f
Bile duct 178f, 193f
   complete duplication of 193f
   partial duplication of 193f
   terminal part of 193f
Biliary apparatus 189
   development of 198fc
Biliary passages 191
Biopsy, endometrial 24
Bipolar cells 312
Bipolar neuroblast 114
Bird beak sign 175
Birth defects 79, 82, 82t, 83
   causes of 80
   functional 79
   structural 79
   types of 79
Bladder
   anomalies of 264f
   trigone of 263
Blastocoele 40

Blastocyst 40, 41f, 45
   formation of 3, 35, 40, 41
   hatching of 40-42, 42f
   penetration of 42, 42f
Blastomeres 39
Blastopore 61f, 62
Bleeding 31
   spontaneous 332
   uterine 24
Blind bronchus 213
Blood
   cells 105f, 115
      formation of 104, 104f
   chimeras 329
   collection, peripheral 10
   culture procedure 10
   groups 331
   island 104, 104f
   pregnancy test 43
   separation 92
   supply 249
   test 45
   vessels 104, 104f, 190f, 230f, 312, 314
      development of 233
      formation of 115
Blue sclera 315
Bochdalek herniae 208
Body
   basic tissues of 101
   cavities 200
   wall 146
Bone 105, 115, 142, 143
   cell of 105
   formation 106, 107f
   lacunae of 105f
   length of 108f, 111f
   marrow 104
   morphogenetic proteins 16
   spicule of 106
   structure 105f
      unit of 105f
Bony labyrinth 317, 319f, 322
   basic structure of 319f
Bony lamellae, formation of 108f
Bowman's capsule 260
Bowman's layer 313
Brachydactyly 145
Brain 284, 303
   anomalies of 299
   development of 283
   flexures, formation of 285
   parts of 284
   ventricles of 286f
   vesicles
      primary 284
      secondary 284
Brainstem 291, 292f
Branchial apparatus 126
Branchial arch 126
   derived musculature 146
Breasts, accessory 123
Bronchi 212, 213
   accessory 213
   extrapulmonary 214
Bronchial tree 215f
   morphology of 215

Bronchioles 214
   terminal 214
Bronchopulmonary segment 214
Brown eyes 328
Buccal smear 327, 328
Bucconasal membrane 155, 155f, 156f
Buccopharyngeal membrane 63, 72f, 73, 74, 162f, 171
Buds
   primary 122
   secondary 122
   stage 163
Bulbar septum 226, 226f, 253
Bulbopontine extension 290
   caudal parts of 290f
Bulboventricular cavity 227f
   formation of 225f
Bulboventricular chamber 225
Bulboventricular sulcus 226, 228, 229f
Bulbus cordis 225, 229f, 253
Burst forming unit 104, 105f

C

Calcification, zone of 110
Calcium wave 38
Canal, central 285, 288
Canaliculi 106
Carcinoma 134
Cardiac muscle 113, 116, 147, 229
Cardiac progenitor cells 219
Cardiac wall, layer of 229
Cardinal veins 247f
Cardiogenic area 65, 219, 253
Cardiogenic plate 65
Cardiovascular system 73, 219
Carotid artery
   external 233, 234, 235, 235f
   internal 235f
Carotid duct 234
Cartilage bones 106
Cartilage
   cell
      enlarged 107f
      hypertrophy 106
   formation of 104
Cartilaginous joints, primary 144
Cartilaginous matrix, vascularization of 107
Cataract, congenital 315
Caudal dysgenesis 60
Caudal pharyngeal complex 132
Caudal pleuroperitoneal fold 201
Caudal segment 178
Caudate nucleus 296, 297f, 298f
Cavity 284
   abdominal 180f
   atresia of 156
Cecal bud 172
Cecum 179
   descent of 181f
   development of 179f
Celiac artery 172
Cell 102, 145
   cords of 276
   cycle 12, 12f

division 12, 17, 32
  types of 114f
Cellular transformation 33
Cementoblasts 164
Cementum 164
Central cytotrophoblast cells 52f
Central nervous system 59, 283
Centrifugation 11
Centromere 9
Centrum 139
Cephalic flexure 285
Cephalothoracopagus 96, 96f
Cerebellar cortex 293
Cerebellar peduncle
  inferior 293
  superior 293
Cerebellum 293, 304
  development of 293f
Cerebral aqueduct 285, 304
Cerebral commissures 298
Cerebral cortex 293, 296
  development of 298f
Cerebral hemisphere 293, 295f, 298f, 303
  development of 294f
Cerebrospinal fluid 285, 303
Cerebrum, white matter of 298
Cervical fistula 131
  embryological basis of 135
Cervical flexure 285
Cervical intersegmental artery 237, 238f, 239
Cervical mucus, observation of 24
Cervical nerves 290
Cervical rib 141
Cervical sinus 131, 131f
  congenital anomalies of 131
Cervicothoracic region, veins of 243
Cervix 267
Cheeks, development of 152
Chemical method 41
Chiasmata 14
Chimerism 329, 334
Chondroblasts 102, 104
Chondrocranium 142, 147
  developmental components of 142f
Chondrocytes 104
Chondro-osteo-dystrophy 140
Chorda tympani 167
Chordoma 60
Chorion 49, 51, 85, 86, 97, 99
  formation of 49, 51
  frondosum 51, 51f, 89
  laevae 51, 51f
  types of 51f
  villi, types of 51
Chorionic cavity 49, 50, 50f, 66
Chorionic plate 49, 89, 90
Chorionic villi 51, 97
  biopsy of 81, 93
  formation 43, 50f, 51
    process of 51
  sampling 81
  secondary 53f
  tertiary 53f

Choroid 312, 313, 322
  fissure 295, 295f, 311, 311f, 313
    formation of 295f
  plexus 295, 296f
Chromaffin
  cells 287
  tissue 308
Chromatids 9
Chromatophores 313
Chromonemata 10
Chromosomes 7, 10, 10f, 17, 32, 326, 332
  classification of 10, 10t
  duplication of 9
  homologous 7
  number of 7f
  pairing of 14
  significance of 7
  typical 9f
Ciliary body 312, 313
Ciliary muscles 312, 313
Circumvallate papillae 167
Cisterna chyli 251
Cleavage 3, 35, 39, 41f, 45
Cleft 145
  bilateral complete 157
  lip 153, 158f, 332
    embryological basis of 158
  nose 156
  palate 157, 332
    complete 157
    embryological basis of 158
    incomplete 157
    varieties of 158f
  scrotum 272f
  unilateral complete 157
Cleidocranial dysostosis 143
Clitoris 269, 270f
Cloaca 258, 259
  dorsal subdivision of 181
  incomplete septation of 181
  parts of 279
  subdivisions of 259f
Cloacal membrane 59f, 60, 63, 72-74, 171, 270f
Club foot 145
Cochlear duct 317
Coelomic epithelium 258, 308f
  invagination of 267f
Collagen 104
Colliculi 304
Coloboma 315
Colon
  ascending 179, 204f
  descending 181, 204f
Colony forming unit 104, 105f
Color
  blindness 331, 333
  vision tests 333
Columnar uterine epithelium 42
Common bile duct 191
Common cardinal vein 243
Common carotid artery 235f, 253
Common hepatic
  duct 192f, 193f
  vein 241

Common iliac vein 246
Compact bone 106
Complete agenesis 193f
Congenital high airway obstruction syndrome 213
Conjoined twins 96f
Conjunctiva 312
Conjunctival sac 314, 314f
Connective tissue 101, 102
  cells 189
Contraception 30, 41, 45
Conus 220, 225
  arteriosus 225
  cordis 225
Cor triloculare biventriculare 225
Cord
  blood therapies 88
  length 88
  prolapse 88
Cordocentesis 81
Cornea 311-313, 315
  anomalies of 315
Corneal epithelium 310
Corniculate cartilages 212
Corona radiata 37
  cells 23
Coronary ligament 189, 209
Coronary sinus 221, 222f, 244, 245f
  derivation of 245f
  valve of 223, 224
Coronary sulcus 269
Corpora atretica 26
Corpus albicans 25
Corpus callosum, development of 299f
Corpus luteum 25, 31
  formation of 25f
Corpus striatum 293, 296, 297f, 303
  deep part of 297f
  early development of 297f
Cortex 307
  congenital hyperplasia of 308
  fetal 307
Corti organ 317
Cortical cords 276
Corticobulbar fibers 291
Costal arch 141
Costal element 139, 141
Costotransverse joint 141
Cranial nerve 291f
  nuclei 291f
    location of 292f
Cranial outflow 302f
Cranial parasympathetic outflow 301
Cranial ventral anastomosis 243f
Craniocaudal axis 59
Craniopagus 96, 96f
Craniopharyngiomas 306
Craniosynostosis 332
Cricoid 212
  cartilage 212
Crista dividens 249
Crista terminalis 222f, 223, 224
Crown-heel length 77
Crown-rump length 68, 78f
Crus cerebri 292

Cryptorchidism 275
Cumulus
    oophoricus 23
    ovaricus 23
Cuneate nuclei 290
Cuneiform cartilages 212
Cuvier duct 243
Cyclopia 315
Cylindrical embryo 69
Cylindrical neural tube 63
Cyst, branchial 131
Cystic duct 191, 192f, 193f
Cystic fibrosis 331, 332
Cytokinesis 12
Cytosine 8
Cytotrophoblast 50f, 51, 91
    cells, intermediate 53f
    shell 66
        formation of 53f

D

Dandy-Walker syndrome 300
Daughter cells 15f
Davidson body 11, 12
Decidua 44, 45, 78f
    basalis 44, 51f, 89
    capsularis 51f
    fate of 44
    plate 89
    subdivisions of 44, 44f
    types of 44
Deep cervical artery 237
Deformities 145
Delivery, expected date of 39
Dendrites 113
Dendritic cells 119
Dental
    cuticle 164
    lamina 162, 162f-164f
        stage of 163
    papilla 163
Dentate 293
Dentin 169
Dentinogenesis imperfecta 165
Deoxygenation, degree of 250f
Deoxyribonucleic acid 8
    structure of 8, 8f
Dermal papillae 119
Dermal root sheath 120
Dermatoglyphics 120
Dermatome 112, 115, 119
Dermis 113f, 119, 124
Dermoepidermal junction 119
Descemet's membrane 313
Dextrocardia 228, 230f
Diaphragm 116, 146, 200, 206, 208f, 209
    accessory 208
    anomalies of 208
    components of 206
    congenital eventration of 208
    crura of 207
    descent of 208
    development of 206, 207f, 208f
    embryological components of 206t
Diaphyseal aclasis 112

Diaphysis 109
Diastematomyelia 140
Diencephalon 283, 286f, 294f, 295, 297f
DiGeorge syndrome 130
Digital arteries 239
Diploid 7
    chromosomes 7
Diplotene 14
Disc
    ectodermal layer of 58, 59
    incomplete duplication of 96
Discus proligerus 23
Dislocation, congenital 145
Dispermic chimeras 329
Disruptions 79
Distal bulbar septa 225
Distal esophagus, atresia of 213f
Diverticula 102, 156, 263, 266
    congenital 179f, 264
Diverticulum 213
    allantoenteric 87
    allantoic 71, 71f, 74, 86, 88, 172
Dizygotic twins 94, 95f, 97, 99, 99t
Dorsal anastomosis 243f
Dorsal aorta 128, 172, 219, 233
    branches of 238f
Dorsal lamina 288
Dorsal mass 286, 304
Dorsal mesentery 172, 203, 207, 209
Dorsal mesocardium 228
Dorsal mesogastrium 175, 176f, 197f, 204f, 209
    fusion of 197f
    parts of 206f
Dorsal nerve root 289
    ganglia 289
Dorsal pancreatic buds 194f, 196f
Dorsal wing 131
Dorsum 155
Double bubble sign 178
Down's syndrome 326, 329
    clinical features of 327f
Drumstick body 11, 12
Duchenne muscular dystrophy 331, 333
Duct system 167
Ductus arteriosus 234, 235, 249, 250, 251
Ductus caroticus 234, 236
    disappearance of 234f
Ductus deferens 273, 277f
Ductus venosus 241, 249, 251
Duodenal atresia 178
Duodenal cap 178
Duodenal diverticulum 178
Duodenal papilla 194
Duodenal stenosis 178
Duodenum 178, 178f, 179f, 186, 204f
    development of 178f
    obstruction of 179f
    parts of 178f
Dwarfism 112
Dysmenorrhea 28
Dysphagia 303
Dysplasia 79, 119
    congenital 145
Dyspnea 303

E

Eardrum 132
Ears 310, 322
    development of 317, 323, 323fc
    external 153, 318
    internal 317, 322
    molecular regulation of development of 321
    ossicles 322
Eccentric implantation 42
Eccrine sweat gland 121
Ectoderm 48, 48f, 59f, 60, 73, 75, 101, 182f, 265f
    surface 59, 73, 118, 310
Ectodermal cells, solid mass of 182f, 320f
Ectodermal cleft 127, 126, 130, 135, 318
    fate of 130
Ectodermal cloaca 73
Ectodermal part, derivation of 162f
Ectopia 275
    cordia 238, 230f
    vesicae 264, 264f
Ectopic pancreatic tissue 195
Ectopic thyroid tissue 134
Ectropion 316, 316f
Edema, angioneurotic 331
Edinger-Westphal nucleus 301
Edward's syndrome 326
Efferent cranial nerve nuclei 304
Ejaculatory ducts 264, 266f, 273, 277f
Elastic cartilage 105
Elastic fibers 104
Emboliform 293
Embryo 50f, 144f
    axes of 59
    body axes of 66
    folding of 69
    genome, genotype of 79
    growth of 68
    head end of 150f
    lateral view of 126f, 201f
    molecular control of development of 15
    primitive veins of 241f
Embryoblast 40, 48
Embryology 1, 5
    basic processes in 4
    molecular aspect of 7
    role of 1
    subdivisions of 1
    systemic 1
Embryonic body 144f
Embryonic disc 58, 59f, 65f, 73f, 174f, 219f
    caudal end of 61f
    duplication of 96
    shape of 58
Embryonic dorsal aorta, basic branching pattern of 237f
Embryonic limb, adduction of 144f
Embryonic period 68, 69
Embryonic stem cells 5t
Embryonic structure 278
    arrangement of 73f
Enamel 169
    organ 169
        formation of 163f

Encephalocele 143, 299, 300f
Enchondromatosis 112
Endocardial cushions 223, 230
Endocardial proliferation 227f
Endocardium 229
Endochondral ossification 106, 107f, 108f, 115, 116fc
Endocrine glands 102
Endoderm 48, 60, 48f, 59f, 74, 75, 101, 182f, 186, 212, 263-265
Endodermal derivatives 136, 161, 266f
Endodermal diverticulum 211
Endodermal origin 132, 211
Endodermal pouches 126, 136fc
    fate of 131
Endolymph 317
Endolymphatic duct 317
Endolymphatic sac, formation of 318f
Endometrium 28, 31, 44, 54
    erosion of 42
Endothelial cells 102, 104
Endothelium 219, 251
Enteric nervous system 301
Enterocystoma 180
Entropion 316, 316f
Enzyme collagenase 24
Epiblast
    ectoderm 48
    formation of 48
Epicanthus 316
Epicardium 229
Epidermal growth factor 16
Epidermis 59, 118, 119f, 124
    development of 119f
Epididymis 273, 277f
    appendix of 277
Epigastric arteries, inferior 237
Epigenital tubules 277
Epiglottis 128, 166, 212
Epimere 113, 145
Epimyocardial mantle 229
Epiphyseal cartilage 109, 111f
    structure of 111f
Epiphyseal plate 109, 115
Epiphysis 109, 115
    cerebri 307
    fusion of 110
Epiploic foramen 203
Epispadias 266, 272
Epithalamic sulci 295
Epithalamus 295
Epithelia 101, 115
Epithelial epithelial interaction 16
Epithelial mesenchymal interaction 16
Epithelial root sheath 120
Epithelial surfaces 102
Epithelial tissue 101
Epitrichium 118
Eponychium 120
Epoophoron 278
Esophageal arteries 237
Esophageal atresia 175
Esophageal stenosis 175
Esophagus 173, 186, 204f, 217f, 237f
    development of 175f
    dorsal mesentery of 207

    mesenteries of 207f
    normal arrangement of 175f
Estradiol 30
Estrogen stimulates uterine growth 93
Ethmoid bone 142
Excretory renal tubules 259
Exocrine glands 102
Exomphalos 180, 180f
Exostosis 112
    multiple 112
Experimental embryology 1
External acoustic meatus 130, 135, 318, 322
    development of 320f
External auditory
    canal, atresia of 322
    meatus, anomalies of 321
External genitalia 279, 280
    development of 269
    female 269
    male 272
Extraembryonic coelom 49, 65f, 93, 94f, 97
    formation of 49, 49f
    obliteration of 94f
Extraembryonic membranes 85, 85f
Extraembryonic mesoderm 49, 53f
    formation of 49, 49f
    lie, cell of 49
    splanchnopleuric 49
Extrahepatic biliary tract 193f
    agenesis of parts of 193f
Extrahepatic duct system, anomalies of 191, 192f
Eyeball 312t
    accessory structures of 314
    anomalies of 315
    blood vessels of 314
    coats of 313f
    derivation of parts of 311
    extraocular muscles of 146, 315
Eyelids 314, 315, 322
    coloboma of 316
    formation of 314f
Eyes 310, 322
    anterior chambers of 313
    development of 152, 310, 323, 323fc
    formation of lens of 312f
    molecular regulation of development of 315
    posterior chambers of 313

F

Face 150
    abnormal 154f
    development of 150, 151f-153f
    developmental anomalies of 153
    different structures of 159fc
    muscles of 152
    parts of 152f
Facial
    cleft, lateral 154
    nerve 130, 152
    skeleton 142
Falciform 189
    ligament 176, 191f, 203, 209
Fallot's tetralogy 227, 228f, 251, 252f

Family planning, rhythm-method of 29
Fastigial nuclei 293
Fat cells 104
Female external genitalia
    anomalies of 269
    development of 269, 270f
Female urethra 265f, 280
    development of 264
Femoral artery 240
Fertility 39
Fertilization 2, 3, 30, 31, 35, 36f, 38, 39, 40t, 41f, 45
    stages of 35
Fertilized ovum, segmentation of 40f
Fetal
    circulation 248, 249, 250f
    cotyledon 53, 90
    fissure 311
    health, assessment of 80
    liver, functions of 190
    membranes 85
        development of 85
    pancreas, functions of 195
    skull 143
    surface 89, 90, 90f
    surgery 82
    therapy 81
    tumors, removal of 82
    umbilical arteries 87
Fetomaternal circulation 91
Fetoscopy 81
Fetus 77
    papyraceous 96, 97f
    prenatal diagnosis of 80
    viability of 3, 5
    viable age of 78, 216
Fibers 102
Fibrils, arrangement of 20f
Fibroblast growth factor 16, 104
    receptor 332
Fibrocartilage 105
Fibrous cords 180
Fibrous joint 144
Fibrous membrane 106
Fibrous pericardium 202, 232
Fifth lumbar intersegmental artery 239
First arch syndrome 154
Fissures 214, 293
    abnormal 216
    absence of 216
Fistula 269f
    branchial 131
Flexures, formation of 285f
Follicles
    differentiation of 22
    growth of 22
    primary 23, 23f
    secondary 23, 23f
    stimulating hormone 29, 30, 30f
    tertiary 23, 23f
Follicular cells 23
Folliculogenesis, formation of 23
Fontanelles 143
Foramen
    cecum 133, 133f, 166

ovale 249, 250, 250f, 253
    premature closure of 225
    primum 222f, 223
    secundum 222f, 223
Foregut 70, 74, 161, 171, 174, 186
Forelimb bud 144, 144f
Fossa ovalis 224
Fraternal twins 94
Frontonasal process 150, 152, 155, 159
    formation of 150f
Fundamental axes 60
Funnel chest 141
Fused heart tube, subdivisions of 220f
Fusion 165

G

Gag reflex 303
Galea capitis 19
Gallbladder 179f, 191, 192f, 193f
    absence of 191f
    anomalies of 191
    duplication of 192f
    transverse 192f
Gametes 2, 19
    formation of 14
    fusion of 37
    release, timing of 33
    viability of 26
Gametogenesis 2, 5, 19, 31, 327
Ganglia 301
    parasympathetic 304
    sympathetic 304, 308
Ganglion cells 312
Gastric glands 176
Gastrointestinal tract 74, 171
Gastrophrenic ligament 205, 209
Gastroschisis 180
Gastrosplenic ligament 176, 195, 205, 206f, 209
Gastrulation 3, 60, 66
Gemination 165
Gene
    expression, regulation of 15
    mutation 334
    polymorphism 328, 334
    therapy 82
General somatic
    afferent 289, 291
    efferent 289, 291
General visceral
    afferent 289, 291
    efferent 289, 291
Genetic 334
    counseling 11, 330, 333
        benefits of 333
    disorders, inheritance of 329, 330
    diversity 14
    factors 80
    information 7
Genital ridge 258, 272, 276
Genital system 266, 278t
    female 266
    formation 258
Genital tubercle 269, 270f, 278

Genitalia
    ambiguous 278, 279f
    external 279, 280
    male 269, 271f
Genotype 329
Germ
    cells 19, 20
    disc 58, 65f
    layers 75
        derivative 68, 73
Germinal matrix 120
Germinal period 46fc
Germline mutations 329
Gestation 2, 5, 39
Gestational age 39, 77f
Gestational sac 50, 69, 87f
Gigantism 112
Glands 2, 102, 121
    parts of 134f
    secretory part of 122
    suprarenal 307
Glans 269
Glaucoma, congenital 316
Glioblasts 114
Globose 293
Globus pallidus 296
Glomerulus 260
Glossopharyngeal nerve 130
Glucose-6-phosphate dehydrogenase deficiency 331
Glycoproteins 40
Gonadal arteries 253
Gonadal differentiation, molecular control of 278
Gonadotropin 39
    releasing hormones 29
Gonads 2, 259, 280, 309
    development of 273f
Gracile nuclei 290
Granulosa cells 23
Great vessels 227
    transposition of 227
Greater curvature 176, 205
Greater omentum 205, 206f, 209
Growth 4, 111f
    abnormal 232
    and development 14
    appositional 111
    differentiation factors 16
    interstitial 111
    regulation of 16
    retardation 79, 326
    umbilical 180f
Guanine 8
Gubernaculum 274, 274f
Gums 161
Gut 70, 74, 115, 171
    arteries of 173
    derivatives of 175f, 187f, 187fc
    duplication of 184, 185f
    fixation of 184
    mesenteries of 202
    parts of 171f, 173
    peritoneal relations of 204f
    rotation of 183
    stenosis of 180f

Gynecomastia 123
Gyri 297

H

Habenular nuclei 295
Hair 120, 124
    distribution abnormalities 120
    follicle 120
        development of 121f
    shaft of 120
Hand-Schuller-Christian disease 143
Haploid 7
    chromosomes 7
    number 17
Hard palate 156
    cleft of 157
Harelip 153
    varieties of 154f
Harlequin fetus 120
Hartmann's pouch 192f
Head and neck, muscles of 116
Heart 72, 219
    arterial end of 220
    conducting system of 231
    congenital anomalies of 228
    defects 327
        congenital 325, 326
    development of various chambers of 220
    develops 253
    exterior shape of 228
    field 219
        primary 219
        secondary 219
    forming plate 65
    tube 219
        development of 219
        endothelial 253
        main subdivisions of 221f
    valve 230
        congenital anomalies of 231
    venous end of 220
Hemangioblasts 104
Hematopoietic cells 189
Hemiazygos
    vein 247
        accessory 247
    vertical parts of 247
Hemiglossia 167
Hemivertebra 140
Hemocytoblasts 102
Hemophilia 331, 332
Hemopoiesis 190
Hemopoietic stem cells 104
Hensen's node 60, 66
Hepatic architecture, formation of 189
Hepatic bud 189
    origin of 190f
Hepatic cells 190f, 192f, 193f
Hepatic ducts 189
Hepatic lobule 189, 190f
Hepatic segment 245, 248f
Hepatic sinusoids 190f
Hepatic trabeculae 189
Hepatocardiac channel 241, 245
Hepatocytes 189

Hermaphrodite
　female 278
　male 278
　true 278
Hernia 276f
　anterior 208
　diaphragmatic 208, 208f
　inguinal 275
　lung 216
　physiological 77, 88, 179
Heterochromatin 11
Heuser's membrane 49
Hindgut 70, 74, 171, 174, 186
　development 181
Hindlimb buds 144
Hippocampal cortex 297
Hippocampus 298
Hirschsprung's disease 181
His copula 166
His furcula 212
Histiocytes 104
Holoprosencephaly 60, 315
Hormonal regulation 33
Hormone
　luteinizing 29, 30, 30f
　placental 93
　synthesis 92
　use of 30
Horseshoe kidney 261, 262f
Hourglass bladder 264, 264f
Human chorionic gonadotropin 43, 93
　qualitative 44
　quantitative 44
Human chorionic somatomammotropin 93
Huntington's chorea 331
Hyaline
　cartilage 105
　membrane disease 216
Hyaloid artery 313f, 314
Hydatidiform mole 54, 55
　embryological basis of 54
Hydrocele 275, 276f
Hydrocephalus 300, 301f
　congenital 143
Hydronephrosis 261
Hydroureter 263
Hyoid arch 127
Hyoid artery 233
Hyoid bone
　greater part of 135
　parts of 135
　superior part of body of 128
Hyperphagia 328
Hyperplasia 261
Hypertelorism 154
Hypertrichosis 120
Hypertrophied cartilage cells, zone of 108
Hypertrophy
　benign 266
　ventricular 252f
Hypoblast 48
Hypobranchial eminence 166, 169
Hypomere 113, 145
Hyponychium 120

Hypophysis
　cerebri 274, 306
　　development of 307f
　pharyngeal 306
Hypoplasia 216, 232, 261, 306
Hypospadias 266, 272, 272f
Hypothalamic sulci 295, 296f
Hypothalamus 293, 295, 296f, 309
　development of 296f
Hypoxia 88

I

Ichthyosis 120
Idiogram 11
Ileum 179
Iliac artery
　external 240
　internal 239, 239f
Iliac vein 246
Immunity transfer 92
Imperforate anus 181
　types of 182f
Implantation 3, 35, 41
　abdominal 43
　abnormal sites of 42, 43
　normal site of 42
　process of 41, 46fc
　stages of 42, 42f
　types of 42, 42f
In vitro fertilization 39, 45
Incisors, germ of 164f
Incus 128, 318, 322
Indusium griseum 298, 298f
Infections 80
　respiratory 332
Inferior parathyroid gland 131, 135
　derivation of 133f
Inferior vena cava 212, 222f, 242f, 243f, 245, 245f-247f, 248, 251f, 253
　anomalies of 248f
　azygos continuation of 248
　development of 246f
　valve of 223, 224
Infertility 39, 44
Infracardiac bursa 204, 204f, 206f
Infrahyoid thyroid 134
Infundibular stalk 306
Infundibulum 225
Inguinal bursa, formation of 273
Inguinal canal 274
Inner cell mass 39
　duplication of 95
Insula, opercula of 297
Integumentary system 118
Interatrial septal defects 224
Interatrial septum, formation of 222, 222f, 223
Intercellular matrix, calcification of 106
Intermediate mesoderm 64-66, 74, 258, 279, 281fc, 307
　location of 258f
Internal thoracic artery 237
　development of 238f, 239
Interneurons 289
Interspinous ligaments 139
Interstitial cells 272

Interstitial gland cells 26, 276
Interstitial implantation 42
Intersubcardinal anastomosis 247f
Interventricular foramen 285
Interventricular septal defects 226
Interventricular septum 225, 226, 226f
　formation of 226
Intervertebral disc 139, 147
Intervillous space 52
Intraembryonic coelom 65, 65f, 74, 200, 200f, 201f
　formation of 65, 65f, 200
　subdivisions of 201f
Intraembryonic mesoderm 59, 60, 61f, 63, 64f, 66, 74
　components of 65
　extensions of 63
　formation of 59f, 63, 65
　splanchnopleuric layer of 211, 214
　spread of 59f
　subdivisions of 64, 64f
Intrahepatic biliary
　apparatus 190f
　atresia 191
　passages 189
　system 189
Intralobular ducts 195f
Intramembranous ossification 106, 107f, 109, 110f, 115, 116fc
Intrapulmonary bronchi 214
　subdivisions of 214
Intratonsillar crypt 132
Intrauterine blood transfusion 82
Intrauterine device, use of 41
Intrauterine life 200, 258, 314
Iridopupillary membrane 314
Iris 310-313
　anomalies of 315
　coloboma of 316f
　muscles of 312
　musculature of 313

J

Jaw 151, 159
Jejunum 179
Joints 93, 144, 332
　cartilaginous 144
Jugular veins
　external 243
　internal 243

K

Karyotype 10, 11, 11f, 17, 45, 328
Keratinization defect 120
Keratinocytes 118
Kidney 261, 262, 280, 281fc, 281t
　anomalies of 261, 262f
　ascent of 261, 261f
　collecting part of 259, 260f
　development of 259
　rotation of 262
　transposition of 262f
Kinetochore 9

Klinefelter syndrome 328, 329
   clinical features of 328f
Klippel-Feil syndrome 140
Labia
   majora 269, 270f
   minora 269, 270f

L

Labiogingival sulcus 161
Lacrimal apparatus 314
   anomalies of 316
Lacrimal canaliculi 314
Lacrimal gland 314, 314f
Lacrimal sac 314, 322
Lactiferous duct 122
Lacunae 105, 105f
   radial arrangement of 52f
Lamella formation 107
Lamellar bone 106
Lamellus 105, 105f, 107
Lamina terminalis 298, 298f
Langerhans cells 118, 119
Lanugo hair 78
Laparoscopy 45
Laryngeal diverticulum 211
Laryngeal nerve
   recurrent 212
   superior 167, 212
Laryngeal web 213
Laryngocele 213
Laryngoptosis 213
Laryngotracheal diverticulum 211
   development of 211, 211f
Laryngotracheal groove 211
   development of 211f
Laryngotracheal tube 212
   separation of 212
Larynx 212
   anomalies of 213
   cartilages of 135
   development of 212
   developmental components of 212
   inlet of 212
   ventricles of 213
Lateral plate mesoderm 64-66, 74, 119
Lateral ventricles 285, 294, 303
   development of 294
Left superior intercostal vein 244
   development of 245f
Lens 310-312, 322
   anomalies of 315
   placode 152, 310, 311, 322
   vesicle 311
      development of 311f
      formation of 310
Lentiform nucleus 296, 297f, 298f
Leptomeninges 115
Leptotene 14
Lesser cornu 128
Lesser curvature 176, 205
Lesser omentum 176, 189, 203, 205, 205f, 209
Lesser sac 176, 204, 205f
   development of 203, 204f, 206f
   inferior recess of 205
   splenic recess of 205

   superior recess of 204
   vestibule of 205
Lid 316f
Lienorenal ligament 176, 195, 197f, 205, 206f, 209
Ligaments, intertransverse 139
Ligamentum
   arteriosum 234
   teres hepatis 241
   venosum 241
Limb
   anomalies of 145
   arteries of 239, 240f
   bones 147
   buds 143, 144f, 147
      development, molecular regulation of 144
      longitudinal axis of 144f
   development of 143
   muscles of 116, 146
Limbic bands, inferior 223
Limbic system 298f
Lingual swellings 166f, 169
Lingual thyroid 134
Lingual tonsil 168
Linguogingival sulcus 161, 162f
Lips 151, 159
   development of 151
   epithelium lining inside of 161
Liver 104, 189, 204
   anomalies of 191f
   cells 189
   congenital anomalies of 191
   development of 190f, 191t, 198fc
   peritoneal folds of 189
   polycystic 191
   sinusoids 189
Lobar bronchi 214
   formation of 211f
Lobes, abnormalities of 216
Lobster claw 145
Long bone, growth of 110
Loose connective tissue, formation of 104
Lower respiratory tract 211
Lumbar
   arteries 237
   intersegmental artery 239f
   rib 141
   vertebra 140, 289
Lung 214
   abnormal lobes of 216f
   accessory lobe of 217f
   anomalies of 216
   azygos lobe of 216, 216f
   bud 217
      invagination of 201
   congenital cysts of 216
   development of 214
   ectopic 216
   maturation of 214, 215f
   molecular regulation of development of 216
   parenchyma 212
   stage of 215
   tissue, sequestration of 216
Luschka foramina 285

Luteal cells 25
Lutein 25
Lymph sacs 251, 251f
Lymphatic duct 251, 251f
Lymphatic system 251
Lymphoblasts 102
Lyon hypothesis 11

M

Macrodactyly 145
Macroglossia 167
Macrostomia 154, 154f
Magendie foramen 285
Male genitalia
   anomalies of 272
   development of 269, 271f
Male urethra 265f
   development of 265
Malformation 79
   congenital 79
Malleus 128, 318, 322
   anterior ligament of 128
Malocclusion 165
Mammary artery 237
Mammary gland 118, 122, 122f, 124
   development 122f, 124fc
   developmental anomalies of 123
Mammary ridge 122, 122f
Mandible 128, 143
Mandibular arch 127, 159
Mandibular nerve 167
Mandibular processes 142, 150, 151, 159, 162f
   formation of 151f
Mandibulofacial dysostosis 143, 153, 321
Marble bone disease 112
Marrow cavity 110
Marshall, oblique vein 244
Mast cells 104
Master gene 16
Mastoid air cells 318
Maternal cotyledons 53f, 89
Maternal genome, genotype of 79
Maternal-fetal circulation 99
Matrix cell layer 113
Maturation, process of 21, 32
Mature graafian follicle 23, 24f
Mature spermatozoon, structure of 19
Maxillae, alveolar parts of 164
Maxillary artery 233
Maxillary nerves 152
Maxillary process 142, 150, 151, 152, 157f, 159, 163f
   formation of 151f
McCune-Albright syndrome 329
Meatal plug 319
Meckel's cartilage 128, 135
Meckel's diverticulum 87, 180, 180f
Median umbilical ligament 72, 263, 239
Medulla
   cell of 308
   oblongata 290, 304
      development of 290f
   white matter of 291
Medullary cords 272, 276
Medulloblasts 114

Megacolon 182f
Meiosis 14, 20, 22, 33
   completion of 32
   stage of 24
Melanoblasts 119
Melanocytes 118, 119
Melanocytic nevi, congenital 120
Membrana granulosa 23
Membrane 64, 94
   bones 106
Membranous labyrinth 317, 319f, 322
Membranous neurocranium 142
Menarche 23, 26
Meningocele 299, 300f
Meningomyelocele 299, 300f
Menometrorrhagia 28
Menopause 23
Menorrhagia 28
Menstrual age 39
Menstrual bleeding 28
Menstrual cycle 19, 23, 28, 31, 26, 27f-30f
   disorders of 28
   phases of 27, 27f
Menstruation 23, 31
   corpus luteum of 25
Merkel cells 118, 119
Mesaxon 115
Mesencephalic flexure 285
Mesencephalon 283, 286f, 292, 303
Mesenchymal cells 103f, 164f
   derivatives of 103f
Mesenchymal condensation 104, 106, 107f, 109
Mesenchyme 102, 115
Mesenteric artery 185f
   inferior 172
Mesoappendix 209
Mesocolon, transverse 184, 204f, 209
Mesoderm 66, 75, 101, 104, 113, 118, 212, 263, 280, 311, 322
   branchial 146
   central extraembryonic 53f
   paraxial 64, 66, 74
   secondary 63
   splanchnic 146
   splanchnopleuric 263
Mesodermal components 206
Mesoduodenum 178, 178f
Mesoesophagus 207
Mesogastrium 177f, 178f, 205f
Mesonephric cap 260
Mesonephric ducts 259, 260, 260f, 262, 263, 263f, 264, 265f, 273, 277, 277f, 278
   fate of 277
   lower parts of 262
   parts of 262
Mesonephric tubules 278
   remnants of 277
Mesonephric vesicle 260
Mesonephros 259, 260f
Mesothelium 200
Messenger ribonucleic acid 8
Metanephric blastema 259, 281
Metanephros 259, 260f, 280
Metaphase 13
Metaphysis 110, 115

Metencephalon 285, 293, 304
   alar lamina of 293f
Metrorrhagia 28
Microcephaly 143
Microglia 114
Microglossia 167
Microphthalmos 315
Microstomia 154, 154f
Microtia 322
Midbrain 292, 304
Middle cerebellar peduncle 291, 293
Middle ear 317, 322
   anomalies of 321
Midgut 70, 74, 171, 174, 186
   development 178
   loop 179f
Miscarriage 43
   recurrent 333
Mitochondria 32
Mitosis 12, 13f, 14, 22
Mitral valves 230
Molar pregnancy 54
Molecular biology, central dogma of 9
Mongolian eye slant 316f
Monochorionic monoamniotic twinning, hazards of 96
Monozygotic twins 95, 95f, 97, 99, 99t
Monro foramen 285
Morgagni hernia 208
Morula 39, 45
   formation 35
Mosaicism 329, 334
Motor nerve 167
Mouth
   development of 161
   roof of 162
Mullerian agenesis 268
Mullerian ducts 266
Multifactorial inheritance 80, 330, 331
Multiple births 94, 97
Mural trophoblast 40
Muscles 116, 130, 146, 332
   group 116, 116t
Muscular derivatives 148, 148t
Muscular system 138, 145
   development of 146
Muscular tissue 101, 111
Mutations 329
   types of 329
Myelencephalon 285, 290, 304
Myelin 304
   sheath, formation of 114
Myelinated nerve fibers 115
Myelocele 299, 300f
Myoblasts 102, 111
Myocardium 229
Myoepicardial mantle 229
Myofibrils 112
Myometrium 26, 266, 267f
Myosin 111
Myotome 112, 113f
Myotomic segment derived muscles of body 146f
Myotubes 111

N

Nail 120
   bed 120
   derivation of 120f
   develop 124
   field, primary 120
   folds 120
   groove 120
   matrix 120
   plate 120
   root of 120
   substance 120
Nasal cavity 155f, 156, 159
   anomalies of 156
   development of 155
   separation of 157f
Nasal concha 155
   inferior 142
Nasal dermoid 156
Nasal fin 155
Nasal glioma 156
Nasal pits 150, 151, 155f
Nasal placodes 150
Nasal sacs 155, 156f
   anterior part of 156f
   posterior part of 156f
Nasal septum 155, 156
   formation of 156f
Nasolacrimal duct 152, 314, 315f, 322
   formation of 315f
Nasolacrimal furrow 315f
   position of 315f
Nasolacrimal sulcus 152
Naso-optic furrow 151f, 152
Natal teeth 165
Neck 20
Neocortex 297
Nephric duct 259
Nephrogenic cord 258, 258f
Nephrons 259, 260
   development of 261f
   formation of 260
Nerve 128, 139f
   arrangement of 128f
   cells 288
   components 136
   fibers, layer of 312
Nervous system 73, 283
Nervous tissue 101, 113, 303
Neural arch 139, 140, 141f
   mesenchymal basis of 133f
Neural crest cell 63, 73, 113, 118, 119, 285, 287, 304, 307, 308f
   derivatives of 286
Neural ectoderm 62
Neural folds 63
Neural groove 63, 283, 303
Neural plate 62, 63, 72, 73, 283, 303
   formation of 283
Neural tissue, formation of 283
Neural tube 62, 113, 113f, 283, 284t, 303
   adult derivatives of 304
   anomalies of 300f
   defects 299
      types of 300f

development of 284f
flexures of 304
formation of 62, 63f, 284f
layer of 113f
outward bulging of 299
parts of 288
subdivisions of 284, 304
Neurectoderm 303
Neurenteric canal 62
Neurilemmal sheaths 304
Neuroblasts 286
multiple 114
Neurocranium 142, 147
cartilaginous 142
Neuroectoderm 59, 63, 73, 113, 283
Neuroepithelium 114f
Neurofibromatosis, multiple 331
Neuroglial cells 113, 114, 116
formation of 113
Neurohypophysis 296f, 306, 309
Neurolemma 114
Neurons 113, 116, 288, 304
formation of 113
parasympathetic 301
sympathetic 301
Neurulation 3, 62, 283
Nipple
crater 123
inverted 123
Nissl's granules 114
Norethisterone acetate 30
Nose 150
alae of 155
anomalies of 156
bridge of 155
development of 155
prominence of 155
Notch signaling 16
Notochord 59
fate of 62
formation of 59, 60, 62f
region of 59f
Notochordal canal 61f, 62
Notochordal plate 62
Notochordal process 61f, 62, 66
Nuclei, functional columns of 291
Nucleotides 8
Nucleus
fusion of 38
pulposus 62, 139

O

Oblique facial cleft 154, 154f, 316
Occipital somites 141
Odontoblasts 164f, 169
Olfactory epithelium 155
Olfactory pits 150
Olfactory sensations 298
Oligodendroblasts 114
Oligodendrocytes 114, 116
Oligohydramnios 86
Oligomenorrhea 28
Olivary nuclei 290, 290f, 304
Olive-shaped mass 177

Omental bursa 176
development of 203
Omphalocele 180, 185, 185f, 186
embryological basis of 185
Omphalomesenteric duct 70
Omphalomesenteric veins 241
Ontogeny 2, 5, 260
Oocytes 2, 32, 38, 276
plasma membrane 38
primary 22
secondary 22
Oogenesis 2, 19, 31, 22, 22f, 32, 32t, 33
Optic cup 311, 311f, 312f
formation of 311
subdivisions of 312f
Optic fissure 311
Optic nerve 310, 312
Optic stalk 310
formation of 311f
Optic sulcus 310
Optic vesicle 310, 315, 322
formation of 310, 310f, 315, 317f
Oral cavity 73, 161, 169
floor of 161
Organogenesis 3, 5, 16
beginning of 3
period of 68
Organs
maturation of 77
regeneration of 5
Ossification 106, 139
center of 106, 109, 109f, 115
Osteoblasts 102, 106f
Osteoclasts 106
Osteocytes 105f, 108
Osteogenesis imperfecta 112, 331
Osteoid 106, 107
Osteopetrosis 112
Osteosclerosis 112
Otic capsule 142, 317
Otic pit 317
Otic placode 317, 322
Otic vesicle 317
Otocyst 317, 318f
Ova 31
Ovarian arteries 237
Ovarian cycles 23, 29, 29f
hormonal control of 29, 30f
Ovarian follicles 31
fate of 26, 26f
formation of 23
Ovarian implantation 43
Ovarian veins 246
Ovary 259, 273f
anomalies of 277
descent of 276
development of 276
ligament of 276
Ovulation 22-24, 29, 31, 41f
time of 24
Ovum 2, 32, 32t, 35, 36f
fate of 25
maturation of 36f
structure of 24, 25f
transport of 36
Oxyntic glands 176

P

Pachytene 14
Palatal process 156
Palate 150, 155
development of 156, 157f, 160fc
embryological subdivisions of 157f
Palatine tonsil 132, 135, 169
development of 132
Palatoglossus 167
Palmar capillary plexus 239
Pancake kidney 261, 262f
Pancreas 189, 192, 195f
annular 195
anomalies of 195, 196f
development of 193f, 198fc
divisum 195
duct system of 194, 194f
endocrine components of 195f
exocrine components of 195f
uncinated process of 194
Pancreatic buds 192, 194f
derivatives of 193
Pancreatic ducts 194
inversion of 195, 196f
Pancreatic tissue, accessory 195
Papilla 120
Paradidymis 277
Parafollicular cells 132, 133
Paragenital tubules 277
Parahippocampal gyrus 298
Paramesonephric ducts 259, 266, 267f, 269, 278, 280
fate of 267f
formation of 267f
Paranasal sinuses 159
development of 156
Parathyroid 133f
gland
development of 132
inferior 131, 135
Parietal pleura 214
Paroophoron 278
Parotid duct 168
Parotid gland 168
Pars cystica 190f
Pars distalis 306
Pars hepatica 190f
Pars nervosa 306
Pars tuberalis 306
Patau's syndrome 325
Patent ductus arteriosus 252f
embryological basis of 252
Patent foramen ovale 224, 225f
Patent truncus arteriosus 227, 228f
Patent vitellointestinal duct 180f
Pectinate line 181
Pectus carinatum 141
Pectus excavatum 141
Pedigree chart 330, 330f, 334
symbols used in 330f
Pelvic kidney 261
Pelvic ligaments 93
Pelvic mesocolon 184, 204f
Pelvic part 259, 279

Pelvic section 264
Pelvic viscera 301
Pelvis 260
Penetration defect, closure of 42
Penile urethra 265f, 271f, 280
    terminal part of 265
Penis 269
    prepuce of 270f
Percutaneous umbilical cord blood sampling 81
Pericardial canals 200f
Pericardial cavity 65f, 70, 72, 74, 200, 201, 209, 230f, 231
Pericardial sac 231f
Pericardioperitoneal canal 201, 214
    enlargement of 202f
Pericardiopleural membrane 202
Pericardium 72f
    congenital anomalies of 232
    oblique sinus of 232, 233f
    transverse sinus of 231f, 232
    visceral layer of 229
Perichondrium 105, 106, 107f
Perichordal disc 139
Periderm 118
Perilymph 317
Perimetrium 26
Periodontal ligament 164
Periosteal bone 110f
Periosteal bud 107
Periosteal collar 109, 109f
Periosteum 109
Peripheral nervous system 283
Peritoneal cavities 201, 202, 202f-204f, 209
Peritoneal fold 209, 209t
Peritoneum
    parietal layer of 202
    visceral layer of 202
Perivitelline space 25
Permanent teeth, germ of 164f
Persistent pupillary membrane 315
Phallus 269
Pharmacologic therapy 81
Pharyngeal apparatus 126
Pharyngeal arch 126, 127f, 128f, 135, 136, 138, 165f, 166f, 320f
    arteries, anomalous development of 236
    cartilages of 129f
    derivatives of 136t
    development, genetic basis of 132
    disorders 130
    formation of 126f, 127f
    nerves of 130t, 135
Pharyngeal cleft 136
    derivatives of 136t
Pharyngeal membrane 132, 136
Pharyngeal pouch 126, 132
    fate of 131f
Pharyngeal tonsils 168
Pharyngotympanic tube 131, 319f
Pharynx 161
    development of 168
    floor of 133f, 165f, 166f, 211f
Phenotype 329
Phenylketonuria 331
Pheochromocytoma 308

Pheromones 122
Philtrum 152
Phimosis 272
Phocomelia 144, 145
Phrygian cap 192f
Phylogeny 2, 5, 260
Pia mater 115
Piebaldism 120
Pierre Robin sequence 130
Pigeon chest 141
Pigment disorders 120
Pineal body 295
Pineal gland 306, 307, 309
    development of 307f
Pinna 130, 153, 319
Piriform cortex 298f
Pituitary agenesis 306
Pituitary gland 306, 307f
    anomalies of 306
Placenta 51, 71, 78f, 85, 88, 88f, 89f, 97, 99, 248
    accreta 93
        spectrum 93
    circumvallate 93
    classification of 92, 92t
    congenital abnormalities of 93t
    development of 98fc
    fenestrate 93
    functions of 92
    increta 93
    measurements of 90
    normal attachment of 89, 89f
    percreta 93
    previa 43, 89, 93
        degree of 89
    structure of 90
    succenturiate 93, 93f
    types of 92
Placental membrane 91
Plagiocephaly 143
Plasma cells 104
Plasmodiotrophoblast 51
Pleura 214
Pleural cavity 201, 202f, 209, 212, 214
    formation of 201, 202f, 214
Pleuropericardial folds 214
Pleuropericardial membrane 201, 202
Pleuroperitoneal canals 200f, 207, 207f
    closure of 207f
Pleuroperitoneal folds 214
Pleuroperitoneal membrane 201, 202, 202f
Pluripotent cells 59, 287
Pluripotent ectodermal cells 62
Polar bodies 45
Polar trophoblast 40
    adhesion of 42
Polycystic kidney, congenital 262, 262f
Polydactyly 145
Polyhydramnios 86
Polymastia 123
Polymenorrhea 28
Polymorphism 328
Polyploidy, prevention of 14
Polyspermy 38
Polythelia 123
Pons 291, 304
    development of 292f

Pontine flexure 285
Pontine nuclei 290f, 291, 304
Popliteal artery 240
Portal triads 189, 190
Portal vein 241, 253
    development of 241, 243f
    left branch of 242
    right branch of 242
    stem of 242
Postarterial segment 178
Postcaval ureter 263
Posterior cardinal vein 243, 245, 245f, 246f
Posterior nasal aperture 155
Posterior sacs 251
Postganglionic parasympathetic neurons 301
    development of 302f
Potter syndrome 261
Prader-Willi syndrome 328
Preantral follicle 23
Preaortic anastomosis 245
Preauricular appendages 321
Prechordal plate, formation of 49, 49f
Preganglionic parasympathetic neurons, development of 302f
Preganglionic sympathetic neurons, development of 302f
Pregnancy 2, 5, 81
    complications, evaluation of 80
    corpus luteum of 26
    ectopic 43
    length of 77
    tests 43
        types of 43
Premature implantation 40
Premaxilla 156
Premuscle cells 111
Presomite 68
Previa 97
Primary villi 51, 52
Primary vitreous humor 313
Primordial follicle 23, 23f, 276
Primordial germ cells 272, 278, 280
    migration of 272f
Primum 253
Proboscis 315
Processus vaginalis 274, 275f
    abnormal persistence of 276f
    anomalies of 275, 276f
Prochordal plate 50, 59, 59f, 72
    region of 72
Proctodeum 73
Progesterone 30f, 93
Pronephric duct 260, 260f
Pronephros 259, 260f
Pronucleus
    female 38
    male 38
Prosencephalon 283, 293, 303
Prostaglandins, concentration of 24
Prostate 280
    development of 266
    endodermal derivatives of 266f
    female homologues of 266
    inner glandular zone of 266
    mesodermal derivatives of 266f
Prostatic urethra 265, 266f, 273, 280

Prostatic utricle 267f
Protein
 inhibin 30
 synthesis of 8
Proximal bulbar septum 227f
Proximal segment 172
Pseudohermaphroditism 278, 308
Ptosis 316
Pulmonary valves 230
 formation of 231f
Pulmonary veins 223f
 absorption of 224, 224f
Pulmonary vessels 251
Pulp 169
Punnett square diagram 329, 329f, 334
Pupil 313
 anomalies of 315
Pupillary membrane 314
Purkinje fibers 231
Putamen 296
Pygopagus 96, 96f
Pyloric stenosis, congenital 177, 178f
Pyramidal lobe 134
Pyriform cortex 297

R

Rachischisis 299, 300f
Radial arteries 239
Radiation 80
Ramuli chorii 53, 53f, 54
Rapid growth 77
Rathke's pouch 306, 307f
 proliferates 306
Rectal fistula 181, 182f
Rectovaginal fistula 182f, 269, 269f
Rectovesical fistula 182f
Rectum 173, 181, 204f, 259
Red blood cells 332
Red nucleus 292, 304
Reichert's cartilage 128
Reidel's lobe 191f
Renal abnormalities 325
Renal agenesis 261
 bilateral 261
Renal artery 253, 262
Renal pelvis 263
Renal segment 245
Renal tubule 260
Renal vein 246
Reproductive cycle 31fc, 32fc
Reproductive period 19, 26
Respiratory bronchioles 214
Respiratory distress syndrome 216
Respiratory diverticulum 211
 derivatives of 212
 development of 211, 211f
 growth 211f
Respiratory system 211
 development of 211, 217fc
Rete-testes 273
Reticular fibers 104
Retina 310, 312
 anomalies of 316
 iridial parts of 312
 optical part of 312
 pigmented layer of 312
Retinal detachment 316
Retinal fissure 311
Retinal vessels 314
Retrogressing veins 244
Retroperitoneal sac 251
Rhombencephalon 283, 303
Rhombic lip 291
Ribonucleic acid 8
Ribs 141
 anomalies of 141
Right atrium, development of 224
Rocker-bottom feet 326
Root, formation of 164

S

Saccule 317
 macula of 317
Sacral parasympathetic outflow 301
Sacral vertebra 140
Sacrococcygeal teratoma 60, 82, 140
Salivary glands 161, 168, 169
 development of 167
Satellite bodies 10
Scala tympani 317
Scala vestibuli 317
Scaphocephaly 143
Schwann cells 114, 116, 304
Sclera 312, 313, 322
 anomalies of 315
Sclerotome 112, 115, 138
 cell of 113f
Scoliosis, congenital 141
Scrotum 274f
Sebaceous gland 121, 124
Sebum 121
Secondary villi 51, 52, 66
Secretory acini 167
Secretory elements 122
Segmental bronchi 214
 formation of 212f
Semicircular canals 317
Semicircular ducts 317, 318f
 cristae of 317
Seminal analysis 44, 45
Seminal vesicle 273, 277f
Seminiferous tubules 272
Seminoma 275
Sensory ganglia 304
Sensory nerve 167
 roots 289
Sensory organs 310
Septa, defective formation of 224, 226
Septum 269
 intermedium 222f, 223, 226
 primum 222f, 223, 224
  defect 225f
 secundum 222f, 223, 224, 253
  defect 225f
  development of 223
 spurium 221
 transversum 65, 70, 72, 74, 189, 190f, 207f
  migrates 207
Serous cavities, formation of 200

Serous pericardium 232
Sex
 chromatin 11, 17
 chromosomes 7, 325
 cords 272, 276, 278
 determination 39
 differences 12
Sex-linked inheritance, pedigree chart of 331f
Sickle cell anemia 331, 332
Sigmoid colon 181
Sigmoid mesocolon 209
Single median eye 154f
Single umbilical artery 88
Sinoatrial orifice 223f
Sinovaginal bulbs 268, 268f
Sinuatrial orifice 220, 222f
Sinus
 branchial 131
 septum 221
 venosus 220, 222f, 254f
Sinusoids 190f
Sirenomelia 60
Situs inversus 184
Skeletal derivatives 148
Skeletal element 127, 135
 derivatives of 128
Skeletal muscle 111, 115, 145, 147
Skeletal system 138
Skene glands 266
Skin 118, 124fc, 141
 anomalies of 119
 appendages of 120
 derivation of components of 118f
 dermis of 113f
 development
  genetic basis of 121
  molecular basis of 121
 disorders, embryological basis of 123
 epidermis of 59
 glands of 121, 121t
Skull
 anomalies of 143
 base of 142
 develops 147
 vault of 142
Small cells 287
Small intestine, mesentery of 184, 209
Smooth muscle 113, 115, 147
Soft bulging 303
Soft palate 156, 157
 cleft of 157
Somatic cell 7f, 328
 normal 328
Somatic mesoderm 146
Somatic veins 240, 242
Somatopleuric extraembryonic mesoderm 49
Somatopleuric layer 66, 74, 138, 214
Somites 64, 115, 68, 74, 130, 130t, 146, 148
 derived skeletal musculature 146
 embryo 69f
 fate of 112
 sclerotomes of 138
 subdivisions of 113f
Somitomere 64, 130, 130t

Sonic Hedgehog
    inhibition of 315
    proteins 16
Special sense organs 73
Speech articulation 161
Sperm 2, 32, 36f
Spermateleosis 20
Spermatic arteries 237
Spermatids 31
Spermatocytosis 20
Spermatogenesis 2, 19-21, 21f, 22, 31, 32, 32t, 33
Spermatogonia 20
Spermatozoa
    capacitation of 21
    maturation of 21
Spermatozoon 2, 31, 32, 32t
    parts of 19f
    penetration of 37f
    transport of 35
    transverse section across principal piece of 20f
Spermiogenesis 20, 21, 21f, 31
Sphenoid 143
    spine of 128
Sphenomandibular ligament 128
Spherical centriole 20
Spider fingers 145
Spina bifida 140, 141f, 299, 300f
    anterior 140, 299, 300f
    aperta 140
    myelomeningocele repair for 82
    occulta 140, 299, 300f
Spinal cord 284, 288, 290, 303
    anomalies of 299
    ascending tracts of 289
    development of 288f
    gray matter of 289
    position of 289
    recession of 289, 289f, 290f
    white matter of 289
Spinal ganglia 289
Spinal nerves 290f
    motor nerve roots of 288
    roots, development of 289f
Spindle 13
Spiral ganglion 317
Spiral septum 225
    defects of 227
Spiral sheath 20
Splanchnic arteries, intermediate 237
Splanchnopleuric layer 66, 74
Spleen 189, 192, 195
    accessory 196
    anomalies of 196
    development of 197f
Splenic notches 195
Spleniculi 195
Spondylolisthesis 140
Spongioblasts 114, 286
Spongy bone 106
Sry gene activation 278
Stapedial artery 233
Stapedius 318
Stem cell 5
    therapy 5

transplantation 82
types of 5
Stenosis 231, 321
    congenital 213, 266
    pulmonary 231
    tracheal 213
Sternal bars 141
Sternum 141, 147
    anomalies of 141
    development of 141f
Stigma 24
Stomach 175, 179f, 186, 187fc, 204, 206f
    position of 177f
    rotation of 176
    shape of 176, 177f
Stomatodeum 73, 126f, 159, 161
Stomodeum 73
Stratum
    basale 27, 28
    compactum 27, 28
    corneum 118
    germinativum 118
    granulosum 118
    lucidum 118
    spinosum 118
    spongiosum 27, 28
Streak 59, 66, 72
Striated muscle 127, 135
Stylohyoid ligament 128
Styloid process 135
Subcardinal veins 245, 246f, 247f
    formation of 246f
Subcardinal-hepatocardiac anastomosis 245
Subclavian artery 235f, 236, 237, 237f, 239, 253
Subclavian veins 243
Subhepatic cecum 180
Sublingual gland 168
Submandibular gland 168
Substance abuse 80
Substantia nigra 292, 304
Substantia propria 313
Sulci 297
Sulcus limitans 288, 289, 304
Sulcus terminalis 166
Superior aberrant ductules 277
Superior intercostal arteries 237
Superior mesenteric artery 172, 183f
Superior parathyroid gland 131135
    derivation of 133f
Superior vena cava 221, 222f, 243, 245f, 248, 248f, 251f, 253
Superior vesical artery 239
Support cells 33
Supracardinal veins 245, 246f
Suprahyoid thyroid 134
Surrogacy 39
Sweat glands 121, 124
    development of 122f
    pore of duct of 122
Swellings, genital 269, 270f, 278
Sylvius aqueduct 285
Sympathoblasts 287
Synapsis 14
Synchondrosis joints 144

Syncytiotrophoblast 50, 50f, 51, 52, 52f, 53f
    formation of 50f
    peripheral 52f
Syndactyly 145
Syndesmosis 144
Synophthalmos 315, 316f
Synovial joint 144
    development of 145f
Synphalangia 145

T

Talipes equinovarus 145
Taste
    buds 167
    perception 161
    sensation 167
Taussig-Bing syndrome 227
Tela choroidea 295
    formation of 296f
Telencephalic flexure 285
Telencephalic vesicles 283, 294f, 298
Telencephalon 283, 286f, 296
    lentiform nucleus 298f
    wall of 297f
Telophase 14
Temporary teeth 164f
Tensor tympani 318
Teratogen 79, 82, 83
Teratogenesis 60
Teratogenic drugs 80
Teratogenicity, theories of 79
Teratology 1
Teratoma 277
Tertiary villi 51, 52, 66
Test tube babies 39
Testicular veins 246
Testis 259, 273f, 276, 277f
    anomalies of 275
    appendix of 267f, 269
    bilateral undescended 275f
    descent of 273, 274, 274f
    development of 272
    duct system of 272, 274f, 275, 280
    ectopic positions of 275f
Testosterone
    deficiency, symptoms of 328
    production 278
Thalamus 293, 295
    development of 296f
Thalassemia 331
Theca externa 24
Theca interna 24, 31
Thecal gland 24
Thoracic artery, internal 237
Thoracic duct 251
    development of 251f
Thoracopagus 96, 96f
Thymic tissue, accessory 132
Thymine 8
Thymocytes endoderm 132
Thymus 131, 135
    development of 132
    fragmentation of cervical part of 132
Thyrocervical trunk 237
Thyroglossal cysts 134

Thyroglossal duct 133, 133f, 166
    path of 134f
Thyroglossal fistula 134
Thyroid 133, 212
    gland 126, 131-133, 135
        anomalies of 134, 134f
        development of 133, 133f
        pyramidal process of 134f
    intrathoracic 134
    tissue 134f
Tissue
    maintenance 14
    maturation of 77
    regeneration of 5
    repair 14
Tongue 131, 161, 166f, 167
    anomalies of 167
    anterior two-third of 166, 169
    components of 167t
    development of 165, 167f
    epithelium of 161
    muscles of 146
    nerve supply of 166
    posterior one-third of 166, 169
    posterior-most part of 166
Tonsillar crypts 132
Tonsils 131
    development of 168
Tooth 161
    development 162
        cap stage of 163
    formation 332
    germ 163
        formation of 163f
    parts of 165t
    supernumerary 165
Torticolis, congenital 141
Trabeculae
    formation of 108
    radial arrangement of 52f
Trachea 212
    agenesis of 213, 213f
    anomalies of 213, 213f
    development of 213
    normal arrangement of 175f
Tracheal bronchus 213
Tracheoesophageal fistula 175, 175f, 213
Tracheoesophageal folds 212
Tracheoesophageal septum 175, 212
Transforming growth factor-beta 16
Transforms bilaminar embryonic disc 60
Transmission genetic disorders, mode of 330
Transverse anastomosis, formation of 246f
Transverse colon 179f, 181
Treacher-Collins syndrome 130, 154
Triangular ligaments 189, 209
Tricuspid atresia 231
Tricuspid valve 227f, 230
Trilaminar germ disc 58, 60
Trisomy 325, 326
Trophoblast 40, 41f, 42, 48, 50, 66
    development of 48
    invasion 43
Truncus
    arteriosus 220, 225, 253, 254t
    chorii 53
    swellings 225

Trunk, pulmonary 234, 253
Tubal implantation 43
Tubal patency, laparoscopy for 45
Tubal tonsils 168
Tubercles 153, 319
Tuberculum 166f
    impar 133, 169
Tubotympanic recess 131, 317
    formation of 319f
Tubules 277
Tunica albuginea 272
Tunica vaginalis 274
Turner syndrome 327, 329
    clinical features of 327f
Twinning 94, 95f
    basis 98fc
    types of 94, 98fc
Twin-to-twin transfusion syndrome 82
Tympanic antrum 131, 318
Tympanic membrane 132, 319
    layer of 130, 321f
Tympanum 320f
Typical gland, development of 102f
Typical long bone, formation of 109f, 110f
Typical neuroblast, formation of 114f

U

Ulnar arteries 239
Ultimobranchial body 131, 133
Ultrasound 186
    fetal 252f
    transvaginal 44, 45
Umbilical artery 88, 239, 239f, 249, 250
    development of 239f
    parts of 239f
Umbilical cord 49, 71, 71f, 72f, 74, 85, 87, 88f, 97
    attachment, types of 88
    formation of 71, 87
Umbilical hernia
    anomalies 180
    congenital 180
Umbilical sinus 180, 180f
Umbilical vein 88, 189, 248, 251
Umbilical vesicle 70, 72, 88
Unipolar neuroblast 114
Unmyelinated nerve fibers 115
Upper eyelid, coloboma of 316f
Upper limb, arteries of 239, 240f
Upper lip 152
    development of 151
    formation of 152f
Upper respiratory tract 211
Upper uterine segment 43f, 89f
Urachal cyst 264
Urachal sinus 264
Urachus 72, 263
    anomalies, congenital 264
Ureter 280
    anomalies of 263, 264f, 267f
    development of 262
    double 263
Ureteric bud 259, 280, 281
Ureterovaginal fistula 269f

Urethra 263, 266, 269f, 272f, 279
    anomalies of 266
    development of 264, 265f
    female 265f, 280
    male 265f
    membranous 265, 265f, 280
    parts of 263f
    penile part of 265
    spongy part of 265
Urethral folds 269, 270, 278
Urethral glands 266
Urethral groove 270
Urethral plate 270
Urinary bladder 265f, 269f, 279, 280
    anomalies of 264
    development of 262
Urinary system 259
    development of 258
Urine pregnancy test 43
Uriniferous tubules 260
Urogenital membrane 173, 270f
Urogenital ridge 258
    formation of 258
Urogenital sinus 172f, 173, 186, 263f, 265f, 259, 263, 264, 270, 279
    phallic part of 270
    subdivisions of 259f
Urogenital system 258, 279, 281fc
    developmental primordia of 280fc
Urogenital tract 115
Urorectal septum 172
    formation of 172f, 173f
Uterine
    blood vessels 52f
    canal 266
    cavity 93, 94f, 97
    cycles 29, 29f
        hormonal control of 29, 30f
    endometrium 48
        components of 27f
    epithelium 28f, 42, 42f
    segment 43
    tubes 266, 267, 280
        anomalies of 268
        development of 266
        fimbriae of 268
Uterovaginal canal 266, 267f, 268f
    formation of 267f
Uterus 266, 280
    anomalies of 268
    arcuate 267f, 268
    bicornis 268
        bicollis 267f
    bicornuate 267f, 268
    development of 266
    didelphys 267f, 268
    endometrium of 44, 54
    fundus of 267, 267f
    round ligament of 276
    septate 267f
    subseptate 267f, 268
    unicornuate 268, 268f
Utricle 317
    macula of 317

V

Vagina 269f
  anomalies of 269
  development of 268
  part of 266
Vaginal fistulae 269f
Vaginal plate 268
  canalization of 268f
Vaginal smear 24
Vagus
  internal laryngeal branch of 213
  nerve 177f
    recurrent laryngeal branch of 130, 213
    superior laryngeal branch of 130
Vasa efferentia 260, 273, 277
Vascular endothelial growth factor 104
Vasculogenesis 104, 233
Veins 254
  anomalies of 248
  azygos system of 247
  brachiocephalic 243
  development of 240
  embryonic 255, 255t
  formation of 244f
  suprarenal 246
Vena cava
  hepatic segment of 248f
  inferior 212, 222f, 242f, 243f, 245, 245f-247f, 248, 251f, 253
  preureteric 248
  superior 221, 222f, 243, 245f, 248, 248f, 251f, 253
Venae advehentes 242
Venae revehentes 242
Ventral aorta 128, 233
Ventral mass 287, 304
Ventral mesentery 172, 189, 203
Ventral mesogastrium 175, 176f, 189, 190f, 203, 204f, 209
Ventral pancreatic buds 194f
Ventral splanchnic arteries 237
Ventral wing 131
Ventricles
  development of 225
  formation of 285
  terminal 285

Ventricular chamber, parts of 225f
Ventricular septal defect 226, 228f, 252f
Ventricular septum, formation of 226f
Vernix caseosa 78, 118
Vertebra 140f, 147
  development 148fc
    molecular regulation of 140
  ossification of 139
Vertebral artery 237
  development of 237, 238f
  stem of 237
Vertebral column 138, 147
  congenital anomalies of 140
Vertical anastomoses, sites of 238f
Vesicourethral canal 259, 262, 264, 265, 265f, 279
Vesicovaginal fistula 259f, 269
Vessels 255
  postnatal occlusion of 255t
Vestibular folds, upper pair of 213
Vestibular ganglion 317
Vestibule 317
Vestigial structures 276
Villi, subdivisions of 53, 53f
Visceral pleura 214
Visceral veins 240, 241
Viscerocranium 142, 147
Visual system 322
Vitamin
  A deficiency 315
  D rickets 332
Vitelline
  arteries 172
  cyst 180
  duct 70
  membrane 25, 37, 38
  veins 189, 190f, 241
Vitellointestinal duct 70, 86, 88, 171, 172f, 178, 180f
Vitiligo 120
Vitreous humor 313
Vocal cords
  false 213
  true 213
Volvulus 184

W

Waardenburg syndrome 120
Waste elimination 92
Wharton's jelly 71, 88
Winslow foramen 203
Wolffian duct 259
Woven bone 106
Wrinkled appearance 78

X

X chromosome 328
  inactivation 11
X-linked dominant inheritance 331, 331f
XXY syndrome 328

Y

Y-linked inheritance 330, 331, 331f
Yolk sac 48f, 49, 62, 69, 70, 85-87, 87f, 97, 99, 104, 171, 172f
  extraembryonic part of 88f
  fate of 87fc
  formation of 49, 86, 87fc
  incorporation of 88f
  neighborhood of 272f
  primary 86
  secondary 49, 50f, 86
Yolk stalk 70

Z

Zenker's diverticulum 175
Zona
  pellucida 37, 38, 41
    glycoproteins 40
    functions of 40
  reaction 21, 38
  reticularis 307
Zygote 2, 5, 31, 95
  formation of 38
Zygotene 14

EU GSPR Authorised Reprsentative
Logos Europe, 9 rue Nicolas Poussin
1700, La Rochelle, France
Phone: +33 (0) 6 67 93 73 78
E-mail: contact@logoseurope.eu

www.ingramcontent.com/pod-product-compliance
Ingram Content Group UK Ltd.
Pitfield, Milton Keynes, MK11 3LW, UK
UKHW050814130226
467992UK00005B/16